Lecture Notes in Artificial Intelligence   1211

Subseries of Lecture Notes in Computer Science
Edited by J. G. Carbonell and J. Siekmann

Lecture Notes in Computer Science

Edited by G. Goos, J. Hartmanis and J. van Leeuwen

Springer
Berlin
Heidelberg
New York
Barcelona
Budapest
Hong Kong
London
Milan
Paris
Santa Clara
Singapore
Tokyo

Elpida Keravnou   Catherine Garbay
Robert Baud   Jeremy Wyatt (Eds.)

Artificial Intelligence in Medicine

6th Conference on Artificial Intelligence
in Medicine Europe, AIME'97
Grenoble, France, March 23-26, 1997
Proceedings

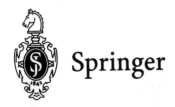

Springer

Series Editors

Jaime G. Carbonell, Carnegie Mellon University, Pittsburgh, PA, USA
Jörg Siekmann, University of Saarland, Saarbrücken, Germany

Volume Editors

Elpida Keravnou
University of Cyprus, Department of Computer Science
75 Kallipoleos Street, P.O. Box 537, CY-1678 Nicosia, Cyprus
E-mail: elpida@turing.cs.ucy.ac.cy

Catherine Garbay
Lab. TIMC/IMAG-Institut Albert Bonniot, Faculté de Medicine
Domain de la Merci, F-38706 La Tronche Cedex, France
E-mail: Catherine.Garbay@imag.fr

Robert Baud
Centre d'Informatique Hospitalière, Hospital Cantonal Universitaire de Genève
CH-1211 Geneva 14, Switzerland
E-mail: baud-robert@diogenes.hcuge.ch

Jeremy Wyatt
Biomedical Informatics Unit, Imperial Cancer Research Fund
Lincoln's Inn Fields, P.O. Box 123, London WC2A 3PX, UK
E-mail: jeremy@biu.icnet.uk

Cataloging-in-Publication Data applied for

Die Deutsche Bibliothek - CIP-Einheitsaufnahme

Artificial intelligence in medicine : proceedings / 6th
Conference on Artificial Intelligence in Medicine Europe,
AIME '97, Grenoble, France, March 23 - 26, 1997. Elpida
Keravnou ... (ed.). - Berlin ; Heidelberg ; New York ;
Barcelona ; Budapest ; Hong Kong ; London ; Milan ; Paris ;
Santa Clara ; Singapore ; Tokyo : Springer, 1997
  (Lecture notes in computer science ; Vol. 1211 : Lecture notes in
  artificial intelligence)
ISBN 3-540-62709-X
NE: Keravnou, Elpida T. [Hrsg.]; ; GT

CR Subject Classification (1991): I.2, I.4, J.3, H.4

ISBN 3-540-62709-X Springer-Verlag Berlin Heidelberg New York

© Springer-Verlag Berlin Heidelberg 1997
Printed in Germany

Typesetting: Camera ready by author
SPIN 10549462   06/3142 – 5 4 3 2 1 0   Printed on acid-free paper

Preface

The European Society for Artificial Intelligence in Medicine in Europe (AIME) was established in 1986 following a highly successful workshop held in Pavia the year before. The aims of AIME are to foster fundamental and applied research in the application of Artificial Intelligence (AI) techniques to medical care and medical research, and to provide a forum for reporting significant results achieved at biennial conferences. In accordance with the latter aim, this volume contains the proceedings of AIME'97, the Sixth Conference on Artificial Intelligence in Medicine Europe, held in Grenoble, 23rd-26th March 1997. AIME'97 follows previous conferences held in Marseille (1987), London (1989), Maastricht (1991), Munich (1993), and Pavia (1995).

In the conference announcement, authors were encouraged to submit original contributions to the development of theory, techniques, and applications of AI in Medicine (AIM). Contributions to theory could include a presentation or an analysis of the properties of novel AI methodologies potentially useful in solving relevant medical problems. Papers on techniques were required to describe the development or the extension of AI methods and their implementation. Also they had to discuss the assumptions and limitations which characterize the proposed methods. Application papers were required to describe the implementation of AI systems in solving significant medical problems, and had to present sufficient information to allow evaluation of the practical benefits of using the system.

The call for AIME'97 resulted in 82 paper submissions and 9 poster submissions which represents a substantial increase over previous AIMEs. Also the geographical scope of the AIME conferences appears to have broadened both within and outside Europe. Overall, the submissions for this conference covered no less that 24 countries and 4 continents.

Each paper submission was evaluated by two independent assessors on the basis of a detailed review form covering relevance, originality, research contribution, quality of research, presentation, and an overall qualitative ranking. Similarly each poster submission was evaluated by two independent assessors on the basis of a similar review form. All submissions in each category (paper or poster) were ranked using a two-level ranking, where the first-level was given by the overall assessments of the two evaluators while the second-level was based on a quantitative score obtained from all the individual aspects of evaluation. The program committee chair and the organizing committee co-chairs met in Cyprus (10-11 November 1996) to make the final selections. In the majority of cases there was close agreement between the two evaluators. For the remaining cases where there appeared to be some disagreement between the original evaluations, all the comments of the evaluators were carefully considered and the given manuscripts were closely reexamined before reaching a final decision. Overall, out of the 82 paper submissions, 33 were selected for oral presentation which represents a 40% acceptance rate for this category of submissions. Each of the selected papers received two positive recommendations, at least one of which was highly positive, and has been allocated a maximum of 12 pages in this volume. In addition another 19 paper submissions, each of which also received two positive recommendations, plus 6 poster submissions, each of which received at least one positive recommendation, were selected for poster presentation. Each of these has been allocated a maximum of 4 pages in this volume. All accepted submissions have been organised in this volume under nine themes, which include classical themes such as Knowledge Acquisition and Learning, Decision-Support Theories, Diagnostic Problem Solving etc., as well as younger, but already firmly established themes such as Protocols and Guidelines, and Hybrid and Cooperative Systems. This volume also includes a full paper and two extended abstracts for the three invited lectures.

We would like to note that the increased interest in the Sixth AIME Conference has resulted in high quality papers making this volume a worthwhile addition to the AIM literature, and supporting the belief stated by the editors of the proceedings of previous conferences, that the quality of papers will steadily improve over the years resulting in establishing the AIME conferences as major events for the consolidation and dissemination of important research results in the AIM field. The effort of organizing the AIME conferences is indeed paying off well.

We would like to finish by thanking all those who contributed to the success of AIME'97: the authors, the members of the program committee as well as the additional reviewers, the members of the organizing committee, the invited speakers Professors Stelios Orphanoudakis, Jean-Raoul Scherrer, and Russell Taylor, the tutorial presenters Anne-Marie Rassinoux and Robert Baud (Natural Language Processing), John Fox and Nicky Johns (Protocols, Guidelines and Clinical Decision Support Systems: A Practical Introduction based on the PROforma Methodology), Charles P. Friedman and Jeremy Wyatt (Evaluation of Artificial Intelligence Systems), and Randolph A. Miller (Development, Evaluation and Dissemination of Diagnostic Decision Support Systems), and last but not least the Institutions that sponsored the conference, namely Université Joseph Fourier, Grenoble, France; CNRS (Centre National de la Recherche Scientifique), France; Grenoble Isère Développement, France; and AFIA (Association Francaise pour l'Intelligence Artificielle).

January 1997

Elpida Keravnou
Catherine Garbay
Robert Baud
Jeremy Wyatt

Program Committe

Chair: Elpida Keravnou, University of Cyprus

Steen Andreassen (Denmark)
Pedro Barahona (Portugal)
Robert Baud (Switzerland)
Jan van Bemmel (The Netherlands)
Enrico Coiera (United Kingdom)
Carlo Combi (Italy)
Luca Console (Italy)
Michel Dojat (France)
Rolf Engelbrecht (Germany)
John Fox (United Kingdom)
Catherine Garbay (France)

Werner Horn (Austria)
Jim Hunter (United Kingdom)
Nada Lavrač (Slovenia)
Stelios Orphanoudakis (Greece)
Alan Rector (United Kingdom)
Costas Spyropoulos (Greece)
Mario Stefanelli (Italy)
Mario Veloso (Portugal)
John Washbrook (United Kingdom)
Jeremy Wyatt (United Kingdom)

Additional Reviewers

Riccardo Bellazzi (Italy)
Marko Bohanec (Slovenia)
Eleni Christodoulou (Cyprus)
Daniele Theseider Dupre (Italy)
Sašo Džeroski (Slovenia)
Liliana Ironi (Italy)
Vangelis Karkaletsis (Greece)
Stavros Kokkotos (Greece)
Igor Kononenko (Slovenia)

Matjaz Kukar (Slovenia)
Silvia Miksch (Austria)
Wolfgang Moser (Germany)
Johann Petrak (Austria)
Silvana Quaglini (Italy)
Marco Ramoni (Italy)
Mathias Scherf (Germany)
Nick Vassilas (Greece)
Blaž Zupan (Slovenia)

Organizing Committee

Chair: Catherine Garbay, Institut Albert Bonniot - Domaine de la Merci
Co-Chair: Robert Baud, Hopital Cantonal Universitaire de Geneve

Jean-Dominique Monet
Georges Weil
Nicole Brochier
Paulette Souillard

Catherine Plottier
Jacques Chevallier
Pierre Kermen

Tutorials

Chair: Jeremy Wyatt, Imperial Cancer Research Fund

Table of Contents

Probabilistic Models and Fuzzy Logic

Temporal Reasoning and Planning

Natural Language and Terminology

Image and Signal Processing

Hybrid and Cooperative Systems

Keynote Lectures

Robots as Surgical Assistants: Where We Are, Wither We Are Tending, and How to Get There

Russell H. Taylor
Computer Science Department
The Johns Hopkins University
3400 N. Charles Street
Baltimore, Maryland 21218

email: rht@cs.jhu.edu; phone: (410)516-6299; fax: (410)516-6134

Abstract: This paper concerns the use of "robotic" technologies and systems to significantly improve the ability of human clinicians to perform surgery and other interventional procedures. We discuss briefly several possible taxonomies and adopt one of them to structure a brief overview of the field, using the different roles that robotic systems can play as an organizing principal. Our discussion emphasizes the complementary capabilities of robots and humans, and includes short sections on "intern replacements", telesurgical systems, robotic navigational aids, precise positioning systems and precise path systems. We conclude with a few remarks on the essential collaboration between clinical end users and robotics technology researchers that is crucial to future progress in this emerging field.

1. Introduction: Taxonomies

Robots are programmable machines that sense and manipulate the physical world in complex ways. Robotics researchers usually tend to describe their field in terms of the underlying technologies and methods used to construct and control robots. Thus, robotics conferences often have sessions on subjects such as "sensors", "mechanisms", "kinematics & dynamics", "control", "dexterous manipulation", "path planning", and so forth. Within "medical robotics" we often also consider more specialized topics such as "sterility & OR compatibility", "image-based anatomical modeling", "image-to-model registration", and the like. The advantages of this approach are that it is convenient for researchers with specialized interests to share and extend techniques within their particular fields of expertise and that it provides a convenient indexing principle for knowledge about particular problems that must be solved in constructing systems for a variety of purposes. One drawback is that technical sub-disciplines are relatively uninteresting to the society at large, which values robots more for what they can do than for what university professors say about them. More seriously, technical subjects often can take on a life of their own, with research effort and attention focused on minutiae and incremental advances far removed from any practical (or even theoretical) importance in the real world.

A second way of thinking about robotics focuses on applications, i.e., on the ultimate end uses for robotic systems. Thus, we also see sessions and specialized conferences on such subjects as "construction robots", "undersea robots", "flexible manufacturing robots", or, indeed, "medical robots". Within medical robotics, we talk about systems for orthopaedics, neurosurgery, laparoscopic general surgery, eye surgery, etc. The great strengths of this approach are that it naturally engages the attention and participation of the end user communities who will apply (and ultimately pay for) our research and, more fundamentally, that it helps insure that research attention is focused on relevant and important topics and that realistic benchmarks are available to assess progress. The drawback, of course, is that purely application-oriented meetings can ignore potentially relevant technology and techniques that have been developed elsewhere, thus leading to considerable duplication of effort.

An intermediate classification focuses on the *role* played by robotic systems, rather than on individual technical components or on end applications themselves. Here, we may talk of the "three *A*'s" of robotics research: *automation, autonomy,* and *augmentation.* The first economically important – and still the most prevalent – use of robotic systems was for industrial automation. Robots were used to *replace* human workers in factories, either because they were cheaper (rare), more reliable in carrying out repetitive tasks (common), or able to do things that humans could not do well, such as manufacture very precise parts or operate in contamination-free environments. The second sort of systems – though perhaps the original motivation for AI-oriented research into robotics – are those that seek to function autonomously in unstructured environments encountered in the "real" world. Examples include home care, cleaning, undersea and planetary exploration, mine field clearing, agriculture, and similar application domains. Such systems are only now becoming technically and economically practical. Usually the motivation is either to replace humans in tasks (such as home care or bathroom cleaning) for which it is difficult to hire people at affordable wages or else to perform tasks in environments into which it is not practical or desirable to send humans at all. A third class – and the one most relevant for medical applications – stresses the role of robots as tools that can work cooperatively with humans in the performance of useful work. We refer to such robots as *augmentative* or *assistive* systems. Although in some cases the goal is to replace work done by human assistants, we often rely upon the robot to provide capabilities that complement those of human surgeons (see Table 1). Thus, medical robotics is primarily concerned with systems that can work cooperatively with human surgeons in the performance of skilled tasks, primarily in surgery and other interventional procedures.

We will use this last organizational method, focusing on the role played by robots, to structure our discussion of medical robots. Broadly, we can identify five classes of system that appear to have significant potential for interventional applications.

1. "Intern replacements",
2. Telesurgical systems,
3. Navigational aids,
4. Precise positioning systems, and
5. Precise path system.

Subsequent sections of this paper will discuss each of these classes in a bit more detail, and will give some examples of each. It is important to note that we are here concerned broadly with "surgical robotics", which we define as the application of computation, sensing, and manipulation to enhance a human's ability to perform surgical procedures, rather than narrowly with anthropomorphic devices that might be called "surgical robots".

	Strengths	Limitations

Humans	Good judgment
	Strong hand-eye coordination
	Integrate extensive & diverse
	   information.
	Very flexible and adaptable.
	Very dexterous at "human" scale
	Able to use qualitative
	   information
	Superb hand-eye coordination
	Highly evolved
	Easy to instruct (except teen-agers)
	Explain themselves (ditto)
		Tremor
		Fatigue
		Limited manipulation ability &
		   dexterity outside natural scale
		Bulky
		Geometric accuracy limited
		Do not use quantitative
		   information naturally
		Hard to keep sterile
		Susceptible to radiation, infection

Robots	Good geometric accuracy
	Untiring & stable
	Potentially constructed in many
	   sizes & immune to infection
	Potentially unaffected by radiation
	Able to incorporate many sensors
	   (chemical, force, acoustic, etc.)
	   into control laws.
		Poor judgment
		Expensive
		Technology is evolving
		Difficult to instruct
		Inscrutable
		Limited ability to do complex
		   control & hand-eye tasks

Table 1: Complementary capabilities of humans and surgical robots [1].

2. "Intern Replacements"

These systems perform assistive tasks that are ancillary to the main surgical procedure and that are frequently performed by surgical interns and other people whose main job is to help the surgeon. Examples include robots for limb positioning (e.g., [2]), retraction (e.g., [3]) and laparoscopic camera holding (e.g.,[4, 5]). The primary justifications for such systems include (a) cost savings by reducing the number of people in the operating room, (b) improved access to the patient, and (c) reduction in problems associated with human fatigue and inattention.

A key challenge for such systems is that they must simultaneously be unobtrusive, responsive to the surgeon's wishes, and inexpensive. If these conditions cannot be met, it is often difficult to justify the additional cost and complexity of a robot, compared either to a very low cost passive clamp or to a very versatile human assistant. The cost-benefit balance can shift significantly in cases where the robotic device does not have to *compete* with a human, but can offer surgically useful capabilities that a human lacks, as we shall see below. Our approach with the IBM/Johns Hopkins LARS system for laparoscopic surgery [6] was motivated in part by these considerations. Although its initial application was laparoscopic camera pointing, the system incorporates some rudimentary image processing capabilities and was designed to be accurate enough to precisely position a surgical instrument onto an interactively designated lesion or anatomical target, as well as to be used in some of the stereotactic applications discussed subsequently. One very important focus for future work in these systems [1] is to increase their "intelligence" by incorporating simple models of surgical procedures and using these models to improve the ease of commanding such systems.

3. Telesurgical Systems

Many of the "intern replacement" systems discussed above are teleoperated. I.e., the robot's motions are specified directly by the surgeon by means of a joystick, control handle, or similar device. Although this interface can be inconvenient if the robot is functioning as a surgical assistant, since the surgeon's attention is divided, this is less a problem in cases where the surgeon is using the robot as an extension of his own direct manipulation capabilities. Indeed, "telepresence surgery" systems [7] have been developed that give the surgeon the sensation of directly controlling surgical instruments, even though the patient is far away. There are two principal advantages offered by telesurgical systems. The first – important in environments such as battlefield or disaster emergency care and for provision of expert care to remote areas -- is the ability to perform surgery on patients who are remote from the surgeon (e.g., [7-9]). A less ambitious, but more immediately practical, use of remote telerobotic systems (e.g.,[10]) permits the surgeon to provide expert consultation and assistance to colleagues at a distant site. The other advantage offered by telesurgical systems is their ability to give the surgeon access to difficult to reach parts of the body or the ability to perform delicate microsurgical tasks without tremor (e.g., [8, 11]). In addition to further progress in the mechanical and sensory capabilities of such systems, an important area of future development is integration with the information infrastructure from presurgical images and models and novel methods of "shared automony" in which the robot acts autonomously under the surgeon's supervision for some aspects of a task and as a teleoperated slave for others.

4. Navigational Aids

Many of the most promising applications of "robotics" to surgery do not involve the use of a moving robot. Instead, the goal is simply to provide the surgeon with accurate positional feedback about the location of surgical instruments relative to the patient's anatomy. These systems are often referred to as Computer-Assisted Surgery, or CAS systems, and typically consist of a 3D localizing device such as an instrumented passive manipulator, ultrasound detector, or 3D optical tracker, together with a computer graphics workstation for displaying positions relative to volumetric medical images. They are widely used in neurosurgery (e.g., [12, 13]) and more recently in orthopaedics (e.g., [14, 15]) and are of interest for more traditional active robots both because they may be used synergistically with such systems and because many of the underlying sensing, registration, and human-machine communication problems are ubiquitous in all aspects of medical robotics. One emerging application for such systems combines an optical navigation aid with a passive manipulation aid decoupling rotational and translational motions for precise osteotomies [16, 17]. Other examples include safety checking of active robots [18] and a variety of calibration and registration schemes.

5. Precise Positioning Systems

One of the earliest uses of active robots in surgery was replacement of stereotactic head frames in neurosurgery (e.g.,[19, 20]). Typically, the robot's coordinate system is registered to presurgical images of the patient using any of a number of techniques [21]. Then, the robot is used to position a tool guide in the desired position and orientation relative to the target anatomy and then turned off. The surgeon then inserts a biopsy needle or other instrument through the guide to perform the procedure. Similar approaches have been proposed for orthopaedic applications (e.g., [22, 23]). For safety reasons, the robot is often turned off during the actual instrument insertion. Although this reduces the chance of unwanted motion at critical times, it does not address the potentially more crucial issue of misregistration. Key research issues include characterization of geometric uncertainties, planning robust sensing and registration strategies, and communication of the limits of accuracy to the surgeon, whose judgment must still control.

The primary advantage gained from use of an active robot rather than a passive frame for most such applications is speed and convenience, which can pay off in reduced operating room charges and possibly fewer errors. Where deformable soft tissues or patient motion (e.g., from respiration) are involved, the ability of a robot to correct its aim very quickly in response to real-time sensing may make a crucial functional difference. For example, at Johns Hopkins, we have been exploring the use of a LARS robot with intraoperative fluoroscopic guidance for precise delivery of percutaneous brachytherapy for the liver and other soft tissue organs [24].

6. Robots as Precise Path Systems

Robots are much better than humans at moving a cutting tool through a numerically defined path, both because of their inherent accuracy and stiffness and because humans have a hard time relating numbers to physical 3D reality. Within orthopaedics, the Robodoc ™ system [18, 25-27] has demonstrated an order-of-magnitude improvement in the accuracy of femoral canal preparation for cementless total hip replacement surgery, and has been followed by a number of other efforts aimed at precise machining of bone (e.g., [23, 28-31]) either using the robot to move the cutting tool or as a means of constraining the surgeon to keep the tool within a predefined volume. Within neurosurgery, there have been several systems, most notably [32], to assist with laser resection of tumors. Other active path systems include a special-purpose robot for transurethral prostate resection [33] and a number of systems for radiation beam therapy (e.g., [34]). As with precise positioning systems, the key challenges for current research in such systems are better integration with preoperative and real-time intraoperative data, extensions to permit working with deformable soft tissues, and means to accommodate patient motion without losing accuracy.

7. Concluding Thoughts: How Should We Proceed?

This brief overview of surgical robots has presented one possible taxonomy based on the *role* such systems play in surgical applications and on what advantages they may offer to the surgeon. It is very unlikely that robots will be much used as *autonomous* agents operating without human supervision or as devices to *automate* surgical procedures, although they may sometimes usefully replace human surgical assistants in performing particular subtasks under the surgeon's supervision. However, robots are machines that have complementary capabilities to those of humans, and may be used in a number of ways to *augment* a surgeon's ability to carry out procedures or, indeed, to provide ways of delivering therapy that cannot be done by unaided humans.

This human-machine partnership has a natural parallel in the clinician-technologist collaboration that is the natural, and probably the only really effective, way to carry out research in this emerging field. For clinicians, robots are surgical tools that can greatly improve their ability to treat patients while also reducing health care costs. For technology researchers, surgical applications provide challenging technology and computational research problems with a very demanding and articulate set of end users to provide focus, relevance, and continual feedback. Our own experience has been that the development of effective communication and collaboration between surgeons and engineering researchers takes a great deal of effort and a willingness on each side to learn a good deal about the other's field of expertise. Especially at first, this can be a very frustrating process, but over time is crucial to success. Sharing of lessons, both between clinicians and engineers and between researchers applying this broadly applicable technology in many different clinical specialties is essential to success.

However, we can look at what has happened over the past few years and believe that this emerging research community is indeed on the road to success. As time goes on, the rather artificial boundaries of any taxonomy such as the one proposed above are certain to break down. We will see the development of a variety of inter-operable technical components, methods, and systems that will be put together in various ways to address particular application requirements. Funding constraints, regulatory concerns, and the long lead times associated with medical technology will remain barriers, but the potential advantages are great. If we pay careful attention to picking problems in which the "leverage" is clear and which encourage the development of key, broadly applicable, components technologies, and if we continue to work together, we can have a significant impact on people's lives and also have a fun time doing it.

8. References

1. Taylor, R.H. and S.D. Stulberg. *Medical Robotics Working Group Section Report*. in *NSF Workshop on Medical Robotics and Computer-Assisted Medical Interventions (RCAMI)*. 1996. Bristol, England: Shadyside Hospital, Pittsburgh, Pa.

2. McEwen, J.A. *Solo surgery with automated positioning platforms*. in *Proc. of NSF Workshop on Computer Assisted Surgery*. 1993. Washington D.C.

3. McEwen, J.A., *et al. Development and initial clinical evaluation of pre-robotic and robotic retraction systems for surgery*. in *Proc. Second Workshop on Medical and Health Care Robotics*. 1989. Newcastle-onTyne.

4. Sackier, J.M. and Y. Wang, *Robotically Assisted Laparoscopic Surgery: from Concept to Development*, in *Computer-Integrated Surgery*, R. Taylor, *et al.*, Editors. 1996, MIT Press: Cambridge, Mass. p. 577-580.

5. Petelin, J.B. *Computer Assisted Surgical Instrument Control*. in *Proc. Medicine Meets Virtual Reality II*. 1994. San Diego.

6. Taylor, R.H., *et al.*, *A Telerobotic Assistant for Laparoscopic Surgery*, in *IEEE EMBS Magazine Special Issue on Robotics in Surgery*. 1995. p. 279-291.

7. Green, P., *et al. Mobile Telepresence Surgery*. in *Proc. 2nd Int. Symp. on Medical Robotics and Computer Assisted Surgery*. 1995. Baltimore, Md.: MRCAS '95 Symposium, C/O Center for Orthop Res, Shadyside Hospital, Pittsburgh, Pa.

8. Mitsuishi, M., *et al. A Telemicrosurgery System with Colocated View and Operation Points and Rotational-force-feedback -free Master Manipulator*. in *Proc. 2nd Int. Symp. on Medical Robotics and Computer Assisted Surgery*. 1995. Baltimore, Md.: MRCAS '95 Symposium, C/O Center for Orthop Res, Shadyside Hospital, Pittsburgh, Pa.

9. Satava, R., *Virtual Reality, Telesurgery, and the New World Order of Medicine*. Journal of Image-Guided Surgery, 1995. **1**(1): p. 12-16.

10. Kavoussi, L., *et al.*, *Telerobotic-Assisted Laparoscopic Surgery: Initial Laboratory and Clinical Experience*. Urology, 1994. **44**(1): p. 15-19.

11. Schenker, P.S. and S.T. Charles. *Development of a Telemantpulator for Dexterity Enhanced Microsurgery*. in *Proc. 2nd Int. Symp. on Medical Robotics and Computer Assisted Surgery*. 1995. Baltimore, Md.: MRCAS '95 Symposium, C/O Center for Orthop Res, Shadyside Hospital, Pittsburgh, Pa.

12. Watanabe, E., *The Neuronavigator: A Computer-Controlled Navigation System in Neurosurgery*, in *Computer-Integrated Surgery*, R.H. Taylor, *et al.*, Editors. 1996, MIT Press: Cambridge, Mass. p. 319-327.

13. Reinhardt, H.F., *Neuronagivation: A ten years review*, in *Computer-Integrated Surgery*, R. Taylor, *et al.*, Editors. 1996, MIT Press: Cambridge. p. 329-342.

14. Nolte, L.P., *et al. A Novel Approach to Computer Assisted Spine Surgery*. in *First Int. Symp. on Medical Robotics and Computer Assisted Surgery (MRCAS 94)*. 1994. Pittsburgh: Shadyside Hospital.

15. Lavallee, S., *et al. Computer-Assisted Knee Anterior Cruciate Ligament Reconstruction First Clinical Trials*. in *First Int. Symp. on Medical Robotics and Computer Assisted Surgery (MRCAS 94)*. 1994. Pittsburgh: Shadyside Hospital.

16. Cutting, C.B., F.L. Bookstein, and R.H. Taylor, *Applications of Simulation, Morphometrics and Robotics in Craniofacial Surgery*, in *Computer-Integrated Surgery*, R.H. Taylor, *et al.*, Editors. 1996, MIT Press: Cambridge, Mass. p. 641-662.

17. Cutting, C., *et al. Optical Tracking of Bone Fragments During Craniofacial Surgery*. in *Proc. 2nd Int. Symp. on Medical Robotics and Computer Assisted Surgery*. 1995. Baltimore, Md.: MRCAS '95 Symposium, C/O Center for Orthop Res, Shadyside Hospital, Pittsburgh, Pa.

18. Taylor, R.H., *et al.*, *An Image-directed Robotic System for Precise Orthopaedic Surgery*. IEEE Transactions on Robotics and Automation, 1994. **10**(3): p. 261-275.

19. Lavallee, S., *et al.*, *Image-Guided Operating Robot: A Clinical Application in Stereotactic Neurosurgery*, in *Computer-Integrated Surgery*, R.H. Taylor, *et al.*, Editors. 1996, MIT Press: Cambridge, Mass. p. 343-352.

20. Kwoh, Y.S., Hou. J., and E.A. Jonckheere, et. al., *A robot with improved absolute positioning accuracy for CT guided stereotactic brain surgery*. IEEE Trans Biomed Eng, 1988. **35**(2): p. 153-161.

21. Lavallee, S., *Registration for Computer-Integrated Surgery: Methodology, State of the Art*, in *Computer-Integrated Surgery*, R.H. Taylor, *et al.*, Editors. 1996, MIT Press: Cambridge, Mass. p. 77-98.

22. Garbini, J.L., *et al. Robotic Instrumentation in Total Knee Arthroplasty*. in *Proc. 33rd Annual Meeting, Orthopaedic Research Society*. 1987. San Francisco.

23. Radermacher, K., G. Rau, and H.-W. Staudte, *Computer-Integrated Orthopaedic Surgery: Connection of Planning and Execution in Surgical Intervention*, in *Computer-Integrated Surgery*, R.H. Taylor, *et al.*, Editors. 1996, MIT Press: Cambridge, Mass. p. 451-463.

24. Anderson, J.P., *et al.*, *Image-Guided Percutaneous Robotic Assisted Therapy*, . 1995, The Johns Hopkins University: Baltimore, Maryland.

25. Mittelstadt, B., *et al.*, *The Evolution of a Surgical Robot from Prototype to Human Clinical Use*, in *Computer-Integrated Surgery*, R.H. Taylor, *et al.*, Editors. 1996, MIT Press: Cambridge, Mass. p. 397-407.

26.   Joskowicz, L., *et al. Computer-Integrated Revision Total Hip Replacement Surgery: Preliminary Results.* in *Proc. 2nd Int. Symp. on Medical Robotics and Computer Assisted Surgery.* 1995. Baltimore, Md.: MRCAS '95 Symposium, C/O Center for Orthop Res, Shadyside Hospital, Pittsburgh, Pa.

27.   Bargar, W., *et al. Robodoc Multi-Center Trial: An Interim Report.* in *Proc. 2nd Int. Symp. on Medical Robotics and Computer Assisted Surgery.* 1995. Baltimore, Md.: MRCAS '95 Symposium, C/O Center for Orthop Res, Shadyside Hospital, Pittsburgh, Pa.

28.   Marcacci, S., *et al., Computer-Assisted Knee Arthroplasty,* in *Computer-Integrated Surgery,* R.H. Taylor, *et al.,* Editors. 1996, MIT Press: Cambridge, Mass. p. 417-423.

29.   DiGioia, A.M., B. Jaramaz, and R.V. O'Toole. *An Integrated Approach to Medical Robotics and Computer Assisted Surgery in Orthopaedics.* in *Proc. 1st Int. Symposium on Medical Robotics and Computer Assisted Surgery.* 1994. Pittsburgh.

30.   Ho, S.C., R.D. Hibberd, and B.L. Davies, *Robot Assisted Knee Surgery.* IEEE EMBS Magazine Sp. Issue on Robotics in Surgery, 1995(April-May): p. 292-300.

31.   Delnondediey, J.Y. and J. Troccaz. *PADyC: A Passive Arm with Dynamic Constraints - A two degree-of-freedom prototype.* in *Proc. 2nd Int. Symp. on Medical Robotics and Computer Assisted Surgery.* 1995. Baltimore, Md.: MRCAS '95 Symposium, C/O Center for Orthop Res, Shadyside Hospital, Pittsburgh, Pa.

32.   Kall, B.A., Kelly, Patrick J., and S.J. Goerss, *Interactive Stereotactic Surgical System for the Removal of Intracranial Tunors Utilizing eh CO2 Laser and CT Derived Database.* IEEE Transactions on Biomedical Engineering, 1985. **February**: p. 112-16.

33.   Nathan, M.S., *et al. Devices for Automated Resection of the Prostate.* in *Proc. 1st International Symposium on Medical Robotics and Computer Assisted Surgery.* 1994. Pittsburgh.

34.   Adler John, *et al., Image-Guided Robotic Radiosurgery.* In the Proceedings of the First International Symposium on Medical Robotics and Computer assisted Surgery, 1994. **2**: p. 291-297.

Intelligent Image Management in an Integrated Telemedicine Services Network

Stelios C. Orphanoudakis

Institute of Computer Science, FORTH
and
Department of Computer Science, University of Crete
Heraklion, Crete, GREECE

email: orphanou@ics.forth.gr; tel: +30 81 391600; fax: +30 81 391601

In recent years, advances in information technology and telecommunications have acted as catalysts for significant developments in the sector of health care, creating the new application domain of health telematics. These technological advances have had a particularly strong impact in the field of medical imaging, where film radiographic techniques are gradually being replaced by digital imaging techniques, and this has provided an impetus to the development of integrated hospital information systems which support the digital transmission, storage, retrieval, analysis and interpretation of medical images [1]. The provision of added-value telemedicine and, in the case of diagnostic imaging, teleradiology services is a natural outcome of the above developments and support the remote access to information contained in the medical record of a patient, remote medical consultation and patient monitoring, and in some cases the remote delivery of health care [2]. All these functions of an integrated telemedicine services network are very important and are currently the subject of vigorous investigation. This presentation is primarily concerned with the first, and implicitly the second. In particular, the presentation will consider issues arising from the need to efficiently and intelligently manage multimedia patient data with emphasis on the management of image data, which constitutes by far the largest volume of data currently generated by different hospital departments. This is a practical issue, whose successful resolution will undoubtedly have a strong impact on the timely and effective delivery of health care services and, therefore, patient outcome.

In the past two decades, diagnostic medical imaging has been revolutionized by a series of developments based on different types of energy used to probe the human body in order to obtain a variety of mostly complementary anatomical and functional images. However, the possibility for yet another type of energy leading to the development of a new medical imaging modality appears to be rather remote. Thus, the main issues and challenges currently confronting the technical and clinical medical imaging community are the following: 1) how to fully exploit in routine clinical practice the wealth of qualitative and quantitative information contained in multimodality medical images; 2) how to facilitate the first by providing effective and intelligent management of multimedia patient data, which is often geographically distributed at a regional, national, and transnational level; and 3) how to use information technology and telecommunications to develop and make available added-value telematics services to health care professionals and citizens, thus making expertise a shared resource, wherever it may exist [2].

Any attempt at meeting the above challenges and providing clinically significant solutions must take into account technical as well as economic issues. The cost of developing and operating an integrated telemedicine services network is high. Therefore, in the context of the much talked about Information and hopefully Informed Society, the question arises of who is going to pay the cost of telematics services in this most important sector of health, so that their provision can by viable in the long term.

This presentation considers the technical choices to be made in the design and implementation of integrated regional, national and transnational telemedicine networks and services with a view toward providing clinically significant and cost-effective added-value telematics services to the health care community. One must also ensure that the potential benefit to be derived from technological advances also finds its way to the scene of an accident and the home of patients and the elderly. Then, the collective effort will have been worth it, whatever the cost. It is important to point out at the outset that connectivity of health care organizations alone is not the issue, neither is the development of a high-end expensive infrastructure, in terms of information and telecommunications technologies, which is underutilized. The conflicting requirements of keeping the operational cost low, while providing a fast system and network response, can be satisfied to a large extent by employing intelligent strategies in the management of large volumes of data, such as images, as well as in the efficient management of other regional resources for the purpose of dealing with pre-hospital health emergencies [3].

The above issues and some answers will be presented and discussed in the framework of the regional health telematics pilot currently being developed on the island of Crete. Systems, which are currently being used in the development of this pilot and employ intelligent strategies and agents which implement such strategies to manage health related information and available physical resources, as well as to facilitate the access to information by various user groups, will also be presented [4-6]. Intelligent agents can also be used and are currently being considered by our group to deal with problems such as: reduction of search space in large image databases, and reduction of work and information overload in the clinical environment, including schemes for presenting information to users which take into account their individual characteristics and preferences.

References

[1]   Orphanoudakis SC: Supercomputing in Medical Imaging. *IEEE Engineering in Medicine and Biology Magazine* (Special Issue on Supercomputing). Vol.7, No. 4, pp. 16-20, December 1988 (Invited Paper).

[2]   Orphanoudakis SC, Kaldoudi E, and Tsiknakis M: Technological Advances in Teleradiology. *European Journal of Radiology*, Vol. 22, June 1996, pp. 205-217 (invited).

[3]   Tsiknakis M, Katehakis DG, and Orphanoudakis SC: Intelligent Image Management in a Distributed PACS and Telemedicine Environment. *IEEE Communications Magazine*, Vol. 34, No. 7, July 1996, pp. 36-45 (invited).

[4]   Orphanoudakis SC, Chronaki C and Kostomanolakis S: I^2C: A System for the Indexing, Storage, and Retrieval of Medical Images by Content. *Medical Informatics*, Vol. 19, No. 2, 1994, pp. 109-122.

[5]   Petrakis EGM and Orphanoudakis SC: A Generalized Approach for Image Indexing and Retrieval Based on 2-D Strings. In *Intelligent Image Database Systems*, Shi-Kuo Chang, Erland Jungert and G. Tortora (Eds.), World Scientific Publishing Company, 1995.

[6]   Orphanoudakis SC, Chronaki CE, and Vamvaka D: I^2Cnet: Content-Based Similarity Search in Geographically Distributed Repositories of Medical Images. *Computerized Medical Imaging and Graphics*, Vol. 20, No. 4, July-August 1996, pp. 193-207 (invited).

AI Technologies : Conditions for Further Impact

Jean-Raoul Scherrer
Geneva State University Hospital, Switzerland
Division of Medical Informatics

Abstract

This paper deals with the impact of some AI technologies expected in the medical domain in the next few years. Many promises have been made already in the past from different research groups, but few have come to fruition. The innate difficulties associated with the explored field, or an underestimation of necessary resources, are the most common causes for delay (up to 200% or more). We will concentrate in this paper on three topics which will lead to clinical applications before the end of the century: Imaging technologies enhanced by expert systems which are already in use today in a few hospitals; Natural Language Processing which is now producing some early results; Knowledge browsers on the Internet that necessitate intelligent processes. For these three situations, this paper presents state-of-the-art prototypes and results which have given a « proof of concept ». Moreover, it evaluates the potential for use in clinics, as well as for taking a position on the software market.

The author and his team would like to emphasise a clear message to researchers: that the main progress of AI techniques in the future will come from field experiments; that only in such a context will theories, principles and algorithms provide their best contributions to the advance of AI technologies. The suggestion: « Come down from the mountains and create pragmatic applications » is certainly a call to be more efficient.

Present Context of AI in Medicine

Since 1970, AI technologies in the medical domain have become quite promising, and there is no need to remind readers that some of the best precursors of expert systems have been in medicine, for example, like MYCIN. However, initial expectations have not been met, one of the main reasons being that, in most practical situations, the AI systems have difficulties in handling a suitable « bunch » of knowledge. Knowledge acquisition has come to be recognised as a bottleneck. Without adequate knowledge, even in a limited domain, a given system is at risk of giving solutions considered too trivial or not « intelligent » enough. A second problem, not recognised in the early 70s, is the handling of « common sense » which has proved much more complicated than expected. The lack of enough visible results has led to a separation between the two worlds, namely: 1) the solution providers, who are AI scientists; 2) the customers involved in clinical practice.

But this schematic point of view should not be considered a pessimistic one. On the contrary, although it is clearly provocative, there is now evidence of new trends from which « proof of concept » is emerging and applications in daily use are not the exceptions anymore. With this in mind, we want to consider in turn three different domains where contributions have been made at the Geneva University Hospital.

Imaging Technologies

These technologies have been boosted by recent advances produced in the computer field, making medium and low-cost platforms suitable for advanced performance and production in a clinical setting. During the last 10 years Multimedia has become widespread. Concurrently, software tools, and the techniques to cope with images, have been strongly developed. Last but not least, information highways (Internet, Netscape, etc.) are now in operation: large hospitals are being equipped with fiber optic LANs; fast communications between hospitals will soon be a reality not just a dream.

AI technologies are the necessary complement to basic imaging software. The main problem with images is not their creation, storage or transport, but clearly their interpretation. Because of their innate limitations, human beings have to be extremely well trained to read images efficiently, and this goal is not often reached in many communities or hospitals. Only an exchange of expertise on the Net may solve this problem. In addition, intelligent tools may be precious for image screening and initial interpretation, before the experts are called in. This will be one of tomorrow's realities for a number of specialised domains. This paper will illustrate this situation by concrete examples taken from our laboratory [1]. [2].

Natural Language Processing

NLP has the worst reputation for making false promises in the AI field. This was not caused by medical applications. In fact, computer translations which were expected to be in use in the 70s are far from even being realised today. There was a huge problem of knowledge representation which was totally underestimated at the time. Even today the modelling in the medical domain is a lengthly task where available resources are limited, and only specific subdomains may bring results within 5 or 10 years.

However, NLP techniques do not need ultimate modelling techniques in order to represent these natural languages being examined. At least, they are in a position to demonstrate practical results using simplified and pragmatic representations of medical concepts. This means that the depth of knowledge representation may be elevated to some intermediate level. Such a level is certainly not superficial, but it prevents the more sophisticated kind of human knowledge in medicine being reached. Such a half-way stop should not be considered against the overall quality, but as an intermediate step before resources, reaching a more detailed representation, are made available.

In the domain of patient encoding, NLP techniques have recently proved themselves to be of benefit in the quality of patient descriptions in our hospital [3], [4]. Discharge summaries are produced on a daily basis by physicians, who build the diagnoses and procedures list using the NLP tools for patient encoding. The leading motivation now is not just for the reimbursement, but also for the patient description, in order to facilitate a possible readmission.

Health Knowledge on Internet

The introduction of Internet on a worldwide basis makes medical knowledge « locally » available to a huge number of people as never before. Rich sources of knowledge are now shared and this movement has only just begun. However, this large amount of information which is supposed to transport a concomitant know-how, despite its new and easy accessibility, may be disappointing. The problem is to qualify any « bunch » of knowledge and to provide navigation guides for (more or less) advanced scientists [5].

Tools have been developed to search the Net and to help comment on the available information. These tools are able to conduct content analyses, full text searches, medical indexing from the content, classification of the sources, and verification of availability and stability of servers. Intelligent agents are the working force for such a task and current experiments raise hope. There is no target in the next 5 years for fully automatized tools, but permanent screening of the Net may help experts with their decisions and final judgements.

Conclusions

Three different domains showing the promise of AI technologies have now been explored. They are not the only domains with the same potential, but are typical of the situation. On the one side we are faced with a problem where classical applications may fail to give an adequate answer; on the other, we have at hand ready-to use technologies, many of which have not yet found a home in a real life application. The next « encounter of the scientist and the clinician » will have the potential of enormous benefits on the condition that the actors demonstrate a great willingness to reach the fixed goals together.

We have learnt that a bright idea and a strong need generally do not match by chance. This means that laboratory-only design, as excellent as it may be, gives poor end-results. The problems to be solved are rarely complicated, although they do necessitate the introduction of new techniques like AI, but they are generally not formulated in a language understandable by a computer scientist or an AI expert. The gap is large and the bridges over it are not numerous. The call to « Come down from the mountains..... » is clearly a solution to this problem. It will not cause an impoverishment to any participating party; on the contrary we can clearly expect new and original developments resulting from initial experiments, and a general progress with the applicativity of AI technologies.

References

[1] Ligier Y, Ratib O, Logean M, Girard C. OSIRIS : A Medical Image Manipulation System. M.D. Computing Journal, July-August 94, Vol. 11. No. 4, pp 212-218. URL: http://expasy.hcuge.ch/UIN/

[2] Appel RD, Bairoch A, Hochstrasser DF. A New Generation of Information Retrieval Tools for Biologists : The Example of the EXPASY WWW Server. Trends in Biomedical Sciences. TiBS June 1994 (222), Vol.19, No.6, pp. 258-260. URL: http://expasy.hcuge.ch/

[3] Baud RH, Rassinoux AM, Wagner JC, Lovis C, Juge C, Alpay LL, Michel PA, Degoulet P, Scherrer JR. Representing Clinical Narratives Using Conceptual Graphs. Meth. Inform. Med. 1995; 34: pp.176-86.

[4] Lovis C, Gaspoz JM, Baud RH, Michel PA, Scherrer JR. Natural Language Processing and Clinical Support to Improve the Quality of Reimbursement Claim Databases. Proceedings SCAMC 1996, Special Issue of JAMIA, 1996.

[5] Boyer C, Baujard V, Aurel S, Selby M, Appel RD. HON : Automated Database of Health and Medical Information. MEDNET 96 : European Congress on the Internet in Medicine, Brighton, UK, Oct. 14-17, 1996. URL: http://www.hon.ch/

Protocols and Guidelines

Protocols for Medical Procedures and Therapies[1]: A Provisional Description of the PRO*forma* Language and Tools

John Fox, Nicky Johns, Ali Rahmanzadeh[2]

Imperial Cancer Research Fund
Lincoln's Inn Fields, London, England, WC2A 3PX
{jf,nj,ahr}@acl.icnet.uk

Abstract

PRO*forma* is a language for describing the actions, information and decisions required in patient care. It is the basis of a method for defining best-practice guidelines, research protocols and other procedures in a form that can be *enacted* by a computer to help clinical professionals comply with preferred practice. Use of the method consists of outlining the clinical tasks required by the procedure, and specifying details using standard templates for each class of task. This paper presents a description of the PRO*forma* language, and associated protocol development and enactment software, illustrated with examples. Our aim is to develop PRO*forma* as a possible standard for representing clinical procedures; the present version (1.5) is presented as a basis for discussion and is subject to revision.

Introduction

Various attempts have been made to design knowledge representation systems which are capable of capturing and supporting clinical procedures. These include flowcharting tools (e.g. ALGO, [17]), data entry and workflow managers (e.g.Protégé [14]) and the Arden syntax, a conventional programming language with facilities for incorporating medical logic modules ([12]). However, the available techniques are widely thought to be insufficiently expressive, versatile or sound for general use. For example, there is often no provision for managing clinical uncertainty, such as the unreliability associated with data and the unpredictability of events. The Arden syntax was a particularly notable attempt to propose a method for representing medical

1 This work was carried out as part of the PROMPT project (PROtocols for medical Procedures and Therapies), project number HC1041 in the EU's Healthcare Telematics Programme and in association with the ACTION cluster of projects funded under this programme.
2 Many people have influenced the development of the concepts and software described here. We would particularly like to thank Subrata Das, David Elsdon, Claude Gierl, Paul Ferguson and Saki Hajnal who made important contributions in earlier projects.

knowledge in a general way but as Musen et al note [14] it „has significant limitations: the language currently supports only atomic data types, lacks a defined semantics for making temporal comparisons or for performing data abstraction, and provides no principled way to represent clinical guidelines that are more complex than individual situation-action rules".

The PRO*forma* method is being developed to address these and other important requirements, including rigorous design and operational safety of applications.

The method assumes that three kinds of knowledge must be used in combination when making patient management decisions: general medical knowledge (of diseases, symptoms, tests, drugs); knowledge of the specific patient (personal details, problems, symptoms, current medications and so forth); and knowledge of best-practice procedures (what should be done when). The PRO*forma* method is primarily focused on the last type of knowledge though it is intended to provide useful constraints for developers of medical knowledge formalisms and clinical data models.

The central element of the method is the PRO*forma* language. This is a *knowledge representation language* in the AI tradition, which is structured around a well-defined ontology of tasks, including decision making and process management tasks. It is also a *specification language* in the sense used in software engineering: a declarative formalism with a clear semantics that can be exploited in rigorous design and the pursuit of high quality and safe software.

The following tools have been developed to implement the method.

(1) A PRO*forma* editor, which provides a set of graphical templates for laying out the tasks that compose a protocol or guideline and the practical and temporal constraints on the execution of those tasks.

(2) A protocol *enactment* engine which takes a PRO*forma* definition constructed with the editor, instantiates it as a care-plan for a specific patient, and assists clinical users to follow the plan.

An Example PRO*forma* Application

The user interface of a decision support application which was implemented with an early version of the PRO*forma* method and tools is shown in figure 1. The application deals with the management of acute asthma in adults based on a guideline published by the British Thoracic Society, which was structured and declaratively specified as a sequence of machine-executable tasks. A graphical representation of this task definition is shown in the background window. Some of these tasks involve advising the user of required actions and some request information; these require additional dialogues, examples of which are shown on the right.

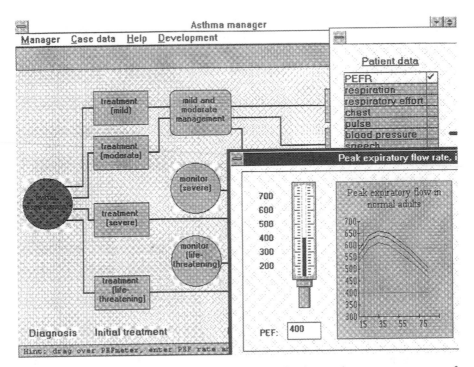

Figure 1: A user display from a computerised guideline/protocol management system for managing acute asthma in adults in the accident and emergency department. The background window shows the guideline published by the British Thoracic Society rendered as a set of tasks in a structured workflow diagram. The first task in this guideline, „initial assessment" requires the user to enter various items of patient data, shown as a prompt list at the top right. The user has selected the peak flow item from this list, and is entering the relevant data using a graphical dialogue shown at the bottom right. As the tasks are executed the graphical interface shows which tasks are pending, which complete and which in various other control states: the task is indicated by dynamic colour coding of the tasks.

The graphical workflow diagram can be used *passively*, to summarise and remind clinical staff of the procedures that need to be carried out, or *actively*, to assist in the correct and timely enactment of specific clinical tasks. In the latter mode the system may prompt users for clinical actions which need to be carried out (taking into account temporal and other constraints), remind them of information that needs to be recorded, and advise on any decisions that need to be taken.

In the example the first task required by the guideline is a patient assessment decision (shown as a circle). The two panels on the right are an *aide memoire* that lists the topics that are relevant to the assessment, and a data entry screen for the user to enter peak flow and associated patient data. Depending upon the assessment (mild, moderate, severe or life threatening) care of the patient will proceed along the appropriate branch of the protocol emerging from the decision. In the centre of the picture are two special decisions: these are „watchdogs" that monitor the patient record in order to detect any adverse events or possible hazards that may occur.

Decision support functions, which are used for the initial classification of the severity of the patient's asthma and the implementation of watchdogs, use a generalised decision procedure that can be used to support most types of clinical decision, including diagnostic, therapeutic and prescribing decisions. A range of different kinds of patient-specific advice can be provided by these functions, including suggesting when a decision is needed; what the decision options are; which information is relevant to making the choice and so on. A particularly crucial piece of advice is whether the decision can (and should) be taken and, if so, which is the best alternative of the available options given what is currently known. The symbolic decision procedure supported in the PROforma language is described below; additional applications and details of the underlying theoretical concepts can be found in [9] and [2].

The enactment engine is written in Prolog. It has a simple default user interface (see below), but it is anticipated that it will often be desirable to embed the engine in locally supplied software that will provide its own interface. Consequently the engine and GUI are run as separate inter-operable processes. In this application the GUI is written in Visual Basic® which permits, for example, use of various visual devices to indicate procedural features of a task, such as colour coding to indicate whether a task is currently scheduled, active, completed, aborted etc., and specialised data entry widgets such as the peak-flow meter. The GUI process sends and receives commands, data and queries to and from the enactment engine via a DDE link.

Computerising a Clinical Procedure with the PROforma Method

Preparation of a computerised care guideline or clinical protocol is a two-step process. In step 1, a high level description of the guideline is developed using a graphical design package. (The source is typically a document which sets out the guideline, ideally one published by an authoritative body.) The resulting diagram shows the clinical tasks required in an easily understood form, together with their logical and temporal interrelationships. In step 2, the graphical outline is converted into a the detailed medical knowledge base required to enact it.

Step 1: Graphical Representation of the high level Structure of a Guideline

The top level structure in PROforma is the *task*. The PROforma language is designed to provide support for a comprehensive range of clinical tasks, such as decision making, scheduling of actions over time, reminders for patient data collection, monitoring adverse events and so forth. Starting from the available knowledge sources, an application designer typically develops the graphical network which summarises the decisions, actions and other tasks recommended by the guideline. PROforma supports four basic classes of task (figure 2):

- A *plan* is a sequence of sub-tasks, or components, which need to be carried out to achieve a clinical objective, such as a therapeutic objective. Plan components are usually ordered, to reflect temporal, logical, resource or other constraints.
- A *decision* task occurs at any point in a guideline or protocol in which some sort of choice has to be made, such as a diagnostic, therapeutic or investigative choice.
- An *action* is a procedure which is to be enacted outside the computer system, typically by clinical staff, such as the administration of an injection.
- An *enquiry* is a task whose objective is to obtain an item of information which is needed in order to complete a procedure or take a decision. The specification of an enquiry includes a description of the information required (e.g. a lab. result) and a method for getting it (e.g. by a query on a local patient record, or a remote laboratory database).

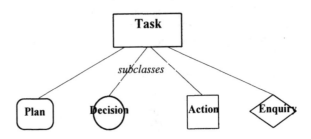

Figure 2: The PROforma task ontology: decisions, actions and enquiries are "atomic" tasks, while plans are compound. Plans can consist of any number of atomic tasks, and subplans. All tasks have a set of common attributes (e.g. goals and preconditions) but each subtype has its own distinguishing attributes (see text).

Figure 3 shows a schematic view of a protocol in the PRO*forma* graphical notation. This figure provides a simplified view of a task network representing a protocol for treatment of limited breast cancer (FB1) used at the Institut Bergonié in Bordeaux (only a subset of decisions and plans is shown here).

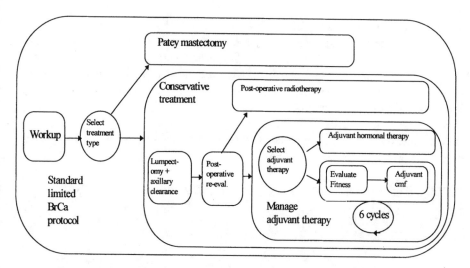

Figure 3: Simplified task analysis for combined therapy protocol for breast cancer. Tasks are represented by simple icons, and the relationships between them by arrows (a circle represents a decision, round-cornered rectangles represent plans, and arrows represent scheduling constraints) A procedure which lies inside another procedure forms a component of that procedure, but may also potentially be reused in other protocols.

This high level diagram shows that the first task to be carried out in FB1 is a plan, the patient workup, followed by a decision about the appropriate treatment type for the patient. Either *Patey mastectomy* may be chosen or, shown here in more detail, *conservative treatment*. Conservative treatment decomposes into a sequence of component tasks, including the task of managing *adjuvant therapy* which itself decomposes into a decision, a cyclical therapy administration task, and so on. Figure 4 shows a screen from the PRO*forma* editor during the creation of a guideline for the management of dyspepsia.

The graphical notation provides an intermediate representation between an informal description of the protocol or guideline (such as a conventional protocol document) and a machine executable knowledge base. The notation provides a succinct and natural summary which can be understood by medical specialists. It also helps to guide the detailed specification of the tasks in Step 2 of the PRO*forma* method, in which the detailed clinical knowledge and other information required to enact the tasks in the network are added.

Step 2: Populating Task Templates

Every clinical task is different, but most can be modelled in terms of a small number of object *classes* which have a common, generic structure, or *template*. Templates guide the application designer in formalising the necessary medical knowledge required by the guideline or protocol. All protocols, for example, have eligibility conditions (preconditions) and conditions under which the protocol should be abandoned (abort conditions). Decisions, actions and enquiries can similarly be modelled as generic tasks; each of the four sub-classes of PRO*forma* task has a common internal structure, but each sub-class also inherits a number of attributes from the general class „tasks". All tasks have a clinical objective (goal), and may have preconditions, post-conditions and so forth. Figure 5 shows two template editing tools provided by the PRO*forma* editor.

The templates for the tasks are based on the constructs supported by the PRO*forma* language, which is described in the next section.

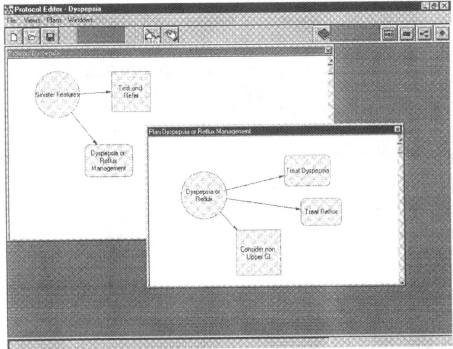

Figure 4: The PROforma editor which provides graphical tools for laying out protocols in terms of four types of task; decisions (circles); plans (round rectangles); actions (square rectangles) and enquiries (diamonds). Arrows are scheduling constraints. The rear window shows component tasks in a guideline for the management of dyspepsia in primary car; the front shows the decomposition for the subplan „dyspepsia and reflux management".

PRO*forma* 1.5 Language Description

PROforma is a declarative language for specifying clinical guidelines and protocols in terms of the generic tasks introduced in the last section. When a collection of tasks is *enacted* by the PRO*forma* engine, the specification attributes determine how and when each task will be carried out. The tables below describe the attributes of the tasks in version 1.5.

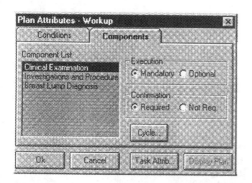 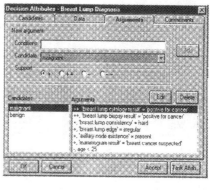

Figure 5: Views of templates for two kinds of PROforma tasks, plans (left) and decisions (right). The plan template shows a view of the components and properties of the components of the „workup" task in the limited breast cancer protocol shown in figure 3. Selecting the „conditions" tab enters a different view in which the designer can attach special conditions to the task, such as termination and abort conditions. The decision template shows a view of the „breast lump diagnosis" decision, which is a component of the workup task. Here we are viewing the specification of the arguments for one candidate diagnosis, malignant tumour, showing the supporting (+) and confirming (++) arguments which are specified for this diagnosis. Selecting the other tabs permits the designer to add alternative candidates, specify other relevant data, or add decision rules by which a diagnosis can be „committed".

The Generic Task

Any task (of type plan, decision, action or enquiry) can have the following attributes.

Attribute	Description
Title	Descriptive title of task
Identifier (= Name(P1,P2,...))	Identifier is name and parameters
Description	Textual description of task
Goal	Purpose of task
Trigger conditions	Conditions necessary to initiate task
Preconditions	Conditions necessary before task may be executed
PostConditions	Conditions true on task completion
Version info	Author, creation date, modifications etc.

The *Identifier* or *TaskName* is a unique identifier for the task. The goal specifies the clinical objective of the task (e.g. diagnose(joint_pain); treat(dyspepsia); investigate(breast_lump). A task's *Preconditions* (if any) must be satisfied before the task can be initiated. *Trigger conditions*, if any, are events that can cause the task to be initiated, but only if the preconditions are satisfied. A task's *Postconditions* are conditions which are always true when the task has been completed.

Plans

A plan has the following specific attributes *in addition to those for the generic task*.

Attribute	Description
Components	List of component subtasks
Scheduling constraints on subtasks	Constraints determining sequencing of tasks
Temporal constraints on subtasks	Constraints determining timing of tasks
Optional tasks	List of tasks which are non-mandatory
Non confirmatory tasks	List of tasks not requiring confirmation
Number of cycles	How many times to repeat a task
Cycle until conditions	When task repetition should stop
Repetition interval	Time interval between task repetitions
Abort Conditions	Conditions causing plan to be abandoned
Terminate Conditions	Conditions indicating completion of plan

Plans have *Components* (subtasks) on which are imposed *Scheduling constraints* which determine the order in which the subtasks may be carried out (although trigger conditions may override scheduling constraints). A scheduling constraint specifies that a particular subtask may not be started until another subtask has been completed. There may also be *Temporal constraints* which determine the timing of the execution of subtasks. For example, a temporal constraint may specify that a particular subtask may not be done until 4 hours after completion of another subtask.

By default all subtasks are considered to be mandatory (i.e. they have to be completed before the plan is considered to be complete), but the *Optional tasks* list allows tasks to be specified as non-mandatory. All subtasks of type *action* or *decision* are assumed by default to require confirmation by the user that they have been carried out, but any tasks listed in the *Non confirmatory tasks* will be completed without confirmation.

If at any time the *Terminate conditions* become true, the plan will be considered complete and no further subtasks within this plan will be activated, but tasks scheduled *after* this plan will then be started. If at any time the *Abort Conditions* become true, the plan (and all its subtasks) will be abandoned. If a task is abandoned, there will be no activation of any of the tasks which follow it.

Any task within a plan may be cyclical, specified by a *Number of cycles* for each such task. If the number of cycles is greater than 1, the task will be repeated until either the number of cycles has been done, or the *Cycle until conditions* are met. The *Repetition interval* specifies the time interval between cycles.

Decisions.

A decision has the following specific attributes in addition to those for general tasks.

Attribute	Description
Candidates	Candidates for result of decision
Arguments	Argument rules for different candidates
Commitment rules	Rules for commitment to a candidate
Sources	Information sources required
Mandatory Info	Information essential for commitment of decision

A decision's *Candidates* represent the possible set of outcomes or choices for a decision. Once a decision becomes active, its candidates are generated: a set of candidates may be an explicit set, or may be defined by rules.

The value of the *Arguments* attribute specifies under what conditions the different candidates should be supported (or excluded): argument rules define the „pros and cons" for each alternative.

A decision's *Commitment rules* specify when the decision may be taken, for example what data must be present and how many of the „pros and cons" must be considered. A commitment rule will usually use the decision's arguments to assess the support for the different candidates: the completion of a decision is when a commitment rule has succeeded.

The *Sources* attribute specifies the information which is needed to make the decision. When this information is required (for example in the evaluation of an argument rule or a commitment rule), and it is not already present in the database, the PRO*forma* engine will issue a request for the data.

Decisions *will not be committed without confirmation from the user*, unless the decision is specified as 'non-confirmatory' in its parent plan.

Actions

An action has the following further specific attributes in addition to those for general tasks.

Attribute	Description
Procedure	Procedure to be carried out
Context	Context, special conditions etc.

When an action is activated, the specified *Procedure* is requested. The PRO*forma* engine assumes that the „outside world" knows how to execute this procedure. The

Context is any extra special conditions or information that may need to be conveyed, such as when, where, how or by whom the procedure should be carried out.

Normally confirmation is required that the action has been done, so an action is only considered to be complete after confirmation has been received. However, if an action is listed as non-confirmatory within the parent plan it will be considered to be complete once its procedure has been requested.

Enquiries

An enquiry has the following further specific attribute in addition to those for general tasks.

Attribute	Description
Data required	Data item(s) needed

An enquiry is similar to an action except that it is expected to return value(s). There may be more than one data item to be returned. An enquiry is complete when all these data items are present in the database. For each data item not already in the database and for which there is no rule defined, the PRO*forma* engine issues a data request.

Oracles and rules

There are two additional PRO*forma* entities which may be used in task specifications, but which
are not tasks (in the sense that they do not lie within the PROforma ontology and do not therefore inherit the generic properties of tasks). These are the *oracle* and the *rule*, which are best viewed as constructs for implementing information acquisition and inference processes.

An oracle has the following attributes.

Attribute	Description
Identifier	Name and parameters
Description	Textual description of oracle
Type	Data type (integer, string, etc.)
Range	Range of allowable values
External call	Procedure for obtaining raw data
Context	Special conditions etc.

A rule describes a relationship between existing data items or knowledge, or describes how to derive new data from existing data. A rule has the following attributes.

Attribute	Description
Identifier	Name and parameters
Description	Textual description of rule

Sources	Data required when executing rule
Rule	Definition of relationship

Any unknown data in the rule definition will be deemed false unless it is included in the *Sources* list, in which case the PRO*forma* engine will issue a data request (as in a decision).

Process Enactment by the PRO*forma* Engine

The purpose of the PRO*forma* engine is to enact the tasks specified by a guideline or protocol, that is to say it issues requests for action, prompts for information and generally assists a user to comply with the protocol in line with medical, procedural and other requirements.

When the engine enacts a protocol, each task in the protocol is "created" as needed as a run-time instance in memory with current time-stamps and other relevant information. The task instances are created as the user progresses through the protocol, and assigned unique runtime „Task IDs" (integers); these identifiers have various uses, such as permitting multiple patients to be managed simultaneously according to a single protocol.

The engine initiates tasks according to their scheduling constraints, preconditions etc., and sends messages to notify that tasks have been activated, inform the user of decisions which need to be made, request data or actions to be carried out etc. Figure 6 shows the engine running a primary care guideline for the management of breast cancer. The user interface shown here is the default interface provided by the engine; the software is designed to be linked to a separate, appropriately tailored application-specific interface, as in the asthma example above. A typical use of the latter capability would be to link the enactment system to an existing patient record system; this would provide the normal interface that is familiar to clinical staff but can call upon the engine to provide decision support or process management advice as needed.

The engine functions reactively, i.e. it responds to messages from external sources (e.g. notifying it of commands from the user interface, updates to the patient record, the completion of time-outs etc.). Any arrival of new data will generally have repercussions throughout the current protocol (e.g. decisions which may now be taken, tasks which may now be started, etc.). The engine's response to the arrival of a message is to propagate all these effects forward until no more changes can be made.

During processing of an incoming message the engine checks

- if there are any tasks to be started or progressed
- if there are any actions to be requested
- if there are any decisions which can now commit

- if there is any data to be requested

For example the arrival of data may mean that a task's preconditions are now met, so that the task can be started. Confirmation that a procedure has been carried out may mean that a subsequent task's scheduling constraints are now satisfied so that this new task may be started, and so on.

These checks (and consequent actions) are repeated until no more can be done, i.e. the engine is once again quiescent. It will then await the arrival of the next message.

Task scheduling and control. Once tasks are created they can pass through different states during the enactment of a PROforma protocol, from being *established* (just created) through to being *performed* (completed). For example, a decision whose commit rules have succeeded becomes *ready to commit.*

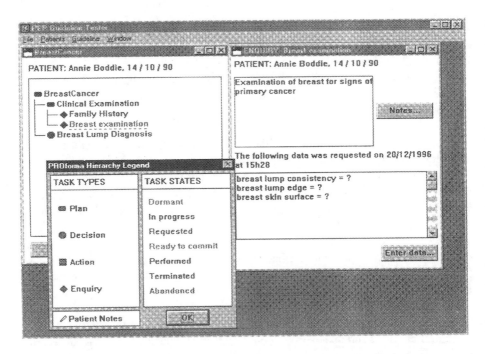

Figure 6: the default interface of the enactment engine, showing the active part of the guideline for the management of breast cancer shown in figure 3 (left), a legend indicating the types of task and colour coding for task states (inset) and a report for a selected task, the diagnosis of a breast lump (right).

Enactment of decisions

The evaluation of decisions in the PROforma engine involves four main functions:

- Generating the candidates for an active decision
- Evaluating the arguments for and against candidates

- Testing the commitment rules for a decision
- Committing to a candidate

Candidates. The PRO*forma* definition of a decision includes a specification of the *candidates*, which represent the options of the decision. Often there will be a fixed set of candidates, but there may also be rules to define candidates, which means that a different set of candidates could be generated for different cases. For example when deciding on a drug to prescribe, the set of „candidate" drugs will obviously depend on the medical problem being treated.

Arguments. A decision also includes *arguments* which specify the „pros and cons" of each possible candidate. An argument rule indicates the „support" for a given candidate, and comprises

- a candidate
- conditions
- support

The default support scheme for arguments uses a semi-qualitative representation or „dictionary" [8]. In this scheme '+' is used to mean the candidate's support is increased by an argument, '-' to mean its support is diminished, '++' to mean the candidate is definitely confirmed, and '—' to mean the candidate is definitely excluded. Arguments can be aggregated to maintain a preference ordering over the candidates using a simple function *netsupport* which assumes that by default all arguments are given equal weight. The netsupport function calculates a simple measure: the number of '+' conditions which are true minus the number of '-' conditions which are true, but with either a '—' or a '++' overriding with values of minus or plus infinity respectively).

Commitment Rules. A decision's *commit rules* define when a decision task may commit to a particular candidate (i.e. when the decision is ready to be taken). Each rule comprises

- a candidate
- a set of conditions which must be true
- a procedure to be executed when the rule succeeds.

Commitment may depend solely on a quantitative argument aggregation function, such as *netsupport*, but provision has been made to evaluate arbitrary conditions, such as safety and other conditions (e.g. [10]). Normally, commitment will also require confirmation from the user, and the user can always select a different candidate from the one suggested by the engine.

Data sources. A decision can specify the data it needs to evaluate its arguments. These are specified as the decision's *sources*, and during the evaluation of conditions in argument rules or commit rules, any source data will be requested if it is not already available.

Discussion

Status of the PRO*forma* Language

The present paper should be viewed as an interim description of the PRO*forma* method and language, rather than a formal definition. Although the technical and theoretical basis of the method are quite well developed (see next section) our experience in building complete applications is too limited to claim that it is definitive. As experience grows, and as we acquire feedback from colleagues in important fields whose developments will impact on the language (such as medical knowledge representation, terminology and patient data modelling etc.) we expect to refine and/or extend the language and associated software.

It is our aim to offer PRO*forma* as a potential standard for representing knowledge of clinical procedures, but at the time of writing we believe this would be premature. Consequently we would encourage readers who share our interest in achieving a knowledge representation and interchange standard for the field to inform us of criticisms or concerns about any aspect of the description. This will help to identify and remedy the method's weaknesses and assure the community that what finally emerges can claim some consensual support.

Ensuring that Clinical Decision Support Systems are Safe and Sound

In an extensively discussed paper Heathfield and Wyatt raised a number of concerns about the many factors which can adversely affect the practical clinical value of even the best motivated and conceived decision support system [11]. They attach particular importance to the need to make use of well established ideas from software engineering, notably the use of a well-defined development methodology, encompassing coherent methods for modelling the clinical problem, judicious use of rapid prototyping, use of application development tools which are appropriate for the domain, and rigorous empirical evaluation.

We support this view, of the need to establish a *quality culture* in medical informatics, and in many ways the development of the PRO*forma* method is an attempt to take seriously the concerns raised by Heathfield and Wyatt. However we also wish to emphasise the importance of a *safety culture* so the PRO*forma* method places great emphasis on achieving *sound design* based on well understood design theories and *safe operation* by providing explicit techniques for managing the hazards that may arise in clinical settings, as is normal in other safety-critical fields, such as aerospace and the nuclear industry [4]. An important element of this concern is to ensure that decision making in particular is carried out in a manner that is mathematically sound and operationally safe.

The PRO*forma* decision procedure was first used in *The Oxford System of Medicine,* a decision support system aimed at general practitioners and a simple task management system was incorporated in the *Bordeaux Oncology Support System* which was aimed at enacting cancer therapy protocols [5]. The general concepts behind the symbolic decision procedure were first described in [7] and an extension to permit task management was outlined in [3]. However, the safety-critical character of medical applications and the need to reassure the user community that the basic concepts are theoretically adequate has since motivated a great deal of work to formalise the underlying concepts and prove the technical soundness of the PRO*forma* approach. The most comprehensive account presents a unified model and semantics covering the whole decision making and plan management scheme represented in PRO*forma* [2].

The topic of uncertainty management is central to medical decision making, and one that attracts particular controversy. The most widely accepted technique for managing uncertainty is to quantify it in terms of prior and conditional probabilities and apply standard methods, such as Bayesian evidence updating methods, to calculate the most preferred clinical option. Unfortunately, as has been observed many times, reliable probabilities are neither easily acquired nor widely accepted by clinicians. A *logic of argumentation* has therefore been adopted in PRO*forma* as an intuitive formalism for the idea of constructing reasons for and against decision alternatives based on qualitative knowledge [8]. Since this is an unorthodox approach we have reported a considerable number of technical results concerning the mathematical and computational properties of the logic [13] as well as a sound formal semantics [1].

In order to take, or commit to, a decision we must combine or *aggregate* arguments in order to establish relative preferences among options. Since clinicians generally have to make decisions in the absence of comprehensive quantitative data PRO*forma* supports the netsupport function, a simple semi-qualitative argument weighting scheme. Perhaps surprisingly there is now considerable evidence that such simple decision functions are highly effective for many clinical applications (e.g. [6,15] The most definitive study to date however is that by Pradhan et al who have rigorously assessed the impact of various evidence aggregation methods in medical decision making [16]. It replicates the earlier findings cited, concluding that the correct qualitative representation of the decision has much more influence on the quality of decision making than the precision of quantitative parameters such as probabilities.

However, we do not doubt that in some application domains precision may be more important than others. Consequently, although the present approach emphasises the representation of arguments and other qualitative aspects of decision making, quantitative argument weighting functions based on various uncertainty calculi are compatible with the approach, including classical probabilities, belief functions, order of magnitude values, qualitative probabilities and so on [13].

In general we believe that although certain theoretical issues remain to be fully addressed the formal soundness of the ideas which underpin the PRO*forma* method has been substantially demonstrated. The approach can be regarded as a flexible, general and safe alternative to more orthodox decision support techniques.

Conclusions

This paper has described a formal knowledge representation language for specifying clinical guidelines and protocols which is believed to be sufficiently expressive, versatile and sound to be used in a wide range of medical applications. The current status of the language and associated software is, however, provisional; a definitive description will be published, when appropriate, in the light of clinical experience and feedback from the medical informatics community.

References

1. Ambler, S „ A categorical approach to the semantics of argumentation" *Mathematical Structures*, 1996.
2. Das S K, Fox J, Krause P J „A unified framework for hypothetical and practical reasoning (1): Theoretical Foundations" in D M Gabbay and H J Ohlbach, *Practical Reasoning*, Berlin: Springer 1996.
3. Fox J, Symbolic Decision Procedures for Knowledge Based Systems, in H Adeli (ed) *Knowledge Engineering, volume 2*, New York: McGraw Hill, 1990.
4. Fox J „On the soundness and safety of expert systems" *Artificial Intelligence in Medicine*, 5, 159-179, 1993.
5. Fox J, Glowinski A J, O'Neil M „The Oxford System of Medicine" *Artificial Intelligence in Medicine*, 1990.
6. Fox J, Barber D C and Bardhan KD „A quantitative comparison with rule-based diagnostic inference" *Meth. Inform. Med.* 19, 210-215, 1980.
7. Fox J, Clark DA, Glowinski A J and O'Neil M „Using predicate logic to integrate qualitative reasoning and classical decision theory, *IEEE Trans. Systems, Man and Cybernetics*, 20(2), 347-357, 1990.
8. Fox J, Krause P J and Ambler S „Arguments, contradictions and practical reasoning" in B Neumann (ed) *Proc. 10th Eur. Conf. On AI*, 623-627, 1992.
9. Fox J and Das S K „A unified framework for hypothetical and practical reasoning (2): Lessons from medicine" in D M Gabbay and H J Ohlbach, *Practical Reasoning*, Berlin: Springer 1996.
10. Hammond P, Harris A L, Das S K and Wyatt J „Safety and decision support in oncology" *Meth. Inform. Med.*, 33 (4), 371-381, 1994.
11. Heathfield H A and Wyatt J „Philosophies for the design and development of clinical decision support systems" *Meth. Inform. Med*, 32, 1-8, 1993.
12. Hripzsak G, Clayton PD, Pryor TA, Haug P, Wigertz OB and Van der Lei J „The Arden Syntax for Medical Logic Modules" in *Proc 14th Annual Symposium on Computer Applications in Medical Care*, Washington: IEEE Press, 200-204, 1990.
13. Krause P, Ambler S, Elvang-Goransson M and Fox J „A logic of argumentation for reasoning under uncertainty" *Computational Intelligence*, 11(1), 1995.

14. Musen M A, Tu S W, Das A K and Shahar Y 'A component based architecture for automation of Protocol-Directed Therapy', in Barahona P, Stefanelli M and Wyatt J (eds) *Proc. AIME95*, Berlin: Springer, 1995.
15. O'Neil M and Glowinski A J „Evaluating and validating very large knowledge based systems" *Medical Informatics*, 15 (3), 237-251, 1990.
16. Pradhan M, Henrion M, Provan G, Del Favero B, Huang K „The sensitivity of belief networks to imprecise probabilities: an experimental investigation" *Artificial Intelligence*, 85, 363-397, 1996.
17. Sitter H, Prunte H, Lorenz „A new version of the Programme ALGO for clinical algorithms" in J Brender et al (eds), *Medical Informatics Europe*, IOS Press, 1996.

Supporting Tools for Guideline Development and Dissemination

Silvana Quaglini[1], Roberta Saracco[2], Mario Stefanelli[1], Clara Fassino[1]

[1] Dpt. Informatica e Sistemistica - *Università di Pavia, Pavia, Italy*
[2] Consorzio di Bioingegneria e Informatica Medica, Pavia, Italy

Abstract. This paper describes a general methodology for specifying clinical practice guidelines, which can be exploited in a WWW environment. The formal representation aims at producing clinical guidelines which 1) can be widely shared between different institutions, 2) can be efficiently shared between human and software agents cooperating inside a clinical context, and 3) are able to deal with patient and organization preferences. Such a formal representation, presenting an expressive syntax and an application-oriented semantics, could facilitate development, implementation and real-time access to the guideline's prescriptions. Moreover, this kind of representation could be crucial for activities such as guideline's validation and modification.

1 Introduction

The aim of this work is to develop a formalism and implement a framework capable of improving guideline-based care at the development, dissemination and use phases.

Today clinical guidelines (GL) are expressed in natural language, but this kind of representation can not be easily transformed into a formal and structured framework required by an information technology approach [1, 2]. In fact, health care delivery is an activity which involves a certain number of different professionals, like clinicians, nurses, laboratory technicians, etc., and the quality of care depends both on their own professional skills, and on the level of cooperation and coordination they reach inside the clinical context. Moreover, health care delivery is a strongly distributed process, i.e. there is expertise, knowledge, physical resources distribution. To realize a shared and distributed medical care, these same characteristics of cooperation, coordination and distribution must be shown by the software tools introduced to support health care delivery, that's why we will often refer to the terminology typical of the *cooperating agent* paradigm [4]. Thus, in our proposal, the GL specification exploits concepts such as negotiation, skill, etc. We propose a formal representation for clinical GLs which can be efficiently shared between human and software agents cooperating inside a clinical context; as a matter of fact, a server of computer-formalized GLs could be a fundamental part of an agent-based Hospital Information System (HIS), given that, capturing the procedural knowledge contained in the GLs, GLs themselves could be seen as algorithms whose elementary steps are tasks, executed by agents, under certain activation conditions and with specific temporal, economic, or other type of constraints (the role of a server of computer-formalized GL within an agent-based health information system is described in [5], while a theory for communication among agents in agent-based HIS can be found in [6]).

2 The Framework Architecture

Figure 1 shows the three fundamental steps of the GL life cycle, that the system is intended to manage: development, implementation, and daily practice.

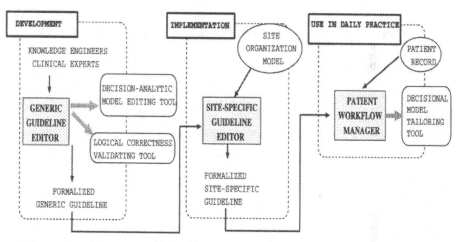

Fig. 1. The framework architecture

Development. To support the clinical expert at specifying the guideline according to a formal specification, we are currently developing a tool called Generic Guideline Editor (GGE). In practice, the GGE should be used by clinical experts and knowledge engineers to encapsulate a traditional guideline into a formal representation meant to be capable of capturing the knowledge contained in the text in a form which can be interpreted by a computer. This formal representation can be produced either starting from an existing textual (or hypertextual) GL, or during the phase of GL production, e.g. during a consensus conference. As a matter of fact, before the text of a GL can be published and disseminated, there must be no doubt about its logical correctness, i.e. the GL must be complete and not ambiguous [3]: verifying the GL's correctness is one of the goals of the GGE. Another tool, a decision model editor, is provided to deal with situations in which a consensus cannot be reached and explicitly declared in the GL: it will help in eliciting and taking into account either the patient preferences or the organization preferences (maybe involving economic evaluations).

Implementation. This point represents the link between GLs and the Hospital Information System (HIS). The GGE has been designed to support, first of all, the development of a *generic* GL, that is the GL as it is provided by national or international health care organizations. Yet, there is a significant gap between the development of such a generic GL and its utilization into a real clinical context. Clinician acceptance and utilization of GLs is hindered by several factors, first of all, very often generic GLs do not consider peculiarities of each organizational context [7] . That's why recent research efforts [13] have been done to build both a generic GL, annotated so as to make explicit criteria and intentions leading each recommendation, and an organizational model of the clinical context, in which roles, resources, policies and preferences must be explicit. The site-specific GL editor should be used by health care professionals in a specific environment, i.e. an hospital, to tailor the generic GL according to organization constraints.

Use in daily practice. In this phase the GL must be linked with the patient record, in such a way that suggestions can be produced by the system. Different tools are useful in this phase. One of them is the monitoring tool, which manages the agents interaction, another one is the decision model tailoring tool, which allows to deal with specific preferences.

3   The Formal Representation of the Guideline

The proposed formal representation is based on a modular, top down structuring of the health care process. Each module is nested in a more general module, which represents the context for its proper use, or, in other words, each module can be decomposed into a certain number of sequential or parallel subtasks. Task which cannot be further decomposed in subtasks are called atomic tasks. When a GL is chosen for a specific patient, the appropriate modules are selected, instantiated and exploded, so as to create, dynamically, a care plan which reflects constraints coming both from the patient status and from current resource availability. For each task in the GL (atomic or not), the GGE provides a Task Frame, storing all the attributes specifying that task. When a GL is accepted in a real clinical context, some attributes are added to the Task Frame, which becomes a Specific Task Frame, while the other attributes are inherited and instantiated. Afterwards, whenever the task is undertaken during a particular care plan, this instance of the task is called Actual Task. Each Actual Task Frame inherits all the attributes in the Specific Task Frame and acquires some further attributes, more directly related to the specific health care plan. This is shown in Table I, where the main distinction between the Task Frame and the Actual Task Frame is that the slots in the former provide a theoretical and pragmatic description of the process, which is completed by the site and patient-related information stored in the latter.

Three main attribute categories may be distinguished: attributes for describing the task (description, type, intention), for allowing the management of the task in an agent-based system (skills, location, time and economic constraints), and for allocating the task within the whole GL (subtasks, next task). The attribute meaning is described in the following:

description: a short description of the task (in natural language);

type: an abstract description of the task. We distinguish between: diagnosis, therapy, monitoring, data collection, financial management;

intention: an explicit description of the aim of the prescription;

manager skill: manager is the agent who is allocating the task to be performed. In the generic GL we just need to specify the professional skills required to assume the role of manager, while the person encharged of the task's performance will be derived from the organizational model;

contractor skill: contractor is the agent who is committed to the task performance. Again, in the Task Frame we just describe the professional skills required to become accountable for a certain task;

location constraints: an abstract definition of the location where the task has to be performed;

activation condition: the set of conditions which must be true before the task can be performed. The domain of all the variables in each activation condition must be explicit;

abnormal termination condition: if the value of this set of conditions becomes true, the task must be abandoned;

iteration condition: it is useful to manage cycle or repetitions;

optimal schedule: this is the first of a set of negotiating parameters, which specify the performed task. The actual value of each parameter will lie inside the range defined by the GL. Other negotiating parameters (like cost, deadline, duration) can be added when necessary;

subtasks: the components of the current task. See below the possible relationships between subtasks;

next task: it is the task following the current one during GL execution;

Table I - Task specification from the generic to the site and patient-specific formulation. Blank cells are meant to be attributes inherited from the left.

TASK FRAME	SPECIFIC TASK FRAME	ACTUAL TASK FRAME
description		
intention		
location constraints	location	
manager skill	manager	
contractor skill	contractor	
activation condition		
abnormal term. cond.		
optimal execution time		
deadline		
		actual execution time
	maximum cost	
		actual cost
subtasks		
next task		
		patient

Each task in the GL is performed if and only if its activation condition is true. And if the generic task T is not atomic, undertaking T means checking the activation conditions of all its subtasks. There are two different relationships between the subtasks of a generic task T, the AND-relation and the XOR-relation. Let us consider a task T with n subtasks. If the relation between the subtasks is AND-relation, T is completed after all the n subtasks are completed. If the relation between the subtasks is XOR-relation, T is completed after one and only one subtask is completed.

Figure 2 shows an example of GL structured in tasks and subtasks, and the different relationships between them. The GL, disseminated by the Center for Disease Control, describes a strategy for eliminating Hepatitis B virus transmission through childhood vaccination [11]. In the figure the four subtasks 2,3,4,5 are in AND-relation. This means that all of them are going to be performed (no particular activation condition is specified, because they are to be considered as mandatory), while the three subtasks 9,10 and 11 are in XOR-relation; let us consider their activation conditions:

task 9: HbsAg test result at delivery time = negative

task 10: HbsAg test result at delivery time = positive

task 11: HbsAg test result at delivery time = missing

for each patient just one of these three activation conditions can be true: one and only one of the three subtasks is going to be performed.

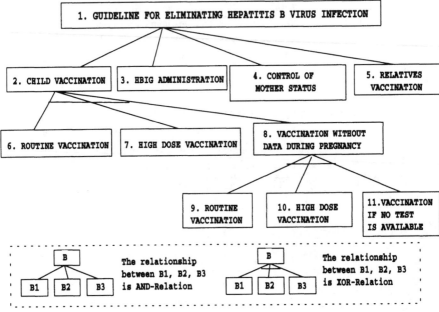

Fig. 2. A graphical layout of the formalized guideline for hepatitis B

3.1 Logical Correctness of the Guideline

Given the modular representation of the GL proposed in the previous section, it is possible to give a formal definition of a logically correct GL:

Def. 1 - A GL is logically correct if and only if it is complete and coherent.

To understand this definition we must, first, give a definition of completeness and coherency related to a single task:

Def. 2 - Let us call

$(S_{i1}, S_{i2}, ..., S_{in})$ the subtasks in XOR-relation of task T_{i-1};

K_i the set of the activation conditions for these subtasks;

$C_j(v_{j1}, v_{j2}, ..., v_{jn_j})$ the activation condition for task j, in the variables $v_{j1}, v_{j2}, ..., v_{jn_j}$;

$d_{j1}, d_{j2}, ..., d_{jn_j}$ the domains of the variables $v_{j1}, v_{j2}, ..., v_{jn_j}$;

$P_j = d_{j1} \times d_{j2} \times d_{jn_j}$;

$p_j \in P_j$ an array of values for the v_j

if C_j is satisfied by p_j, we write $C_j \backslash p_j$ = true.

K_i is complete if and only if $\forall p_j \in P_j \; \exists! \; C_j \backslash p_j$ = true.

Def. 3 - a GL is complete if and only if

∀ set of subtasks $(S_{i1}, S_{i2}, ..., S_{in})$ in XOR-relation in the GL K_i is complete.

Def. 4 - Let us call
$(S_{i1}, S_{i2}, ..., S_{in})$ the subtasks in AND-relation for task T_{i-1}
C_ij the activation condition for subtask S_{ij};
the task T_{ij} is coherent if and only if $C_ij \neq not(C_{ij}) \forall j \neq k$ i+1, ..., n

Def. 5 - A GL is coherent if and only if all the tasks in the GL are coherent.

As shown in next paragraphs, the GGE uses this formal definition to validate automatically the GL, before its publication.

4 The Editor

The GGE has been developed using HTML and JAVA languages. Figure 3 shows an interactive session to formalize one of the GLs which were considered for the system's testing, namely the above mentioned GL for hepatitis vaccination in pregnancy.

TELEMATIC GUIDELINE IMPLEMENTATION

Part 1 – STRUCTURE OF THE GUIDELINE

TASK DESCRIPTION:

1. What kind of task is it?
☐THERAPY ☐DIAGNOSIS ☐MONITORING
■DATA COLLECTION
☐FINANCIAL MANAGEMENT

2. Provide a brief description:

Early pregnancy HbsAg TEST

GO TO INFLUENCE DIAGRAM EDITOR

3. Describe the intention leading this task:

Screening mother for virus infection

4. Where is it located?   hospital

5. Who is the Task Manager?   specialist

6. Who is the Task Contractor?   laboratorist

TEMPORAL CONSTRAINTS

7. Describe the activation condition for the present task:

(PATIENT-PREGNANT T)

Fig. 3. Introducing some tasks of a guideline through the GGE

45

This formalized GL becomes the input for the program checking the logical constraints. Figure 4 shows the result of this check: there is a possible combination of variables which was not considered during GL development. No action is described to consider the case of a high risk mother, negative at the early pregnancy test, but who does not perform further controls.

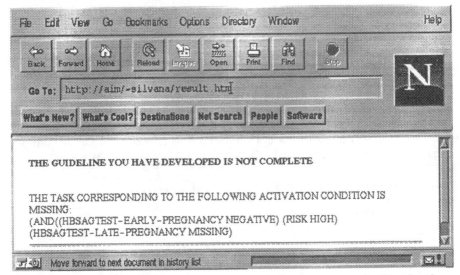

Fig. 4. The guideline has been tested for logical correctness and a bug has been found

Another important issue, that a guideline editor has to take into account, concerns the ontological and terminological definitions related to the application domain. When several guidelines are implemented in the same clinical environment, they should share the same conceptual model of the domain and the same terminology for at least two reasons: 1) for facilitating the user acceptance of the system, and 2) for allowing the communication between guidelines (several) and the electronic patient record (unique). Thus, it is necessary that both the data and knowledge models, on top of which databases and guidelines are built, refer to specific ontology and terminology servers [12].

4.1 Dealing with Uncertainty

If we consider methodologies for GLs production (consensus conferences, for examples), it could be argued that each prescription suggested by the GL should be justified, on the basis of some evidence. In general, the best (in the sense of the most objective) evidence arises from controlled clinical trials, eventually elaborated through meta-analysis tools. Other evidence, unfortunately less reliable, derives from literature revision on retrospective studies, or, when no study is available, on subjective opinions expressed by experts, until consensus is reached [9]. In this latter situation, the prescription suggested by the GL may be interpreted as obtained from a certain model, which takes into account subjective probabilities about different events and opinions about how a patient (or a population, or a society) feels about a certain condition. Finally, there are situations in which, either because of lack of information, or because of lack of consensus, the published GL itself outlines the absence of any possible suggestion. Often these are cases in which the patient's own preferences become crucial to decide between the possible alternatives. As an example, let us consider the GL diffused by the Italian Minister for Health Care Policies, suggesting the surgical choice between radical and conservative treatment for women affected by breast cancer[10]. This GL describes the proper actions in a certain number of clinical situations, but it also highlights cases in which no univocal prescription is available, because of lack of evidence. Table II summarizes the GL indications concerning the main decision between the two kind of surgical interventions.

Table II - The guideline for breast cancer surgery.

CONDITIONS	SUGGESTION
tumor size $<= 3cm$, one only lesion non infiltrating margins, no other pathologies, radiotherapy opportunity	conservative surgery
tumor size $> 3cm$ or multiple lesions or infiltrating margins	radical surgery
tumor size $<= 3cm$, one only lesion non infiltrating margins, other pathologies, no radiotherapy opportunity	uncertain situation no suggestion

In the cases like the last one in the previous table, it could be quite useful to provide tools to support decision making, so that all the interesting variables and the dependencies between them can be properly considered: as a matter of fact, GGE provides a link to a Java applet, which has been developed to build the decision model (influence diagram or decision tree) specific for each situation. Figure 5 shows such an interactive session with the GGE, where the clinical experts ask to enter the Influence Diagram Editor because no categorical prescription is possible corresponding to the given set of Activation Conditions. It can be imagined that the model shown in the figure represents the experts' consensus about the relationships existing between the domain variables; this model becomes part of the GL, it should explicit both the probability and outcome parameters useful for quantifying these dependencies (like the probability of relapse, the median survival, etc., either given as point values or as value ranges), while more subjective and personal parameters, normally related to the quality of life, are left blank, and will be filled at the moment of GL consultation for a specific case.

4.2   Site Specification

Modifications needed to make a generic GL *site-specific* [13] can be very different in entity: it could be just a change in the time schedule of controls and drug delivery, but it could also be necessary to alter a recommendation dramatically, for example because the required resources are not available at the site. Making a generic GL site-specific is crucial to solve the problem of compliance, but it points out several other problems, first of all, how to know when a certain modification is consistent with the intentions leading the generic GL. These two components and a set of rules specifying the legal modifications are the input of a tool capable of developing site-specific GLs in a semi-automatic way. In this way each institution could develop its own GLs, perfectly consistent with the intentions of the *official* generic GL, but which introduce different methods to satisfy the same goals. The organizational model of the site is very important for the purpose of modifying the generic GL: for example, the latter specifies just the professional skills required for a certain task, while the specific agent performing this task is decided by taking in account the organizational model. We propose an ontological description of the health care unit organization, linked to Databases storing details for each relevant entity and entity-relationship. A description of the preliminary version of this ontology can be found in [8].

5 GL's Use in Daily Practice

5.1 The Patient Record

After having developed a site-specific GL, the next step to realize a GL-based care environment, is to make the recommendations *patient- specific*: i.e., the recommendations must be integrated with a Patient Workflow Management Module, which has to consider data stored in the patient record before indicating the next tasks to be performed. The Workflow Management Module is crucial, also, to coordinate activities and to manage patients following more than one protocol at the same time.

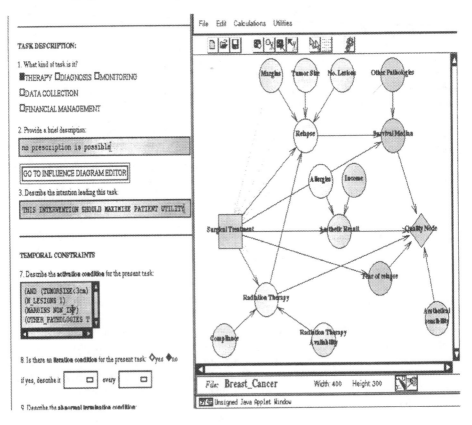

Fig. 5. Interaction with the influence diagram editor

A further goal is to make it easy to share and reuse the procedural knowledge contained in the patient-specific GL, and to share it not only between human experts, but also involving software agents supporting the health care process in order to assist the medical staff in complying with the GL's prescriptions.

So far, we have implemented a Monitoring Software Agent that manages follow-up of HIV+ patients according to AHCPR prescriptions [5].

5.2 The Patient Preferences

Another example of a tool to support GL-based daily practice, is strictly connected to the considerations reported in section 3.1 about the problem of uncertainty. We have shown why and how the clinical expert should develop an influence diagram describing all the interesting variables and their dependencies. In daily practice, this influence diagram should be instantiated taking in account patient's personal opinions or local constraints, so that the utility associated by the diagram resolution to each treatment could reflect in a proper way all the peculiarities regarding both the patient and the setting. In our example, the patient's preferences in terms of fear for relapse or aesthetic considerations are part of the influence diagram and can be adequately weighted, so that the utility of the two different surgical interventions can be evaluated considering the quality of life. It is interesting to see how things could change when the diagram is solved for a real situation, and not just with average population values: while running the model with average values for these variables could lead to no difference between alternatives, the sensitivity analysis in Figure 6 shows that in some cases, these personal preferences can change dramatically the utility of radical versus conservative surgery. The figure refers to a hypothetical patient who is not very interested in aesthetical aspects (utility coefficient of living with aesthetical damage near to 1), but is very worried about living with the fear of relapse (utility coefficient near 0.7). We assumed that the woman convincement is that a radical surgery is more protective against relapse. In this case, as shown by the sensitivity analysis, the suggested choice is the radical surgery, and this result is quite *robust*, given that it holds for a wide area around the nominal point.

6 Conclusion

We propose a formalism for specifying clinical guidelines, so as to make them sharable by human and software agents acting in a distributed health care environment. The main effort of guideline development is to provide specific prescriptions, whenever there is consensus about them. Some supporting tools have been briefly described, that allow to encapsulate the procedural knowledge stored in a guideline and to use it in daily practice. Nevertheless, apart from this typical interpretation of guideline-based care, we would like to introduce a slightly different point of view, related to the problem of uncertainty. The proposed framework embeds also tools for an explicit description of the knowledge used to develop the guideline, or a part of it, so that, even when the guideline cannot give specific prescriptions, each decision can be based on a well-agreed model. If this model is able to manage patient preferences, it could help to smooth dissimilarities in treatment whenever the patient itself should play a fundamental role in addressing the decision.

Acknowledgments The authors thank Dr. Douglas Fridsma, from the Section on Medical Informatics, Stanford University School of Medicine, for helpful discussion on guideline representation.

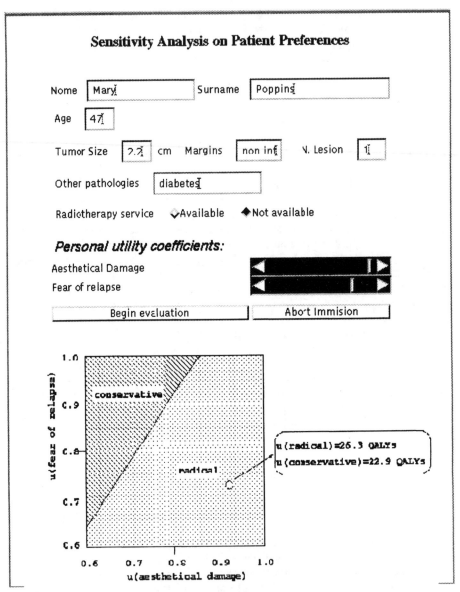

Fig. 6. A sensitivity analysis on patient preferences. The analysis refers to a 45 aged woman, showing the clinical condition which the guideline is unable to face. Utilities are measured by Quality Adjusted Life Years (QALYs).

References

1. Herbert SI. Informatics for Care Protocols and Guidelines: Towards a European Knowledge Model. Health Telematics for Clinical Guidelines and Protocols. (C. Gordon and J.P. Christensen, Eds.) , IOS Press, 1994.

2. Lobach DF. Electronically Distributed, Computer-Generated, Individualized Feedback Enhances the Use of a Computerized Practice Guideline, Proceedings of the 1996 AMIA Annual Fall Symposium (J.J. Cimino, Ed), Washington DC, October 26-30, 493-497, 1996.

3. Shiffman RN, Greenes RA. Improving Clinical Guidelines with Logic and Decision Table Techniques. Medical Decision Making, 14: 245-254, 1994.

4. Lanzola G, Falasconi S, Stefanelli M. Cooperating agents implementing distributed patient management. In Agents Breaking Away, Lecture Notes in Artificial Intelligence 1038 (Van de Velde and Perram Eds) Springer Verlag Berlin 218-232, 1996.

5. Saracco R, Campagnoli M, Quaglini S. A Multi-Agent System for Cooperative Working in Clinical Environments. Congresso Associazione Italiana per l'Intelligenza Artificiale, Napoli, Italy,1996.

6. Lanzola G, Campagnoli M, Falasconi S, Stefanelli M. Cooperating Agents in Intelligent Medical Applications. Accepted for presentation at AIME97 Conference, Grenoble, France, march 23-26, 1997.

7. Purves I. Computerized Guidelines in Primary Health Care: Reflections and Implications. Health Telematics for Clinical Guidelines and Protocols. (C. Gordon and J.P. Christensen Eds.), IOS Press, 1994.

8. Quaglini S, Dazzi L, Falasconi S, Marchetti M, Stefanelli M, Barosi G. An Ontology-Based Framework for Building Economic Evaluation Models in Health Care. Proc. of Medical Informatics Europe '96, (J. Brender, J.P. Christensen, J.R. Scherrer, P. McNair Eds) IOS Press, 930-934, 1996.

9. Woolf SH. Practice Guidelines, a New Reality in Medicine: II. Methods of Developing Guidelines. Archives of Internal Medicine, 152:946-952, 1992

10. Ministero della Sanita'-Regione Lombardia-Unita' Operativa Area Bresciana Istituto di Ricerche Farmacologiche 'Mario Negri'. Linee Guida per il trattamento chirurgico del carcinoma della mammella, Progetto Oncologia Femminile.

11. Center for Disease Control. Hepatitis B Virus: a Comprehensive Strategy for Eliminating Transmission in the United States Through universal Childhood Vaccination. MMWR, 40: 1-25, 1991.

12. Falasconi S, Lanzola G and Stefanelli M. Using ontologies in multi-agent systems, accepted for presentation at the KAW'96 Workshop, Banff, Canada, november 9-14, 1996.

13. Fridsma DB, Gennari JH, Musen MA. Making Generic Guidelines Site-Specific. Proceedings of the 1996 AMIA Annual Fall Symposium (J.J. Cimino, Ed.), Washington DC, October 26-30, 597-601, 1996.

A Task-Specific Ontology for the Application and Critiquing of Time-Oriented Clinical Guidelines

Yuval Shahar[1], Silvia Miksch[2], Peter Johnson[1]

[1] Section on Medical Informatics, Medical School Office Building, x215
Stanford University, Stanford, CA 94305–5479, USA
Email: {shahar,pdj}@smi.stanford.edu

[2] Vienna University of Technology
Department of Software Technology
Resselgasse 3/E188, A-10140 Vienna, Austria
Email: silvia@ifs.tuwien.ac.at

Abstract: Clinical guidelines reuse existing clinical procedural knowledge while leaving room for flexibility by the care provider applying that knowledge. Guidelines can be viewed as generic skeletal-plan schemata that are instantiated and refined dynamically by the care provider over significant periods of time and in highly dynamic environments. In the Asgaard project, we are investigating a set of tasks that support the application of clinical guidelines by a care provider other than the guideline's designer. We are focusing on application of the guideline, recognition of care providers' intentions from their actions, and critique of care providers' actions given the guideline and the patient's medical record. We are developing methods that perform these tasks in multiple clinical domains, given an instance of a properly represented clinical guideline and an electronic medical patient record. In this paper, we point out the precise domain-specific knowledge required by each method, such as the explicit intentions of the guideline designer (represented as temporal patterns to be achieved or avoided). We present a machine-readable language, called Asbru, to represent and to annotate guidelines based on the task-specific ontology. We also introduce an automated tool for acquisition of clinical guidelines based on the same ontology; the tool was developed using the PROTÉGÉ-II framework's suite of tools.

Categories: Knowledge Representation and Acquisition; Planning; Temporal Reasoning; Clinical Guidelines

1. Clinical Guidelines and Protocols

Clinical guidelines are a set of schematic plans for management of patients who have a particular clinical condition (e.g., insulin-dependent diabetes). The application of clinical guidelines by care providers involves collecting and interpreting considerable amounts of data over time, applying standard therapeutic or diagnostic plans in an episodic fashion, and revising those plans when necessary. Guidelines often involve implicit assumptions about the knowledge of the provider executing the plans. *Skeletal plans* are plan schemata at various levels of detail that capture the essence of a procedure, but leave room for execution-time flexibility in the achievement of particular goals (Friedland and Iwasaki, 1985). Thus, they are usually reusable in different contexts. Clinical guidelines can be viewed as reusable skeletal plans that need to be refined by a reactive planner over significant time periods when applied to a particular patient (Tu et al., 1989).

1.1. Automated Support to Guideline-Based care

During the past 15 years, there have been several efforts to support guideline-based care over time in automated fashion. Examples of specialized architectures include ONCOCIN (Tu et al., 1989), T-HELPER (Musen et al., 1992), DILEMMA (Herbert et al., 1995), EON (Musen et al., 1996), and the European PRESTIGE project. Other approaches to the support of guideline-based care encode guidelines as elementary state-transition tables or as situation-action rules dependent on the electronic medical record (Sherman, et al. 1995), but do not include an intuitive representation of the guideline's clinical logic, and have no semantics for the different types of clinical knowledge represented. Several approaches permit hypertext browsing of guidelines via the World Wide Web (Barnes and Barnett 1995) but do not use the patient's electronic medical record.

None of the current guideline-based-care systems have a sharable representation of guidelines that (1) has knowledge roles specific to the several guideline-based-care tasks, (2) is machine and human readable, and (3) allows data stored in an electronic patient record to invoke an application that directly executes the guideline's logic and related tasks, such as critiquing. A task-specific human- and machine-readable representation of clinical guidelines, that has an expressive syntax and semantics, combined with the ability to interpret that representation in automated fashion, would facilitate guideline dissemination, real-time accessibility, and applicability. *Task-specific architectures* (Eriksson et al., 1995) assign problem-solving *roles* to domain knowledge and facilitate acquisition and maintenance of that knowledge. Such a representation also would support additional reasoning tasks, such as automated critiquing, quality assurance (Grimshaw and Russel 1993), and guideline evaluation, and would facilitate authoring and modifying clinical guidelines.

1.2. Support to Application of Clinical Guidelines as an Interactive Process

Application of guidelines involves an interpretation by the care provider of skeletal plans that have been designed by the guideline's author. Providing automated support implies an interactive process. Typical tasks include assessment of the applicability of the guideline to the patient, guidance in proper application of a selected guideline, monitoring of the application process, assessment of the results of the guideline, critiquing the application process and its results, and assistance in the modification of the original guideline. For instance, clinical guidelines often have an inherent ambiguity or incompleteness. To increase flexibility, an automated assistant should recognize cases in which the care provider's actions, although different from the guideline's prescribed actions, adhere to the overall intentions of the guideline's designer, and should adjust accordingly its critique. To be useful, the language in which clinical guidelines are represented needs to be temporally expressive and should enable designers to express complex sequential, parallel, and cyclical procedures in a manner akin to a programming language (although typically on a higher level of abstraction). The language also requires well-defined semantics for both the prescribed actions and the task-specific annotations, such as the guideline designer's intentions. Thus, the care-provider's actions can be better supported, leading to a more flexible dialog and to a better acceptance of automated systems for support of guideline-based care. Having clear semantics for the task-specific knowledge roles also facilitates acquisition and maintenance of these roles.

Given these requirements, we have developed a text-based, machine-readable language, called *Asbru*. The Asbru language is part of the *Asgaard[*)]* project, in which we are developing task-specific problem-solving methods that perform execution and critiquing tasks in medical domains. In the following sections, we introduce the design-time and execution-time model, the required knowledge roles, the guideline-application support tasks, and the overall architecture we are developing. The syntax and the semantics of the Asbru language will be explained using as illustration a guideline for controlled observation and treatment of gestational diabetes mellitus (GDM) Type II. We also mention a graphical tool for acquisition of annotated clinical guidelines.

2. A Design-Time versus Execution-Time Intention-Based Model

During *design time* of a clinical guideline, an *author* (or a committee) designs a guideline (Figure 1). The author prescribes (1) *actions* (e.g., administer a certain drug in the morning and in the evening), (2) an *intended plan*—the intended intermediate and overall pattern of actions, which might not be obvious from the description of the prescribed actions and is often more flexible than prescription of specific actions (e.g., use some drug from a certain class of drugs twice a day), and

---

[*)] In Norse mythology, Asgaard was the home and citadel of the gods, corresponding to Mount Olympus in Greek mythology. It was located in the heavens and was accessible only over the rainbow bridge, called Asbru (or Bifrost).

(3) the intended intermediate and overall pattern of *patient states* (e.g., morning blood glucose should stay within a certain range). Intentions are temporal patterns of provider actions or patient states, to be achieved, maintained, or avoided.

During *execution time*, a *care provider* applies the guideline by performing *actions*, which are recorded, observed, and abstracted over time into an *abstracted plan* (see Figure 1). The *state* of the patient also is recorded, observed, and abstracted over time. Finally, the *intentions of the care provider* might be recorded too—inferred from her actions or explicitly stated by the provider.

2.1. The Guideline-Design And -Application Tasks

Given the intention-based model of clinical guidelines, we can describe a set of tasks relevant to the design and execution of these guidelines and analyze the knowledge requirements of problem-solving methods that perform these tasks (Table 1). The verification and validation tasks are relevant only during design time; the rest of the tasks are relevant during execution time. Each task can be viewed as answering a specific question (see Table 1). Each task can be performed by a problem-solving method (Eriksson, et al. 1995) that has an *ontology*—a set of entities, relations, and domain-specific knowledge requirements assumed by the method. Since knowledge requirements (*roles*) are often common to several of the problem-solving methods, we combine them into a task-specific *knowledge cluster*. Examples of knowledge roles include plan intentions, several types of preferences, and state-transition conditions. The semantics of the specific knowledge roles used in the Asbru language are discussed in the Section 3. Given these knowledge roles, we can define what knowledge is required to solve each task (see Table 1).

Table 1: Several guideline-support tasks and the knowledge required to solve them. Common knowledge roles can be viewed as shareable by the methods requiring them.

Task	Questions to be answered	Required Knowledge
Verification of a guideline	Are the intended plans achievable by following the prescribed actions? (*a syntactic check*)	Prescribed actions; intended overall action pattern (i.e., the plan)
Validation of a guideline	Are the intended states achievable by the prescribed actions and intended plan? (*a semantic check*)	Prescribed actions, intended overall action pattern; intended states; action/plan effects
Applicability of guidelines	What guidelines or protocols are applicable at this time to this patient?	Filter and setup preconditions; overall intended states; the patient's state
Execution (application) of a guideline	What should be done at this time according to the guideline's prescribed actions?	Prescribed actions and their filter and setup preconditions; suspension, restart, completion, and abort conditions; the patient's state
Recognition of intentions	Why is the care provider executing a particular set of actions, especially if those deviate from the guideline's prescribed actions?	Executed actions and their abstraction to executed plans; action and state intentions; the patient's state; action/plan effects; revision strategies; preferences
Critique of the provider's actions	Is the care provider deviating from the prescribed actions or intended plan? Are the deviating actions compatible with the author's plan and state intentions?	Executed actions and their abstraction to plans; action and state intentions of the original plan; the patient's state; action/plan effects; revision strategies; preferences
Evaluation of a guideline	Is the guideline working?	Intermediate/overall state intentions; the patient's state; intermediate/overall action intentions; executed actions and plans
Modification of an executing guideline	What alternative plans are relevant at this time for achieving a given state intention?	Intermediate/overall state intentions; action/plan effects; filter and setup preconditions; revision strategies; preferences; the patient's state

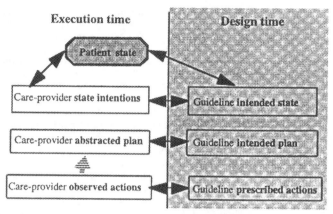

Figure 1. The design-time versus execution-time intention-based model of a clinical guideline. Double-headed arrows denote a potential axis of comparison (e.g., for critiquing purposes) during runtime execution of the clinical guideline. Striped arrows denote an abstracted-into relationship.

A subtask implicit in several of the tasks in Table 1 is the abstraction of higher-level concepts from time-stamped data during the execution of the skeletal plan. Possible candidates for solving this subtask include the RÉSUMÉ system and the temporal data-abstraction component in the VIE-VENT system. The *RÉSUMÉ* system (Shahar and Musen 1996) is an implementation of a formal, domain-independent problem-solving method, the *knowledge-based temporal-abstraction method* (Shahar, in press) and has been evaluated in several clinical domains (Shahar and Musen 1996). *VIE-VENT* is an open-loop knowledge-based monitoring and therapy planning system for artificially ventilated newborn infants, which includes context-sensitive and expectation-guided temporal data-abstraction methods (Miksch et al., in press).

2.2 Plan Recognition and Critiquing in the Application of Clinical Guidelines

The following example demonstrates the tasks of plan-recognition and critiquing in the domain of monitoring and therapy of patients who have insulin-dependent diabetes.

During therapy of a diabetes patient, hyperglycemia (a higher than normal level of blood glucose) is detected for the second time in the same week around bedtime. The diabetes-guideline's prescribed action might be to increase the dose of the insulin the patient typically injects before dinner. However, the provider recommends reduction of the patient's carbohydrate intake during dinner. This action seems to contradict the prescribed action. Nevertheless, the automated assistant notes that increasing the dose of insulin decreases the value of the blood-glucose level directly, while the provider's recommendation *decreases* the value of the same clinical parameter by *reducing* the magnitude of an action (i.e., ingestion of carbohydrates) that *increases* its value. The assistant also notes that the state intention of the guideline was "avoid more than two episodes of hyperglycemia per week." Therefore, the provider is still following the intention of the protocol. By recognizing this high-level intention and its achievement by a different plan, the automated assistant can accept the provider's alternate set of actions, and even provide further support for these actions.

We consider a *plan-recognition* ability, such as demonstrated in the example, an indispensable prerequisite to the performance of *plan critiquing*. Such an ability might increase the usefulness of guideline-based decision-support systems to clinical practitioners, who often follow what they consider as the author's intentions rather than the prescribed actions. Note that we assume knowledge about the *effects of interventions* on clinical parameters, and knowledge of legitimate domain-independent and domain-specific *guideline-revision strategies*. Both intervention effects and revision strategies can be represented formally (Shahar and Musen 1995).

Intentions have been examined in philosophy (Bratman, 1987) and in artificial intelligence (Pollack, 1992). As we explain in more detail in Section 3.2, we are viewing intentions formally as temporally extended goals, comprising action or state patterns, at various abstraction levels.

The example also demonstrates a specific *execution-critiquing* model. In this model, five comparison axes exist: the guideline's prescribed actions versus the provider's actual actions; the guideline's intended plan versus the provider's (abstracted) plan; the guideline's intended patient state versus the provider's state intention; the guideline's intended state versus the patient's (abstracted) actual state; and the provider's intended state versus the patient's (abstracted) actual state. Combinations of the comparison results imply a set of different *behaviors* of the guideline application by the provider. Thus, a care provider might not follow the precise *actions*, but still follow the intended *plan* and achieve the desired states. A provider might even not follow the overall plan, but still adhere to a higher-level *intention*. Alternatively, the provider might be executing the guideline correctly, but the patient's state might differ from the intended, perhaps indicating a complication that needs attention or a failure of the guideline. In theory, there might be up to 32 different behaviors, assuming binary comparisons along five axes. However, the use of consistency constraints prunes this number to approximately 10 major behaviors. (We also are investigating the use of continuous, rather than binary, measures of matching).

2.3 The Conceptual Architecture

In the Asgaard project, we are developing different task-specific reasoning modules that perform the guideline-support tasks shown in Table 1. Figure 2 presents the overall architecture. The task-specific reasoning modules require different types of knowledge, often outside of the scope of the guideline-tasks ontology. For instance, the knowledge-based temporal-abstraction method implemented by the RÉSUMÉ module requires knowledge about temporal-abstraction properties of measurable clinical parameters, such as persistence of their values over time when these values are not recorded (Shahar, in press). These properties exist in the domain's *temporal-abstraction ontology* (Shahar and Musen 1996).

Similarly, the plan-recognition and critiquing methods require generic and domain-specific plan-revision knowledge (Shahar and Musen 1995); much of that knowledge might not be part of the guideline specification, but can represented in a separate knowledge base accessible to the appropriate problem-solving methods (reasoning modules). Effects of specific interventions, such as insulin administration (and, in general, of guidelines) can be represented as part of the guideline, but can also be viewed as a separate knowledge base (Figure 2). The specifications of clinical guidelines and of their independent components (we refer to either of these entities as *plans* in this

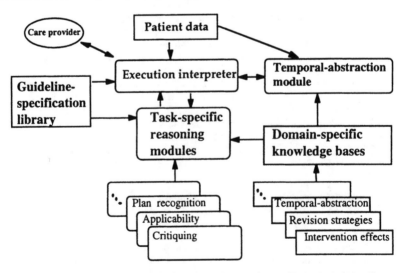

Figure 2. The guideline–support architecture. Arrows denote data or knowledge flow.

paper) are all represented uniformly and organized in a *guideline-specification library*. The library is a set of execution plans expressed in our task-specific language. During the guideline-execution phase, an applicable guideline plan is instantiated with runtime arguments.

3. Asbru: A Global Ontology For Guideline-Application Tasks

We have developed a language specific to the set of guideline-support tasks and the problem-solving methods performing these tasks, which we call *Asbru*. Asbru enables a designer to represent a clinical guideline, including all of the knowledge roles useful to one or more of the problem-solving methods performing the various tasks supporting the application of clinical guidelines. The major features of Asbru are that prescribed actions can be continuous; plans might be executed in parallel, in sequence, in a particular order, or every time measure; temporal scopes and parameters of guideline plans can be flexible, and explicit intentions and preferences can underlie the plan. These features are in contrast to traditional plan-execution representations, which assume instantaneous actions and effects. Interventions often are continuous and might have delayed effects and temporally-extended goals. The requirements of plan specifications in clinical domains (Tu, et al. 1989) are a superset of the requirements of typical toy domains used in planning research. We have defined a formal syntax for the Asbru language in Backus-Naur form. The Asbru language combines the flexibility and expressivity of procedural languages (e.g., the Arden syntax (Hripcsak, et al. 1994)) with the semantic clarity of declaratively expressed knowledge roles. These roles (e.g., preferences and intentions) are specific to the ontology of the methods performing the guideline-support tasks.

3.1. Time Annotation

The time annotation we use allows a representation of uncertainty in starting time, ending time, and duration (Dechter, Meiri, and Pearl 1991; Rit 1986). The time annotation supports multiple time lines by providing different *reference annotations*. The reference annotation can be an absolute reference point, a reference point with uncertainty (defined by an uncertainty region), a function (e.g., completion time) of a previously executed plan instance, or a domain-dependent time point variable (e.g., CONCEPTION). Temporal shifts from the reference annotation represent uncertainty in the starting time, the ending time, and the overall duration (Figure 3).

To allow temporal repetitions, we define sets of cyclic time points (e.g., MIDNIGHTS, which represents the set of midnights, where each midnight occurs exactly at 0:00 A.M., every 24 hours) and cyclic time annotations (e.g., MORNINGS, which represents a set of mornings, where each morning starts at the earliest at 8:00 A.M., ends at the latest at 11:00 A.M., and lasts at least 30 minutes). In addition, we allow certain short-cuts such as for the current time, whatever that time is (using the symbol *NOW*), or the duration of the plan (using the symbol *). Thus, the Asbru notation enables the expression of interval-based intentions, states, and prescribed actions with uncertainty regarding starting, finishing, duration, and the use of absolute, relative, and even cyclical (with a predetermined granularity) reference annotations.

3.2. The Semantics of the Asbru Task-Specific Knowledge Roles

A (guideline) *plan* in the guideline-specification library is composed of a set of plans with arguments and time annotations. A decomposition of a plan into its subplans is attempted by the execution interpreter, unless the plan is not found in the guideline library, thus representing a nondecomposable plan. This can be viewed as a "semantic" halting condition, which increases runtime flexibility. A nondecomposable plan is executed by the user or by an external call to a computer program. The library includes a set of *primitive plans* to perform interaction with the user or to retrieve information from the medical patient record (e.g., OBSERVE, GET-PARAMETER, ASK-PARAMETER, DISPLAY, WAIT)). All plans have return values.

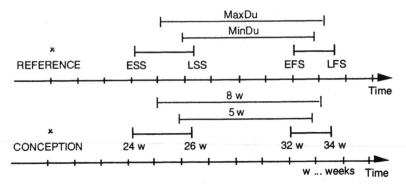

Figure 3. A schematic illustration of the Asbru time annotations. The upper part of the figure presents the generic annotation. The lower part shows a particular example representing the time annotation [[24 WEEKS, 26 WEEKS], [32 WEEKS, 34 WEEKS], [5 WEEKS, 8 WEEKS], CONCEPTION]), which means "starts 24 to 26 weeks after conception, ends 32 to 34 weeks after the conception, and lasts 5 to 8 weeks." REFERENCE = reference annotation, ESS = earliest starting shift, LSS = latest starting shift, EFS = earliest finishing shift, LFS = latest finishing shift, MinDu = minimal duration, MaxDu = maximal duration. The annotation is thus ([ESS, LSS], [EFS, LFS], [MinDu, MaxDu], REFERENCE).

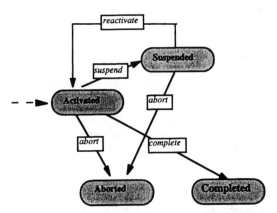

Figure 4. Plan-instance states and associated state-transition conditions in Asbru.

At execution time, a *ready* plan is instantiated. A set of mutually exclusive *plan states* describes the actual status of the plan instance during execution. Particular *state-transition criteria (conditions)* specify transition between neighboring plan-instance states. Thus, if a plan is activated, it can only be completed, suspended, or aborted depending on the corresponding criteria; the suspended state is optional and available for complex plans (Figure 4). State-transition conditions are explained below. Generic library plans also have states (considered, possible, rejected, and ready), that determine whether the plan is applicable and whether a plan instance can be created. A plan consists of a name, a set of arguments, including a time annotation (representing the temporal scope of the plan), and five (optional) components: *preferences, intentions, conditions, effects*, and a *plan body* which describes the actions to be executed. All components are optional. Every subplan has the same structure. Thus, a sequential plan can include several potentially decomposable concurrent or cyclical plans.

We now examine in more detail each of the knowledge roles represented in Asbru.

Preferences: Preferences bias or constrain the selection of a plan to achieve a given goal. Examples include: (1) *Strategy*: a general strategy for dealing with the problem (e.g., aggressive, normal); (2) *Utility*: a set of utility measures (e.g., minimize the cost or the patient inconvenience); (3) *Select-method*: a matching heuristic for the applicability of the whole plan (e.g., exact-fit); (4) *Resources*: a specification of prohibited or obligatory resources (e.g., in certain cases of treatment of a pulmonary infection, surgery is prohibited and antibiotics must be used); and (5) *Start-conditions*: an indication whether transition from a ready state of the generic plan to an activated state of the plan instance is automatic or requires approval of the user.

Intentions: Intentions are high-level goals at various levels of the plan, an annotation specified by the designer that supports special tasks such as critiquing and modification. Intentions are temporal patterns of provider actions and patient states, at different levels of abstraction, that should be maintained, achieved, or avoided. We define four categories of intentions: (1) *Intermediate state:* the patient state(s) that should be maintained, achieved, or avoided during the applicability of the plan (e.g., weight gain levels are slightly low to slightly high); (2) *Intermediate action:* the provider action(s) that should take place during the execution of the plan (e.g., monitor blood glucose once a day); (3) *Overall state pattern:* the overall pattern of patient states that should hold after finishing the plan (e.g., patient had less than one high glucose value per week); and (4) *Overall action pattern:* the overall pattern of provider actions that should hold after finishing the plan (e.g., patient had visited dietitian regularly for at least three months).

Conditions: Conditions are temporal patterns, sampled at a specified frequency, that need to hold at particular plan steps to induce a particular state transition of the plan instance. They are used for actual execution (application) of the plan. We do not directly determine conditions that should hold during execution; we specify conditions that activate the change of a particular plan state (see Figure 4). A plan instance is completed when the complete conditions become true, otherwise the plan instance's execution suspends or aborts (often, due to failure). Conditions are optional. We distinguish between: (1) *filter-preconditions*, which need to hold initially if the plan is applicable, but should not be achieved (e.g., patient is a pregnant female), and are necessary to achieve a possible state; (2) *setup-preconditions*, which need to be achieved to enable a plan to start (e.g., patent had a glucose-tolerance test) and allow a transition from a possible plan to a ready plan; (3) *suspend-conditions*, which determine when an active plan instance has to be suspended (e.g., blood glucose has been high for four days); these are informally the inverse of *protection* conditions in the planning literature, which have to hold during certain time periods; (4) *abort-conditions*, which determine when an active or suspended plan has to be aborted (e.g., there is an insulin-indicator condition: the patient cannot be controlled by diet); (5) *complete-conditions*, which determine when an active plan is completed, typically, but not necessarily, successfully (e.g., delivery has been performed); (and 6) *reactivate-conditions*, which determine when a suspended plan has to be reactivated (e.g., blood glucose level is back to normal or is only slightly high);

Effects: Effects describe the functional relationship between either (1) each of the relevant plan arguments and measurable parameters it affects in certain contexts (e.g., the *dose* of insulin is inversely related in some fashion to the level of blood glucose) or (2) the overall plan and the clinical parameters it is expcted to effect (e.g., the insulin-administration plan decreases the blood-glucose level). Effects can have a likelihood annotation—a probability of occurrence. Effects can be part of the guideline library (when they annotate plans) and can also be stored in a domain-specific knowledge base (especially for common plans, such as administration of drugs).

Plan-Body: The plan body is a set of plans to be executed in parallel, in sequence, in any order, or in some frequency. We distinguish among three types of plans: *sequential, concurrent,* and *cyclical.* Only one type of plan is allowed in a single plan body. A sequential plan specifies a set of plans that are executed in sequence; for continuation, all plans included have to be completed successfully. Concurrent plans can be executed either together, in parallel, or in any order. We distinguish two dimensions for classification of sequential or (potentially) concurrent plans: the number of plans that should be completed to enable continuation and the order of plan execution. Table 2 summarizes the dimensions of the two plan types. Using the two dimensions, we define the plan subtypes DO-ALL-TOGETHER, DO-SOME-TOGETHER, DO-ALL-ANY-ORDER, DO-SOME-ANY-ORDER, DO-ALL-SEQUENTIALLY. The continuation condition specifies the names of the plans that must be completed to proceed with the next steps in the plan.

A cyclical plan (a DO-EVERY type) includes a plan that can be repeated, and optional temporal and continuation arguments that can specify its behavior. *Start* and *end* specify a starting and ending time point. *Time base* determines the time interval over which the plan is repeated and the start time, end time, and duration of the particular plan instance in each cycle (e.g., starting with the first Monday's morning, until next Tuesday's morning, perform plan A every morning for 10 minutes). The *times-completed* argument specifies how many times the plan has to be completed to succeed and the *times-attempted* argument specifies how many attempts are allowed. Obviously, number of attempts must be greater or equal to the number of successful plans. A temporal pattern can be used as a stop condition of the cyclic plan. Finally, the plan itself is associated with its own particular arguments (e.g., dose). The start time, the time base, and the plan name are mandatory to the specification of a cyclic plan; the other arguments are optional.

Table 2: Categorization of plan types by continuation conditions and ordering constraints

Continuation condition --> Ordering Constraints	All plans should be completed in order to continue	Some plans should be completed in order to continue
Start together	DO-ALL-TOGETHER (no continuation-condition; all plans must complete)	DO-SOME-TOGETHER (continuation-conditions specified as subset of plans)
Execute in any order	DO-ALL-ANY-ORDER (no continuation-condition; all plans must complete)	DO-SOME-ANY-ORDER (continuation-conditions specified as subset of plans)
Execute in total order	DO-ALL-SEQUENTIALLY (no continuation-condition; all plans must complete)	————

3.3. Example: A Gestational Diabetes Mellitus Guideline

We represented in Asbru a Stanford University guideline for controlled observation and treatment of gestational diabetes mellitus (GDM) type II (non insulin dependent). The guideline prescribes several concurrent monitoring and management plans following a glucose tolerance test (GTT) between 140 and 200 mg/dl (Figure 5). The plan body consists of three plans that are executed in parallel (*glucose monitoring*, *nutritional management*, and *monitoring for insulin indication*), exist in the guideline-specification library, and are decomposable into other library plans.

4. Summary and Discussion

Representing clinical guidelines and the intentions underlying them in a standard, machine-readable, and machine-interpretable form is a prerequisite for sharing clinical guidelines and for useful, flexible automated assistance in the execution of these guidelines. The task-specific representation we suggest supports several different *knowledge roles* that can be used by multiple reasoning modules, for direct execution of a guideline and for related tasks such as recognition of care providers' intentions and critiquing their actions. In addition, the Asbru language places a particular emphasis on an expressive representation for time-oriented provider actions and patient states. Temporal reasoning is important for many clinical domains and needs to be supported.

Expert physicians need not have familiarity with the Asbru syntax to author clinical guidelines. We used the *PROTÉGÉ-II* framework (Tu, et al. 1995)) to develop an Asbru-like object-oriented guideline ontology and to generate a graphical knowledge-acquisition tool automatically from the ontology. The tool acquires instances of guidelines modeled in an object-oriented Asbru version.

Acknowledgments

This work has been supported by grants LM05708 and LM06245 from the National Library of Medicine, IRI-9528444 from the National Science Foundation, and DARPA Grant N66001-94-D-6055. Computing resources were provided by the Stanford CAMIS project, funded under Grant No. LM05305 from the National Library of Medicine. Silvia Miksch is supported by "Erwin Schrödinger Auslandstipendium, Fonds zur Förderung der wissenschaftliche Forschung", J01042-MAT.

```
(PLAN observing-GDM
;; the following time-annotations are local to the GDM example
(DOMAIN-DEPENDENT TIME-ASSIGNMENT
    (SHIFTS DELIVERY <- 38 WEEKS) ;; domain-specific time shift from the CONCEPTION point
    (POINT CONCEPTION <- (ask (ARG "what is the conception-date?"))))
(ABSTRACTION-ASSIGNMENT
    (CYCLIC
       MIDNIGHTS <- [0, 0 HOURS, 24 HOURS]
       BREAKFAST-START-TIME <- [0, 7 HOURS, 24 HOURS]))
(PREFERENCES
    (SELECT-METHOD EXACT-FIT)    ;; The match in the filter conditions needs to be exact
    (START-CONDITION AUTOMATIC)) ;; the plan starts as soon as it is ready, no user input
(INTENTION:INTERMEDIATE-STATE
    (MAINTAIN blood-glucose-post-meal (<= 130) GDM-Type-II
       [[24 WEEKS, 24 WEEKS], [DELIVERY, DELIVERY], [_,_], CONCEPTION])
    (MAINTAIN blood-glucose-fasting (<= 100) GDM-Type-II
       [[24 WEEKS, 24 WEEKS], [DELIVERY, DELIVERY], [_,_], CONCEPTION])
(INTENTION:OVERALL-STATE
    (AVOIDED STATE(blood-glucose) HIGH GDM-Type-II
       [[24 WEEKS, 24 WEEKS], [DELIVERY, DELIVERY], [7 DAYS,_], CONCEPTION]))
    ;; avoid, throughout the guideline, a period of high blood-glucose level lasting more than 7 days

(SETUP-PRECONDITIONS
    (PLAN-STATE one-hour-GTT COMPLETED
       [[24 WEEKS, 24 WEEKS], [26 WEEKS, 26 WEEKS], [_,_], CONCEPTION])
    ;; The patient must have completed a glucose-tolerance test (another plan in the library)
(FILTER-PRECONDITIONS
    (one-hour-GTT (140, 200) pregnancy
       [24 WEEKS, 24 WEEKS], [26 WEEKS, 26 WEEKS], [_,_], CONCEPTION])
(SUSPEND-CONDITIONS (OR STARTED RESTARTED)
    (STATE(blood-glucose) HIGH GDM-Type-II
       [[24 WEEKS, 24 WEEKS], [DELIVERY, DELIVERY], [4 DAYS,_], CONCEPTION]
    (SAMPLING-FREQUENCY 24 HOURS)))
    ;; suspend if high blood-glucose level exists for at least 4 DAYS
(ABORT-CONDITIONS (OR STARTED SUSPENDED RESTARTED)
    (insulin-indicator-conditions TRUE GDM-Type-II *
       (SAMPLING-FREQUENCY 24 HOURS)))
(COMPLETE-CONDITIONS (OR STARTED RESTARTED)
    (delivery TRUE GDM-Type-II * (SAMPLING-FREQUENCY 24 HOURS)))
(RESTART-CONDITIONS
    (STATE(blood-glucose) (OR NORMAL SLIGHTLY-HIGH) GDM-Type-II
       [[24 WEEKS, 24 WEEKS], [DELIVERY, DELIVERY], [_,_], CONCEPTION]
    (SAMPLING-FREQUENCY 24 HOURS)))

(DO-ALL-TOGETHER
    (glucose-monitoring)
    (nutrition-management)
    (observe-insulin-indicators)))
    ;; the plan body is a concurrent one; the three plans start together and all need to complete
```

Figure 5. A small portion of the representation of the guideline for management of non-insulin-dependent gestational diabetes mellitus (GDM) type II. Double colons are followed by comments.

References

Barnes, M. and Barnett, G. O. (1995). An Architecture for a Distributed Guideline Server. In Gardner, R. M. (Ed.) *Proceedings of the Annual Symposium on Computer Applications in Medical Care (SCAMC-95)*, New Orleans, Louisiana, 233–237. Hanley & Belfus.

Bratman, M.E. (1987). *Intention, Plans and Practical Reason.* Cambridge, MA: Harvard University Press.

Dechter, R., Meiri, L., and Pearl, J. (1991). Temporal Constraint Networks. *Artificial Intelligence, Special Volume on Knowledge Representation,* 49(1-3):61–95

Eriksson, H., Shahar, Y., Tu, S. W., Puerta, A. R., and Musen, M. A. (1995). Task Modeling with Reusable Problem-Solving Methods. *Artificial Intelligence,* 79(2):293–326.

Friedland, P., and Iwasaki, Y. The Concept and Implementation of Skeletal Plans. *Journal of Automated reasoning,* 1(2):161–208.

Grimshaw, J. M. and Russel, I. T. (1993). Effects of Clinical Guidelines an Medical Practice: A Systematic Review of Rigorous Evaluation. *Lancet,* 342:1317–1322.

Herbert, S. I., Gordon, C. J., Jackson-Smale, A., and Renaud Salis, J-L. (1995). Protocols for Clinical Care. *Computer Methods and Programs in Biomedicine,* 48:21–26.

Hripcsak, G., Ludemann, P., Pryor, T. A., Wigertz, O. B., and Clayton, P. D. (1994). Rationale for the Arden Syntax. *Computers and Biomedical Research,* 27:291–324.

Miksch, S., Horn, W., Popow, C., and Paky, F. (in press). Utilizing Temporal Data Abstraction for Data Validation and Therapy Planning for Artificially Ventilated Newborn Infants. *Artificial Intelligence in Medicine,* forthcoming.

Musen, M. A., Carlson, C. W., Fagan, L. M., Deresinski, S. C., and Shortliffe, E. H. (1992). T-HELPER: Automated Support for Community-Based Clinical Research. In Frisse, M. E. (Ed.) *Proceedings of the Sixteenth Annual Symposium on Computer Applications in Medical Care (SCAMC-92),* 719–723. McGraw Hill, New York, NY.

Musen, M.A., Tu, S.W., Das, A.K., and Shahar, Y. (1996). EON: A Component-Based Approach to Automation of Protocol-Directed Therapy. *Journal of the American Medical Information Association,* 3(6):367–388.

Pollack, M. (1992). The Use of Plans. *Artificial Intelligence,* 57(1):43-68.

Rit, J.-F. (1986). Propagating Temporal Constraints for Scheduling. *Proceedings of the Fifth National Conference on Artificial Intelligence (AAAI-86),* 383–388. Morgan Kaufmann, Los Altos, CA.

Shahar, Y. and Musen, M. A. (1995). Plan Recognition and Revision in Support of Guideline-Based Care. *Notes of the AAAI Spring Symposium on Representation Mental States and Mechanisms,* Stanford, CA, 118–126.

Shahar, Y. and Musen, M. A. (1996). Knowledge-Based Temporal Abstraction in Clinical Domains. *Artificial Intelligence in Medicine* 8(3):267–298.

Shahar, Y. (in press). A Framework for Knowledge-Based Temporal Abstraction. *Artificial Intelligence,* forthcoming.

Sherman, E. H., Hripcsak, G., Starren, J., Jender, R. A., and Clayton, P. (1995). Using Intermediate States to Improve the Ability of the Arden Syntax to Implement Care Plans and Reuse Knowledge. In Gardner, R. M. (Ed.) *Proceedings of the Annual Symposium on Computer Applications in Medical Care (SCAMC-95),* New Orleans, LA, 238–242. Hanley & Belfus.

Tu, S. W., Eriksson, H., Gennari, J. H., Shahar, Y., and Musen, M. A. (1995). Ontology-Based Configuration of Problem-Solving Methods and Generation of Knowledge-Acquisition Tools: Application of PROTÉGÉ-II to Protocol-Based Decision Support. *Artificial Intelligence in Medicine,* 7(3):257–289.

Tu, S. W., Kahn, M. G., Musen, M. A., Ferguson, J. C., Shortliffe, E. H., and Fagan, L. M. (1989). Episodic Skeletal-Plan Refinement on Temporal Data. *Communications of ACM,* 32:1439–1455.

User-Adapted Multimedia Explanations in a Clinical Guidelines Consultation System

Berardina De Carolis[*], *Gianni Rumolo*[*], *Vincenzo Cavallo*[o]

[*]Dipartimento di Informatica ed Automazione
Università di Roma Tre - Rome, Italy
tel. +39-6-55177049 email: {decarol, rumolo}@inf.uniroma3.it
[o]Dipartimento di Medicina Sperimentale e Patologia, I Cattedra di Radiologia
Università "La Sapienza" di Roma, Italy
tel. and fax: +39-6-4456695;.

Abstract

In consulting a multimedia information system the user may need an explanation about a particular topic. When users of the system belong to different categories, with different characteristics, and cultural background, their information needs are different. In addition, when dealing with multimedia messages, it becomes important to achieve an effective integration of media by synchronizing in time and space heterogeneous objects of the message. This paper describes how we combined user modelling and Petri nets in order to achieve an effective integration of media and to generate user-adapted multimedia explanations in a system supporting clinical guidelines consultation.

Keywords: Multimedia explanations, user modelling, Petri nets

1.   Introduction

In a multimedia information system different media strictly 'cooperate' in presenting information to the user. This 'cooperation' is expressed through an effective integration and synchronization in time and space of the multimedia objects in the message. This process requires an additional effort when what is *relevant* in the explanation message and which presentation form is *appropriate* depend on the user characteristics. Adapting the information content and the presentation style of the multimedia message can be a solution to meet the user requirements [2]. The approach presented in this paper is based on a combination of user modelling and Petri nets to specify and generate user-adapted multimedia explanations. This method has been used to generate explanations in a multimedia system for clinical guidelines consultation whose users belong to different categories and have different information needs. We have identified the followings categories of potential users of such a system: i) students, who can use the system to learn about the most effective diagnostic and therapeutic procedures; ii) General Practitioners, who can use the system to keep up-to-date on recent diagnostic and therapeutic procedures; iii) patients, who can keep informed about their disease, about the efficacy and entity of the diagnostic examinations and therapies. It is evident that the need to receive explanations on a particular topic during the consultation it is not homogeneous for all these categories of users, but it varies according to the knowledge degree and to the information needs, cultural background, job, and so on. Figure 1 illustrates the system architecture.

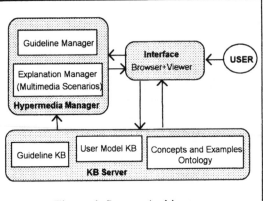

The KB Server provides the services necessary to manage the knowledge bases of the system; in particular, the Concept and Example Ontology and the User Model KB modules are relevant to the generation of explanations.

The Hypermedia Manager allows to build the hypermedia corresponding to the guideline consultation structure, and to generate explanations using what we called *Multimedia Scenarios*.

Figure 1. System Architecture

2. Multimedia Scenarios

The specification and automatic generation of multimedia explanation is adapted to the characteristics and knowledge of the user by means of "Multimedia Scenarios" [1]. In our case a multimedia scenario is a formal and executable specification based on Petri nets [3,4] that models how the attributes of concepts and examples are integrated and synchronized in the net taking into account the user model settings in order to adapt the net semantics and therefore the generation process. A Petri net based model allows: i) to formalize the concurrency and synchronization of events; ii) to adapt the scenario to user characteristics, and to different interaction contexts; iii) to formalize temporal and spatial constraints in order to achieve an effective integration of different media (for instance, the synchronization between a set of images and the correspondent textual comments). Therefore, it is possible to specify effectively different configuration of multimedia messages, according to the user model settings.

A simple example of a multimedia scenario is described in Figure 2 that represent the specification of the explanation of the concept *Sonographic Guidance*.

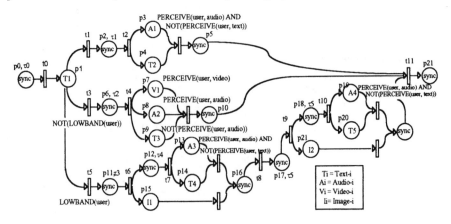

Figure 2. Petri Net corresponding to the multimedia scenario

The appropriate setting in the net of the parameters τ_i related to the synchronization places (i.e. p_0, p_2, ...) allows to synchronize the sequence and/or the simultaneous display of texts, images, audio and videos. The colours related to places and transitions enable to model how different media are used in different context to communicate the same information; for instance, the comment to an image can be expressed as audio or text according to the capability of the user to perceive sounds or to see texts (i.e. p_3, p_{13}, ...), or the colours related to t_3, t_4 allows to use a video only for users with a high-bandwidth network connection.

Tables 1 and 2 represent a partial description of the mappings from net places into information items and net transitions into user/system action according to the user model settings. The *Multimedia Information Content* column expresses which concept attributes (***C.attribute***) are associated to a particular place under the conditions expressed in the *Colours* column. It is also possible to provide the user with the essential description (M) of the attribute or with one or more additional details (Di). E_i denotes one of the examples related to the concept; it is also described by a set of attributes expressed by different types of media. The *Layout* column links an information content to a particular physical layout.

P_i	Colours	Multimedia Information Content	Layout
p_1		Explanation Title (C.name)	T1 in Fig.3 and 4
...	...	...	...
p_3	Type(user, General Practitioner) AND NOT(KNOW (user, C))	C.purpose(M) + C.tools(M) + C.constraints(M) + C.description(M)	A1
	Type(user, Patient) AND NOT(KNOW(user, C))	C.purpose(M) + C.constraints(M) + C.description(M)	A1
	...	...	...
p_4	Type(user, General Practitioner) AND NOT-KNOW (user, C))	C.purpose(M) + C.tools(M) + C.constraints(M) + C.description(M)	T2 in Fig.3
	Type(user, Patient) AND NOT(KNOW(user, C))	C.purpose(M) + C.constraints(M) + C.description(M)	T2 in Fig.4
	...	...	...
p_{15}	Type(user, General Practitioner) AND NOT(KNOW (user, C))	E_1.result	I1 in Fig. 3
	Type(user, Patient) AND NOT(KNOW(user, C))	E_1.description	I1 in Fig. 4
	...	...	...

Table 1. Part of the projection related to places of the net in Figure 2.

t_i	Task	Spatial Relations
t_0	Show title	
...	...	
t_2	Present the explanation about concept C	On(p1, p4)
t_3	Present more details and an example related to the concept C	On(p4, p7, p9)ˆLeft(p7,p9)
.....	.....	

Table 2. Part of the projection related to transitions of the net in Figure 2.

The following figures represent the explanations generated from this scenario addressed to two different users: the general practitioner and the patient.

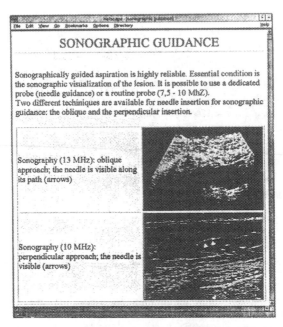

Figure 3. Explanation of .Sonographic Guidance. addressed to General Practitioners.

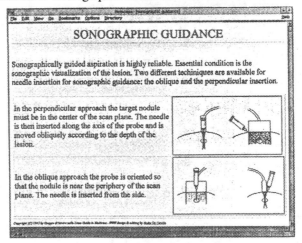

Figure 4. Explanation of .Sonographic Guidance. addressed to Patients.

REFERENCES

1. F. de Rosis, B. De Carolis, S. Pizzutilo. User Tailored Hypermedia Explanations. In the Adjunct Proceeding of INTERCHI 93 (ACM). Amsterdam 24-29 of April, 1993.
2. De Carolis, B. Formal Specification of Multimedia Interfaces. In the Proceedings of CHI'95 Research Symposium. Denver Colorado, 6-7 of May 1995.
3. Lin,C-C., Xiang, J., Chang, S-K.: Transformation and Exchange of Multimedia Objects in Distributed Multimedia Systems. Multimedia Systems, 4:12-19, 1996
4. Stott, P.D., Furuta, R.: Petri-Net based hypertext, document structure with browsing semantics. ACM Transactions on Information Systems, 7, 1, 1989.

Algorithm and Care Pathway: Clinical Guidelines and Healthcare Processes

Colin Gordon[1], Peter Johnson[2,] Chris Waite[3], Mario Veloso[4]

1 Royal Brompton Hospital. 2 Sowerby Unit for Primary Care Informatics, University of Newcastle.
3 Siemens Nixdorf Health Solutions. 4 CENTIS, Lisbon.

Abstract. This paper reports ongoing work in the project *PRESTIGE*: Guidelines in Healthcare. An approach has been developed to representing the knowledge content of clinical guideline and protocols, using a declarative model incorporating a lifecycle model of clinical acts and activities. We also encountered the need to analyse and model the healthcare processes in which the use of a clinical guideline is embedded. A business process re-engineering (BPRE) methodology, developed in the previous AIM programme project SHINE, has been used for this purpose, enabling the mapping of the knowledge components of a clinical guideline to the specific healthcare processes where they are applicable. We review the need for a combination of algorithmic and process-oriented views of guideline knowledge in order to enable effective delivery of guideline-based clinical decision support.

The task of supporting the dissemination and application of clinical practice guidelines and protocols has been identified as a promising field for the practical application of AI methods in healthcare.[1,2] We have developed a generic model for representing the knowledge content of clinical guidelines and protocols.[3] A generic modelling approach offers great potential benefits for the efficient electronic communication of the clinical knowledge which is most relevant to clinical practice, from the various national and international bodies which define best practice guidelines to the clinical users of patient record and care planning systems implemented in varying software platforms and architectures.

A widely accepted definition given by Field and Lohr of clinical practice guidelines is "Systematically developed statements to assist practitioner and patient decisions about appropriate health care for specific clinical circumstances".[4] Efforts are in progress by the USA National Institute of Health and other national bodies to promulgate standards for the development of sound guidelines, and instruments for their appraisal and validation.[5] At the same time, the processes by which clinical guidelines are actually applied, and the properties which make them successfully and effectively applicable, are still poorly understood. Two recent reviews of randomised controlled trials of guideline implementations have, however, identified a number of proven success factors [6,7]:

- in guideline development: User involvement in guideline development
- in guideline implementation: Patient-specific reminder at time of consultation
- in guideline dissemination: Specific education intervention

At least one of these success factors, the need for patient-specific prompts, is clearly amenable to efficient computerised delivery, given access to an adequate electronic patient record and terminology, which could be consulted by a decision support tool to identify the specific guideline recommendations applicable to the individual patient. In the (few) clinical settings where such EPRs exist - notably the HELP system at the University of Utah/LDS Hospital in Salt Lake City [8] - some impressive results have been reported in the delivery of a variety of simple protocol-based advice and reminder services to clinicians.

As was pointed out in the EPISTOL study [1], the interest among medical informaticians in supporting clinical guideline implementation is linked to a certain shift of paradigm in medical knowledge-based systems.[9,10] Some objections to medical experts systems are avoided by the focus on guideline implementation:

- Firstly, in the - explicit - view of their authors, clinical guidelines are not intended to abolish uncertainty: they are intended for decision *support*.
- Secondly, guidelines are not intended to mechanise care: they explicitly allow for modification of their recommendation in cases which present atypical factors not addressed in the guideline.
- Thirdly, guidelines are designed for use within a complex, open-ended healthcare process: many guidelines concern themselves with care planning and management over time, not (just) the single big decisions.

We are interested especially here in the implications of this third point.

PRESTIGE's approach

The *PRESTIGE*: Guidelines in Healthcare project, part of the Healthcare sector of the current European Commission (DGXIII) Telematics Applications Programme [12], is creating implementations of guidelines for several medical specialties as telematics applications in real clinical settings. In one of these, a guideline for the diagnosis and management of angina, the healthcare processes and agents supported extend across the whole range of primary, secondary and tertiary healthcare. Indeed the adoption of practice standards to improve communications and co-operation by these different actors (for example to collect and communicate certain core datasets) is a major explicit goal of the guideline. Guideline authors are alert to these organizational needs and generally address them in their recommendations, but when working at a national and international level they are inevitably required to take a somewhat abstract view of detailed workflows within the healthcare system. In *PRESTIGE* we have sought to identify and model these flows or care pathways in order to determine clearly where (and whether) specific recommendations of a guideline become relevant and usable. A business process re-engineering (BPRE) methodology, developed in the previous AIM programme project SHINE, has been used for this purpose, enabling the mapping of the knowledge components of a clinical guideline to the specific healthcare processes where they are applicable and the agents by whom they can be used. We here concur with the view expressed by Kibbe et. al.

that: "A clinical guideline is not a substitute for the analysis of an actual process...Guidelines look like process maps... in fact, guidelines are idealised decision flows. Process maps trace the actual steps in a process as they take place in an organization" [13]

Algorithmic formats and their limitations

The clinical guideline movement and its extensions in medical informatics has developed in parallel with several initiatives for standardised and formal representation of medical knowledge: the Arden Syntax for Medical Logic Modules, the Clinical Algorithm Standards proposed by Margolis et al. for the Society for Medical Decision Making Committee on Standardization of Clinical Algorithms [14], and developments in the use of decision table techniques. Can this work be applied to the computerised representation of clinical guidelines?

When closely examined, the flowcharts shown in clinical guideline documents often prove to be either high-level overviews, or simplified idealisations which reduce a range of alternative decision-making pathways in a single normative sample. These flowcharts are not intended to be literally and directly applied - they express a mixture of procedural and criterion-based knowledge, which the clinicians is tacitly expected to adjust and adapt according to the specific of a case; they are an effective way of conveying the gestalt of idealised care which in such a graphical form can be quickly assimilated. At present, *the concept of clarity of content in clinical guideline has no clear operational definition* in the healthcare community, largely because there is no single shared or standard understanding of what it is to use or apply a guideline.

Modelling the Guideline

In our approach to the generic modelling of clinical guideline knowledge in the DILEMMA and PRESTIGE projects [3], we follow the prevailing view within the KBS community [15] in adopting a declarative rather than a procedural representation style. For example, we favour the explicit and separate representation of definitional information (e.g. a definition of 'good glycaemic control'), to allow this information to be consulted both in a clinician-patient negotiation on individual management targets, and in periodic monitoring assessments of current controls performance.

Our experience indicates that a typical guideline for the management of a chronic problem contains information which may need to be decomposed along at least three independent axes:

- activities and tasks (such as: diagnosis, treatment planning, monitoring)
- units of care process (such a: annual review; daily ward round)
- care strategies, regimens and process states (such as: diet alone; oral medication; insulin)

In some guidelines, the second of the above categories - the workflow or care-pathway dimension, which, as Kibbe et al correctly note, is often elided in algorithmic guideline constructs, is explicitly acknowledged and addressed. This point is particularly plain in primary care, where the problem covered by a specific guideline may be only a part of the care business transacted between a GP and a patient, and where a reason for a specific encounter may or may not correspond to any task or factor covered by the guideline. Primary care professionals need to operate over time, in their successive encounters with an individual patient, a flexible and pragmatic management - in negotiation with the patient - of the encounter agenda.

Current work in PRESTIGE is addressing the appropriate generic format for the modelling of these interactive elements of guideline use. A satisfactory solution here will bring significantly closer to realisation the attractive goal of a 'plug-and-play' technology for the dissemination of clinical guidelines across a range of different medical software platforms.

References

[1] P. Barahona and J. Christensen (eds.), Knowledge and Decision in Health Telematics, IOS Press, 1994.

[2] C. Gordon and J.P. Christensen (Eds.), Health Telematics for Clinical Guidelines and Protocols. IOS Press, 1995.

[3] C Gordon, SI Herbert, P Johnson, Knowledge Representation and Clinical Practice Guidelines: the DILEMMA and PRESTIGE projects. Medical Informatics Europe '96, IOS Press 1996, 511-515.

[4] Institute of Medicine (M. J. Field and K. N. Lohr Eds.) Guidelines for Clinical Practice. From Development to Use. National Academy Press, Washington DC 1992.

[5] F Cluzeau, P Littlejohns, JM Grimshaw, A Hopkins, Appraising clinical guidelines and the development of criteria - a pilot study. Journal of Interprofessional Care. 9:3, 227-235, 1995.

[6] J. M. Grimshaw, I. T. Russell, "Effect of clinical guidelines on medical practice: a systematic review of rigorous evaluations" (Lancet 1993, Vol 342342 27 Nov 1993 p 1317-1322).

[7] Effective Health Care Bulletin. Implementing clinical practice guidelines: can guidelines be used to improve clinical practice? Leeds: University of Leeds, 1994

[8] Haug PJ, Gardner RM, Tate KE et al. Decision support in medicine: examples from the HELP system. Computers and Biomedical Research 1994: 27: 396-418.

[9] Johnson PE What kind of system should an expert be? Journal of Medicine and Philosophy 7, 77-97 1983

[10] C Gordon, May we support your decision? Journal of Health Services Research and Policy. 1:3, 175-7 July 1996.

[11] C Gordon and M Veloso, The PRESTIGE Project: Implementing Guidelines in Healthcare. Medical Informatics Europe '96, IOS Press 1996, 887-891.

[12] D Pitty, P Reeves, C Gordon, Z Ilic, A Rickards, Telematics Support for the Shared Care Management of Coronary Artery Disease in the *Prestige* Project. Medical Informatics Europe '96, IOS Press 1996, 925-929.

[13] David C Kibbe et al, Integrating Guidelines with Continuous Quality Improvement, Joint Commission Journal on Quality Improvement 20:4; p181ff, 1994.

[14] Society for Medical Decision Making Committee on Standardization of Clinical Algorithms, Proposal for Clinical Algorithm Standards. Medical Decision Making 12, 149-154, 1992.

[15] MA Musen, Dimensions of knowledge sharing and reuse. Computers and Biomedical Research 25: 435-467.

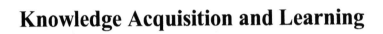

Knowledge Acquisition and Learning

Detecting Very Early Stages of Dementia from Normal Aging with Machine Learning Methods

William Rodman Shankle[1], Subramani Mani[2], Michael J. Pazzani[2] and
Padhraic Smyth[2]

[1] Departments of Neurology and Information and Computer Science, University of
California at Irvine, Irvine CA 92697-5100 *rshankle@uci.edu*
[2] Department of Information and Computer Science, University of California at
Irvine, Irvine CA 92697-3425 *(mani,pazzani,smyth)@ics.uci.edu*

Abstract. We used Machine Learning (**ML**) methods to learn the best
decision rules to distinguish normal brain aging from the earliest stages
of dementia using subsamples of 198 normal and 244 cognitively impaired
or very mildly demented (Clinical Dementia Rating Scale=0.5) persons.
Subjects were represented by their age, education and gender, plus their
responses on the Functional Activities Questionnaire (FAQ), the Mini-
Mental Status Exam (MMSE), and the Ishihara Color Plate (ICP) tasks.
The ML algorithms applied to these data contained within the electronic
patient records of a medical relational database, learned rule sets that
were as good as or better than any rules derived from either the literature or from domain specific knowledge provided by expert clinicians.
All ML algorithms for all runs found that a single question from the
FAQ, *the forgetting rule*, ("Do you require assistance remembering appointments, family occasions, holidays, or taking medications?") was the
only attribute included in all rule sets. CART's tree simplification procedure always found that just the forgetting rule gave the best pruned
decision tree rule set with classification accuracy (93% sensitivity and
80% specificity) as high as or better than any other decision tree rule-
set. Comparison with published classification accuracies for the FAQ and
MMSE revealed that including some of the additional attributes in these
tests actually worsen classification accuracy. Stepwise logistic regression
using the FAQ attributes to classify dementia status confirmed that *the
forgetting rule* gave a much larger odds ratio than any other attribute and
was the only attribute included in all of the stepwise logistic regressions
performed on 33 random samples of the data. Stepwise logistic regression
using the MMSE attributes identified two attributes which occurred in
all 33 runs and had by far the highest odds ratio. In summary, ML methods have discovered that the simplest and most sensitive screening test
for the earliest clinical stages of dementia consists of a single question,
the forgetting rule.

1 Introduction

In this paper, we apply ML methods to the detection of the earliest stages of
dementia due to Alzheimer's disease and other causes. Machine learning (**ML**)

can generate classification rules where the data include the known classification of each case. The application of ML methods in the domain of medicine has been relatively infrequent because of difficulty in accessing medical data electronically. Artificial intelligence approaches to medicine started with knowledge-based systems, which learn from human experts, not data. Beginning with the expert systems of the seventies (MYCIN [28], PUFFS), followed by Bayesian systems of the late eighties and early nineties (ACORN [12], PATHFINDER [5]), these knowledge-based systems generated much enthusiasm and hope. But there are very few such actual systems in routine clinical use. Another approach starting in the mid eighties, sought to make use of real data and a domain model for knowledge acquisition and rule learning[3],[18], [15]. KARDIO[20] is an expert system for evaluation of electrocardiograms based on this approach. With increasing availability of electronic medical records, machine learning has the potential to become a valuable adjunct to clinical decision-making. There has been some recent effort in this direction[2].

Dementia is defined as multiple cognitive impairments with loss of related functional skills without altered consciousness. Most demented patients do not see a physician for the problem of memory loss until four years after symptom onset [7], which usually relates to the patient's social embarrassment about having a memory problem. Additionally, community physicians commonly do not detect dementia [10] or misidentify it [21] in its earliest stages when patients are seeing them for other reasons. At the mid stages of the disease, physicians are less able to slow the progression and minimize debilitating behavioral effects of the dementia. As an example of an intervention which might have greater value if started earlier in the disease, Lubeck et al. [16] reported a 17% reduction in the $200,000 cost of AD patient care using central cholinergic agonists (Tacrine). A simple, unobtrusive method for detecting dementia early in the disease's course would help get patients to seek early evaluation and treatment, resulting most probably in preserved quality of life and reduced financial burden to family and health care providers. The Agency for Health Care Policy Research (**AHCPR**) clinical practice guidelines for the assessment and recognition of Alzheimer's disease and related disorders [30] recommends two simple tests, the Functional Activities Questionnaire (**FAQ** [24]), and the six-item Blessed Orientation, Memory and Concentration test (**BOMC** [8]), to screen for dementia after excluding delirium and depression. We recently reported that the use of Machine Learning (**ML**) methods in conjunction with the FAQ and the BOMC markedly improved sensitivity in detecting dementia in a sample of 609 normal, cognitively impaired, and demented subjects when compared with published scoring criteria [27].

In this paper, we focus on discriminating the effects of normal aging on cognition from the very early stages of dementia because early detection is potentially very important for improving quality of life, and reducing total health care costs to family and society. To do this, we used the AHCPR-recommended screening instrument, the FAQ, plus the Folstein Mini-Mental Status Exam [9] and two items from the BOMC (**MMSEPLUS**) and Ishihara Color Plates (**ICP** [11]) in conjunction with several ML methods, and compared these results to those using published scoring criteria for the same set of data from the same set of subjects. Other items of the BOMC did not need to be considered in addition to the MMSE since the rest of the BOMC is a subset of the MMSE.

2 Methods

2.1 Sample Description

The total sample consisted of the initial visits of 198 cognitively normal and 244 cognitively impaired or very mildly demented (Clinical Dementia Rating Stage ≤ 0.5) subjects seen at the University of California, Irvine Alzheimer's Disease Research Center (ADRC). Patients received a complete diagnostic evaluation consisting of patient and caregiver interviews, general physical and neurological exam, two hours of cognitive testing including the CERAD [29] neuropsychological battery and other selected tests, routine laboratory testing for memory loss, and magnetic resonance neuroimaging with or without single photon emission with computed tomography. Control subjects were either community volunteers or unaffected spouses of patients, and received an abbreviated, 45 minute version of the patient cognitive battery, which consisted of the CERAD plus measures of activities of daily living. They did not receive a medical exam, laboratory testing or neuroimaging unless cognitive or functional testing suggested an impairment. The number of subjects available for the various analyses varied because of missing data. We also performed logistic regressions of the MMSEPLUS and FAQ attributes. The sample sizes for each screening test appears in Table 1.

Table 1. Characteristics of the UCI ADRC Sample of this study

Attribute	Normal			Impaired			Total		
	N	Mean	Std.	N	Mean	Std.	N	Mean	Std
Age*	196	67.2	11.8	278	68.2	10.9	474	67.6	11.3
% Female*	198	71	46	274	43	50	472	59	49
Education(yrs)	140	15.0	2.7	274	15.3	3.2	414	15.2	3.0
FAQ	137	0.2	0.8	211	7.6	6.2	348	5.1	6.1
MMSEPLUS	198	29.2	0.9	227	24.8	5.5	425	26.6	4.8
ICP	133	13.7	1.7	179	11.1	4.1	312	11.9	3.7

* T-test unpaired sample with unequal variance was significant at $P < 0.001$

Classification of Dementia Status

The diagnosis of dementia status, using DSM-IV criteria [1], was based on a review of all the data by the neurologist and neuropsychologist during their diagnostic review session. Each subject was categorized as either unimpaired, cognitively impaired but not meeting criteria for dementia, or demented. A classification of *dementia* required the presence of multiple cognitive impairments plus functional impairments resulting from the cognitive impairments in the absence of delirium or other non-organic etiologies such as major depression. They were also classified by dementia severity using standard criteria for the Clinical Dementia Rating Scale (**CDRS** [19]), in which 0 = normal, 0.5 = questionably or very mildly demented, and 1-5 indicate increasing severity of dementia. Control subjects showing cognitive impairment or very mild dementia (CDRS ≤ 0.5) were included in the cognitively impaired/very mildly demented sample, which we will refer to as the *impaired* group from here on; patients who tested normally were included in the cognitively normal sample; subjects with delirium were excluded from the analysis. Table 1 shows the sample characteristics.

FAQ, MMSEPLUS, and ICP tests

The FAQ (total score ranges from 0 (normal) to 30 (severely disabled)) consists of ten questions about basic and more complex activities of daily life. The answers to these questions were extracted from the UCI ADRC relational database of over 1,200 variables per subject-visit to compute the FAQ total and item scores. The AHCPR recommends using total FAQ scores of 9 or higher for detecting impairment. Pfeffer[24] found a total FAQ score of 5 or higher to be most sensitive as a second stage screen in discriminating normal vs. questionably demented subjects. We examined the sensitivity and specificity of total FAQ scores from 1 to 30 without ML methods. With ML methods, we used age, sex, education, and all FAQ attributes with and without the FAQ total score. The description for how these runs were performed is in the Machine Learning Methods section.

The MMSEPLUS consists of 19 questions from the MMSE regarding orientation for time and place, registration, attention, short-term recall, language, and drawing, plus two attributes from the BOMC test (recall of an address and number of trials to correctly repeat the address twice), which were added because of potential sensitivity in detecting early dementia. The MMSE ranges from 0 (severely impaired) to 30 (no impairment). The occurrence of dementia increases with advancing age and decreases with increasing educational level. Depending upon a subject's age and education, a total MMSE score of 24 or higher is used to classify a subject as normal [22, 4]. We examined the sensitivity and specificity of total MMSE scores from 1 to 30 without ML methods. We then aggregated the individual MMSE attributes reflecting short-term recall, orientation to time, and orientation to place into three aggregate attributes respectively. The MM-SEPLUS attributes therefore consisted of the three MMSE aggregate attributes, individual MMSE attributes reflecting registration, attention and drawing, and the two BOMC attributes. These attributes plus age, sex and education were used with ML methods to classify normal and impaired subject samples.

The ICP consists of 21 pseudoisochromatic plates, 15 with noisy numbers and 6 with noisy trails embedded in a noisy background. The subject reads the number or traces the trail and is scored by the examiner as correct (1) or incorrect (0). The instruction for the number-naming task is, "If you see a number on the plate, tell me what it is", and that for the trail-tracing task is, "If you see the trail, trace it from beginning to end." Because it is such a simple task and it appears to discriminate among Alzheimer's, Vascular dementia and Normal aging subjects [17], we included it as a potential screening test. However, examination of the ML classification results with the 21 ICP attributes (see Table 2), showed that it is not sufficiently sensitive for detecting very mild dementia. Therefore, the ICP was removed from further consideration as a candidate for screening.

2.2 Machine Learning Methods

Specific algorithms We concentrated on decision tree learners, rule learners and the Naive Bayesian classifier. Decision trees and rules generate clear descriptions of how the ML method arrives at a particular classification. The Naive Bayesian classifier was included for comparison purposes. MLC++(Machine Learning in C++) is a software package developed at Stanford University [26] which implements commonly used machine learning algorithms. It also provides standardized methods of running experiments using these algorithms. C4.5 is a decision tree generator and C4.5rules produce rules of the form, *if..then* from the decision tree [25]. Naive Bayes is a classifier based on Bayes Rule. Even though it makes the assumption that the attributes are condtionally independent of each other given the class, it is a robust classifier and serves as a good comparison in terms of accuracy for evaluating other algorithms [6]. FOCL [23] is a concept learner which can incorporate a user provided knowledge of two types. First, when provided with a guideline or protocol directly, FOCL has the capacity for revision if the guidelines produce better classification rules than that produced from exploration of the data. Second, FOCL can accept information on each nominal variable indicating which values of the variable increase the probability of belonging to a class (such as impaired) and information on each continuous variable on whether higher or lower values of the variable increases the probability of belonging to a class. We call this, "constrained FOCL", in the experimental results. FOCL can also learn from the data only, without an initial input of constraints or guidelines. We call this, "unconstrained FOCL", in the experimental results. CART [13] is a classifier which uses a conservative tree-growing algorithm that minimizes the standard error of the classification accuracy based on a particular tree-growing method applied to a series of training subsamples. We ran CART 10 times on randomly selected 2/3 training sets and 1/3 testing sets. For each training set, CART built a classification tree where the size of the tree was chosen based on cross-validation accuracy on this training set. The test accuracy of the chosen tree was then evaluated on the unseen test set.

2.3 Treatment of missing data

We used each ML's method for handling missing data. In C4.5 missing attributes are assigned to both branches of the decision node, and the average of the classification accuracy is used for these cases. In the Naive Bayesian Classifier, missing values are ignored in the estimation of probabilities. In FOCL, any test on a missing value is treated as false. Therefore, it attempts to learn a set of rules that tolerates missing values in some variables. CART uses surrogate tests for missing values.

2.4 Training and Testing Samples

We ran experiments in which data from the FAQ, MMSEPLUS, and ICP tests were used separately by each learning algorithm. The samples for the FAQ, MMSEPLUS, and ICP ML analyses mostly overlapped but the sizes differed due to different patterns of missing data. For the FAQ there were 348 instances— 137 cognitively normal and 211 impaired; for the MMSEPLUS there were 425 instances—198 normal and 227 impaired; for the ICP there were 312 instances— 133 normal and 179 impaired. We cross-validated the results in the following manner. The complete sample of each screening test was used to generate 20 non-overlapping training and testing sets in a 2/3 to 1/3 ratio, with random sampling of the training set. The algorithms were trained on the training set and the resulting decision tree then classified the unseen testing set. The classification accuracy is hence the mean of the accuracies obtained for the twenty runs of the testing set. An example of one decision tree rule-set appears in figure 1.

Rule 1: age > 56 *and* job $> 2 \Rightarrow$ class **impaired**
Rule 2: money > 0 *and* forget $> 0 \Rightarrow$ class **impaired**
Rule 3: gender $= 0$ *and* age > 56 *and* forget $> 0 \Rightarrow$ class **impaired**
Rule 4: age > 56 *and* age ≤ 64 *and* forget $> 0 \Rightarrow$ class **impaired**
Rule 5: age > 73 *and* forget $> 0 \Rightarrow$ class **impaired**
Rule 6: forget $\leq 0 \Rightarrow$ class **normal**
Rule 7: Default $\Rightarrow$ class **impaired**

Fig. 1. A C45rule Set

Nonsense Rules It is possible for ML methods to generate a rule which makes no domain sense (**nonsense rule**). The rule sets generated by the various ML methods were inspected for their clinical sense by an ADRC staff neurologist. After identifying the nonsense rules, we used FOCL to incorporate domain-specific knowledge that would prevent (constrain) such rules from occurring. We then compared classification performance of the constrained vs. unconstrained runs using FOCL to see how performance was affected. An example of a decision tree with a nonsense component follows:

```
forget > 0 (having trouble):
|   age <= 52 :
|   |   edulevel > 16 : normal (4.0)
|   |   edulevel <= 16 :
|   |   |   SHOP <= 0 (no trouble shopping): impaired (5.6)
|   |   |   SHOP > 0 (having trouble shopping): normal (2.0)
```

In this example, eight persons (5.6+2.0) were forgetful, 52 years old or younger, and had 16 or fewer years of education. Among them, those who could shop were classified as impaired while those who required assistance to shop were classified as normal: this is a *nonsense rule*, which arises because of insufficient examples covering the circumstances specified by the nonsense rule. As becomes apparent later, the appearance of such nonsense rules should encourage one to gather more data, to constrain the ML method with domain-specific knowledge, or to search for a reduced rule-set using pruning techniques.

2.5   Logistic Regression Methods

50% random samples of each class were selected 33 times, and analyzed with stata's stepwise logistic regression, which estimates the odds ratios that independently contribute to the model for each run. The FAQ and MMSE were separately regressed against dementia status, and the attributes with the largest odds ratios in each run were identified.

3   Results

We examined the sensitivity (probability of correctly classifying an impaired subject) and specificity (probability of correctly classifying a cognitively normal subject) for each ML run of the testing samples. The same statistics were generated for each run of the cutoff scores of the total FAQ and MMSE without the use of ML methods, and for the stepwise logistic regression. Figures 2 and 3 respectively show the receiver operating characteristic (ROC) curves for the FAQ and MMSE total scores without ML methods, as well as the performance of the best results using various ML algorithms. Table 2 shows the classification results of each ML method and of published criteria for total MMSE and FAQ scores. A number of strategies were used to select an optimal decision tree for clinical use. We ordered pruned decision tree rule-sets by their frequency of occurrence across the different ML methods and runs. We examined the cross-validation procedure of CART, which selects the best single decision tree for a specified number of runs; we repeated this procedure 10 times. Each time, CART selected the same best decision tree. We also ran forward-stepping logistic regression on the dependent variable, *Dementia Class*, against the independent variables of the FAQ attributes (F-to-enter = 0.4, F-to-remove = 0.2) to identify the attributes which made statistically significant independent contributions to prediction of dementia status. For the demographic attributes (Table 1), only age and sex

Table 2. Sensitivity and Specificity of each Screening test by algorithm and published scoring criteria

	CART	C45	C45Rules	FOCL	Naive Bayes	FAQ >8	FAQ >4
FAQ (Normal = 137, Impaired = 211)							
% Sensitivity	93	92	89	94	67	20	49
% Specificity	80	78	79	80	97	99	96
% Accuracy	88	88	85	89	83	51	68

		C45	C45Rules	FOCL	Naive Bayes	MMSE >24	MMSE >27
MMSEPLUS (Normal = 198, Impaired = 227)							
% Sensitivity		77	70	79	66	30	62
% Specificity		80	86	70	87	100	81
% Accuracy		79	77	75	75	63	71

		C45	C45Rules		NAIVE BAYES		
Ishihara Color Plates (Normal = 133, Impaired = 179)							
% Sensitivity		68	68		73		
% Specificity		55	52		52		
% Overall		66	63		64		

showed statistically significant differences between normal and impaired subjects. However, the age difference between normal and impaired subjects was less than one year, which is not a clinically significant difference. Therefore, only gender showed a clinically significant difference, with a preponderance of females in the normal group. The ICP attributes with ML methods resulted in at best a 73% sensitivity (52% specificity) using the Naive Bayes method and were not considered further. For the FAQ test, figure 2 shows that the FAQ with ML methods out-performed the best of the published cutoff criteria for the total FAQ score. It is interesting to note that the cutoff score of 9 or higher, recommended by the AHCPR, has a considerably poorer sensitivity for discriminating very mildly demented from normal subjects (20%) than that obtained for the ML methods, FOCL, C4.5, C4.5Rules, and CART (93%). One should also note that the number of questions needed to achieve these results with ML methods is markedly reduced. In the case of CART, only one question is required (*"Do you require assistance remembering appointments, holidays, family occasions, or taking medications?"*). For the MMSEPLUS test, figure 3 shows that, when used with ML methods, classification accuracy is always higher than when any total MMSE score is used as a cutoff criterion without ML methods. Using constrained vs. unconstrained analysis of the data with FOCL, there did not appear to be a significant improvement in classification accuracy, but no nonsense rules were generated when constraining FOCL with domain-specific knowledge. Given the various search strategies for finding the best decision tree or rule-set for clinical use, all approaches converged on one main conclusion: the response to a single question from the FAQ test gave classification accuracy as good as any other rule set and better than any published criteria. This question, *"Do you require assistance remembering appointments, family occasions, holidays or tak-*

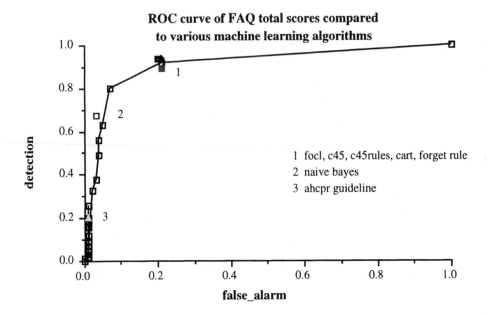

Fig. 2. FAQ ROC

ing medications?", we call the **forgetting rule**. All runs for all ML algorithms studied included this rule in the decision tree/rule-set; no other attribute was included in every decision tree/rule-set. Using CART's cross-validation procedure, this single rule decision tree was selected as the best tree on 10 out of 10 runs. Finally, forward-stepping logistic regression was used to identify the most important attributes in each run. These attributes were compared to those selected by the ML methods. For the FAQ, the forgetting attribute had the largest odds ratio on 32 of 33 runs (11.9 ± 7.6), and was the only attribute included in all 33 models. Job performance (odds ratio = 4.2 ± 4.2) was the 2nd most frequently selected attribute, occurring in 20 of 33 runs. For the MMSEPLUS, the attribute, *# of trials to obtain 2 correct repetitions*, had overwhelmingly the highest odds ratio (90 ± 59), and was the first attribute entered for all 33 runs. The only other attribute included in all 33 runs was the *delayed recall attribute* ($1 \div oddsratio = 2.3 \pm 0.4$).

4   Discussion

There are four main findings of the present analysis. *First*, the ML methods can be interfaced with an electronic medical record system to learn directly from the data. The feasibility of this is also demonstrated by the work described in for example [2] and [14]. This feature contrasts with that of knowledge-based

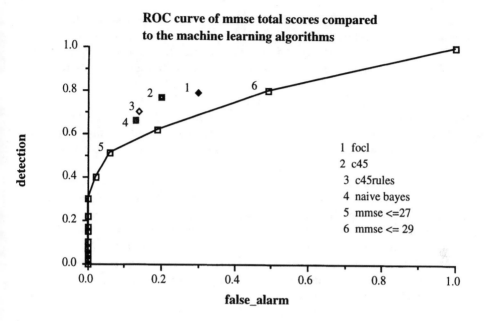

Fig. 3. MMSE ROC

systems, in which human experts design the decision rules and then test the data. Whereas humans usually select a few rules by which they make decisions, a machine can consider a larger number of rules. This is a specific advantage of ML methods. When supplemented by a review of the ML-generated rules or by incorporation of domain-specific knowledge into the ML algorithm, specific rules that violate domain knowledge can be minimized, thus enhancing the power of ML methods. This approach also identifies subtle logical errors in the electronic medical record that could be overlooked. For example, after reviewing a nonsense rule using job performance as a criterion, we discovered that some normal subjects had misinterpreted the question about their ability to perform a job, answering that they could no longer perform their job because they had retired. In fact, they were fully able to perform their job given the need to do so. The inconsistency in the attribute values was discovered, and corrected. Re-running the ML algorithm verified that the nonsense rule had been eliminated by this correction of the data. The *second* important finding of this paper is that ML methods used in conjunction with the MMSEPLUS test attributes outperform any published criteria for using total MMSE score to classify normal and cognitively impaired or very mildly demented subjects. They also do much better than any cutoff possible using the ROC curve. This supports the idea that some attributes of the MMSEPLUS are more important than others, and that the less important attributes may actually confuse classification. The findings of the logistic regression analyses did not substantially alter these conclusions. Two attributes, trials to learn address and recall of address performed as well as any other combination of MMSEPLUS attributes. The *third* important finding of this paper is clinical: when used with ML methods, a single question from the FAQ (the forgetting question) classifies normal cognitive and the mildest stages of a dementia as well as or better than any other combination of attributes from the FAQ, the MMSEPLUS and the ICP with and without total score, and outperforms any of the recommended scoring criteria for the FAQ or the MMSE total scores. The results of the logistic regression analyses confirmed the importance of the forgetting question. For screening purposes, we think that the tradeoff for higher sensitivity is preferable given the ease and applicability of the forgetting attribute as a screening test.

It is interesting to note that the AHCPR-recommended criteria for impairment using a total FAQ score of 9 or higher, is much higher than the score of a person answering positively only to the forgetting question (their FAQ total = 1-3 in that case). The higher total FAQ score recommended by the AHCPR is based on studies which included all levels of dementia severity. Using this criterion for the very mildly demented subjects in the present study resulted in only a 20% sensitivity, which implies that responses to other questions of the FAQ actually reduce the sensitivity for detecting very mild stages of dementia (compared to the forgetting rule alone). This is why inclusion of the total FAQ score as an attribute in the ML runs reduced the specificity and sensitivity when compared with the results obtained from analyses of the FAQ item attributes alone. The FAQ attributes therefore contribute unequally to dementia classification, with the forgetting question being the most contributory. This is our *fourth* significant finding.

4.1 Limits on Accuracy

Sample bias: The only demographic variable which differed to a clinically significant extent between normal and cognitively impaired subjects was gender. Since the decision rule sets rarely included gender in any of the ML runs and methods, we conclude that the findings presented here are not due to sample biases in age, education or gender. The findings are, however restricted to the population represented, which consists of individuals, mostly over 65 years and with more than a high school education. However, previous studies showing the insensitivity of the FAQ to educational level suggests that the results of this study apply to persons 65 or over, regardless of education.

5 Conclusions

We have successfully applied ML methods to increase sensitivity and specificity of commonly used dementia screening tests plus reduce the information required to make this decision. Additionally, ML methods can identify subtle errors in the electronic medical record which are due to misinterpretation of what is being asked of the subject. The rule set derived from the full data can be used on paper or as software in various clinical settings to enhance the detection of very early stages of a dementing illness. This should result in less disability per patient and better quality of life for both caregiver and patient through early intervention. The utility of ML-derived protocols with some human supervision has general applicability to many important medical areas, including cancer, heart disease, and stroke.

5.1 Acknowledgements

We thank professor Carl Cotman for helping establish a working relation with the AHCPR. This work was supported by the Alzheimer's Association Pilot Research Grant, PRG-95-161, *The Alzheimer's Intelligent Interface: Diagnosis, Education and Training.*

References

1. American Psychiatric Association, Washington, D. C. *Diagnostic and Statistical Manual of Mental Disorders*, 4 edition, 1994.
2. Ohmann C, Yang Q, Moustakis V, Lang K, and PJ van Elk. Machine learning techniques applied to the diagnosis of acute abdominal pain. In Pedro Barahona and Mario Stefanelli, editors, *Lecture Notes in Artificial Intelligence: Artificial Intelligence in Medicine AIME95*, volume 934, pages 276–281. Springer, 1995.
3. Cestnik G, Konenenko I, and Bratko I. Assistant-86: A knowledge-elicitation tool for sophisticated users. In Bratko I and Lavrac N, editors, *Progress in Machine Learning*, pages 31–45. Sigma Press, 1987.
4. Crum R.M, Anthony J.C, Bassett S.S, and Folstein M.F. Population-based norms for the mini-mental state examination by age and educational level. *JAMA*, 269(18):2386–2390, May 1993.
5. Heckerman D.E, Horvitz E.J, and Nathwani B.N. Towards normative expert systems: Part i the pathfinder project. *Methods of Information in Medicine*, (31):90–105, 1992.
6. Duda R.O and Hart P.E. *Pattern Classification and Scene Analysis.* John Wiley, New York, 1973.
7. Ernst R.L and Hay J.W. The u.s. economic and social costs of alzheimer's disease revisited. *American Journal of Public Health*, 84(8):1261–4, Aug 1994.
8. Fillenbaum G.G, Heyman A, Wilkinson W.E, and Haynes C.S. Comparison of two screening tests in alzheimer's disease—the correlation and reliability of the mini-mental state examination and the modified blessed test. *Archives of Neurology*, 44(9):924–7, Sep 1987.
9. Folstein M.F, Folstein S.E, and McHugh P.R. Mini-mental state–a practical method for grading the cognitive state of patients for the clinician. *Journal of Psychiatric Research*, 12(3):189–98, Nov 1975.
10. Hoffman R.S. Diagnostic errors in the evaluation of behavioral disorders. *JAMA*, 248:225–8, 1982.
11. Shinobu Ishihara. *Ishihara Tests for Colour-Blindness.* Kanehara Shuppan, Ltd., Tokyo Japan, 1994.
12. Wyatt J. Lessons learned from the field trials of acorn, a chest pain advisor. In Barber B, Cao D, Qin D, and Wagner F, editors, *Proceedings MedInfo*, pages 111–115. Elsevier Scientific, 1989.

13. Brieman L, Friedman J.H., Olshen R.A., and Stone C.J. *Classification and Regression Trees.* Wadsworth, Belmont, 1984.

14. Gierl L. and Stengel-Rutkowski S. Integrating consultation and semi-automatic knowledge acquisition in a prototype-based architecture: Experiences with dysmorphic syndromes. *Artificial Intelligence in Medicine*, 6:29–49, 1994.

15. Nada Lavrac and Igor Mozetic. Second generation knowledge acquisition methods and their application to medicine. In Keravnou E, editor, *Deep Models for Medical Knowledge Engineering*, pages 177–198. Elsevier, New York, 1992.

16. Lubeck D.P, Mazonson T and Bowe P.D. Potential effect of tacrine on expenditures for alzheimer's disease. *Medical Interface*, 7(10):130–8, Oct 1994.

17. McCleary R, Shankle W.R, Mulnard R.A, and Dick M.B. Ishihara test performance and dementia. *Journal of the Neurological Sciences*, in press 1996.

18. R.S. Michalski, Mozetic I, Hong J, and Lavrac N. The multi-purpose incremental learning system aq15 and its testing application to three medical domains. In *In Proceedings of the Fifth National Conference on Artificial Intelligence*, pages 1041–1045, Philadelphia, PA, 1986. Morgan Kaufmann.

19. Morris J.C. The clinical dementia rating (cdr): current version and scoring rules. *Neurology*, 43(11):2412–4, Nov 1993.

20. Igor Mozetic and Bernhard Pfahringer. Improving diagnostic efficiency in kardio: Abstractions, constraint propagation and model compilation. In Keravnou E, editor, *Deep Models for Medical Knowledge Engineering*, pages 1–25. Elsevier, New York, 1992.

21. O'Connor D.W, Fertig A, Grande M.J, Hyde J.B, Perry J.R, Roland M.O, Silverman J.D and Wright S.K. Dementia in general practice: the practical consequences of a more positive approach to diagnosis. *Br J Gen Pract*, 43:185–8, 1993.

22. Oconnor D.W, Pollitt PA, Treasure F.P, Brook C.P.B, and Reiss B.B. The influence of education, social class and sex on mini-mental state scores. *Psychological Medicine*, 19:771–776, 1989.

23. Michael Pazzani and Dennis Kibler. The utility of knowledge in inductive learning. *Machine Learning*, (9):57–94, 1992.

24. Pfeffer R.I, Kurosaki T.T, Harrah C.H, Chance J.M, and Filos S. Measurement of functional activities in older adults in the community. *J Gerontology*, 37:323–9, 1982.

25. Quinlan J.R. *C4.5: Programs for Machine Learning.* Morgan Kaufmann, Los Altos, California, 1993.

26. Kohavi R, George John, Richard Long, David Manley, and Karl Pfleger. Mlc++: A machine learning library in c++. In *Tools with Artificial Intelligence*, pages 740–743. IEEE Computer Society Press, 1994.

27. Shankle W.R, Datta P, Dillencourt M, and Pazzani M. Improving dementia screening tests with machine learning methods. *Alzheimer's Research*, 2(3), Jun 1996.

28. Shortliffe E. *Computer-Based Medical Consultations: MYCIN.* Elsevier/North Holland, New York, 1976.

29. Welsh K.A, Butters N, Mohs R.C, Beekly D, Edland S, and Fillenbaum G. The consortium to establish a registry for alzheimer's disease (cerad. part v. a normative study of the neuropsychological battery. *Neurology*, 44(4):609–14, Apr 1994.

30. Williams T.F and Costa P.T. Recognition and initial assessment of alzheimer's disease and related dementias: Clinical practice guidelines. Technical report, Department of Health and Human Services, 1995.

Acquiring and Validating Background Knowledge for Machine Learning Using Function Decomposition

Blaž Zupan and Sašo Džeroski

Department of Intelligent Systems, Jožef Stefan Institute
1000 Ljubljana, Slovenia (E-mail: Blaz.Zupan@ijs.si, Saso.Dzeroski@ijs.si)

Abstract. Domain or background knowledge is often needed in order to solve difficult problems of learning medical diagnostic rules. Earlier experiments have demonstrated the utility of background knowledge when learning rules for early diagnosis of rheumatic diseases. A particular form of background knowledge comprising typical co-occurrences of several groups of attributes was provided by a medical expert. This paper explores the possibility to automate the process of acquiring background knowledge of this kind. A method based on function decomposition is proposed that identifies typical co-occurrences for a given set of attributes. The method is evaluated by comparing the typical co-occurrences it identifies, as well as their contribution to the performance of machine learning algorithms, to the ones provided by a medical expert.

1 Introduction

When applying machine learning to learn medical diagnostic rules from patient records, it may be desirable to augment the latter with additional diagnostic knowledge about the particular domain, especially for difficult diagnostic problems. In machine learning terminology, additional expert knowledge is usually referred to as *background knowledge*. While most machine learning approaches have only limited capabilities of taking into account such knowledge, inductive logic programming [12] systems can handle different types of background knowledge.

A particular type of medical expert knowledge specifies which combinations of values (co-occurrences) of a set (grouping) of attributes have high importance for the diagnostic problem at hand. These combinations of values are called typical co-occurrences. A medical expert would specify the groupings as well as the typical co-occurrences associated with them.

Typical co-occurrences are used in expert diagnosis. When asked for some additional knowledge about the difficult problem of early diagnosis of rheumatic diseases, a medical expert provided typical co-occurrences for several groupings of attributes. These were then used by the LINUS [12] system for inductive logic programming in the domain of early diagnosis of rheumatic diseases [14] from anamnestic data. In this domain, the task here is to diagnose into one of eight diagnostic classes, given sixteen anamnestic attributes. The difficulty of the diagnostic problem itself and noise in the data make this a very hard problem for machine learning approaches. A more detailed description of the domain can be found in Section 3.

The medical expert provided six groupings (pairs or triples of attributes) and their typical co-occurrences (characteristic combinations of values). These are given in Table 4 in Section 3. For each grouping, LINUS introduces a new attribute which is considered in the learning process. For a particular patient record (example) this attribute has as value the typical co-occurrence observed for the patient, if one was indeed observed, or has the value "irrelevant" otherwise. A rule induction system, such as CN2 [3], or any attribute-value learning system can then be applied to the extended learning problem.

To illustrate the concept, let us consider Grouping 2. It relates the attributes "Spinal pain" and "Duration of morning stiffness" and the typical co-occurrences are: no spinal pain and morning stiffness up to 1 hour, spondylotic pain and morning stiffness up to 1 hour, spondylitic pain and morning stiffness longer than 1 hour. An example rule that uses this grouping and the second co-occurrence is given in Table 1. This rule was induced by LINUS using CN2 [14].

Table 1. A rule that makes use of a typical co-occurrence in the domain of early diagnosis of rheumatic diseases

```
IF    Duration_of_present_symptoms > 6.5 months
AND   Duration_of_rheumatic_diseases < 5.5 years
AND   Number_of_painful_joints > 16
AND   grouping2(Spinal_pain,Duration_of_morning_stiffness) =
                'spondylotic & up to 1 hour'
THEN  Diagnosis = Degenerative_spine_diseases
```

The background knowledge in the form of typical co-occurrences was shown to have positive effect on rule induction in several respects. First, rules induced in the presence of background knowledge performed better in terms of classification accuracy and information content [14]. Second, it substantially improves the quality of induced rules from a medical point of view as assessed by a medical expert [14]. Finally, it reduces the effects of noisy data on the process of rule induction and nearest neighbor classification [7].

The motivation for our work is based on the following line of reasoning: It is very desirable to have and use background knowledge in the form of typical co-occurrences in rule induction, as it can greatly improve performance. Typical co-occurrences are also a natural and useful human concept used by the medical expert. However, it is well-known that direct knowledge acquisition from experts is an arduous and error-prone process [9]. This paper therefore proposes a method for automated acquisition of background knowledge in the form of typical co-occurrences. The expert need only specify the groupings, while the associated co-occurrences are determined automatically.

Before proceeding further, let us briefly mention related work. The domain of early diagnosis of rheumatic diseases has been first treated with a machine learning approach by Pirnat et al. [16]. Decision tree based approaches have been further applied to this domain by Karalič and Pirnat [10]. The use of background knowledge in this domain has been investigated by Lavrač et al. in combination with a decision tree approach [13] and in combination with a rule induction approach [14] and by Džeroski and Lavrač [7] in combination with nearest neighbor classification.

The typical co-occurrence acquisition method proposed in this paper uses several fundamental algorithms from function decomposition. The pioneers of this field are

Ashenhurst [1] and Curtis [5]. They have used function decomposition for the discovery of Boolean functions. Its potential use within machine learning was first observed by Samuel [17] and Biermann [2]. A recent report of Perkowski et al. [15] provides a comprehensive survey of the literature on function decomposition. In this paper we refer to the decomposition algorithms which use decision tables with multi-valued attributes and classes and were developed by Zupan and Bohanec [20].

The remainder of the paper is organized as follows. Section 2 describes the method for acquisition of typical co-occurrences. Section 3 describes the domain of early diagnosis of rheumatic diseases, and the background knowledge provided by the expert. Taking the groupings provided by the expert, we apply the proposed method to determine the typical co-occurrences. The results of these experiments are also given in Section 3 and discussed in Section 4, where the typical co-occurrences provided by the expert and the ones generated by the proposed method are compared. The latter are quite similar to the former, but mostly have higher mutual information with the diagnostic class. Section 5 outlines some prospects for further fork and Section 6 concludes.

2 The method

This section formally and through an example introduces the method that, given a set of examples represented as attribute-value vectors with assigned classes, derives typical co-occurrences for a given set of attributes. The overall data-flow of the method is shown in Figure 1. The method first converts the set of examples to a decision table (Step 1). Next, decision table decomposition methods are used to derive a so-called partition matrix (Step 2). Finally, the typical co-occurrences for a given set of attributes are derived (Step 3), using an approach based on coloring the incompatibility graph of the partition matrix.

We first give an example of decision table decomposition and introduce the required decomposition methodology. The description of the method to acquire a set of typical co-occurrences is given next. For machine learning in medical domains, the data is usually represented as a set of examples, and we propose a technique to convert this representation to a decision table, a representation required by the proposed method. The section concludes with a brief note about the implementation.

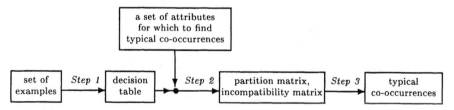

Fig. 1. The entities used and derived by the typical co-occurrence derivation method

2.1 Decision table decomposition: an example

Suppose we are given a *decision table* $y = F(X) = F(x_1, x_2, x_3)$ (Table 2) with three attributes x_1, x_2, and x_3, and class y, and we want to decompose it to decision tables G

89

and H, such that $y = G(x_1, c)$ and $c = H(x_2, x_3)$. For this decomposition, an initial set of attributes X is partitioned to a *bound set* $\{x_2, x_3\}$ used with H and a *free set* $\{x_1\}$ used with G. Decomposition requires the introduction of a new attribute c which depends only on the variables in the bound set.

Table 2. A small decision table

x_1 x_2 x_3	y		
lo lo lo	lo	med med lo	med
lo med hi	med	med hi lo	med
lo hi lo	lo	med hi hi	hi
lo hi lo	lo	hi lo lo	hi
lo hi hi	hi	hi hi lo	hi

To derive G and H from F, we first need to represent a decision table with a *partition matrix* (Table 3). This uses all possible combinations of attribute values from the bound set as column labels and from the free set as row labels. Each column in a partition matrix specifies a behavior of the function F when the attributes in the bound set are constant. Two elements of a partition matrix are compatible if they are the same or at least one of them is unknown (denoted by "-"). Two columns are compatible if all of their elements are pairwise compatible: these columns are considered to represent the same behavior of the function F.

Table 3. Partition matrix for the decision table from Table 2, free set $\{x_1\}$, and bound set $\{x_2, x_3\}$

	x_2	lo	lo	med	med	hi	hi
x_1	x_3	lo	hi	lo	hi	lo	hi
lo		lo	-	-	med	lo	hi
med		-	-	med	-	med	hi
hi		hi	-	-	-	hi	-
color		3	3	3	2	3	1

The problem is now to assign labels to the columns of the partition matrix so that only groups of mutually compatible columns have the same label. Columns with the same label exhibit the same behavior in respect to F and can use a single value of the new concept c. Label assignment involves the construction of a *column incompatibility graph*, where columns of the partition matrix are nodes and two nodes are connected if they are incompatible. Column labels are then assigned by coloring the incompatibility graph. For our example, the incompatibility graph with one of the possible optimal colorings is given in Figure 2.

For better comprehensibility, we interpret the column labels "1" as hi, "2" as med, and "3" as lo. These labels and the partition matrix straightforwardly determine the function $c = H(x_2, x_3)$. To determine the function $G(x_1, c)$, we lookup the annotated partition matrix for all the possible combinations of x_1 and c. The final result of the decomposition is represented as a hierarchy of two decision tables in Figure 3. If we further examine the discovered functions G and H we can see that $G \subset \text{MAX}$ and $H \subset \text{MIN}$.

2.2 Acquiring typical co-occurrences from a decision table

In the above example, different colors can be assigned to the same column of a partition matrix while retaining the minimal number of colors. For example, the column

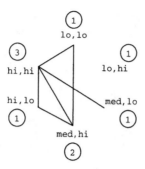

Fig. 2. Incompatibility graph for the partition matrix in Table 3

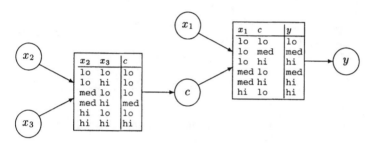

Fig. 3. The result of decomposing the decision table from Table 2

(med,lo) could be assigned either color 2 or 3, and the column (lo,hi) could be assigned any of the three colors used. On the other hand,, the column (lo,lo) could be assigned just a single color because of the incompatibilities with (med,hi) and (hi,hi) which are assigned different colors. While there exists just one distinct behavior for (lo,lo) with respect to F, there exist several for (med,lo) and (lo,hi). The combination (lo,lo) of attributes x_2 and x_3 thus tells more about the behavior of the function F and is therefore more typical. Moreover, the columns that can be assigned only one color form a foundation for such color assignment and will be called *typical columns* of the partition matrix (*typical nodes* of the incompatibility graph) and will further indicate for *typical co-occurrences* of attributes in the bound set.

Therefore, for a given set of attributes for which we want to derive the typical co-occurrences (bound set) and for a given decision table, we have to first derive a corresponding partition matrix and its incompatibility graph. The algorithms for the construction of the partition matrix and incompatibility graph are described in detail in [20]. The typical co-occurrences derivation method then uses the incompatibility graph and discovers the typical co-occurrences through coloring. Since graph coloring is an NP-hard problem, the computation time of an exhaustive search algorithm is prohibitive even for small graphs with about 15 nodes. Instead, we use the simple Color Influence Method of polynomial complexity [15]. The Color Influence Method sorts the nodes to color by their decreasing connectivity and then assigns to each node a color that is different from the colors of its neighbors so that a minimal number of colors is used. In this way, the coloring can have a single or several candidate colors for each node. The number of these candidate colors is used to determine the typicality of the node. We use the following definition:

Definition (Typical node n of incompatibility graph IG) *A node $n \in IG$ is typical if and only if in the process of coloring using the Color Influence Method it has only one candidate color to be assigned to.*

The above definition is then used to augment the Color Influence Method to both color the incompatibility graph and discover typical co-occurrences (Algorithm 1).

Input: incompatibility matrix IG
Output: typical co-occurrences for attributes in bound set

while there are no uncolored nodes in IG **do**
    select the uncolored node $n \in IG$ with highest connectivity
    if there are no colored non-adjacent nodes
      or all colored non-adjacent nodes have the same color
    then n is typical **else** n is not typical **endif**
    color n with the first free color different from the colors of adjacent nodes
endwhile

Algorithm 1: Coloring of an incompatibility graph and selection of typical nodes

Let us illustrate the use of Algorithm 1 on the incompatibility graph from Figure 2. The nodes sorted by decreasing connectivity are
(hi,hi), (med,hi), (lo,lo), (hi,lo), (med,lo), (lo,hi)
First, the node (hi,hi) is selected, determined to be typical (no other nodes have been colored yet), and assigned the color 1. Next, the node (med,hi) is considered. There are no colored nodes non-adjacent to it and so this node is typical. Since the adjacent node (hi,hi) has color 1, the color 2 is assigned to (med,hi). Similarly, (lo,lo) is also typical and colored with 3 because the colors 1 and 2 have already been used for the adjacent nodes (hi,hi) and (med,hi). Next, the node (hi,lo) has a single colored non-adjacent node (lo,lo) and is thus typical and colored with the same color 3. The first non-typical node is (med,lo): it has three nodes (med,hi), (lo,lo), and (hi,lo) that are non-adjacent to it and use different colors 2 and 3. Among these, the color 3 is then arbitrarily chosen for (med,lo). Similarly, the node (lo,hi) is found not to be typical and among three candidate colors the color 3 is arbitrarily assigned to it. Therefore, among six possible combinations of attribute values the algorithm found four typical co-occurrences: (hi,hi), (med,hi), (lo,lo), and (hi,lo).

The described method finds a possible set of typical nodes but it does not guarantee that this is the only such set. An alternative method that would search more exhaustively and possibly evaluate all different coloring of the incompatibility graph may be more complete and propose different sets of typical co-occurrences, but its (possibly exponential) complexity would limit its applicability.

2.3 Derivation of a decision table from a set of examples

The typical co-occurrence derivation method requires domain data in the form of a decision table. Decision tables require nominal attributes and for a specific combination of attribute values define at most one class. However, the data sets from medical domains often include continuous attributes and may use several examples with the same attribute values but possibly different classes. Therefore, we need a method that, given a set of domain examples, would derive a corresponding decision table. For all continuous attributes, we assume that a discretization is given or can be derived from the examples.

Input: Set of examples $E = \{e_i\}$, Discretization for continuous attributes
Output: Decision table DT

while $E \neq \emptyset$ **do**
    find all $E' = \{e_k; e_k \in E\}$ such that
        1) for all discrete attributes, e_k has the same value as e_j
        2) for all continuous attributes, e_k's discretized value is the same as e_j's
    $E' \leftarrow E' \cup \{e_j\}$
    $c \leftarrow$ a majority class value of examples in E'
    add e_j with discretized continuous values and with class c to DT
    $E \leftarrow E \setminus E'$
endwhile

Algorithm 2: Derivation of a decision table from a set of examples

The method is given in Algorithm 2. It searches through the set of examples E whose attribute values are the same if nominal or discretize to the same value if continuous. For such sets of examples E', a majority class value is found and a corresponding entry is added to the decision table. The examples from E' are then removed from E and the process repeated until there are no more examples in E.

2.4 Implementation

The typical co-occurrences extraction method was implemented as HINT$_{TCO}$, an extension of the Hierarchy Induction Tool HINT [20] for learning concept hierarchies from examples by decision table decomposition. Both HINT and HINT$_{TCO}$ run on a variety of UNIX platforms, including HP/UX, SunOS and IRIS.

3 Extracting and validating background knowledge in early diagnosis of rheumatic diseases

3.1 The domain

The data used originate from the University Medical Center in Ljubljana [16] and comprise records on 462 patients. The multitude of over 200 different diagnoses have been grouped into three, six, eight or twelve diagnostic classes. Our study uses eight diagnostic classes: degenerative spine diseases, degenerative joint diseases, inflammatory spine diseases, other inflammatory diseases, extraarticular rheumatism, crystal-induced synovitis, non-specific rheumatic manifestations, and non-rheumatic diseases.

For each patient, sixteen anamnestic attributes are recorded: sex, age, family anamnesis, duration of present symptoms (in weeks), duration of rheumatic diseases (in weeks), joint pain (arthrotic, arthritic), number of painful joints, number of swollen joints, spinal pain (spondylotic, spondylitic), other pain (headache, pain in muscles, thorax, abdomen, heels), duration of morning stiffness (in hours), skin manifestations, mucosal manifestations, eye manifestations, other manifestations, and therapy. The continuous attributes (age, durations and numbers of joints) have been discretized according to expert suggestions. For the continuous attributes that appear in groupings, the discretizations can be read out from Table 4. For example, from Table 4.1 we can see that the attribute "Duration of morning stiffness" has been discretized into two intervals: up to 1 hour and longer than 1 hour.

3.2 The background knowledge

In an earlier study [13], a specialist for rheumatic diseases has provided his knowledge about typical co-occurrences of six groupings of attributes. The groupings and the co-occurrences are given in Table 4, where a dot in the row marked "specialist" and the column marked X means that tuple X is a typical co-occurrence for the corresponding Grouping. For example, Table 4.1 specifies Grouping 1, which relates the attributes "Joint pain" and "Duration of morning stiffness", with typical co-occurrences suggested by HINT$_{TCO}$: no joint pain and morning stiffness up to 1 hour, arthrotic pain and morning stiffness up to 1 hour, arthritic pain and morning stiffness up to 1 hour.

3.3 The experiments

To evaluate our method for typical co-occurrences acquisition, we took the dataset and the six groupings described above, the latter without the typical co-occurrences provided by the expert. We then applied our method to produce the typical co-occurrences. For each grouping, the typical co-occurrences produced by HINT$_{TCO}$ are listed in the row labeled "HINT$_{TCO}$" of the corresponding table. For example, HINT$_{TCO}$ suggests that the typical co-occurrences for Grouping 1 should be: no joint pain and morning stiffness up to 1 hour, arthrotic pain and morning stiffness up to 1 hour, arthritic pain and morning stiffness up to 1 hour.

The groupings with the new typical co-occurrences suggested by HINT$_{TCO}$ are then provided as background knowledge to LINUS [12] in addition to the 462 training examples (patient records). LINUS then introduces a new attribute for each grouping (as explained in the introduction). The 462 examples augmented with the six new attributes (thus having in total 22 attributes) are then fed to the rule induction system CN2 [3] and to a nearest neighbor classifier [19, 8, 4]. The goal of this was to evaluate the usefulness of the new attributes and in this way the usefulness of the typical co-occurrences proposed by HINT$_{TCO}$.

The number of occurrences of each grouping (i.e., the new attribute corresponding to that grouping) in the set of rules induced by CN2 is listed in the column marked f_{CN2}. The mutual information between the grouping and the diagnostic class, calculated as a weight for nearest neighbor classification [19] is listed in the column marked f_{NN}. The mutual information [18] between an attribute and the class tells us how useful the attribute is for classification. The two measures have been used in earlier experiments to assess the utility of background knowledge in machine learning [14, 7].

Table 4. The six groupings and their typical co-occurrences

Joint pain, Morning stiffness	specialist	HINT_TCO
No pain, ≤ 1 hour	•	•
Arthrotic, ≤ 1 hour	•	•
Arthritic, ≤ 1 hour		•
No pain, > 1 hour		
Arthrotic, > 1 hour		
Arthritic, > 1 hour	•	
f_{CN2}	2	1
f_{NN}	0.345	0.353

1)

Spinal pain, Morning stiffness	specialist	HINT_TCO
No pain, ≤ 1 hour	•	•
Spondylotic, ≤ 1 hour	•	•
Spondylitic, ≤ 1 hour		•
No pain, > 1 hour		
Spondylotic, > 1 hour		
Spondylitic, > 1 hour	•	
f_{CN2}	3	3
f_{NN}	0.545	0.643

2)

Sex, Other pain	specialist	HINT_TCO
male, no		•
male, muscles		•
male, thorax	•	
male, heels	•	
male, other		•
female, no		•
female, other		•
other 7 combinations		
f_{CN2}	1	4
f_{NN}	0.080	0.096

3)

Joint pain, Spinal pain	specialist	HINT_TCO
No pain, No pain	•	•
Arthrotic, No pain	•	•
Arthritic, No pain	•	•
No pain, Spondylotic	•	
Arthrotic, Spondylotic		•
Arthritic, Spondylotic		
No pain, Spondylitic	•	
Arthrotic, Spondylitic		
Arthritic, Spondylitic	•	
f_{CN2}	9	8
f_{NN}	0.908	0.743

4)

Joint pain, Spinal pain, Painful joints	specialist	HINT_TCO
No pain, No Pain, 0	•	•
No pain, No Pain, 1≤joints≤5		•
No pain, Spondylotic, 0	•	•
No pain, Spondylitic, 0	•	•
Arthrotic, No pain, 1≤joints≤5	•	•
Arthrotic, No pain, 5<joints≤30	•	
Arthrotic, Spondylotic, 1≤joints≤5		•
Arthrotic, Spondylotic, 5<joints≤30		•
Arthritic, No pain, 1≤joints≤5	•	•
Arthritic, No pain, 5<joints≤30	•	•
Arthritic, Spondylitic, 1≤joints≤5	•	
other 25 combinations		
f_{CN2}	7	9
f_{NN}	0.757	0.834

5)

Swollen joints, Painful joints	specialist	HINT_TCO
0, 0	•	•
0, 1≤joints≤5	•	•
0, 5<joints≤30	•	
0, 30<		•
1≤joints≤10, 0	•	•
1≤joints≤10, 1≤joints≤5	•	
1≤joints≤10, 5<joints≤30	•	•
1≤joints≤10, 30<		
10<, 0		
10< 1≤joints≤5,		
10<, 5<joints≤30		
10<, 30<		
f_{CN2}	1	1
f_{NN}	0.331	0.392

6)

4 Discussion

For groupings 1, 2, 5, and 6, the typical co-occurrences derived by HINT_TCO correspond reasonably well to those proposed by the specialist for rheumatic diseases. For these groups, while using the same (groupings 1, 2, and 6) or slightly higher number of co-occurrences (grouping 5), two thirds or more of the co-occurrences originally proposed by the specialist were discovered by HINT_TCO. This is different to grouping 4, where less than one half of the co-occurrences match and to grouping 3, where there are no matches.

In terms of the mutual information evaluation metrics f_{NN}, the co-occurrences derived by HINT_TCO score higher for all but the grouping 4. A similar behavior is observed when the number of appearances in CN2 induced rules f_{CN2} is used as an evaluation metrics. There, HINT$_{TCO}$ scores equal or higher for all but the groupings 1 and 4.

Overall, compared to the co-occurrences proposed by the specialist, HINT$_{TCO}$ performed well for groupings 1, 2, 5, and 6. There are slight differences in the proposed co-occurrences, which, in turn, contribute to higher values of the evaluation metrics. For grouping 3, there is a complete mismatch between the co-occurrences proposed by the specialist and those derived by HINT$_{TCO}$. The co-occurrences derived by HINT$_{TCO}$ score higher on both metrics (4 to 1 on f_{CN2}). However, the weights assigned by mutual information suggest that this grouping might be substantially less important for classification than the others (f_{CN2} of 0.096 and 0.080).

It is grouping 4 where the of co-occurrences derived by HINT$_{TCO}$ seem to be less appropriate than those proposed by the specialist. However, note that for this grouping the specialist proposed six co-occurrences while HINT$_{TCO}$ discovered only four. Instead of using HINT$_{TCO}$ to derive only the typical co-occurrences for which the corresponding number of colors in the partition matrix is one, we can use this number as a measure of appropriateness for a certain combination of attribute values to be used as a typical co-occurrences. The lower the number of colors, the better the corresponding combination. For grouping 4, the number of possible colors for the columns in the partition matrix is shown in Table 5. It indicates that (No pain, Spondylotic) and (No pain, Spondylitic) are the next best candidates for typical co-occurrences. Interestingly, both are also proposed by the specialist. Their inclusion to the set of typical co-occurrences derived by HINT$_{TCO}$ makes this set very similar to that of the specialist, and also increases the mutual information weight from 0.743 to 0.887.

Table 5. Number of possible colors for columns of partition matrix of Grouping 4

Joint pain, Spinal pain		No pain, No pain	Arthrotic, No pain	Arthritic, No pain	No pain, Spondylotic	Arthrotic, Spondylotic	Arthritic, Spondylotic	No pain, Spondylitic	Arthrotic, Spondylitic	Arthritic, Spondylitic
# colors		1	1	1	2	1	3	2	3	4

With the above extension, we can therefore conclude that HINT$_{TCO}$ discovered typical co-occurrences that were comparable to those proposed by the expert both in terms of similarity and usefulness as background knowledge for machine learning. This is important since HINT$_{TCO}$ is not meant to be a stand-alone tool for unsupervised discovery of background knowledge, but should rather provide support to the expert by (1) proposing a set of co-occurrences and (2) weighting different combinations of attribute values to indicate how important it is that they are included in such a set. It would then be up to the expert to decide which of the proposed co-occurrences are meaningful and should be used.

As an overall evaluation of the typical co-occurrences suggested by HINT$_{TCO}$, let us consider the performance and size of the rules induced by CN2 from the dataset generated by LINUS. The accuracy and information content [11, 6] (as measured on the training set) of the rules induced (using the significance test in CN2) are 56.5% and 31%, respectively. For comparison, those obtained with the expert-proposed co-occurrences are 52.4% and 30%, respectively. The co-occurrences proposed by $HINT_{TCO}$ yield 35 rules with 106 conditions, while the expert-proposed ones yield 38 rules with 120 conditions. CN2 without background knowledge performs worse than with either of the two sets of co-occurrences: the accuracy and information content are 51.7% and 22%, while the rule set contains 30 rules and 102 conditions.

5 Further work

Currently $HINT_{TCO}$ assumes the set of attributes for which to derive typical co-occurrences are given in advance. We envision an extension of this approach to propose not only co-occurrences but also the set of attributes for which the background knowledge in the form of co-occurrences should be defined. The idea is straightforward and is illustrated with Algorithm 5. The implementation would require the integration of $HINT_{TCO}$ with the machine learning tools that evaluate and use the groupings.

Input: set of examples
Output: sorted list of attribute groupings with assigned weights

derive a decision table from the set of examples
for all the pairs and triples of attributes **do**
    derive the typical co-occurrences
    derive the corresponding weight
endfor
sort the groupings by descending weights and present them to the user

---

Algorithm 3: Derivation of groups of (two and three) attributes for which background knowledge in the form of typical co-occurrences might be useful for machine learning

A more careful evaluation of the background knowledge acquired through using our method is needed. This should include an evaluation of the quality of induced rules from a medical point of view. An evaluation of the performance in terms of classification accuracy on unseen cases is also desirable, but requires a slightly more complicated experimental setup: typical co-occurrences would have to be determined for each partition of the dataset into training and testing cases. An alternative is to have a medical expert assess the co-occurrences suggested by $HINT_{TCO}$, which is the most desirable option.

6 Conclusion

Background knowledge in the form of typical co-occurrences has positive effect on machine learning results in terms of performance and the quality of induced rules from a medical point of view. We have developed a method that proposes typical co-occurrences through functional decomposition of a given set of examples. While medical diagnosis background knowledge of this type has been previously completely specified by a medical expert, our approach offers the possibility to automate the background knowledge acquisition process by proposing typical co-occurrences to the expert, who would then consider them in the light of his expert knowledge.

References

1. Ashenhurst, R.L. (1952). The decomposition of switching functions. Technical report, Bell Laboratories BL-1(11): 541–602.
2. Biermann, A.W., Fairfield, J., and Beres, T. (1982). Signature table systems and learning. *IEEE Trans. Syst. Man Cybern.*, 12(5): 635–648.
3. Clark, P., and Boswell, R. (1991). Rule induction with CN2: Some recent improvements. In *Proc. Fifth European Working Session on Learning*, pages 151–163. Springer, Berlin.
4. Cover, T.M., and Hart, P.E. (1968). Nearest neighbor pattern classification. *IEEE Transactions on Information Theory*, 13: 21–27.
5. Curtis, H.A. (1962). *A New Approach to the Design of Switching Functions*. Van Nostrand, Princeton, N.J.
6. Džeroski, S., Cestnik, B., and Petrovski, I. (1993). Using the m-estimate in rule induction. *Journal of Computing and Information Technology*, 1: 37–46.
7. Džeroski, S., and Lavrač, N. (1996). Rule induction and instance-based learning applied in medical diagnosis. *Technology and Health Care*.
8. Fix, E., and Hodges, J.L. (1957). Discriminatory analysis. Nonparametric discrimination. Consistency properties. Technical Report 4, US Air Force School of Aviation Medicine. Randolph Field, TX.
9. Harmon, P., Maus, R., and Morrissey, W. (1988). *Expert systems: Tools & Applications*. John Wiley, New York.
10. Karalič, A., and Pirnat, V. (1990). Machine learning in rheumatology. *Sistemica* 1(2): 113–123.
11. Kononenko, I., and Bratko, I. (1991). Information-based evaluation criterion for classifier's performance. *Machine Learning*, 6(1): 67–80.
12. Lavrač, N., and Džeroski, S. (1994). *Inductive Logic Programming: Techniques and Applications*. Ellis Horwood, Chichester.
13. Lavrač, N., Džeroski, S., Pirnat, V., and Križman, V. (1991). Learning rules for early diagnosis of rheumatic diseases. In *Proc. Third Scandinavian Conference on Artificial Intelligence*, pages 138–149. IOS Press, Amsterdam.
14. Lavrač, N., Džeroski, S., Pirnat, V., and Križman, V. (1993). The utility of background knowledge in learning medical diagnostic rules. *Applied Artificial Intelligence*, 7:273–293.
15. Perkowski, M.A., and Grygiel, S. (1995). A survey of literature on function decomposition. Techical report, Dept. of Electrical Engineering, Portland State University.
16. Pirnat, V., Kononenko, I., Janc, T., and Bratko, I. (1989). Medical analysis of automatically induced rules. In *Proc. 2nd European Conference on Artificial Intelligence in Medicine*, pages 24–36. Springer, Berlin.
17. Samuel, A. (1967). Some studies in machine learning using the game of checkers II: Recent progress. *IBM J. Res. Develop.*, 11:601–617.
18. Shannon, C.E. (1948). A mathematical theory of communication. *Bell. Syst. Techn. J.*, 27: 379–423.
19. Wettschereck, D. (1994). A study of distance-based machine learning algorithms. PhD Thesis, Department of Computer Science, Oregon State University, Corvallis, OR.
20. Zupan, B., and Bohanec, M. (1996). Learning concept hierarchies from examples by function decomposition. Technical report, IJSDP-7455, J. Stefan Institute, Ljubljana. URL ftp://ftp-e8.ijs.si/pub/reports/IJSDP-7455.ps.

Automated Revision of Expert Rules for Treating Acute Abdominal Pain in Children

Sašo Džeroski[1,2], Giorgos Potamias[1], Vassilis Moustakis[1,3], Giorgos Charissis[4]

[1] FORTH-ICS, P.O.Box 1385, 711 10 Heraklion, Greece
[2] Department of Intelligent Systems, Jožef Stefan Institute
Jamova 39, 1000 Ljubljana, Slovenia (Email: Saso.Dzeroski@ijs.si)
[3] Department of Production and Management Engineering,
Technical University of Crete, 73100 Chania, Greece
[4] Director, Pediatric Clinic, University Hospital, Medical School,
University of Crete, Heraklion, Greece

Abstract. Decision making knowledge acquired directly from a medical expert is often incorrect and incomplete. Another source of knowledge about a decision making problem are examples of expert decisions in situations that have occurred in practice, stored in patient records of clinical information systems. Such examples can be used to revise the expert-provided knowledge, i.e., to discover and repair its deficiences. The revised knowledge performs better than the original one and often better than rules learned from examples alone. In addition, it inherits parts of the original expert knowledge and is thus easier to understand and accept for the expert. We present an application of the machine learning approach of theory revision to the problem of revising an expert-provided theory for treating children with acute abdominal pain.

1 Introduction

One of the most difficult problems in the development of intelligent systems is the construction of the underlying knowledge base. Normal knowledge acquisition can be divided into two phases: an initial phase in which a knowledge engineer extracts a rough set of rules from an expert and knowledge base refinement, in which the initial knowledge is refined to improve its performance. Performance improvement is also divided into two phases: the first establishes the correctness of the knowledge base and the second improves efficiency.

There exists a variety of machine learning tools that deal with improving the performance of a given rough set of rules. Explanation-based learning (De Jong and Mooney 1986) improves the efficiency of a correct domain theory. Theory refinement or theory revision (Ourston and Mooney 1994) deals with repairing a domain theory which is incorrect (incomplete and/or inconsistent). Examples are used to guide the theory revision process.

In this paper, we describe an application of a theory revision system to refine a knowledge base for treating children with acute abdominal pain. A rough set of rules was provided by the domain expert (G. Charissis). A set of patient records from the same domain was also available. The rough domain theory was then refined by the theory revision system NEITHER (Baffes and Mooney

1993), using a subset of the patient records available. The revised knowledge base performs much better than the original one and slightly better than rules learned from examples alone. In addition, it inherits parts of the original expert knowledge and is thus easier to understand and accept for the expert.

The remainder of the paper is organized as follows. The theory revision system used is briefly described in Section 2. Section 3 describes the medical domain of acute abdominal pain in children (AAPC). A general description is followed by a description of the patient records available and a decision making theory provided by the medical expert. Section 4 describes experiments designed to investigate the properties of the revised theory as the number of examples used for revision increases. This enables us to choose a subset of the available cases of an appropriate size, with which to perform revision. Section 5 describes the resulting revised theory and compares it to the original theory and a theory learned only from the examples used for revision. Section 6 first summarizes the contributions of the paper, then discusses related and further work.

2 The theory revision system NEITHER

The problem of theory revision (or knowledge base refinement) can be defined as follows: **Given** an imperfect domain theory (knowledge base) in the form of classification rules and a set of classified examples, **find** an approximately minimal syntactic revision of the domain theory that correctly classifies all of the examples.

A representative recent system that addresses this problem is EITHER (Ourston and Mooney 1994). EITHER refines propositional Horn-clause theories using a suite of abductive, deductive and inductive techniques. Deduction is used to identify the problems with the domain theory, while abduction and induction are used to correct them.

Two kinds of problems are encountered within imperfect domain theories: over-generality occurs when an example is classified into a class other than the correct one, while over-specificity occurs when an example cannot be proven to belong to the correct class. Note that a single example can be misclassified both ways at the same time. Overly general rules are either specialized by adding new conditions to their antecedents or are deleted from the knowledge base. Problems of over-specificity are solved by generalizing the antecedents of existing rules, e.g., by removing conditions from them, or by the induction of new rules.

The basic algorithm used by EITHER has three steps.

1. It first computes all possible repairs for each misclassified example.
2. It then enters a loop to select a subset of these repairs that can be applied to the theory to fix the misclassified examples. Repairs are ranked according to a benefit-to-cost-ratio between the number of examples fixed and the size of the repair and the number of new misclassifications it creates. The best repair is added at each iteration.
3. Finally, the selected subset of repairs is applied to the theory.

Any remaining misclassifications are solved by applying induction.

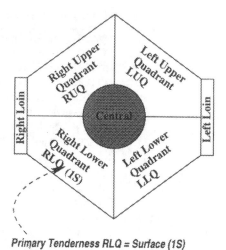

Primary Tenderness RLQ = Surface (1S)

Fig. 1. A geometrical representation of the abdomen areas (de Dombal 1991).

The process of computing all possible repairs for each example is very costly: it can be exponential in the size of the theory. A new version of EITHER, called NEITHER (Baffes and Mooney 1993) has been thus implemented which adopts a greedy approach. Its main loop computes a single repair for each example, applies the best repair to the theory removing all examples fixed by the repair, and repeats until all examples are fixed. In contrast to EITHER, NEITHER's algorithm is linear in the size of the theory.

In our experiments, we used the theory revision system NEITHER. Both EITHER and NEITHER can introduce intermediate concepts during the revision process. NEITHER, however, has an option to avoid the introduction of new intermediate concepts, which we employed in our experiments.

3 Acute abdominal pain in children

The domain of acute abdominal pain in children (AAPC) encompasses a set of symptoms that cause severe pain, discomfort and increased tenderness in the abdomen of the child. AAPC originates from disorders either in the intra-abdominal or the extra-abdominal areas (Waldschmit and Charissis 1990).

Management of patients is based on an explicit protocol by de Dombal (1991) that captures pain specifics, related symptoms and results of laboratory tests. The attending physician needs to diagnose the cause of pain and then make one of the following mutually exclusive treatment decisions: **1)** discharge the child (in case the cause of the pain is not pathologic), **2)** proceed to immediate operation, or **3)** follow-up the case for a period of six to eight hours at the end of which patient condition is re-assessed and the child is either discharged or admitted for operation.

In case an operation decision is adopted, the physician should already have in mind a spectrum of different potential causes which are to be confirmed or rejected and treated accordingly during the surgery operation.

Table 1. The original attributes. The short and long names of each attribute are listed.

AGE_GROUP (age)	ANALGET (on_analgetics)
P_DUR (pain_duration)	ANTIAC (on_antiacid)
P_START (pain_started)	ANTIEPIL (on_antiepileptics)
TYPE (type_of_pain)	ANTIBRO (on_antibrochial)
SEVERITY (severity_of_pain)	CHEMOTH (on_chemotherapy)
MOVE (movement)	MOOD (mood)
COUGH (coughing)	COLOR (color)
RESPIR (respiration)	PULSEQ (pulse)
EATING (eating)	D_PRESQ (diastolic_pressure)
R_R_SHOULD (rebound_right_shoulder)	S_PRESQ (systolic_pressure)
R_L_SHOULD (rebound_left_shoulder)	TEMPQ (temperature)
R_LOIN (rebound_loin)	DISTENS (distension)
SITE_{LUQ,RUQ,LLQ,RLQ,CENTRAL,LLO,RLO}	TENDER_
(site_of_pain_at_onset_at_	{LUQ,RUQ,LLQ,RLQ,CENTRAL,LLO,RLO}
{LUQ,RUQ,LLQ,RLQ,Central,LLo,RLo})	(primary_tenderness_
ANOREXIA (anorexia)	{LUQ,RUQ,LLQ,RLQ,Central,LLo,RLo})
NAUSEA (nausea)	REBOUND (rebound)
VOMITING (vomiting)	RIGIDITY (rigidity)
BOWELS (bowels)	GUARDING (guarding)
BLOOD_STOOLS (blood_in_stools)	B_SOUNDS (bowel_sounds)
MUCUS_STOOLS (mucus_in_stools)	RECTAL (rectal)
MICRUR (micrurition)	HT (hematocrit)
HAEMATUR (haematuria)	W_CELLS (white_cells)
RESPIRATORY (respiratory)	NEUTRO (neutrophiles)
HEART (heart_disease)	LEUCO (leucocytes)
ABDO (abdominal)	ERYTHRO (erythrocytes)
HAEMATOL (haematologic)	BACTERIA (bacteria)
ANTIBIOT (on_antibiotics)	PROTEIN (protein)

3.1 The patient records

A total of 312 AAPC patient records have been selected from a database installed and running at the Pediatric Surgery Clinic of the University Hospital at Heraklion, Greece. These are described with 63 attributes, which are listed in Table 1. Two groups of attributes refer to the site of pain at onset and primary tenderness. Both derive from a geometrical model of the abdominal area (see Figure 1), originally introduced by de Dombal (1991), that facilitates accurate capturing of expert assessment with respect to the area of tenderness and the site of pain at onset.

Five attributes are continuous (age, pulse, diastolic pressure, systolic pressure, and temperature). These have been discretized into two intervals each according to the suggestions of the domain expert (G. Charissis). Of the 312 patients, 144 have been discharged, 80 operated, and 88 assigned for follow up after their first examination.

3.2 The expert domain theory

The medical expert has formulated a theory that encompasses his theoretical decision making knowledge about this domain. The theory, given in Table 3,

Table 2. Attributes introduced for the expert rules and their definitions in terms of the original attributes.

```
COUGH_CHANGE: YES IF (COUGHING GETTING_WORSE) OR (COUGHING GETTING_BETTER)
FEVER_OR_VOMITING: YES IF (TEMPQ GREQ_37) OR (VOMITING YES)
NAUSEA_VOMITING: YES IF (NAUSEA YES) OR (VOMITING YES)
RIGIDITY_OR_GUARDING: YES IF (RIGIDITY YES) OR (GUARDING YES)
URINE_TEST_ABNORMAL: YES IF (NOT (LEUCO NORMAL)) OR (NOT (ERYTHRO NORMAL))
                 OR (NOT (BACTERIA NORMAL)) OR (NOT (PROTEIN NORMAL))
TENDER_YES: YES IF for ANY X of [LUQ,RUQ,LLQ,RLQ,CENTRAL,LLO,RLO]
            (NOT (TENDER_X NONE))
TENDER_SHALLOW_DEEP: YES IF for ANY X of [LUQ,RUQ,LLQ,RLQ,CENTRAL,LLO,RLO]
            (TENDER_X SHALLOW) OR (TENDER_X DEEP)
TENDER_SHALLOW: YES IF for ANY X of [LUQ,RUQ,LLQ,RLQ,CENTRAL,LLO,RLO]
            (TENDER_X SHALLOW)
TENDER_EVERYWHERE_SHALLOW_OR_DEEP:
            YES IF for ALL X of [LUQ,RUQ,LLQ,RLQ,CENTRAL,LLO,RLO]
            (TENDER_X SHALLOW) OR (TENDER_X DEEP)
TENDER_CENTRAL_SHALLOW_OR_DEEP: YES IF (TENDER_CENTRAL SHALLOW)
                 OR (TENDER_CENTRAL DEEP)
TENDER_RLQ_SURFACE_SHALLOW: YES IF (TENDER_RLQ SURFACE)
                 OR (TENDER_RLQ SHALLOW)
TENDER_LLQ_SURFACE_OR_SHALLOW: YES IF (TENDER_LLQ SURFACE)
                 OR (TENDER_LLQ SHALLOW)
TENDER_LUQ_SURFACE_OR_SHALLOW: YES IF (TENDER_LUQ SURFACE)
                 OR (TENDER_LUQ SHALLOW)
```

comprises 22 rules that prescribe patient treatment scenarios based on the 63 attributes listed in Table 1. The expert provided rules make use of 13 additional attributes, defined in terms of original attributes. These new attributes and their definitions are listed in Table 2. They have been defined in order to keep the expert provided rules in the form of conjunctions.

Each of the rules has one of the three possible treatments in the conclusion part: 6 rules recommend operate, 5 discharge, and 11 follow up. The antecedent of each rule is a list or conjunction of attribute value pairs. For example, rule 01 of Table 3 recommends the treatment operate if the attribute RIGIDITY has the value YES.

The theoretical expert knowledge encompassed in the rules of Table 3 is not entirely consistent with the treatment decisions taken in practice. In fact, when tested on the 312 cases provided, the rules prescribe a unique treatment that agrees with the actual one in only 50 cases: a correct treatment is only prescribed in 16% of the cases.

The poor performance of the rules should not be perceived as a consequence of poor expert performance. The main reason for the poor performance of the rules is that the expert is not accustomed to expressing his medical knowledge in terms of rules. For instance, with rule 01 of Table 3 the expert actually meant that the occurrence of RIGIDITY is a necessary, but not a sufficient condition to operate.   This has serious implications for the effectiveness of using a rule

Table 3. The original theory as provided by the expert. Annotations indicate what happened to each rule during theory revision. The Ri's refer to Table 4.

```
01: OPERATE <- (RIGIDITY YES) :specialized into R6 and R7
02: OPERATE <- (ANTIBIOT YES) (ABDO YES) (TEMPQ GR_37)
               (TENDER_RLQ_SURFACE_SHALLOW YES) :unchanged
03: OPERATE <- (TYPE STEADY) (TEMPQ GR_37) (TENDER_RLQ SHALLOW)
               (NOT (ERYTHRO NORMAL)) :unchanged
04: OPERATE <- (ABDO YES) (NAUSEA_VOMITING YES)
               (TEMPQ GR_37) (REBOUND YES) :unchanged
05: OPERATE <- (AGE_GROUP LESS_4) (TYPE STEADY) (NAUSEA_VOMITING YES)
               (P_DUR TODAY) (TEMPQ GR_37)
               (TENDER_RLQ_SURFACE_SHALLOW YES) :unchanged
06: OPERATE <- (AGE_GROUP GREQ_4) (TYPE STEADY) (NAUSEA_VOMITING YES)
               (TEMPQ GR_37) (W_CELLS INCREASED) (NEUTRO INCREASED)
               (TENDER_RLQ_SURFACE_SHALLOW YES) :unchanged
07: FOLLOW_UP <- (TEMPQ GR_37) (COUGH_CHANGE YES) :unchanged
08: FOLLOW_UP <- (NAUSEA YES) (ANOREXIA YES) (AGE_GROUP LESS_4) :deleted
09: FOLLOW_UP <- (B_SOUNDS INCREASED)
                 (TENDER_SHALLOW_DEEP YES) :specialized into R14
010: FOLLOW_UP <- (VOMITING YES) (BOWELS DIARRHEA)
                  (TENDER_SHALLOW_DEEP YES) :unchanged
011: FOLLOW_UP <- (HAEMATUR YES) (NAUSEA_VOMITING YES) :unchanged
012: FOLLOW_UP <- (W_CELLS INCREASED) (NEUTRO INCREASED)
                  (TENDER_YES YES) :specialized into R15
013: FOLLOW_UP <- (TENDER_YES YES) :deleted
014: FOLLOW_UP <- (BOWELS CONSTIPATION) :deleted
015: FOLLOW_UP <- (NAUSEA_VOMITING YES) (URINE_TEST_ABNORMAL YES) :deleted
016: FOLLOW_UP <- (NAUSEA_VOMITING YES) (MICRUR DYSURIA)
                  (TENDER_SHALLOW_DEEP YES) :unchanged
017: FOLLOW_UP <- (NAUSEA_VOMITING YES) (TENDER_SHALLOW YES) :deleted
018: DISCHARGE <- (TENDER_LUQ_SURFACE_OR_SHALLOW YES)
                  (RIGIDITY_OR_GUARDING YES) :deleted
019: DISCHARGE <- (TENDER_LLQ_SURFACE_OR_SHALLOW YES)
                  (RIGIDITY YES) (GUARDING YES) :deleted
020: DISCHARGE <- (TYPE COLICKY) (BOWELS CONSTIPATION)
                  (VOMITING YES) (TEMPQ LEQ_37) :unchanged
021: DISCHARGE <- (TENDER_CENTRAL_SHALLOW_OR_DEEP YES)
                  (FEVER_OR_VOMITING YES) :deleted
022: DISCHARGE <- (TENDER_EVERYWHERE_SHALLOW_OR_DEEP YES) (RIGIDITY NO)
                  (GUARDING NO) (VOMITING NO) (TEMPQ LEQ_37) :unchanged
```

based representation and poses challenges for further research on the interaction between a human expert and a revision system. On the technical level, there are several reasons for this poor performance. To start with, the set of rules as a whole sometimes prescribes two or even three conflicting treatments at the same time. For example, whenever rule 019 recommends the treatment discharge, the rule 01 will recommend the treatment operate. For some patients, only one inappropriate treatment is recommended. Finally, no treatment is recommended for some patients.

In any case, the expert provided rules obviously need to be revised if they are to be used for any practical purpose. In the remainder of the paper, we describe the application of the theory revision system NEITHER, described in Section 2, to revise the expert provided rules using (a subset of) the provided patient records.

4 The AAPC learning curve for theory revision

This section describes the experiments designed to investigate how the accuracy of the revised theory on unseen cases and the size of the revised theory behave as the number of examples used for revision increases. This in order to enable us to choose an appropriately sized subset of the available patient records for revision.

The first experiment was designed as follows. Ten different partitions of the 312 cases into a training R_i and testing Ei ($i = 0..9$) set (sized roughly 281 and 31 cases, respectively) were created using the ten-fold cross-validation method. Stratified cross-validation was used, making an effort to preserve the relative proportions of treatment decisions from the entire set of cases. For example, a training set R_i would have roughly 72 ($281 * 80/312$) cases to which treatment operate was prescribed.

For each of the ten partitions, the following actions were taken: ten different subsets of R_i were created such that $R_{i0} \subset R_{i1} \subset \ldots \subset R_{i9} = R_i$, where R_{ij} is of size approximately $(j + 1) * 0.1 * |R_i|$. Again, an effort was made to preserve the relative proportions of treatment decisions. The original theory from Table 3 was revised using NEITHER and the cases from R_{ij} yielding a revised theory T_{ij}. T_{ij} was then tested on the unseen cases from Ei and its accuracy A_{ij} recorded. The accuracies A_{ij} are averaged over the ten splits to yield A_j. It is these averages that are shown in Figure 2a): the first point represents the accuracy of the original theory, while the last point represents A_9, the accuracy of the theory revised with approximately 280 examples.

In the second experiment, the behavior of the size of the revised theory was investigated. Ten different partitions of the entire dataset R were created into training sets P_i and testing sets Q_i ($i = 0..9$), such that $P_i \cup Q_i = R$, $P_0 \subset P_1 \subset \ldots \subset P_9 = R$ and $|P_i| \approx (i+1) * 0.1 * |R|$. Again, an effort was made to preserve the relative proportions of the three different treatment decisions as in the entire dataset.

The original theory from Table 3 was revised using NEITHER and the cases from P_i to yield a revised theory S_i. The sizes of these theories, measured as $|S_i|$, i.e., the number of rules in S_i, are shown in Figure 2b).

To summarize the results of the two experiments, as the number of examples used for revision increases, the accuracy on unseen cases increases at first, but levels off quickly at roughly 100 examples. The size of the revised theory, however, grows more or less monotonically with the number of examples used for revision. The latter result suggests that we should use as small a set of cases for revision as possible, provided this is not at the expense of the accuracy of the revised theory. As accuracy levels off at 100 examples, this seems to be an appropriate number of cases to use for theory revision in the AAPC domain.

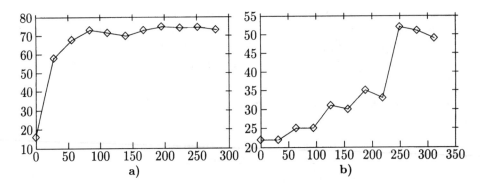

Fig. 2. Learning curves for theory revision in the domain of acute abdominal pain in children. The x-axes show the number of examples used to revise the theory provided by the expert. For graph **a)** the y-axis shows the accuracy of the revised theory on unseen cases. For graph **b)**, the y-axis shows the number of rules in the revised theory.

5 The revised AAPC theory

Having determined the appropriate number of examples to perform revision with, we conducted the following experiment. The whole dataset of 312 samples was split into a training/revision set of size 30% (95 examples) and a testing set of 217 examples. The relative proportions of the treatment decisions were preserved: the training set contains 24 operate cases, 26 follow up and 45 discharge cases. The original theory (Table 3) was then given to NEITHER to revise using the 95 cases of the revision set.

The revised theory produced by NEITHER is given in Table 4. NEITHER was also given the empty theory to revise, which causes it to construct a theory in an entirely inductive way, i.e., by learning from the 95 examples only. This learned theory is shown in Table 5.

The accuracies of all three theories (original, revised and learned from examples only) were measured on both the training/revision set and on the unseen cases from the testing set and are shown in Table 6. The original theory performs poorly on both the training and the testing set (19% and 15%, respectively). After revision, its performance is drastically improved. It is now 100% accurate on the training set and 75% accurate on the unseen cases. The theory learned from examples only is 100% accurate on the training cases and 73% on the testing cases. Thus, the revised theory performs much better than the original theory and slightly better than the theory learned from examples only.

To highlight the effects of theory revision on the original theory, the rules in the original theory and the revised theory have been labeled and annotated. For example, rule O1 of the original theory was specialized, resulting into rules R6 and R7 of the revised theory. Rule O2 has been left unchanged as rule R1 of the revised theory, and rule O8 has been deleted. On the other side, rule R11 of the revised theory is a copy of rule O16, rules R12 and R13 are entirely new, while rule R14 is a specialization of the rule O9.

Table 4. The revised theory. The comments provided indicate the origin of each rule.

```
R1:  OPERATE  <- (ANTIBIOT YES) (ABDO YES) (TEMPQ GR_37)
                 (TENDER_RLQ_SURFACE_SHALLOW YES) :unchanged O2
R2:  OPERATE  <- (TYPE STEADY) (TEMPQ GR_37) (TENDER_RLQ SHALLOW)
                 (NOT (ERYTHRO NORMAL)) :unchanged O3
R3:  OPERATE  <- (ABDO YES) (NAUSEA_VOMITING YES)
                 (TEMPQ GR_37) (REBOUND YES) :unchanged O4
R4:  OPERATE  <- (AGE_GROUP LESS_4) (TYPE STEADY) (NAUSEA_VOMITING YES)
                 (P_DUR TODAY) (TEMPQ GR_37)
                 (TENDER_RLQ_SURFACE_SHALLOW YES) :unchanged O5
R5:  OPERATE  <- (AGE_GROUP GREQ_4) (TYPE STEADY) (NAUSEA_VOMITING YES)
                 (TEMPQ GR_37) (W_CELLS INCREASED) (NEUTRO INCREASED)
                 (TENDER_RLQ_SURFACE_SHALLOW YES) :unchanged O6
R6:  OPERATE  <- (RIGIDITY YES) (TYPE STEADY) (SITE_RUQ NO) :specializes O1
R7:  OPERATE  <- (RIGIDITY YES) (TENDER_RLQ SURFACE) :specializes O1
R8:  FOLLOW_UP <- (TEMPQ GR_37) (COUGH_CHANGE YES) :unchanged O7
R9:  FOLLOW_UP <- (VOMITING YES) (BOWELS DIARRHEA)
                 (TENDER_SHALLOW_DEEP YES) :unchanged O10
R10: FOLLOW_UP <- (HAEMATUR YES) (NAUSEA_VOMITING YES) :unchanged O11
R11: FOLLOW_UP <- (NAUSEA_VOMITING YES) (MICRUR DYSURIA)
                 (TENDER_SHALLOW_DEEP YES) :unchanged O16
R12: FOLLOW_UP <- (TENDER_YES NO) :new
R13: FOLLOW_UP <- (TEMPQ GREQ_37) (COLOR NORMAL)
                 (TENDER_SHALLOW_DEEP YES) (COUGH GETTING_WORSE) :new
R14: FOLLOW_UP <- (B_SOUNDS INCREASED)
                 (TENDER_SHALLOW_DEEP YES) (SITE_LUQ NO) :specializes O9
R15: FOLLOW_UP <- (W_CELLS INCREASED) (NEUTRO INCREASED) (TENDER_YES YES)
                 (SITE_CENTRAL NO) (RIGIDITY NO) :specializes O12
R16: FOLLOW_UP <- (TENDER_SHALLOW YES) (TENDER_LLQ NONE)
                 (SITE_RUQ YES) :new
R17: FOLLOW_UP <- (TENDER_SHALLOW YES) (TENDER_LLQ NONE)
                 (P_DUR DAYS_1_3) :new
R18: FOLLOW_UP <- (TENDER_SHALLOW YES) (TENDER_LLQ NONE) (PULSEQ LESS_100)
                 (RIGIDITY NO) :new
R19: DISCHARGE <- (TYPE COLICKY) (BOWELS CONSTIPATION)
                 (VOMITING YES) (TEMPQ LEQ_37) :unchanged O20
R20: DISCHARGE <- (TENDER_EVERYWHERE_SHALLOW_OR_DEEP YES) (RIGIDITY NO)
                 (GUARDING NO)(VOMITING NO)(TEMPQ LEQ_37) :unchanged O22
R21: DISCHARGE <- (TENDER_RUQ DEEP) (P_START SUDDENLY) :new
R22: DISCHARGE <- (TENDER_CENTRAL_SHALLOW_OR_DEEP YES) (SITE_LUQ YES) :new
R23: DISCHARGE <- (TENDER_RLQ_SURFACE_SHALLOW NO) (SITE_RUQ NO)
                 (PULSEQ GREQ_100) (SITE_LLQ YES) :new
R24: DISCHARGE <- (TENDER_RLQ_SURFACE_SHALLOW NO) (SITE_RUQ NO)
                 (NEUTRO NORMAL) (TENDER_LUQ NONE)
                 (RESPIR GETTING_WORSE) :new
R25: DISCHARGE <- (TENDER_RLQ_SURFACE_SHALLOW NO) (SITE_RUQ NO)
                 (NEUTRO NORMAL) (TENDER_LUQ NONE) (COUGH NO_CHANGE) :new
```

Table 7 gives several statistics on the numbers of rules in the three theories and also summarizes the changes made to the original theory during the revision process. The first four rows of the table pertain to the original theory, the next four to the revised and the last row to the theory learned from examples only. The latter is the shortest with 15 rules, the revised the longest with 25 rules.

Table 5. The theory learned from examples only.

```
L1:  OPERATE <- (RIGIDITY YES) (TYPE STEADY) (SITE_RUQ NO)
L2:  OPERATE <- (TENDER_RLQ SURFACE)
L3:  FOLLOW_UP <- (TENDER_SHALLOW YES) (NEUTRO INCREASED) (TYPE COLICKY)
L4:  FOLLOW_UP <- (W_CELLS INCREASED) (TENDER_SHALLOW_DEEP YES)
                  (TENDER_SHALLOW NO) (ANTIBRO NO)
L5:  FOLLOW_UP <- (PULSEQ LESS_100) (D_PRESQ GREQ_120) (SITE_LUQ YES)
L6:  FOLLOW_UP <- (PULSEQ LESS_100) (W_CELLS INCREASED) (NAUSEA NO)
L7:  FOLLOW_UP <- (SITE_RUQ YES) (TENDER_LLQ NONE) (TYPE COLICKY)
L8:  FOLLOW_UP <- (TENDER_RLQ SHALLOW) (ERYTHRO RARE)
L9:  FOLLOW_UP <- (TENDER_SHALLOW YES) (TENDER_LLQ NONE)
                  (TYPE INTERMITTENT)
L10: DISCHARGE <- (TENDER_CENTRAL DEEP) (COUGH NO_CHANGE)
L11: DISCHARGE <- (ANTIBRO YES)
L12: DISCHARGE <- (TENDER_RLO SURFACE)
L13: DISCHARGE <- (TENDER_RLQ_SURFACE_SHALLOW NO) (TENDER_SHALLOW NO)
                  (W_CELLS NORMAL) (TENDER_RLQ DEEP)
L14: DISCHARGE <- (NEUTRO NORMAL) (TENDER_LLQ SHALLOW)
L15: DISCHARGE <- (W_CELLS NORMAL) (SITE_RUQ NO) (TEMPQ LESS_37)
```

We can see that the revised theory has three rules more than the original theory. In the original theory, half of the rules were left unchanged during the revision process, 8 rules were deleted (of which none recommended **operate**, 5 recommended **follow up**, and 3 recommended **discharge**), and 3 were specialized (resulting in 4 rules in the revised theory). No new rule was created for recommendation **operate** in the revised theory, while 5 new rules were created for each of **follow up** and **discharge**. The specialist provided rules recommending **operate** are thus much more consistent with actual clinical practice than is the case with the other two recommendations.

Table 6. The accuracies of the original, revised and learned theory on the training and testing sets of examples.

Accuracy of _ theory on _	Training set (95 examples)	Testing set (217 examples)
Original	19%	15%
Revised	100%	75%
Learned	100%	73%

Finally, let us consider the number of attributes that appear in the three theories. The revised theory uses 37 attributes, of which 25 are used in the original theory (which uses 33 attributes): 8 attributes are thus deleted from the original theory and 12 other added during the theory revision process. The theory learned from examples only uses 20 attributes, of which 10 are used in the original theory and 14 in the revised theory.

Table 7. Statistics on the number of rules of the original, revised and learned theory.

Number of rules	Total	Operate	Follow up	Discharge
Original	22	6	11	5
unchanged	11	5	4	2
deleted	8	0	5	3
specialized	3	1	2	0
Revised	25	7	11	7
old	11	5	4	2
specializations	4	2	2	0
new	10	0	5	5
Learned	15	2	7	6

Nine attributes are used in all three theories. One might say that these 9 attributes are essential for appropriate treatment of children with acute abdominal pain. The 9 attributes are as follows: type of pain, temperature, primary tenderness at right left quadrant (RLQ), rigidity, white cells, neutrophiles, erythrocytes, tenderness shallow or deep (anywhere), and tenderness surface or shallow at RLQ. This is in agreement with existing expert knowledge.

6 Discussion

We have presented an application of theory revision techniques from the field of machine learning in the domain of acute abdominal pain in children (AAPC). The expert provided domain knowledge turns out to disagree with actual cases that appear in clinical practice. We have first determined the appropriate number of cases to be used for revision and then revised the expert provided domain knowledge using patient records. The revised knowledge performs much better than the original knowledge and slightly better than the knowledge learned from patient records alone. In addition, the revised knowledge inherits parts of the original expert knowledge and is thus easier to understand and be used in practice by the expert.

One of the reasons for the ppor performance of the initial set of rules provided by the expert is the fact that they have not been validated prior to evaluating their performance. If they had been validated, the improvement in performance may have been less drastic. However, this rises the point that theory revision can be used to both validate and refine a set of rules provided by an expert.

Potamias et al. (1996) have preliminary applied theory revision techniques in the AAPC domain. The expert provided theory there consists of the operate and follow up rules of the theory considered here. The interactive knowledge revision tools of MOBAL (Morik et al. 1993) are used to revise the restricted domain theory. Revisions to the theory have to be approved by a human supervisor of the revision process, who has also to provide rule schemata (templates) that the revised rules have to match. MOBAL allows a first-order logic representation of rules and second-order logic representation of rule templates.

There are obviously arguments for and against each of the two approaches. NEITHER uses a propositional representation and requires essentially no human intervention during the revision process. It is consequently faster and easier to apply. MOBAL, on the other hand, uses a more powerful representation and allows tight control of the revision process by a human supervisor. It is consequently much slower and more difficult to apply. In any case, the experiments conducted in this study are more complete, as a theory with rules for all three decisions is used and revised. In further work, we plan to apply MOBAL and other theory revision systems that use more powerful formalisms, such as FORTE (Richards and Mooney 1991) on the problem studied here and compare the advantages and disadvantages of each approach.

Acknowledgements

At the time of writing this paper, S. Džeroski was supported through an ERCIM fellowship by the Foundation of Research and Technology - Hellas. This work was partially supported by the research grant PENED 1248 from the Ministry of Development of Greece (V. Moustakis). The AAPC database development and maintenance was done by the Pediatric Clinic, University Hospital, Heraklion, Greece (G. Charissis), in the context of the STAR 1045 European Health Telematics project. Thanks go to an anonymous referee for the useful comments provided.

References

1. Baffes, P.T., and Mooney, R.J. (1993). Symbolic revision of theories with M-of-N rules. In *Proc. Thirteenth International Joint Conference on Artificial Intelligence*, pp. 1135-1140. Chambery, France, 1993.
2. de Dombal, F.T. (1991). *Diagnosis of abdominal pain*. Churchill Livingstone, Singapore.
3. De Jong, J.F., and Mooney, R.J. (1986). Explanation based learning: an alternative view. *Machine Learning*, 1(2): 145-176.
4. Morik, K., Wrobel, S., Kietz, J.-U., and Emde, W. (1993). *Knowledge Acquisition and Machine Learning - Theory, Methods, and Applications*. Academic Press, London.
5. Potamias, G., Moustakis, V., and Charissis, G. (1996). Iterative knowledge construction and maintenance. In *Proc. ICML'96 Workshop Machine Learning Meets Human Computer Interaction*. Bari, Italy, 1996.
6. Richards, B.L., and Mooney, R.J. (1991). Refinement of first-order Horn-clause domain theories. *Machine Learning*, 19(2): 95-131.
7. Ourston, D., and Mooney, R.J. (1994). Theory refinement combining analytical and empirical methods. *Artificial Intelligence*, 66: 273-309.
8. Waldschmit, J., and Charissis, G. (1990). *Das akute Abdomen im Kindesalter. Diagnose und Differentialdiagnose*. Edition Medezin, New York.

Evaluation of Automatic and Manual Knowledge Acquisition for Cerebrospinal Fluid (CSF) Diagnosis

A. Ultsch[1], T.O. Kleine[2], D. Korus[1], S. Farsch[1], G. Guimarães[1], W. Pietzuch[2], J. Simon[2]

[1] Neuroinformatics and Artificial Intelligence, Dep. of Mathematics, University of Marburg, D-35032 Marburg, Germany

[2] Dep. of Neurochemistry, Medical Centre of Nervous Diseases, University of Marburg, D-35033 Marburg, Germany

Abstract

Neural Network technology for knowledge acquisition appears to be promising. Neural Networks alone, however, are insufficient for a medical domain, because of their inability to explain decisions. Knowledge conversion procedures from neural networks to symbolic knowledge are necessary. As a first milestone of the MEDWIS project NELA a knowledge conversion algorithm, called *sig**, was tested. We compared a knowledge base generated by *sig** with a first prototype of a manually built knowledge base for the diagnosis of cerebrospinal fluid. We have found the performance of the automatically build knowledge base to be quantitatively comparable to the manually acquired knowledge base. The quality of the extracted rules with respect to human understanding and medical plausibility was evaluated by use of a questionnaire. A low number of missing parameters found together with a correct choice of parameters in most cases indicated that the extracted rules correspond well to knowledge expressed by a medical expert. The results presented here confirm that a part of our automatic knowledge acquisition procedure, that is conversion of knowledge from subsymbolic representation to a rule based representation of knowledge, performed comparably, proved to be superior to manual knowledge acquisition with some respects.

1. Introduction

In a medical laboratory the supervising doctor has continuously to do with data which are characterised by the property that often one single element does not have a meaning (interpretation) of itself alone. Trying to support the doctor in interpreting the data, optimising the laboratory routine and providing better diagnostic results leads naturally to the idea of using knowledge based systems in laboratory medicine. The advantage of minimising the costs of laboratory medicine by a ready knowledge based system will be counterbalanced, however, by the high costs, in time and personnel work, of manual knowledge acquisition in the development process. Therefore procedures are sought that make knowledge acquisition more efficiently[7].

For a special laboratory medicine domain, the cerebrospinal fluid diagnosis, the project MEDWIS NELA („Neuronal unterstütztes Expertensystem zur Liquoranalytik") aims at the production of a high quality knowledge base using a combination of self-organising neural networks and symbolic knowledge bases [27]. Automatic knowledge acquisition for CSF diagnosis in the NELA project will be performed in three phases: unsupervised neural network learning, knowledge conversion and integration of medical knowledge. In the first phase self-organising neural networks will adapt to structures inherent in laboratory data. The next step is to express the knowledge learned by the neural network in an understandable form. This is performed by a special designed knowledge conversion algorithm called *sig** [30, 31]. In this paper we investigate the performance of this algorithm. We compare *sig** with a first prototype of a manually built knowledge base for some central problems of CSF diagnosis.

This paper is organised as follows: chapter 2 sketches the problem domain, chapter 3 describes the data sets used. Chapter 4 gives an overview on the structures of both, the manually and the automatically acquired knowledge base. Sections 5 and 6 present a quantitative and qualitative evaluation. In chapter 7 these results are discussed.

2. Cerebrospinal fluid diagnosis

The analysis of cerebrospinal fluid (CSF) is the only way to investigate the state of the human central nervous system. Imaging procedures and clinical findings have to be confirmed by cerebrospinal fluid diagnosis with respect to different inflammations, haemorrhages etc. Therefore, a complete CSF diagnosis has to consider and to combine clinical findings, findings of imaging procedures and laboratory data to the final medical diagnosis. Special knowledge is required in the field of clinical chemistry, cytology, immunology, neuropathology, and neurology to interpret and to diagnose laboratory parameters correctly. There are only few experts in cerebrospinal fluid diagnosis on the world.

Different steps in the process of diagnosis finding have to be considered with respect to high efficiency and low costs:

- In emergency situations an CSF analysis has to be performed quickly only with few significant laboratory parameters for screening the most important central nervous system diseases with laboratory diagnosis;

- A basis diagnostic program is necessary to complete the emergency diagnosis program and to confirm the laboratory diagnosis indicated by the first program;

- An extended, more time and cost intensive program confirms further the diagnosis found by the former programs, if necessary. With such an analysis it is possible to explore special diagnosis by applying highly specified methods.

Cerebrospinal fluid diagnosis is complex because it has to consider simultaneously cellular and blood parameters from cerebrospinal fluid and blood as well. CSF diagnosis has to discriminate the portion of measured quantities penetrating the blood-brain-barrier (bbb) from the brain and CSF constituents. Moreover, the CSF sample establishing a cerebrospinal fluid diagnosis system by using simple statistical evaluation between two parameters [11, 12], test combinations of two parameters [11,15] or cluster analysis of several parameters [18] were only able to differentiate between two laboratory symptoms (parameters) to some extent but they were insufficient in considering the complexity of the CSF diagnosis.

Therefore, a knowledge base of cerebrospinal fluid routine diagnosis is desired to provide it to medical doctors who are involved with this kind of diagnosis and as tutorial for postgraduates and medical students as well.

3. Patients and Laboratory Data

The data used in this study were derived from 727 manually selected cases of patients attending the Medical Centre of Nervous Diseases of the University of Marburg. The laboratory data were determined by EU standardised methods [9, 10, 11, 13, 16, 17] in lumbar cerebrospinal fluid (CSF) and venous blood serum simultaneously collected. The data contained in total 25 laboratory parameters in two diagnosis programs:

- The emergency program consisted of 9 parameters: leukocyte and erythrocyte counts [11, 21], free haemoglobin [11, 12], total protein in CSF and blood serum [12, 19], glucose in CSF and blood plasma [11, 12], glucose concentration ratio: [glucose in plasma]/[glucose in CSF], L-lactate in CSF [15, 11, 14]);

- The *basis program* completed the emergency program with the 16 additional parameters: CSF protein electropherogramm [11, 12], serum protein electropherogramm [11, 12], granulocytes, lymphocytes, and monocytes as % of total leukocytes [11, 21]).

The data were checked for plausibility by applying parameter specific limits and plausibility checks especially developed for this purpose. Each case was classified by the CSF expert. Five laboratory diagnosis in the parameter space of the emergency and basis programs mentioned above were assigned: "*controls*" ("normal"), "*acute bacterial meningitis*", "*acute abacterial meningitis*", "*haemorrhage into CSF*", "*artificial bleeding*". Per diagnosis class, between 29 and 78 cases were classified.

The data set was divided into a *development set* (n=533) and an *assessment set* (n=194). The development set included manually selected, exemplary cases of the laboratory diagnosis under investigation. It was used for developing and optimising the knowledge bases. The assessment set contained much more cases with multidiagnosis to fit the requirements of laboratory routine. Both data sets contained a nearly equal distribution of sex and age. This was checked by applying standard statistical methods [26]. In the development set the control group consisted of over 50% of the cases where the other classes were of nearly equal size (9-14%). For the assessment set a nearly equal distribution of all diagnosis classes was intended resulting in sizes of 14–34% with a mean of 20%.

4. The Knowledge Bases

In order to compare the quality of different knowledge bases, a rapid-prototype of a diagnostic expert system was realised using the expert system shell Nexpert Object [2]. The implemented expert system is able to operate as well on knowledge bases build with conventional knowledge acquisition methods as also on knowledge bases that are generated with the aid of automatic, i.e. neuronal, methods. In this paper two knowledge bases, the „Manually Acquired Knowledge Base" and the „Automatically Generated Knowledge Base", are compared.

The Manually Acquired Knowledge Base (MKB)

For this knowledge base the acquisition of knowledge was performed using standard knowledge engineering procedures involving interview techniques, presentations of the expert, medical textbooks, statistical analysis and case studies [3,6,11,13]. 40% of the laboratory parameters were used. Diagnosis using the manually acquired knowledge base was guided by establishing so called „laboratory symptoms" like "pleocytosis", "granulocytic reaction", "mixed-cell reaction", "blood-brain-barrier (bbb) disturbance" etc. The manually acquired knowledge base used 24 formal hypotheses and consisted of a total of 121 rules. The majority of these, 84 rules, were necessary in order to guide the inference process. 37 rules dealt with specialised medical knowledge. Laboratory diagnoses were established as follows: First, certainty factors were calculated for each hypothesis as a measure for the possibility of a positive result. Secondly, each hypothesis was evaluated using weighted alternatives, weighted parameter conditions and weighted hypothesis conditions. Each parameter condition consisted of the parameter value, an operator and two operands to build a rating function that was evaluated according to Dempster-Shafer-theory [24].

The Automatically Generated Knowledge Base (AKB)

The machine learning algorithm called $sig*$ operates on the weights of self-organised neural networks [20] together with the cluster information found with the *U-matrix* method [30] and produces rules to be used in a knowledge base of an expert system. In order to test the operational capabilities of this knowledge conversion algorithm separately from the clustering abilities of a self organising neural network, the diagnoses assigned to the development set by the expert was used as cluster information [4,8]. The rules generated by $sig*$ come in two types: so called characterising and differentiating rules. Characterising rules model the primary characteristics of a data cluster. Differentiating rules are used to differentiate between clusters. They are used to distinguish cases that would be subsumed under two different diagnoses. A detailed description of $sig*$ can be found in [28,31]. For the automatically generated knowledge base $sig*$ produced five characterising rules corresponding to the five laboratory diagnoses. With the parameter set of the emergency diagnosis program $sig*$ generated 20 differentiating rules. The parameter set of the basis diagnosis program led to 18 differentiating rules.

Both the automatically generated knowledge base and the manually acquired knowledge base were integrated into the expert system. Both knowledge bases were tested and improved using the development set until a satisfactorily performance was reached.

5. Quantitative Evaluation

In the following we compared the quality of finding a cerebrospinal fluid diagnosis of a knowledge base, obtained by manual knowledge acquisition (MKB), with one obtained by automatic knowledge acquisition with SIG* (AKB). We used the quality measures „accuracy", „sensitivity", „specificity", and „predictive value" according to [22] in order to compare the different methods of knowledge acquisition.

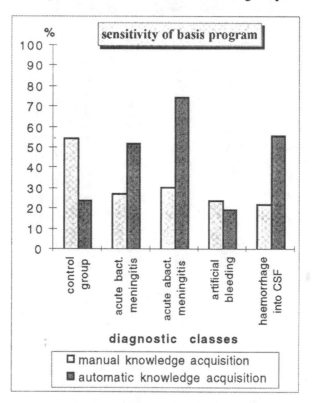

Fig. 1: Sensitivity of diagnosis classes in percentage of each diagnosis class.

Figure 1 gives the percentages of cases of the assessment set (n=194) that were assigned any of the five laboratory diagnoses. Roughly 60% of all cases could not be treated by the manually acquired knowledge base. The automatically generated knowledge base, however, assigned a diagnosis to about 60% of all cases. For both knowledge bases the overall accuracy, i.e. the number of correct diagnosed cases per diagnosed cases, was 71%. This means that the automatically generated knowledge base produced about 10% more correct diagnoses than the manually acquired knowledge base.

The *sensitivity* measure of a diagnosis gives the number of cases that are correctly diagnosed by the system in percentage of the total number of cases with this diagnosis. The percentage of diagnosed cases in the Assement Set is 43.3 for the manual knowledge acuisition, 57.7 for the automatic knowledge acuisition.

Specificity of a class is the number of cases that do not belong to the class and are not diagnosed by the system to be in the class per the number of cases that do not belong to the class. If specificity is high then very few cases are wrongly classified. Figure 2 gives the specificity achieved with the assessment set.

Both the manually acquired knowledge base and the automatically generated knowledge base show high specificity (>90%) (see Fig 2.). Comparable results were found with the parameters of the „emergency diagnosis program".

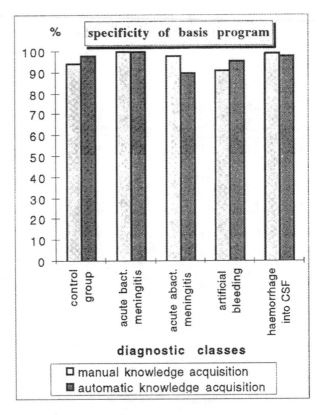

Fig. 2: Specificity of diagnosis classes in the assessment set

The average sensitivity for the manually acquired knowledge base was 30,9%, for the automatically generated knowledge base 41,2% (see Figure 2). Sensitivity exhibited higher values with the automatically generated knowledge base for three diagnosis classes and lower ones for the control group and artificial bleeding.

6. Qualitative Evaluation

In order to judge the plausibility and understandability as well as the medical adequacy and consistency with medical knowledge we designed a questionnaire[1,5,23]. In this questionnaire the expert had to judge each rule generated by **sig*** under the following aspects:

- the correct choice of the characterising parameters (correct choice),
- the detection of new parameters that have not been considered before by the expert (missing variables),
- the elimination of irrelevant parameters (irrelevant variables) and
- the inclusion of parameters, that were not used by the expert before but could be used, if their diagnosis power is significant (new variables).

	normal	*haem-orrhage into CSF*	*artificial bleeding*	*acute bacterial meningitis*	*acute abacterial meningitis'*
parameters used	14	7	6	16	7
correct choice	11	6	6	12	7
missing variables	0	1	0	1	1
irrelevant variables	3	1	0	4	0
new variables	0	0	2	0	1

Tab. 1: Qualitative evaluation of the automatically acquired knowledge base (AKB)

Table 1 shows the results obtained for all diagnosis classes. More than 85% of the parameters chosen by sig* were judged to be correct for the particular diagnosis. In two of five laboratory diagnoses even all of the parameters were found to be correct. In two laboratory diagnoses 12 to 14 per cent of the variables were missing according to the expert. For the diagnosis "artificial bleeding" one third of the variables used in sig*s rules made the expert think that these parameters might prove new insights into the diagnostic process. One such parameter has been identified also for „acute abacterial meningitis".

In summary, the machine learning algorithm *sig** showed an average performance of 93% for the selection of the most significant parameters for each diagnostic class. Rarely one parameter was found to be missing.

7. Discussion

Considerable effort in manpower involving a medical expert and a knowledge engineer was spent in the manual development of a knowledge base (MKB). Rigorous testing with a number of cases not used during the development process (assessment set) showed, however, that only 40% of cases new to the system could be treated at all. It has to be considered, however, that the experimental setting for testing acquisition procedures in this work is a tough one. For the data set used for the development of both knowledge bases hand selected „prototypical" cases were used. In contrast to this for the assessment set cases from every day routine including cases with more than one laboratory diagnosis were considered. The performance of manually acquired knowledge base can be explained by the well known observation in knowledge acquisition, that human experts are very good in producing rules for „normal" situation but perform poor if asked for exceptions or special cases.

The knowledge base generated automatically by **sig*** (AKB) showed a considerable improvement of more than 14% over MKB in the treatment of new cases. Overall correctness achieved by both methods is 71%. For this hard test this is a fairly good result. In particular it is remarkable that the performance of the automatic knowledge acquisition procedure is about the same as the performance of the manual knowledge base.

Considering the results under medical aspects, it may be stated that the sensitivity of diagnosing haemorrhages into CSF was higher than that of diagnosing artificial bleedings. This is desired from the medical point of view because haemorrhages have to be diagnosed further in order to be treated optimally. The sensitivity of diagnosing acute bacterial meningitis has to be improved to be at least 70% which may be sufficient for the daily routine. A high specificity for the differential diagnose "meningitis" is required from the diagnostic point of view because the acute bacterial meningitis has to be treated specifically as soon as possible to prevent a bad medical outcome of the patient. This is not the case with the acute abacterial meningitis. A sufficient specificity of about 90% was obtained for all types of acute meningitis by both knowledge bases.

A drawback of automatic generated knowledge bases is often that such methods produce rules which are implausible or hardly understandable by a human expert. ID3, for example, tries to minimise the number of decisions necessary for a diagnosis [25]. This is clearly an unsuitable approach in the medical problem domain. Human diagnosis follows much more criteria such as complexity or severity of the case taking also risks of a misdiagnosis into account. Minimality of diagnostic decisions is certainly not a primary goal in this domain.

Quality of the extracted rules with respect to human understanding and medical plausibility was tested to give an average performance of 93% for the selection of the most significant parameters for each diagnostic class. The selected attributes of the data were found to be significant to characterise each class appropriately. Some new attributes were found to describe a certain diagnostic class. This may provide new information for the description of the laboratory diagnosis artificial bleeding. In summary the rules generated by the SIG* algorithm showed a remarkable expressive power and were judged to be compatible with medical knowledge.

8. Conclusion

One of the major aims of the MEDWIS project NELA is to show the feasibility and effectiveness of self-organising neural networks as a tool for automatic generation of knowledge bases in medicine. The automatic knowledge acquisition procedure that will be developed in NELA for a special domain of medical laboratory diagnosis involves both, neural networks and symbolic knowledge representations [27].

As a first milestone of the project a knowledge conversion algorithm, called *sig** [28, 31], that will be used in the project NELA for the extraction of knowledge from self-organising neural networks, was tested. We compared a knowledge base, automatically generated by *sig** (AKB) to a first prototype of a manually built knowledge base for the diagnosis of cerebrospinal fluid. We have found that the performance of the

AKB built with *sig** was quantitatively comparable to the manually acquired knowledge base. Slight improvements in accuracy, sensitivity, specificity and number of diagnosed cases can be stated for the automatically generated knowledge base.

The quality of the extracted rules with respect to human understanding and medical plausibility was evaluated by use of a questionnaire. The low number of missing parameters found together with the correct choice of parameters in most cases indicated that the extracted rules correspond well to knowledge expressed by a medical expert. The results presented here confirm that one part of our automatic knowledge acquisition procedure, the conversion of knowledge from subsymbolic representation to a rule based representation of knowledge, performed comparably, proved to be superior to manual knowledge acquisition with some aspects.

Next milestones of the NELA projects are the expansion of the data bases to include more special cases [10]. Furthermore unsupervised neural networks will be trained in order to show properties inherent in the data base, that were not readily known in beforehand [27, 29, 32, 33, 34].

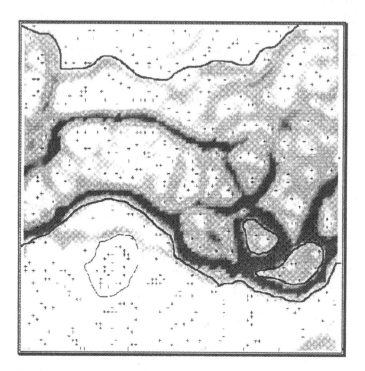

Fig. 3: Visualisation by a *U-matrix* method of a self-organised neural network with data from the development set. Exemplary some borders were drawn to elucidate the structure (see text).

Figure 4, for example, gives a special representation of a toroid self-organised neural network with 6400 neurons, called *U-matrix* [30]. The crosses are data points that the neural network ordered according to similarity. The sector below the top thick line and above the bottom thick line is occupied by the data of the control group. Subclasses of a collective that have common properties can be detected by this method. In Figure 4, for example, some clearly visible clusters are marked. The small sectors surrounded by thick lines belong both to the diagnosis class of bacterial meningitis. If such subclasses are identified on a *U-matrix*, the *sig** algorithm is used in order to produce rules understandable by the expert. The generated rules represent, as shown in this work, central properties of the chosen subgroup. They can be used for an effective procedure to build a knowledge base even for difficult diagnostic problems such as cerebrospinal fluid analysis.

Neural network technology for knowledge acquisition appears to be promising. Neural networks alone, however, are not suited for a medical domain, because of their inability to explain decisions. Knowledge conversion procedures such as the one tested here are necessary. Moreover, neural networks learn by numbers. I.e. cases that are rarely presented in a data collective because they correspond to rare diseases will not be treated correctly by such systems. For this respect an integrated knowledge based system such as it is being developed by the NELA project is necessary.

Acknowledgement

This research was supported in part by the German Bundesminister für Bildung, Wissenschaft, Forschung und Technologie (BMBF) with MEDWIS-Vorhaben Az. 103/1/2 „NELA".

9. References

[1]   Beach, S. S., Gevarter, W.: Standarts for Evaluating Expert System Tools. in: Expert Systems with Applications, Vol. 2, 1991, 259-267.

[2]   Bense, H., Bodrow, W. (Eds.) (1995) *Objektorientierte und regelbasierte Wissensverarbeitung*, Spektrum Akademischer Verlag GmbH, Heidelberg.

[3]   Berlit, P (1992) *Klinische Neurologie*. VCH Weinheim.

[4]   Deichsel, G., Trampisch, H.J.: Clusteranalyse and Diskriminanzanalyse. Gustav Fisher Verlag, Stuttgart, 1985.

[5]   Engelbrecht, R., Rector, A., Moser, W.: Verification and Validation. in: Assessment and Evaluation of Information Technologies, E.M.S-J- van Gennip and J.L. Talmon (eds.), IOS Press, 1995, 51-66.

[6]   Felgenhauer, K. (1988, 1992) Liquordiagnostik. In: L. Thomas: *Labor und Diagnose*. S. 1403-1423. Medizinische Verlagsgesellschaft Marburg, 1403–1423.

[7]   Gallant, S.I.: Neural Network Learning and Expert Systems, MIT Press, Cambridge, MA, 1993.

[8]   Hartung, J.: Statistik, 8. Aufl., Oldenbourg Verlag, 1991.

[9]   Kleine, T. O. (1979) New developments in the diagnosis of cerebrospinal fluid. Report on the Workshop Conference of the German Society for Clinical Chemistry. *J. Clin. Chem. Clin. Biochem.* 17, 505-511

[10] Kleine, T. O. :(1989) New diagnostic methods for inflammation of the human central nervous system by cerebrospinal fluid analysis. Workshop Conference of the German Society for Clinical Chemistry. J. Clin. Chem. Clin. Biochem. 27, 895-932

[11] Kleine, T.O. (1980) *Neue Labormethoden für die Liquordiagnostik.* Thieme, Stuttgart 1980

[12] Kleine, T.O. (1984): Diagnostische Untersuchungen im Liquor cerebrospinalis. In: L. Thomas: *Labor und Diagnose.* S.937-965. Medizinische Verlagsgesellschaft Marburg

[13] Kleine, T.O. (1989): Nervensystem. In: H.Greiling, A.M. Gressner: *Lehrbuch der Klinischen Chemie und Pathobiochemie,* Schattauer Stuttgart, 859-893.

[14] Kleine, T.O. (1991): D-Lactat und L-Lactat im Liquor cerebrospinalis bei akuten entzündlichen Erkrankungen des Zentralnervensystems. *Lab. med.* 15, (114-116.

[15] Kleine, T.O., Baerlocher, K., Niederer, V., Keller, H., Reutter, F., Tritschler, W., Bablok, W. (1979) Diagnostische Bedeutung der Lactatbestimmung im Liquor der Minigitis, *Dtsch. Med. Wschr.* 104(15), 553-557

[16] Kleine, T.O., Hackler, R., Lehmitz, R., Meyer-Rienecker, H. (1994): Liquordiagnostik: Klinisch-chemische Kenngrößen - eine kritische Bilanz. DG *Klinische Chemie Mitteilungen 25,* 199-214.

[17] Kleine, T.O., Hackler, R., Lütcke, A., Zöfel, P., Albrecht, J., Rumpl, E., Meyer-Rienecker, H.J. (1994) Laboratory diagnosis of radicular and pseudoradicular Syndromes in Cerebrospinal Fluid (CSF): Reliability of methods in consideration of pathogenetic aspects, *Eur.J.Clin.Chem.Clin.Biochem.* 32, 45-52.

[18] Kleine, T.O., Weber, L., Zöfel, P. (1987) Diagnostische Aussage eines Basis-Liquor-Programmes bei Erkrankungen des Zentralnervensystems (ZNS), *Lab. med.* 11, 175-176

[19] Kleine, T.O., Wittmann, M. (1995): Protein determination in urine and cerebrospinal fluid (CSF) with the pyrogallol red molybdate method compared with the biuret method. Abstract SEPaC Congress Vienna 1995. *Wien. Klin. Wschr.* 107 Suppl. 199, 10.

[20] Kohonen, T.: Self-Organizing Maps. Springer, Berlin, 1995.

[21] Lehmitz, R., Kleine, T.O. (1994): Liquorzytologie: Ausbeute, Verteilung und Darstellung von Leukozyten bei drei Sedimentationsverfahren im Vergleich zu drei Zytozentrifugations-Modifikationen. *Lab. med.* 18, 91-99.

[22] Michaelis, J., Wellek, S., Willems, J.L. (1990) Reference Standards for Software Evaluation, *Methods of Information in Medicine* 29, F. K. Schattauer Verlagsgesellschaft mbH, 289-297.

[23] Ohmann, C., Belenky, G.: Leitfaden zur Evaluierung von Wissensbasen. MEDWIS-Arbeitskreis Evaluation, 1996.

[24] Puppe, F. (1991) *Einführung in Expertensysteme,* 2. Auflage, Springer Verlag, Berlin.

[25]   Quinlan, J.R. (1984) Learning Efficient Classification Procedures and their Application to Chess End Games, in: Michalski, R.; Carbonell, J.G.; Mitchell, T.M. (Eds.) *Machine Learning - An Artificial Intelligence Approach*, Berlin, 463-482.

[26]   Sax, L. (1992) *Angewandte Statistik*, 7. Auflage, Springer-Verlag, Berlin.

[27]   Ultsch, A, Korus, D., Kleine, T.O. (1995) Integration of Neural Networks and Knowledge-Based Systems in Medicine, 5th. Conf. Artificial Intelligence in Medicine Europe AIME'95, Pavia, Italy, June 1995, in: Barahona, P.; Stefanelli, M.; Wyatt, J. *Artificial Intelligence in Medicine*, Lecture Notes in Artificial Intelligence 934, Springer, 425-426.

[28]   Ultsch, A. (1993) Knowledge Extraction from Self-organizing Neural Networks, in O. Opitz, B. Lausen and R. Klar, (Eds.) *Information and Classification*, Berlin: Springer, 301-306.

[29]   Ultsch, A. (1993) Self-Organized Feature Maps for Monitoring and Knowledge Acquisition of a Chemical Process, in Gielen, S., Kappen, B. (Eds.): *Proc. Intl. Conf. on Artificial Neural Networks* (ICANN), Amsterdam, Sep. 1993, Springer, 864-867.

[30]   Ultsch, A. (1993) Self-organizing Neural Networks for Visualization and Classification, in O. Opitz, B. Lausen and R. Klar, (Eds.) *Information and Classification*, Springer-Verlag, Berlin 307-313.

[31]   Ultsch, A. (1994) The Integration of Neural Networks with Symbolic Knowledge Processing, in: Diday et al.: *New Approaches in Classification and Data Analysis*, Springer, 445-454.

[32]   Ultsch, A., Korus, D. (1995) Erwerb von Fuzzy-Wissen aus Selbstorganisierenden Neuronalen Netzen, *Proc. 3. Workshop Fuzzy-Neuro-Systeme'95*, Darmstadt/F.R.G, Nov. 15-17, 1995, 325-332.

[33]   Ultsch, A., Korus, D. (1995) Integration of Neural Networks with Knowledge-Based Systems, *Proc. IEEE Int. Conf. on Neural Networks, IEEE-ICNN'95*, Perth/Australia, Nov./Dec. 1995, Vol. 4, 1828-1838.

[34]   Ultsch, A., Mantyk, R., Halmans, G. (1993) A Connectionist Knowledge Acquisition Tool CONKAT, in D. J. Hand (Ed.) *Artificial Intelligence Frontiers in Statistics*, Chapman & Hall 1993, 256–263.

Knowledge Acquisition by the Domain Expert Using the Tool HEMATOOL

Johan P Du Plessis and C Janse Tolmie
Dept. of Computer Science and Informatics, University of the Free State
PO Box 339, Bloemfontein 9300
SOUTH AFRICA

1 Introduction

Knowledge Acquisition (KA) is a crucial activity in the development of knowledge-based systems (KBSs). It is a complex and tedious task to perform, often causing the failure of a KBS project, if not performed properly. A KBS is regarded as successful if the system is put into routine use. Currently the knowledge engineer (KE) is responsible for KA, using the tools available to him. Development of KBSs is hindered by the well-known knowledge acquisition bottleneck - a major cause of unsuccessful projects. The more failures the more scepticism and "resistance" from potential users/domain experts. The use of proper KA tools is an attempt to improve the development of KBSs, which would result in more routinely used systems, and reduce the scepticism and resistance of the users.

Many of the commercial tools currently available to the KE fall in the category of first generation KA tools. Certain aspects of the development process are well-supported, e.g. ways of representing knowledge, the implementation of the knowledge base, etc., but some aspects, e.g. knowledge acquisition, are still poorly supported. Since these tools are oriented towards the KE, it makes the development of the KBS heavily dependant on the skills and availability of the KE. A possible solution is to develop tools for the domain expert, allowing him to construct a significant proportion of the knowledge base (KB) without KE interference.

We propose a practical realisable solution with the emphasis on ease of use by the domain expert. It is based on objects, which makes the implementation of the tool in an object-oriented programming language possible. Explicit models of the domain and the task are constructed, which forms the base of the knowledge acquisition tool. The tool called HEMATOOL, assists a Hematologist in the development of a knowledge base for the interpretation of Complete Blood Count (CBC) results, and for the diagnosis of possible causes (a differential diagnosis), should an abnormality be found. It is a prototype system implemented in the object-oriented environment KAPPA-PC.

2 Modelling with Objects in HEMATOOL

We suggest a partially automated model-based approach that relies heavily on the OO paradigm. We identified task and domain model skeletons for diagnosis performed by a pathologist in a clinical lab.

In order for the expert to perform KA activities a knowledge representation method is necessary which is simple enough for a (non-AI specialist) expert to comprehend and

Tel: + 27 - 51 - 4012754   Fax: + 27 - 51 - 4474152
Email: johan@wwg3.uovs.ac.za

express himself in, is powerful enough for the chosen domain, and is easily mapable onto a knowledge-based language. The KA tool forms a kind of KA interface between the expert and the KB. The knowledge provided by the expert should therefore, easily be converted to the required KB format, and the KB format should also easily be converted to a form understandable by the expert. This ability is dependant on the knowledge representation scheme(s) applied. Our approach is to apply essentially the same knowledge representation scheme in both the tool and the KB, but with the difference that in the tool the expert will be freed from syntactic detail of the scheme, e.g. instead of typing text the expert chooses from menus.

We chose the OO paradigm to represent the knowledge in both the tool and the KB. This has several benefits:

➣ As the idea of objects was drawn from the metaphor of real life, the expert might intuitively grasp the concept. This is important for the expert's interaction with the tool. For mapping the knowledge onto the KB this is ideal, because there are numerous commercial shells that support the OO paradigm.

➣ The object concept provides a natural way to give structure to a domain. This is accomplished by decomposing a body of knowledge into knowledge units, and by representing the knowledge units as objects (classes and instances). This feature provides a mechanism for the knowledge engineer to develop a domain model skeleton, i.e. an object hierarchy, for the domain.

➣ Once a task model skeleton is intact, the knowledge engineer can identify the knowledge units (objects) that fall within the scope of the domain expert, and hand these units over to the expert for completion. The feature of the OO paradigm (encapsulation) which allows an entity to be considered on its own, allows the knowledge engineer/expert to focus on only one knowledge unit at a time - thus preventing the expert to get lost in an ever-growing labyrinth of knowledge.

2.1 The Task Model

The task model is based on the reasoning process of a hematologist in a clinical lab. The two main tasks performed are identified as Interpretation and Diagnosis, both involves a generate-and-test strategy or problem-solving method. For each task, interpretation and diagnosis, we can identify three substeps: Abstraction, Generate Hypotheses and Test Hypotheses.

If an expert is responsible for knowledge acquisition he should be familiar with the reasoning process applied to the knowledge. As generate-and-test is a fairly simple and straight-forward approach that is widely employed by medical professionals, an expert will feel comfortable with this.

2.2 The Domain Model

The domain knowledge is modelled as objects in an object world, where each object represents a real-world entity in the problem domain. An object (which can be considered as a knowledge unit) is seen as a micro-world. In other words, each object "acts" in its own (micro) world, but also interacts with the other objects. The interaction between objects is based on the relationships that exist between the different objects. The task model is constructed in such a way that it makes use of the objects and their relationships to perform the interpretation and eventually provides a final diagnosis.

In the case of HEMATOOL, we have an object class, called Parameters, to represent the test results in an abstracted form, e.g. the hemoglobin (HGB) content of the blood which can be Normal, High or Low.

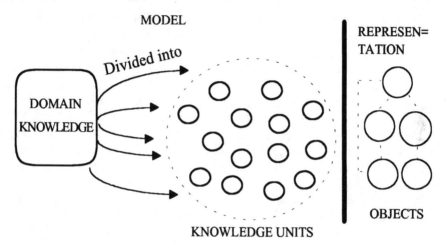

Figure 1: Representation of the domain using Objects.

An Interpretation Class defines the possible interpretations. An example of an interpretation is Hypochromic-Microcytic-Anemia. The parameters HGB, MCV (Mean red Cell Volume) and MCHC (Mean Corpuscular Hemoglobin Content) play a role in the determination of this interpretation. In its micro-world this interpretation instance is aware of the values the different parameter objects must have in order for the interpretation instance to be valid. This is a fact considered by the generate-and-test problem-solving method when applied to the generation of possible interpretations.

A Diagnosis Class defines the possible diagnoses or causes, e.g. Iron-Deficiency. A diagnosis is valid given a certain context(s). A diagnosis is influenced by the presence of certain parameters and/or a certain combination of interpretations. Different contexts under which the validity of a diagnosis is defined, are constructed by the domain expert while using HEMATOOL.

3 Discussion

The task and domain models provide a base for knowledge acquisition. The domain is seen as a body of knowledge which consists of various knowledge units. These knowledge units are related to one another in the domain. In modelling these units as separate units, we need to make these relationships explicit. Objects are used in the modelling process to encapsulate the knowledge units of the domain. Figure 1 gives a schematic overview of the main ideas behind our approach.

The micro world of the objects representing the domain is a feature that we are now only beginning to explore. Each object instance is provided with the knowledge in order for the object to determine its own applicability in the current context of the full blood count results. In the case of Thalassemia, for example, this feature is further explored in the sense that the validity of this diagnosis are based, amongst others, on the calculation of a certain formula. This formula is easily incorporated into the diagnosis object to provide the knowledge for the object to determine its applicability.

Both the task and domain models can easily be adapted for other domains. It is the task of the knowledge engineer to model the task and the domain knowledge, according to the domain of interest, when development starts. The knowledge engineer will construct the task model for the application, based on the skeleton task model provided. The same is done for the domain model - the knowledge engineer based the domain model on the skeleton domain model provided and alter it according to the current domain of interest. Thus, as is the case with CBC interpretation, the use of the tool in other areas will be based on the task and domain models with the aim of assisting the domain expert in the filling (instantiation) of the model, i.e. the domain expert fills the knowledge base by creating the object instances of the domain.

The basis of the tool is provided by the task and domain models. A suitable user interface built around these models will provide the basic essentials of the tool. The expert can now interact with the tool, filling the objects (viewed by the expert as parameters, interpretations and diagnoses (diseases)) in a way he sees best.

The main attractions of this approach are:
- The knowledge engineer is less involved in the knowledge acquisition process and can devote more time and effort to other important aspects of expert systems development.
- The domain expert is more involved in the process, but should feel more in control, and can do knowledge acquisition at his own pace in his own time.
- Knowledge base maintenance is done by the expert.
- Objects are used in the modelling process - an object-oriented programming language is therefore needed to start implementation, and not an expensive tool.
- A reusable toolkit can be constructed for further use.

4 Conclusion

The commercial expert system tools do not provide enough support for knowledge base construction and maintenance with respect to KA tools provided. HEMATOOL provides an easy way to overcome some of the problems of KA and knowledge base maintenance. HEMATOOL allows the domain expert to concentrate on various parts of the domain, e.g. parameters, one at a time. As new knowledge becomes available, the expert is in the position to maintain, to a certain extent, the knowledge base. However, in some situations the knowledge engineer will be still be required to render assistance. HEMATOOL is a prototype system which is currently being evaluated.

In this paper we suggest an Object-Oriented approach towards KB modelling. Not all the domains are best modelled by the OO paradigm. The applicability of this approach, therefore, depends on the nature of the knowledge in the domain.

Application of Inductive Logic Programming for Learning ECG Waveforms

Gabriella Kókai[1], Zoltán Alexin[2], and Tibor Gyimóthy[3]

[1] Institute of Informatics, József Attila University
[2] Department of Applied Informatics, József Attila University
Árpád tér 2, H-6720 Szeged, Hungary
e-mail: alexin@inf.u-szeged.hu

[3] Research Group on Artificial Intelligence
Hungarian Academy of Sciences,
Aradi vértanuk tere 1, H-6720 Szeged, Hungary
e-mail: gyimi@inf.u-szeged.hu.

Abstract. In this paper a learning system is presented which integrates an ECG waveform classifier (called PECG) with an interactive learner (called IMPUT). The PECG system is based on an attribute grammar specification of ECGs that has been transformed to Prolog. The IMPUT system combines the interactive debugging technique IDT with the unfolding algorithm introduced in SPECTRE. Using the IMPUT system we can effectively assist in preparing the correct description of the basic structures of ECG waveforms. [4]
Keywords: inductive logic programming, program specialization, syntactic pattern recognition

1 Introduction

In this paper a complex system is presented that is able to classify ECG waveforms described as a combination of primitives. The system helps the user to improve the classifier program if it cannot recognize correctly the given input waveforms.

The system integrates an ECG waveform classifier (called PECG) with an interactive learner (called IMPUT).

The PECG system is based on an attribute grammar specification of ECG waveforms published by Skordalakis et al [9]. The basic idea of PECG, introduced in [3], is to integrate the ECG classifier program (implemented in Prolog) with the Interactive Diagnosis and Testing (IDT) module [7] and a graphic viewer. This integrated tool can recognize whether any modification in the classifier program is needed. If the system cannot analyze the input then the user is helped by the built-in IDT debugger to find the false clause. The learning part of the new system is based on an Inductive Logic Programming (ILP) [4, 5] method (called IMPUT) introduced in [1].

[4] This work was supported by the grant OTKA T14228 and the project PHARE TDQM 9305-02/1022 ("ILP2/HUN").

In the PECG system the ECG waveforms are described in Definite Clause Grammars (DCGs). The construction of these grammars for different waveforms is a very sophisticated task, therefore a tool which can assist in this work would be very useful. That was the reason for us to develop an extended version of the PECG system.

The user of this system has to prepare an *over-generalized* grammar in the first step. This grammar may accept not only correct but many incorrect waveforms as well. Of course it is much more easier to prepare such *over-generalized* initial grammar than the correct one. The inputs of the extended PECG system are this initial grammar, some background knowledge, positive and negative examples of ECG waveforms to be inferred. The system uses an ILP learning method to improve the inital grammar such that the modified grammar accepts each positive example but no negative ones.

In Section 2 we briefly describe the integrated system Sections 3 contains a brief summary and comments on possible future studies.

2 The architecture of the learning system

In this section we give a overview of the extended PECG system which involves an integration of PECG with the IMPUT interactive learning system. The structure of the system can be seen in Figure 1.

The main parts comming from the PECG are the following:

- *the ECG processing module:* this part of the system uses a syntactic approach to recognize an electrocardiographic pattern. In this part Skordalaki's work was used to decompose the waveform, to select the peaks and present the waveform as a string from a alphabet. The classifier module recognizes the ECG waveforms from their linguistic representation

- *the IDT module:* this part is an interactive debugging and testing tool that is based on the Shapiro's Interactive Diagnosis Algorithm [8] and Category Partition Testing Method (CPM) [6]. It can be divided into three submodules. The *test database* module generates the initial test database from a CPM specification. In the *testing* part a predicate can be chosen and the user can give a representing element of the testframe generated for this predicate. Then he or she can decide whether, for the given input, the output is correct or not. The *debugging* part is based on the idea that if the program has already been tested then the test results can be directly applied without asking the user *difficult* questions.

- *the graphic viewer module:* this part makes visible the current subpatterns being analyzed.

The learning part of the new system consists of two main parts. The specialization algorithm comes from the SPECTRE [2] system while the interactive debugger part is imported from the IDT.

The main idea of IMPUT is that the identification of the next clause to be unfolded has a crucial importance in the effectiveness of the specialization

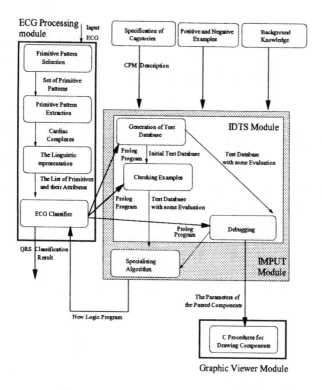

Fig. 1. The structure of the extended PECG system

process. The specialization steps are invoked by the negative examples that are covered by the target predicate. We assume that when a negative example is covered by the current version of the program, then there is at least one clause which is responsible for this incorrect covering. IMPUT uses the IDT debugging algorithm to identify a buggy clause of the program. The clause identified in this process will be unfolded in the next step of the specialization algorithm.

3 Conclusion, Further Work

In this paper an integrated system has been presented which can classify and learn ECG waveforms. Combining the IMPUT method with the PECG system the integrated system was able to suggest correct clauses to replace the *buggy* clauses recognized during the debugging process. In general the graphic viewer helps to find bugs, and in our case shows the ECG subpattern is currently being analyzed.

The main advantage of our system comparing with Skordalakis' approach is that our integrated tool can positively assists the developer (user) working with the ECG classifier program because the program itself is "self-correcting".

Applying the IMPUT learning method to the ECG domain we found that correct DCG programs can be inferred for the basic structures of complex ECG waveforms. In these approaches the user only needs to prepare very general initial DCG programs. The extended PECG system is able to specialise these programs into the correct ones in a very effective way. .

The current version of the PECG system is about 3500 lines in SICStus Prolog, and 500 lines written in C for the implementation of the graphic viewer. The IDT module is about 1400 Prolog lines, containing 150 predicates while the classifier program is more than 2000 lines in Prolog. The IMPUT system itself contains more than 800 lines without the IDT module. [5]

At present the PECG system does not contain any preprocessing module for the linguistic representation of ECG waveforms. To make our system a complete ECG recognizer we plan to implement these preprocessing modules. We also plan to ensure an interactive connection between the graphic viewer and the user. It means that the user may control the analyzing process from the graphic window by marking the subparts of the waveforms to be analysed.

References

1. Alexin, Z., Gyimóthy, T., Boström, H.: Integrating Algorithmic Debugging and Unfolding Transformation in an Interactive Learner in Proceedings of the 12th European Conference on Artificial Intelligence ECAI-96 ed. Wolfgang Wahlster, Budapest, Hungary (1996) 403–407 John Wiley & Son's Ltd. 1996.
2. Boström, H., Idestam-Almquist, P.: Specialization of Logic Programs by Pruning SLD-trees., Proc. of the Fourth International Workshop on Inductive Logic Programming (ILP-94) Bad Honnef/Bonn Germany September 12-14. (1994) 31–47
3. Kókai, G., Alexin, Z., Gyimóthy, T.: Classifying ECG Waveforms in Prolog Proc. of the Fourth International Conference on The Practical Application of PROLOG (PAP96) London, United Kingdom April 23-25, (1996) 193–221
4. Lavrač, N., Džeroski, S.: Inductive Logic Programming: Techniques and Applications Ellis Horwood, (1994)
5. Muggleton, S., De Raedt, L.: Inductive Logic Programming: Theory and methods, Journal of Logic Programming 19 (20) (1994) 629–679
6. Ostrand, T. J., Balker, M. J.: The Category-Partition Method for Specifying and Generating Functional Tests CACM 31:6 June (1988) 676–686
7. Paakki, J., Gyimóthy, T., Horváth T.,: Effective Algorithmic Debugging for Inductive Logic Programming. Proc. of the Fourth International Workshop on Inductive Logic Programming (ILP-94) Bad Honnef/Bonn Germany September 12-14. (1994) 175–194
8. Shapiro, E. Y.: Algorithmic Program Debugging MIT Press (1983)
9. Skordalakis, E.: ECG Analysis in Syntactic and Structural Pattern Recognition Theory and Applications ed. Bunke, H. and Sanfeliu, A. World Scientific (1990) 499–533

---

[5] The implementation language currently is SICStus Prolog Version 3.0 #3 running on a SUN SPARCStation.

Knowledge Discovery from a Breast Cancer Database

Subramani Mani[1], Michael J. Pazzani[1] and John West MD[2]

[1] Department of Information and Computer Science, 444 Computer Science Building,
University of California at Irvine, Irvine, CA 92697-3425 *(mani,pazzani)@ics.uci.edu*
[2] Breast Care Center, 1140 W.La Veta, Orange CA 92668

Abstract. We report on the use of various Machine Learning algorithms on an electronic database of breast cancer patients. The task was to predict breast cancer recurrence using a short subset of clinical attributes such as tumor presence, tumor size, invasive nature of tumor, number of lymph nodes involved, severity of lymphedema and stage of tumor. The predictive accuracy over fifty runs employing test sets not used to build the model were 63.4%(Cart), 63.9%(C45), 62.5%(C45rules), 66.4%(FOCL) and 68.3%(Naive Bayes). An extension of the model using additional features and larger datasets is contemplated.

1 Introduction

Breast cancer affects approximately ten per cent of women in US. Much of the research effort has been focussed on early detection for better treatment of the condition. Breast cancer *staging* and TNM(Tumor, Node, Metastasis) classification were applied for devising optimal treatment plans. In spite of the advances made, relapse or recurrence of the malignancy continues to be a significant problem. Tumor characteristics, extent of lymph node involvement and patient parameters have been postulated to be predictors of prognosis. The primary treatment selected for the condition also plays a modifying role.[1] Machine Learning(ML) methods have been employed in many domains including some medical domains for induction of useful rules from data. ML algorithms have been used successfully to classify benign and malignant tumors from histological data.[2] There has also been earlier attempts at application of these techniques to the problem of relapse but they emphasized development of ML methods to noisy data.[3]

2 Aim of the Study

In this work we explore the use of various machine learning techniques to identify with a high degree of certainty the tumor characteristics responsible for recurrence of carcinoma of the breast.

131

3 Methods

3.1 Database

For this study we used the electronic medical record database of Breast Care Center, Orange, CA. Data consisted of demographic factors, clinical features, tumor parameters(macroscopic and microscopic), investigative procedures performed, diagnostic variables, treatment given and follow up measures. There were 887 patients.

3.2 Attribute Selection

Six attributes were identified by the surgeon Dr. John West for usefulness in predicting recurrence. The features considered for evaluation were presence of tumor, size of tumor, whether the tumor was of invasive nature, number of lymph nodes involved, severity of lymphedema and stage of tumor. The class variable was recurrence(coded yes and no).

3.3 Datasets for ML Runs

Out of the total sample of 887, 802(90%) did not develop recurrence during follow up and 85(10%) had relapse. To eliminate the bias of class distribution(90% versus 10%), the major class was randomly partitioned and six datasets created with class proportions of approximately 60% and 40%(total n = 233). Each algorithm was run fifty times on all the datasets. The datasets were randomly split into a two-third *training* set and a one-third *testing* set. The accuracies reported are of the test set.

3.4 Machine Learning Algorithms

Machine Learning algorithms which generate classification trees and rules are of particular importance in our context. The rules and trees provide necessary explanation for their predictions. The tree classifiers (C4.5[4] and CART[5]) and rule inducers (C4.5rules and FOCL[6]) were tried for this work. The results were compared in terms of prediction accuracy with a robust classifier *Naive Bayes* which assumes that the attributes are conditionally independent given the class. Nevertheless, it gives a good baseline performance.

4 Results

The comparative results of the different ML algorithms on these six datasets are shown in Table 1. An example of a rule set from C45rules run and a Cart induced tree are given in subsection 4.1 and subsection 4.2.

Table 1. Recurrence Prediction with Various ML Algorithms

Algorithm	Accuracy averaged over fifty runs						Mean
	dataset1	dataset2	dataset3	dataset4	dataset5	dataset6	
Cart	63.3	64.2	62.6	60.1	65.9	64.5	63.4
C45	66.7	73.6	62.5	62.5	54.2	63.9	63.9
C45rules	56.9	69.4	66.7	62.5	54.2	65.3	62.5
FOCL	68.7	66.0	67.0	65.6	66.4	64.7	66.4
Naive Bayes	73.6	76.4	62.5	66.7	65.3	65.3	68.3

4.1 C45 Rule Set

The following rules generated by C45rules are ordered with their accuracies given in braces.

1. if stage > 3 ⇒ recurrence class (71%)
2. if number_nodes_involved > 8 ⇒ recurrence class (68%)
3. if lymphedema ≤ 0 and tumor_size > 120mm ⇒ recurrence class (62%)
4. if tumor_size ≤ 120mm and number_nodes_involved ≤ 1 ⇒ no_recurrence class (74%)
5. if lump = 0 and stage ≤ 2 ⇒ no_recurrence class (74%)
6. default class ⇒ no_recurrence class

4.2 Cart Induced Tree

Cart generated a simplified decision tree for most of the runs.

− if stage ≤ 1 ⇒ no_recurrence class
− if stage ≥ 2 ⇒ recurrence class

5 Discussion

In terms of prediction accuracy Naive Bayes and FOCL stood out from the other algorithms. All the ML algorithms performed better than chance. Examination of the generated rules and trees showed that most of them reflected domain knowledge. Compared to C45, Cart notably produced much smaller trees. We consider the results encouraging but further evaluation on larger datasets is required.

6 Future Work

We propose to constrain the learning algorithms with prior knowledge to generate more meaningful rules. FOCL will be used for this purpose. For example Rule # 3 is inadequate. Prior knowledge will improve or suppress such rules. Other attributes covering patient factors, primary treatment variables and clinical features could be tried. It would be interesting to learn Bayesian Networks also.

References

1. Fentiman IS and Gregory WM. "The Hormonal Milieu and Prognosis in Operable Breast Cancer" In: *Cancer Surveys–Breast Cancer vol 18 pp149-163* Guest ed. Fentiman IS and Taylor-Papadimitriou J. Cold Spring Harbor Laboratory Press. 1993.
2. Wolberg W.H and Mangasarian O.L. "Computer-Designed Expert Systems for Breast Cytology Diagnosis" *Analytical and Quantitative Cytology and Histology, vol 15, pp67-74, Feb 1993.*
3. Tan M and Eshelman L. "Using weighted networks to represent classification knowledge in noisy domains. *Proceedings of the Fifth International Conference on Machine Learning, pp121-134* Ann Arbor, MI.
4. Quinlan, JR. "C4.5: Programs for Machine Learning" Morgan Kaufmann 1993 Los Altos, California.
5. Brieman L, Friedman J.H., Olshen R.A. and Stone C.J. "Classification and Regression Trees" Wadsworth 1984 Belmont.
6. Pazzani, Michael and Dennis Kibler. "The Utility of Knowledge in Inductive Learning" Machine Learning 9:57-94, 1992

An Adaptive Two-Tier Menu Approach to Support On-Line Entry of Diagnoses

Sugath K. Mudali, James R. Warren, and Susan E. Spenceley

Advanced Computing Research Centre, School of Computer and Information Science
University of South Australia, The Levels, SA 5095, Australia
Email: {s.mudali, j.warren, s.spenceley}@unisa.edu.au

Abstract

We demonstrate how a task model derived from data mining techniques could be used to anticipate diagnosis codes from patient complaints for improved data entry efficiency. The anticipated diagnoses are presented to the user in a two-tier fashion with the first tier presenting the most likely diagnoses based upon the complaints which the second tier refines. A success rate of 70% was obtained in anticipating patient diagnosis.

Category: knowledge acquisition & learning

1 Introduction

An interface that changes according to user requirements, known as an adaptive interface, is particularly important to physicians who will typically vary both in their own individual practice styles and the context of practice. To adapt effectively, the interface requires information on how the user performs their task: a *task model*. This task model could be supplied either by an expert providing rules (a formidable job that also assigns the knowledge about data entry to the experts idealised case) or by machine learning techniques. The latter, a branch of Artificial Intelligence involved with mechanising the acquisition of knowledge from experience, is a more practical technique that can be applied directly to learn the patterns of different physicians. There is also a precedence for adaptive interfaces that successfully employ machine learning techniques to anticipate data entry in the domain of medicine. Canfield [1] has observed an estimated two to five times less effort in data entry for echocardiography records based on the analysis of frequencies of occurrences of terms in existing data.

The interface described here demonstrates anticipation of data entry requirements with a series of short dynamic menus hereafter known as hot lists. These hot lists are presented to the user as a two-tier menu as shown in figure 1. The hot list on left, known as the *main list*, contains the most likely diagnosis codes based upon the complaints for the case at hand. The hot list next to the main list, known as the *associate list*, contains the most highly associated diagnosis codes for the presently selected diagnosis from the main list.

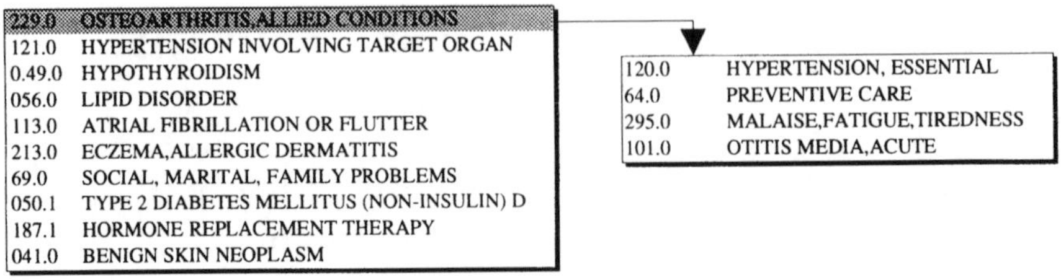

229.0	OSTEOARTHRITIS,ALLIED CONDITIONS
121.0	HYPERTENSION INVOLVING TARGET ORGAN
0.49.0	HYPOTHYROIDISM
056.0	LIPID DISORDER
113.0	ATRIAL FIBRILLATION OR FLUTTER
213.0	ECZEMA,ALLERGIC DERMATITIS
69.0	SOCIAL, MARITAL, FAMILY PROBLEMS
050.1	TYPE 2 DIABETES MELLITUS (NON-INSULIN) D
187.1	HORMONE REPLACEMENT THERAPY
041.0	BENIGN SKIN NEOPLASM

120.0	HYPERTENSION, ESSENTIAL
64.0	PREVENTIVE CARE
295.0	MALAISE,FATIGUE,TIREDNESS
101.0	OTITIS MEDIA,ACUTE

Fig. 1. Two-tier menu approach

2 Description of Data

The work presented here is based on an analysis of 3085 anonymous primary care SOAP [2] (Subjective, Objective, Analysis, and Plan) notes from a single physician general practice in Adelaide, South Australia. The diagnosis component (Analysis) is coded using a proprietary coding system while the subjective component (presenting complaint) is given in free text. To facilitate the application of data mining techniques to this data, we used the *Codes Finder* [3] to convert 800 first encounters to the ICPC Plus (8/95) [4] classification system. Encounters with no diagnoses or complaints were removed thereby providing a database of 560 patients for the analysis.

3 Methods

The main list contains the k most likely diagnosis codes based upon the presenting complaints of the case at hand. The conditional probability underlying the Bayesian formalism was used to formulate the list. A matrix giving the posterior probability for each diagnosis given each complaint is formulated from a sample of cases. This matrix constitutes our task model. Two approaches were considered to resolve different complaints suggesting a common diagnosis. The first approach resolves the conflict by assigning the responsibility to the complaint that has the *maximum* conditional probability. The second approach adopts the *combination method* in MYCIN [5], where the probability is computed by combining data from two or more observations using the amount from one observation plus some increment from the other(s).

The associate hot list contains the most likely k diagnoses associated with the selected code in the main list. Unlike the main list, only the selected diagnosis in the main list determines the contents of the associated list. Two different methods are explored for the creation of the list. The first method uses the conditional probabilities between diagnoses while the second method uses the similarities between diagnoses based upon a distance metric.

4 Evaluation

The main metric to evaluate the task model anticipation is the hit rate which ranges between 0 and 1 indicating respectively that none of the diagnoses and all of the diagnoses were correctly anticipated for a given case. For example, a hit rate of 0.50 is given if 2 out of 4 codes are found in the hot lists. Two different strategies were adopted to compute the hit rates: optimum and realistic. The optimum strategy assumes that a physician would fully consider both the main and associate lists. In contrast, the realistic strategy assumes that a physician would explore the associate list only as a result of selection made with the main list. The results from experiments performed under the optimum strategy provide the benchmarks for their corresponding experiments under the realistic strategy. For all the experiments, sample sets of 6 different sizes (100, 200, 300, 400, 500, and 560) were constructed with each set consisting of randomly selected records. Each set is then divided into 90% training data and the remaining 10% as unseen testing data. Ten different random sets and task models were generated for each sample set. A list length of 12 was chosen as it represents a reasonable maximum size without being too difficult to mange on the screen and also because of its use in prior research [1].

As expected, the average hit rates for the experiments performed under the optimum category out-performed the corresponding experiments under the realistic category. In general, the experiments using the conditional probability approach provided better results than experiments based on the distance. The conditional probabilities in conjunction with the combination approach (to resolve conflicts in the main list) achieved marginally better results than the maximum approach. The average hit rates of both strategies for the combination approach over various sample sizes are shown in figure 2. In general, performance is improved as the size of the sample training set increases although a levelling off at about 70% for the realistic strategy and 78% for the optimum category is observed.

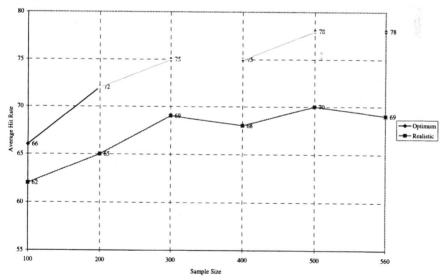

Fig. 2. Comparison of hit rates for the experiment using the combination approach

It is possible for the results to be improved by an enhancement to the task model with information such as a patient's sex or age. For instance, there is no need to include any diagnoses related to cervix if the patient is a male or a child. Other information which might be relevant to use include the longitudinal aspect to patient data and the negative correlations (i.e. facts that contradict one another).

5 Conclusion

In summary, we have proposed a mechanism to assist a physician in the creation of a complete, precise, and accurate, on-line medical record by providing appropriate interface technology for data entry. The principles of the machine learnt adaptive interface have been demonstrated by simulated data entry of the diagnosis component of a SOAP note. A task model was used to anticipate data entry requirements and was based upon the complaint codes and other diagnosis codes.

A task model put into long term usage provides a number of opportunities. First, the data mining approach has captured a lot of information about the relationships between complaints and diagnoses without having assumed any background knowledge or the causalities between the two components. Second, the abstraction of knowledge about the diagnosis in the task model creates a portable package of information that could be used for the anticipation of data entry by other modes such as the recognition of handwriting or speech. Third, the portable nature of the task model suggests that it might become an important World Wide Web resource. Sites with task models could act as servers for remote physicians' (clients') queries. Securing an existing task model could provide a useful start up for a small site while other task models could be built to serve to medical specialities. Finally, the task model may reveal some interesting patterns that are difficult to notice with human judgement alone and provides a source of verification for human decisions

References

1. Canfield, K. (1995) Primary intelligent split menus with text corpora for computerised patient record data-entry. *International J. Bio-Medical Computing*, Vol. 39, 263-273.
2. Weed, L.L. (1969) *Medical Records, Medical Education, and Patient Care.* Press of the Case Western Reserve University.
3. Mudali, S.K., Warren, J.R., Spenceley, S.E., and Kirkwood, I (1996) Toward an Intelligent Interface for Clinical Data Capture: Probabilistic Analysis of the Subjective Component. *Proceedings of the Fourth National Health Informatics Conference (HIC96)*, B. McGuiness and T. Leeder (eds), Melbourne, August 19-21, 57-62.
4. ICPC (1987) *International Classification of Primary Care.* H. Lamberts and M. Wood (eds.), Oxford University Press, Oxford.
5. Shortliffe, E.H. (1976) *Computer-Based Medical Consultations: MYCIN.* New York, Elsevier.

Acknowledgment

Thanks are owed to Dr Helena Britt for providing the ICPC Plus classification system; physicians Ian Kirkwood, Don Walker, and Oliver Frank, for their guidance on medical matters.

Machine Learning Applied to Diagnosis of Sport Injuries

Igor Zelič[1], Igor Kononenko[2], Nada Lavrač[3], Vanja Vuga[4]

[1] INFONET, Planina 3, 4000 Kranj, Slovenia
[2] Faculty of Computer and Information Science, Tržaška 25, Ljubljana, Slovenia
[3] J. Stefan Institute, Jamova 39, Ljubljana, Slovenia
[4] Center for Sport Medicine, Celovška 25, Ljubljana, Slovenia
igor.zelic@infonet.si, igor.kononenko@fri.uni-lj.si, nada.lavrac@ijs.si

Abstract. Several machine learning algorithms were used in the development of an expert system for diagnosing sport injuries. The applied methods include variants of the Assistant algorithm for top-down induction of decision trees, and variants of the Bayesian classifier. Since the available dataset turned out to be insufficient for reliable diagnosis of selected sport injuries, expert-defined diagnostic rules were added and used in combination with classifiers induced by machine learning systems. Experimental results show that the classification accuracy and the explanation capability of the naive Bayesian classifier with the fuzzy discretization of numerical attributes was superior to other methods and therefore the most appropriate for practical use in our application.

1 Introduction

Machine learning technology is well suited for the induction of diagnostic and prognostic rules. Data about correct diagnoses and prognoses is often made available from archives of specialized hospitals and clinics, where the number of stored cases grows daily. Such data gathering occurs also in the Center for Sport Medicine of the Ljubljana University Medical Center, where records of patients with sport injuries are collected daily. This work is limited to data analysis of patient records with injuries in athletics and handball. The aim of our work is to provide systematic computer-supported data gathering and storing, intelligent analysis of stored data, support of diagnostic decisions, and the transfer of expert diagnostic knowledge from the experienced specialist to young inexperienced medical doctors. An important aspect which has motivated this study is also to reveal the unclear influence of individual anamnestic and clinical parameters for individual diagnoses. Moreover, to support the diagnostic decisions, reasonably high diagnostic accuracy has to be achieved, as well as the transparency of proposed decisions.

2 Machine learning systems

In this study we used machine learning systems that are able to explain their decisions. The selection of systems was limited to variants of the Assistant top-down decision tree learner and to variants of the Bayesian classifier that have proved to be well suited for supporting diagnostic decision making in numerous medical domains [2, 3]. The explanation capabilitity of decision tree learners is based on the induced decision trees themselves: an explanation is a path from the root to a leave of the tree, corresponding to attribute values of the instance to be classified. On the other hand, an explanation of the Bayesian classifiers consists of the sum of information gains of all attribute values describing the instance. The value of an attribute can be in favour of the proposed diagnosis (positive information gain) or can be againsts it (negative information gain).

The variants of Assistant (Assistant-I, Assistant-R and Assistant-R2) [3] implement several extensions of the original Assistant algorithm for top-down induction of decision trees [1]. The main difference between the algorithms lies in their heuristics for attribute selection: Assistant-I uses informativity whereas Assistant-R and Assistant-R2 use the algorithm ReliefF [3]. Assistant-R2 is a variant of Assistant-R that generates separate decision trees for each class (diagnosis), and combines these into a classifier for the entire domain. This is in contrast with Assistant-I and Assistant-R that build one general decision tree for the whole domain.

We used two variants of the Bayesian classifier with extensions for handling continuous attributes: the naive Bayesian classifier and the semi-naive Bayesian classifier. The semi-naive Bayesian classifier is an extension of the naive Bayesian classifier that explicitly searches for dependencies between values of different attributes [2]. Both systems require the pre-discretization of continuous attributes. The problem of (strict) pre-discretization is that minor changes in values of the continuous attributes (or, equivalently, minor changes in boundaries) may have a drastic effect on the probability distribution and therefore on the classification. In order to avoid this problem, the naive Bayesian classifier with the fuzzy discretization of continuous attributes was also used [2].

3   Diagnostic problem

The current database of athletic and handball injuries consists of 118 patient records, described by the values of 49 attributes. Diagnoses are grouped into 30 diagnostic classes. The most frequent diagnosis is the injury of ligamentary insertions (16% of patients have this diagnosis), thus the majority class is not significantly larger than other classes. Eleven diagnostic classes are represented by a single training instance, and four classes with two training instances each.

For the given large number of diagnostic classes, the number of recorded training instances is much too small to result in reliable diagnostic decisions. This was (temporarily) solved by providing a combined expert system—machine learning interaction when classifying new cases. The system supports the input of expert-defined rules in the form identical to the training examples themselves, except that the expert defines only those attribute values that are characteristic for the diagnosis, leaving unimportant attributes undefined (value 'unknown'). Expert-defined diagnostic rules can be used in two ways: as pre-classifiers or as generators of additional training instances. In pre-classification mode, rules are fired in preprocessing, before using a learner's classification mechanism. In example-generation mode, rules can be used to 'artificially' generate new training examples.

4 Experiments and results

Since the ultimate test of the quality of learners is their performance on unseen cases, experiments were performed on ten different random partitions of the data into 70% training and 30% testing examples. Results of the experiments in terms of the classification accuracy and information score are outlined in Table 1.

Classifier	accuracy (%)		inf. score (bits)		leaves (#)
	$\bar{x}$	σ	$\bar{x}$	σ	
Assistant-I	58.2	5.8	2.19	0.28	20.9
Assistant-R	62.9	5.7	2.25	0.21	26.3
Assistant-R2	61.7	6.2	2.22	0.06	3.2
naive Bayes - strict	59.4	4.9	1.83	0.15	/
naive Bayes - fuzzy	69.4	3.0	2.32	0.19	/
semi-naive Bayes - fuzzy	59.4	4.8	1.82	0.15	/

Table 1. The performance of various systems.

All the algorithms were used with the default values of their parameters. The three variants of Assistant achieve approximately the same accuracy and absolute information score (Assistant-R being just slightly better). However, the comparison of decision trees reveals that Assistant-I selects substantially different attributes than the other two algorithms. It also generates slightly smaller decision trees than Assistant-R (notice that the number of leaves for Assistant-R2 is measured as the average of 30 trees, therefore the results can not be compared).

The best results are acieved by the naive Bayesian classifier that uses the fuzzy discretization of continuous attributes. Although the number of these attributes is relatively small, the strict pre-discretization of continuous attributes overestimates the importance of these attributes (according to the physician's opinion) and leads to less favourable results. The use of the semi-naive Bayesian classifier turns out to be inappropriate for this domain. Joining of values of attributes causes the accuracy to drop. Consequently, the result suggests that in this domain the attributes are relatively conditionaly independent.

Results of experiments using expert-defined rules are as follows. In the pre-classification mode we compared the performance of a combined classifier by including or excluding the training examples covered by the expert-defined rules. The exclusion of these training instances does not change the classification accuracy significantly, whereas the generated decision trees are much smaller. This suggests that excluding the instances covered by expert-defined rules drasticaly simplifies the model for other diagnoses. In the example-generation mode, where additional training instances are generated, no significant change in the classification accuracy is achieved.

According to the physician's assessment, the classification accuracy achieved by the naive Bayesian classifier is acceptable. Also the explanation of decisions provided by the naive Bayesian classifier is acceptable, since the sum of information gains in favour/against a given diagnosis and the explanation in terms of all the available attributes seem to be close to the way how physicians actually diagnose patients. On the other hand, the small number of attributes used in the decision trees was estimated as insufficient for reliable classification, since a decision tree tends to ignore significant information about the patient. Despite this deficiency, the decision tree of Assistant-R successfully replicates the physician's knowledge about the most important attributes and their logical relations, whereas the decision tree generated by Assistant-I is non-logical.

5 Discussion and further work

The best classification accuracy achieved (nearly 70%) is high if we take into the account the large number of different diagnoses and attributes and the fact that only 118 training instances are available. The study suggests that the good result is due to the appropriate selection of attributes describing the diagnoses.

The naive Bayesian classifier uses all the available attributes, achieves the highest classification accuracy, and provides transparent explanations of its decisions. Therefore, it was estimated as the learner (classifier) that can best support physicians' decisions in this stage of our application. On the other hand, decision trees were estimated as less apropriate since their decisions and explanations are based on few attributes only. These conclusions are in agreement with previous studies of machine learning applications in medicine [2]. In the future, the number of training instances will increase since the physicians are planning to input data of new patients on-line using the expert system shell developed for this application. With new training instances we are expecting to build a more accurate and robust diagnostic system. We are also planning to extend the current expert system to support the diagnosis of other sport injuries.

References

1. Cestnik, B., Kononenko, I., and Bratko, I. (1987). ASSISTANT 86: A knowledge elicitation tool for sophisticated users. In I. Bratko and N. Lavrač, editors, *Progress in Machine Learning*, pages 31–45. Sigma Press, Wilmslow.
2. Kononenko, I. (1993). Inductive and Bayesian learning in medical diagnosis. *Applied Artificial Intelligence*, 7:317-337.
3. Kononenko, I. and Šimec, E. (1995). Induction of decision trees using RELIEFF. In: G. Della Riccia, R. Kruse and R. Viertl (eds.), *Proc. of ISSEK Workshop on Mathematical and statistical methods in Artificial Intelligence*, (Udine, September 1994), Springer Verlag, pp.199-220.

Decision-Support Theories

A Theoretical Framework for Decision Trees in Uncertain Domains: Application to Medical Data Sets

B. Crémilleux

GREYC, CNRS - UPRESA 1526
Université de Caen
Esplanade de la Paix
F-14032 Caen Cédex France
cremilleux@info.unicaen.fr

C. Robert

Institut de Recherche
en Mathématiques Appliquées
Université Joseph Fourier
BP 53 X
F-38041 Grenoble Cédex France
crobert@mail-serv.inrialpes.fr

Abstract. Experimental evidence shows that many attribute selection criteria involved in the induction of decision trees perform comparably. We set up a theoretical framework that explains this empirical law. It furthermore provides an infinite set of criteria (the C.M. criteria) which contains the most commonly used criteria. We also define C.M. pruning which is suitable in uncertain domains. In such domains, like medicine, some sub-trees which don't lessen the error rate can be relevant to point out some populations of specific interest or to give a representation of a large data file. C.M. pruning allows to keep such sub-trees, even when keeping the sub-trees doesn't increase the classification efficiency. Thus we obtain a consistent framework for both building and pruning decision trees in uncertain domains. We give typical examples in medicine, highlighting routine use of induction in this domain even if the targeted diagnosis cannot be reached for many cases from the findings under investigation.

1. Introduction

Decision trees have been used successfully for many different decision making and classifications tasks. Medicine is an important application domain for such methods (see for example [1], [21] and [13]). Broadly speaking, a decision tree is built from a set of training data having attribute values and a class name. The result of the process is represented as a tree in which nodes specify attributes and branches specify attribute values. Leaves of the tree correspond to sets of examples with the same class or to elements in which no more attributes are available. Construction of decision trees is described, among others, by Breiman *et al.* [2] who present an important and well-known monograph on classification trees. A number of standard techniques have been developed in the machine learning community, like the basic algorithms ID3 [32] and CART [2]. A survey of different methods of decision tree classifiers and the various existing issues are presented in Safavian and Landgrebe [36].

In induction of decision trees various attribute selection criteria are used to estimate the quality of attributes in order to select the best one to split on. We will see in Section 2 that considerable research effort has been directed towards comparison of different attribute selection criteria in real world domains ([29] and [5]). It appears that most commonly used criteria perform comparably: this is an empirical law. We cannot escape from setting up a theoretical framework that explains this empirical law. To achieve this, we write down (in Section 2) the basic constraints of the problem. We derive from them an infinite set of criteria which we call C.M. criteria (concave-maximum or convex-minimum criteria). We will see that the most commonly used criteria which are the Shannon entropy (in the family of ID3 algorithms) and the Gini criterion (in CART algorithm), are C.M. criteria; we can predict at a theoretical level that all C.M. criteria yield similar trees.

In medicine, as in many areas, we are sure a priori that it is impossible to build a tree that correctly classifies all the examples. In such situations, decision tree algorithms tend to divide nodes having few examples and a main drawback appears (see [2], [31], [6] and [37]): the resulting trees tend to be very large and overspecified. Some branches, especially towards the bottom, are due to sample variability and are statistically meaningless (one can also say that they are present due to noise in the sample). Such branches must either not be built or be pruned. If we do not want to build them, we have to set out rules to stop the building of the tree. We know it is better to generate the entire tree and then to prune it (see for example [2] and [16]). In Section 3, we propose a pruning method (called C.M. pruning) suitable in uncertain domains. C.M. pruning builds a new attribute binding the root of a tree with its leaves, the attribute's values corresponding to the branches leading to a leaf. It permits computation of the global quality of a tree. The best sub-tree for pruning is the one that yields the highest quality pruned tree. This pruning method is not tied to the use of the pruned tree as a classifier. Thus we have a consistent framework for both building and pruning decision trees.

In Section 4, we present examples in medical domains where we routinely use decision trees either as a statistical descriptive tool allowing a representation of a large data set, or to point out some populations of specific interest. We compare trees pruned with C.M. pruning to hand-made pruned trees.

2. Building Decision Trees

One can find many experiments in the literature that compare several criteria with the intention of giving prominence to the suitable ones (see [26], [14], [27] and [25]). Mingers [29] compares the trees induced by ten selection criteria using data sets corresponding to four fields. These ten criteria all comply either with functions using impurity measures or with χ^2. He notes that the trees constructed with χ^2 seem to be a little more dense, but without being able to give any satisfactory explanation. Further we recall he notes that by choosing at random one attribute for each node, the induced trees hold around twice the amount of nodes as trees produced with other classical criteria. In a more recent paper, Buntine and Niblett [5] present additional results. They conclude that "the entropy criterion is statistically indistinguishable from the Gini criterion" ([5], p. 82).

Let us formulate the question of the attribute selection criterion. Let us consider a node Ω and let $Y_1,...,Y_p$ be the attributes under study. An attribute selection criterion consists in looking for an extremum of a function ψ; let us formulate it as a minimum search problem:

$$\psi(Y_{i_0}) = \min\{\psi(Y_i); i = 1..p\}$$

where Y_{i_0} denotes the attribute selected by the criterion ψ.

We present a straightforward sensible set of constraints. Let D be the class that we want to explain, with values $d_1,...,d_k$, and let Y be any attribute defined on the node Ω, with values $y_1,...,y_m$ (see Fig. 1).

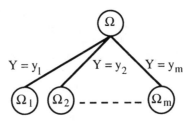

Fig. 1. Splitting of a node Ω using an attribute Y.

i)   The minimum value of ψ is reached if and only if the sub-nodes induced by Y are pure with respect to D, that is if and only if two examples with the same value of Y imply that they have the same value of D.

ii)   Let P (respectively P_i, i = 1...m) be the frequency distribution of D in Ω (respectively on the set Y = y_i, i = 1..m). ψ has its maximum value if and only if $P_1 = ... = P_m$ (which implies that P = P_i for all i).

iii) ψ (Y) can be viewed as a combined measure of impurity of the sub-nodes induced by Y. If we want ψ to take into account the respective sizes of the sub-nodes Ω_i (which is necessary in real world applications), the simplest form for ψ is:

$$\psi \, (Y) = \sum_{i}^{m} \alpha_i \, \varphi \, (\Omega_i) \text{ where } \Omega_1,...,\Omega_m \text{ are the sub-nodes yielded by Y, } \alpha_i \text{ is the rate}$$

of Ω_i in Ω, and φ is a function that quantifies the impurity of D in the node Ω_i.

Thus we are led to address the question of defining an impurity measure. A minimal set of constraints is:

(1) The impurity of D in Ω depends only on the frequency distribution $P = (p_1,...,p_k)$ of D in Ω. Thus a measure of impurity is a function φ defined on the set of k-uples with positive coordinates, the sum of which is 1. We will note either φ (P) or φ (Ω) the impurity of a node Ω.

(2) φ doesn't depend on the way we code D. Thus φ has to be equal over all permutations of the components of P. The mathematical term for this is: φ is a symmetric function.

(3) φ reaches its minimum value minφ if and only if D is a constant function on Ω.

(4) φ reaches its maximum value maxφ if all values of D are equally frequent.

(5) Combining groups tends to increase the impurity. For example, when we combine r groups Ω_i, D might be constant on each of them, while D might not be constant on the whole group; from i) φ (Ω_i) = minφ and φ (Ω) $\geq$ minφ with $\Omega = \Omega_1 \cup ... \cup \Omega_r$.

We have to translate this into a mathematical form and for that, we suggest to refer to current considerations in the fields of statistics (and particularly in ANOVA). We define an intra-group impurity by $\sum \alpha_i \, \varphi \, (\Omega_i)$ where α_i is the rate of Ω_i in Ω; we suppose φ can be linearly split into an intra-group impurity component and an inter-groups impurity component:

$$\varphi \, (\Omega) = \text{inter-groups impurity} + \sum \alpha_i \, \varphi \, (\Omega_i)$$

Since the inter-groups impurity is a positive quantity, φ has to satisfy the constraint:

$$\varphi \, (\Omega) \geq \sum \alpha_i \, \varphi \, (\Omega_i)$$

which can be written:

$$\varphi\ (P) \geq \sum \alpha_i\ \varphi\ (P_i)$$

where P (resp. P_i) is the frequency distribution of D in Ω (resp. in Ω_i).

Let us remark that the selection criterion ψ (Y) satisfying iii) is simply the intra-group impurity of the partition of Ω yielded by Y and that the impurity of Ω is greater than or equal the average impurity of the sub-nodes. We can also say that this condition states that splitting nodes does not increase impurity.

But since $P = \sum \alpha_i\ P_i$, the condition $\varphi\ (P) \geq \sum \alpha_i\ \varphi\ (P_i)$ means that φ is concave. One can then show [7], that if φ is strictly concave (i.e. $\varphi\ (P) = \sum \alpha_i\ \varphi\ (P_i)$ only if $\alpha_i = 1$ for some i, or if $P = P_1 =...= P_m$) and is symmetric, then it satisfies constraints (1) to (5). Finally, any element of the set $\mathcal{C}$ of symmetric strictly concave functions is a proper function to define an impurity measure. The most commonly used concave functions and their properties are described for example in Rockafellar [35]. Furthermore, the intra-group impurity ψ defined by iii) satisfies i) and ii).

Finally we have a whole set of possible criteria, which will be called concave minimum criteria. If we had considered a maximum search criterion (replacing ψ by $-\psi$) then we would have had to define purity measures and the proper set would have been the set of symmetric strictly convex functions which would have yielded "convex maximum criteria". We choose to introduce the attribute selection question with impurity, since the notion of impurity is usual in artificial intelligence and it is close to the notion of variance. It is clear that concave minimum criteria and convex minimum criteria are the same, up to a sign -. We will speak of C.M. criteria for both concave-minimum and convex-maximum criteria.

Which C.M. criterion should we choose? The involved impurity (or purity) functions of C.M. criteria have the same concave (or convex) shape and reach their extrema for the same arguments; thus:
1-If ψ_1 and ψ_2 are two C.M. criteria, Y and Y' are two attributes, then:
$\Delta = [\psi_1\ (Y) - \psi_1\ (Y')] \times [\psi_2\ (Y) - \psi_2\ (Y')]$ will be positive in most cases and both criteria select the same attribute. Experiments (see Section 4) show that when a criterion ψ_1 selects Y, while a second criterion ψ_2 selects Y', it appears that $\Delta_1 = [\psi_1\ (Y) - \psi_1\ (Y')]$ and $\Delta_2 = [\psi_2\ (Y) - \psi_2\ (Y')]$ are small. Thus with a reasonable precision we can consider that $\Delta_1 \approx \Delta_2 \approx 0$ and that the choice between Y and Y' is actually random.
2- We cannot give any theoretical simple condition implying that Δ is positive.

Let us now consider some commonly used selection criteria.
The most commonly used criterion [32] is that of entropy (which is also called information gain), coming from $\varphi\ (P) = - \sum p_i \log p_i$ with $P = (p_1,...,p_k)$, which is an impurity measure. It is a C.M. criterion.
The Gini criterion [2] uses $\varphi\ (P) = 1 - \sum_i p_i^2$ and is also a C.M. criterion.

The χ^2 criterion (examples are described in [18], [28] and [15]) selects the attribute Y, the chi-square value χ^2 (D,Y) of which is maximum. But χ^2 (D,Y) can be written in the form iii), up to a multiplicative constant N which is the number of elements in the considered node. Thus, using the previous notations,

$$\psi(Y) = \chi^2(D,Y) = \sum \alpha_i \, \varphi(P_i)$$

where $\varphi(P_i) = N \, || \, P_i - P \, ||^2_{(P)}$ Here $|| \, ... \, ||_{(P)}$ denotes the metric defined by the

diagonal matrix $\begin{pmatrix} 1/p_1 & & 0 \\ & \ddots & \\ 0 & & 1/p_k \end{pmatrix}$.

It appears that $-\varphi$ is a strictly concave function which is not symmetric; $-\varphi(P)$ has its maximum value when $P_1 = ... = P_m = P$, and its minimum value when all leaves induced by Y are pure. $-\varphi$ is not an impurity measure and the χ^2 criterion is not a C.M. criterion.

The ratio criterion, deriving from the entropy criterion, is customized to avoid favouring attributes with many values. Actually, in some situations, to select an attribute essentially because it has many values might jeopardize the semantic acceptance of the induced trees ([40] and [24]). The ratio criterion proposed by Quinlan [32] consists in maximizing $\psi(Y) = \dfrac{\varphi(P) - \sum \alpha_i \, \varphi(P_i)}{\varphi(P_Y)}$ where $\varphi(P)$ is the entropy

of P, ψ the associated function and $\varphi(P_Y)$ the entropy of the frequency distribution of Y in the node. It appears that ψ doesn't satisfy condition i) since it can reach its maximum value ($\psi(Y) = 1$) when the sub-nodes yielded by Y are not pure. One example is where D has three values, Y two values and if $Y = y_1$ implies $D = d_1$, while $Y = y_2$ implies $D = d_2$ or $D = d_3$. The ratio criterion is not a C.M. criterion.

Let us note that other selection criteria such as the J-measure [17] are related to other specific issues. The J-measure is the product of two terms that are considered by Goodman and Smyth as the two basic criteria for evaluating a rule: one term is derived from the entropy function and the other measures the simplicity of a rule. Quinlan and Rivest [33] were interested in the minimum description length principle to construct a decision tree minimizing a false classification rate when one looks for general rules and their case's exceptional conditions. This principle has been resumed by Wallace and Patrick [39] who suggest some improvements and show they generally obtain better empirical results than those found by Quinlan. Buntine [4] presents a tree learning algorithm stemmed from Bayesian statistics whose main objective is to provide outstanding predicted class probabilities on the nodes. Kira and Rendell [22] define the algorithm RELIEF for estimating the quality of attributes. The key idea of RELIEF is to assess attributes according to how well their values distinguish among instances that are near to each other. RELIEF is extended by Kononenko [23] to deal with noisy, incomplete, and multi-class data sets. Kononenko shows that, with some assumptions, the estimates of RELIEF are highly correlated with the Gini criterion. We can also address the question of deciding which sub-nodes have to be built. For a splitting, the GID3* algorithm [12] groups in a single branch the values of an attribute which are estimated meaningless compared to its other values. For building of binary trees, another criterion is twoing [2]. Twoing groups classes into two superclasses so that considered as a two-class problem, the greatest decrease in node impurity is realized. Some properties of twoing are described in Breiman [3]. Always for binary trees, Fayyad and Irani [11] propose the ORT measure. ORT favours attributes that simply separate the different classes without taking into account the number of examples of nodes so that ORT produces trees with small pure (or nearly pure) leaves at their top more often than C.M. criteria. Nevertheless, in uncertain domains, such leaves may be irrelevant and it is difficult to prune them without destroying the tree.

3. Pruning Decision Trees

The principal methods for pruning decision trees are examined in [30], [10] and [8]. Most of these pruning methods are based on minimizing a classification error rate when each element of the same node is classified in the most frequent class in this node. These pruning methods are inferred from situations where the built tree will be used as a classifier and they systematically discard a sub-tree which doesn't improve the used classification error rate. We will see that the resulting pruned tree produced by C.M. pruning could be different.

Let us now consider a C.M. criterion. The value of the criterion in a node reflects how appropriately the chosen attribute divides the data. If we consider impurity measures, the smaller the value of ψ, the better the split. The value of a criterion permits comparison of divisions of a node, but not of the whole sub-tree built below the node. Fortunately, theoretical considerations embedding C.M. criteria consistently yield a global quality index which will be used for pruning (see [8] for more details). Let us note I (T) the global quality index of the tree T. I (T) measures the difference between the impurity of the root of T and the mean impurity of its leaves, this difference being normalized to a value in [0,1]. I (T) = 1 if and only if all the leaves are pure, and I (T) = 0 if and only if the frequency distributions of D (the class) in the root and in all leaves of T are identical. I (T) doesn't actually depend on which C.M. criterion is used. Moreover if two trees T_1 and T_2 have the same mean impurity of their leaves but the impurities of their roots are not the same, I (T_1) and I (T_2) are different. So we can compare two trees built from two different samples of the same population (we will see examples in Section 4).

A straightforward pruning method (that we call C.M. pruning because it goes with using a C.M. criterion to build the tree) perfectly coherent with the building of the tree, consists in pruning the sub-tree T' of T such that T without T' has the highest quality [8]. C.M. pruning produces a family of nested trees spreading from the initial large tree to the tree restricted to its root. We will see in Section 4 that the curve of the global quality index as a function of the number of pruned tree gives a pragmatic method to stop the pruning process. The computational cost of C.M. pruning is particularly low and it is tractable even with large databases.

As previously mentioned, most pruning methods consist of pruning the sub-tree which minimizes a classification error rate. The resulting pruned tree is different from that produced when one uses C.M. pruning. For example C.M. pruning doesn't systematically discard a sub-tree, the classification error rate of which is equal to the rate of the root. In Fig. 2, D is bivalued and in each node the first (resp. second) value indicates the number of examples having the first (resp. second) value of D. This sub-tree doesn't lessen the error rate, which is 10% both in its root or in its leaves; nevertheless the sub-tree is of interest since it points out a specific population with a constant value of D while in the remaining population it's impossible to predict a value for D. The global quality index of this sub-tree is 0.55, which means that it explains 55% of the initial impurity.

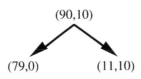

(90,10)

(79,0)   (11,10)

Fig. 2. A tree which could be interesting although it doesn't decrease the number of errors.

4. Experiments

We have designed induction software called ARBRE, (which means "tree" in French) which produces decision trees using C.M. criteria and which prunes trees with the C.M. pruning method. In this section we describe the results obtained by running ARBRE on two medical data sets. We have seen in the introduction that data sets from the medical domain are frequently used to test induction systems. Uncertainty (i.e. randomness) is basically unavoidable in the medical field. In some domains such as those in the examples below, one knows that the diagnosis is in most cases hardly feasible from the attributes under study. However an appropriately pruned tree may suggest how to separate some sub-populations where the diagnosis is feasible with the involved attributes from the sub-populations where no diagnosis decision can be made without further information. In such situations the tree cannot be used as a classifier; its quality will be poor yet it yields interesting results. Let us remark that in any case pruning is a key point the role of which is to discard the part of the tree that is essentially due to sample variation.

4.1. Data Sets

We consider the following two examples:
• *venous thrombo-embolism:* venous thrombosis is a common pathology which can lead to a pulmonary embolism thereby endangering the life of the patient [20]. Among patients having a deep venous thrombosis some will be suffering from pulmonary embolism and others will not. Pulmonary embolism diagnosis rests on more or less complex paraclinical findings and at present it is impossible to accurately predict the risk of this pathology. It is thus impossible to produce any tree which would permit classification of a reasonable part of the examples used to build it. The main aim of this study is to identify high risk populations to whom complementary examinations would be proposed. Physicians are aware that once these populations, if they exist, are considered aside, it is impossible to predict whether there will or will not be embolism in the remaining population; in other words they are aware that there is no hope of using the tree as a classifier for the whole population of patients with deep venous thrombosis.

This data set TE (thrombo-embolism data set) is composed of all the 1063 patients with deep venous thrombosis treated in the angiology department of the University Hospital at Grenoble (France) and for whom data are reliable. Around fifty percent of these cases were affected by pulmonary embolism (see Table 1). D (the class) is bivalued (embolism versus no-embolism).
• *genetic abnormalities:* genetic abnormalities touch about 1 couple in 600 [19]. Couples with chromosomal segregation allow for two possibilities in their descendants: alternate segregation (the child will be either normal or a healthy carrier)

or no-alternate segregation (which implies death or severe handicaps). The genetic cytology department of the Faculty of Medicine in Grenoble has at its disposal the largest European data set on these genetic abnormalities. This data set is constituted of two files:
- the first file G1 is composed of data coming from 86 European Medical Centers and collected from 1975 to 1986.
- the second file G2 is composed of cases published in the medical literature from 1971 to 1984.

Table 1. Details of the data files used. "No. of Attributes" indicates the number of attributes including D. "Values / Attributes" are the numbers of values of the attributes; "D" is the number of examples in each class determined by a value of D: in TE (resp. in G1 and G2), the first value is the number of patients who have suffered a pulmonary embolism (resp. alternate segregation) and the second value is the number of patients who never had a pulmonary embolism (resp. no-alternate segregation).

Data file	No. of Examples	No. of Attributes	Values / Attributes	D
TE	1063	7	2 - 3 - 4	528 - 535
G1	2993	15	2 - 3	2646 - 347
G2	3247	15	2 - 3	2456 - 791

The two files G1 and G2 involve the same attributes. Unlike in the TE set, the frequency distribution of D (alternate segregation versus no-alternate segregation) is highly unsymmetric (see Table 1). The two files were both completely unknown to expert physicians in the domain (such lack of prior knowledge is unusual in medicine but will become more common in the future, due to patient-data management systems). Decision trees provide them with the possibility of acquiring a valuable knowledge of these files. Indeed a decision tree represents all information contained in the data set and oriented by the evolution of the disease towards alternate segregation or no-alternate segregation.

4.2. Experimental Procedure

For each data set, we induced both trees using the two C.M. criteria available with ARBRE (entropy and Gini). We performed C.M. pruning with entropy criterion since it is stemmed from the most commonly used impurity measure (see for example [34] and [38]). We pruned each tree until the root was reached. Thus, we obtained a family of nested trees spreading from the initial large tree to the tree restricted to its root. It happens that considering the sequence of quality of these trees allows definition of a pragmatic method to choose a best pruned tree.

We also presented to expert physicians the initial large trees and we asked them to prune these trees; we call this method semantic pruning. We then compared C.M. pruning with semantic pruning.

4.3. Results and Discussion

We have predicted in Section 2 that C.M. criteria coming from functions with a common shape and common extrema should to a large extent be interchangeable. This prediction is verified in the three files. For each file, the trees obtained with entropy and with Gini criteria are very similar. For example, the TE tree produced with the entropy criterion is distinguished from the TE tree built with Gini criterion by only two inversions of attributes, but the close values of the criteria for these two attributes explain this phenomenon. Table 2 presents the characteristics of the initial large trees built with entropy criterion.

Table 2. Details of the initial large trees built with entropy criterion.
The number of nodes includes the leaves.

	Depth	No. of Nodes	No. of Leaves
TE	6	83	59
G1	12	88	48
G2	14	160	86

The TE tree exhibits some large leaves with a high embolism risk. These leaves were given confirmation by angiologists though most of them had not been previously brought to light. The trees built from G1 and G2 trees also exhibited relevant leaves with high frequency of alternate segregation. Let us remark that given the large number of attributes and the dissymmetry of the distribution of D, it would have been difficult to use other classical statistical descriptive methods. Finally it happened that though the data in the G1 and G2 files had not been collected in the same way, they yield trees with a close resemblance where the same attributes are selected at the same level of each tree. Here, trees used as descriptive tools yielded the conclusion that the two files could be combined.

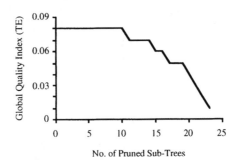

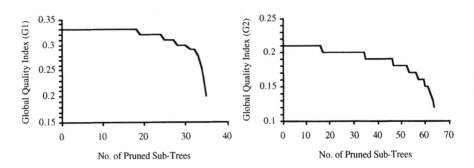

Fig. 3. For each tree, advancement of the global quality index according to the number of pruned sub-trees.

Let us now come back to the pruning stage. Fig. 3 is the graphical representation of the global quality index as a function of the number of pruned sub-trees. The global quality index of the TE tree is low (8% of the impurity of the root is explained by the considered attributes). As previously stated, this value is not so surprising given the great difficulty of pulmonary embolism diagnosis.

Let us now consider the global quality index as a function of the number of pruned trees. We see on the graphical representations in Fig. 3 that several sub-trees can be pruned without lessening the global quality index. In the three files considered, the shape of the curves in Fig. 3 indicates that the knowledge which is supplied by the induced trees is essentially at their tops [9]; thus only the highest parts of these trees are reliable. Furthermore, these curves indicate the relevant stages where pruning can be stopped; more precisely since these curves present flat or nearly flat parts, we can stop pruning when the number of pruned sub-trees is a number ending a flat segment of the curve.

The experts for their part pruned the tree until it was around two times smaller than the original tree. Moreover the trees obtained with semantic pruning were very close or identical to one of the trees provided by C.M. pruning. That is: for each family of nested trees, there is always a tree which is very similar (and even identical in the case of G1) to the tree provided by the semantic pruning. More precisely the trees provided by C.M. pruning which are the nearest to the trees given by semantic pruning all have their global quality index reduced by 1%.

5. Conclusion

The C.M. attribute selection criteria and the C.M. pruning can be performed consistently within the same theoretical framework. It contains the most commonly used criteria and it explains why these criteria perform comparably. It is a general framework since on the one hand there are no specific conditions on the attributes and on the other hand it doesn't rely on any specific use of the pruned tree. C.M. pruning allows to keep sub-trees with leaves yielding the determination of relevant decision rules, even when keeping the sub-trees doesn't increase the classification efficiency.

The use of a tree as a classifier is highlighted in the artificial intelligence field. In this paper, we stress on some other aspects of the use of decision trees which are, from our point of view, as important as the first, especially with the development of data collection in hospitals. More precisely, a tree built from a data set is an efficient description oriented by an a priori classification of its elements. Pruning the tree discards overspecific information to get a more legible description. A tree can also be built to distinguish some sub-populations of interest in large populations. Here only some leaves of the pruned tree will be considered for further investigation. Let us note that in all the situations described above, pruning is a key point.

Further work has to be done to compare more precisely C.M. pruning with other pruning techniques on consistent data sets. Let us remark that a limit of the global quality index is that its definition doesn't take into account the size of the tree hence the risk associated with the leaves. Another direction is to include such parameters.

References

[1]   Babic, A., Krusinska, E., & Strömberg, J. E. (1992) Extraction of diagnostic rules using recursive partitioning systems: a comparison of two approaches. *Artificial Intelligence in Medicine 4*, 373-387.

[2]   Breiman, L., Friedman, J. H., Olshen, R. A., & Stone, C. J. (1984) Classification and regression trees. Wadsworth. Statistics probability series. Belmont.

[3]   Breiman, L. (1996) Some properties of splitting criteria (technical note). *Machine Learning 21*, 41-47.

[4]   Buntine, W. (1992) Learning classification trees. *Statistics and Computing 2*, 63-73

[5]   Buntine, W., & Niblett, T. (1992) A further comparison of splitting rules for decision-tree induction. *Machine Learning 8*, 75-85.

[6]   Catlett, J. (1991) Overpruning large decision trees. *In proceedings of the Twelfth International Joint Conference on Artificial Intelligence IJCAI 91.* (pp 764-769). Sydney, Australia.

[7]   Crémilleux, B. (1991) Induction automatique : aspects théoriques, le système ARBRE, applications en médecine. Ph D thesis. Joseph Fourier University. Grenoble (France).

[8]   Crémilleux, B., & Robert, C. (1996) A Pruning Method for Decision Trees in Uncertain Domains: Applications in Medicine. *In proceedings of the workshop Intelligent Data Analysis in Medicine and Pharmacology, ECAI 96.* (pp 15-20). Budapest, Hungary.

[9]   Crémilleux, B., & Zreik, K. (1996) Le rôle de l'interaction personne-système lors de la production d'arbres de décision. *In proceedings of the international Conference on Human-System Learning CAPS 96.* (pp 20-31). Caen, France.

[10]   Esposito, F., Malerba, D., & Semeraro, G. (1993) Decision tree pruning as search in the state space. *In proceedings of European Conference on Machine Learning ECML 93.* (pp 165-184). Vienna (Austria), P. B. Brazdil (Ed.). Lecture notes in artificial intelligence. N° 667. Springer-Verlag.

[11]   Fayyad, U. M., & Irani, K. B. (1992) The attribute selection problem in decision tree generation. *In proceedings of Tenth National Conference on Artificial Intelligence.* (pp 104-110). Cambridge, MA: AAAI Press/MIT Press.

[12]   Fayyad, U. M. (1994) Branching on attribute values in decision tree generation. *In proceedings of Twelfth National Conference on Artificial Intelligence.* (pp 601-606). AAAI Press/MIT Press.

[13]   File, P. E., Dugard P. I., & Houston, A. S. (1994) Evaluation of the use of induction in the development of a medical expert system. *Computers and Biomedical Research 27*, 383-395.

[14]   Gams, M., & Petkovsek, M. (1988) Learning from examples in the presence of noise. *In proceedings of Eighth International Workshop Expert Systems and Their Applications.* (pp 609-624). Avignon, France.

[15]   Gascuel, O., & Caraux, G. (1992) Statistical significance in inductive learning. *In proceedings of the Tenth European Conference on Artificial Intelligence ECAI 92.* (pp 435-439). Vienne, Austria.

[16]   Gelfand, S. B., Ravishankar, C. S., & Delp, E. J. (1991) An iterative growing and pruning algorithm for classification tree design. *IEEE Transactions on Pattern Analysis and Machine Intelligence 13(2)*, 163-174.

[17]   Goodman, R. M. F., & Smyth, P. (1988) Information-theoretic rule induction. *In proceedings of the Eighth European Conference on Artificial Intelligence ECAI 88.* (pp 357-362). München, Germany.

[18] Hart, A. (1984) Experience in the use of an inductive system in knowledge engineering. In M. Bramer (Ed.), *Research and development in expert systems.* Cambridge University Press.

[19] Jalbert, P., Jalbert, H., & Sele, B. (1988) Types of imbalances in human reciprocal translocations: risks at birth. The cytogenetics of mammalian rearrangements, Alan R. Liss. 267-291.

[20] Janssen, F., Schachner, J., Hubbard, J., & Hartman, J. (1987) The risk of deep venous thrombosis: a computerized epidemiologic approach. *Surg. Am.*

[21] Kern, J., Dezelic, G., Dürrigl, T., & Vuletic, S. (1993) Medical decision making based on inductive learning method. *Artificial Intelligence in Medicine 5*, 213-223.

[22] Kira, K., & Rendell, L. (1992) A practical approach to feature selection. *In proceedings of the International Conference on Machine Learning.* (pp 249-256). Aberdeen, D. Sleeman & P. Edwards (Eds). Morgan Kaufmann.

[23] Kononenko, I. (1994) Estimating attributes: analysis and extensions of RELIEF. *In proceedings of European Conference on Machine Learning ECML 94.* (pp 171-182). Catania (Italy), F. Bergadano & L De Raedt (Eds.). Lecture notes in artificial intelligence. N° 784. Springer-Verlag.

[24] Kononenko, I. (1995) On biases in estimating multi-valued attributes. *In proceedings of the Fourteenth International Joint Conference on Artificial Intelligence IJCAI 95.* (pp 1034-1040). Montréal, Canada.

[25] Liu, W. Z., & White, A. P. (1994) The importance of attribute selection measures in decision tree induction. *Machine Learning 15*, 25-41.

[26] Lopez de Mantaras, R. (1991) A distance-based attribute selection measure for decision tree induction. *Machine Learning 6*, 81-92.

[27] Marshall, R. (1986) Partitioning methods for classification and decision making in medicine. *Statistics in Medicine 5*, 517-526.

[28] Mingers, J. (1986) Expert systems - experiments with rule induction. *Journal of the Operational Research Society 37(11)*, 1031-1037.

[29] Mingers, J. (1989) An empirical comparison of selection measures for decision-tree induction. Machine Learning 3, 319-342.

[30] Mingers, J. (1989) An empirical comparison of pruning methods for decision-tree induction. *Machine Learning 4*, 227-243.

[31] Niblett, T. (1987) Constructing decision trees in noisy domains. *In proceedings of 2nd European Working Sessions on Learning EWSL 87.* (pp 67-78). Bled (Yugoslavia), Sigma Press. Wilmslow.

[32] Quinlan, J. R. (1986) Induction of decision trees. *Machine Learning 1*, 81-106.

[33] Quinlan, J. R., & Rivest, R. L. (1989) Inferring decision trees using the minimum description length principle. *Information and Computation 80(3)*, 227-248.

[34] Quinlan J. R. (1993) C4.5 Programs for Machine Learning. San Mateo, CA. Morgan Kaufmann.

[35] Rockafellar, R. T. (1970) Convex analysis. Princeton University Press. Princeton. New Jersey.

[36] Safavian, S. R., & Landgrebe, D. (1991) A survey of decision tree classifier methodology. *IEEE Transactions on Systems, Man, and Cybernetics 21(3)*, 660-674.

[37] Schaffer, C. (1993) Overfitting avoidance as bias. *Machine Learning 10*, 153-178.

[38] Taylor, C. C., Michie D., & Spiegelhalter, D. J. (1994) Machine learning, neural and statistical classification. Ellis Horwood Series in Artificial Intelligence.

[39] Wallace, C. S., & Patrick, J. D. (1993) Coding decision trees. *Mach. Learn.11*, 7-22.

[40] White, A. P., & Liu, W. Z (1994) Bias in Information-Based Measures in Decision Tree Induction. *Machine Learning 15*, 321-329.

Developing a Decision-Theoretic Network for a Congenital Heart Disease[*]

Niels Peek[1] and Jaap Ottenkamp[2]

[1] Dept. of Computer Science, Utrecht University, P.O. Box 80.089, 3508 TB Utrecht,
e-mail: niels@cs.ruu.nl
[2] Dept. of Paediatric Cardiology, Academic Medical Centre, University of
Amsterdam, Meibergdreef 15, 1105 AZ Amsterdam

Abstract. To support paediatric cardiologists in prognostic assessment and treatment planning, a decision-theoretic network for congenital heart disease is being constructed. The network is built in collaboration with a domain expert, using modelling methods commonly advocated in the literature. Although these methods prove to be useful in many cases, it was found that in some situations their applicability falls short. These situations and their associated problems are described. Techniques that have been developed to effectively deal with the problems are presented.

1 Introduction

Recent work in the fields of artificial intelligence and statistical decision theory has yielded the framework of decision-theoretic networks [15]. The framework combines explicit, declarative domain models known from artificial intelligence with normative theories of decision making under uncertainty. In contrast with the classical decision-theoretic and knowledge-based approaches employed in the past two decades to decision making under uncertainty, the framework of decision-theoretic networks couples expressiveness to mathematical correctness. The framework is therefore especially suited as a basis for decision-theoretic expert systems.

In building a decision-theoretic network, the origins of the framework are reflected [13]. As with any expert system, knowledge has to be acquired from domain experts, literature and databases. As such, the knowledge-acquisition process accords with the methodologies for knowledge engineering proposed in recent years (cf. [16]). These knowledge-engineering methods have to be supplemented with modelling techniques from decision analysis and statistics. However, due to the often large size and complex dependence structure of network models, application of the latter techniques is not straightforward in the context of decision-theoretic networks [4]. It is also not apparent how knowledge-engineering techniques and statistical methods must be combined. Although

[*] The investigations were (partly) supported by the Netherlands Computer Science Research Foundation with financial support from the Netherlands Organization for Scientific Research (NWO).

considerable effort is being spent on developing and maintaining network models (e.g., [1, 5, 6, 8, 9]), detailed methodologies for building decision-theoretic networks are currently lacking.

The Tetrade project aims at the development of methods and tools for knowledge acquisition for decision-theoretic network-based systems, tailored to the problem class of prognostic assessment and treatment planning in medicine. The field of *paediatric cardiology* was chosen as a test bed for gaining experience in building decision-theoretic networks. *Ventricular septal defect* is the most common disorder that the paediatric cardiologist is confronted with. It is therefore relatively well-understood, and comparatively large amounts of data on the disorder are available. As these circumstances render good opportunities for network construction and validation, ventricular septal defect was chosen as the first problem domain to be examined.

In this paper, we describe the building of the qualitative part of a network model for ventricular septal defects. In the next section, we briefly review the theory of decision-theoretic networks. Section 3 addresses the aspects of ventricular septal defects that are relevant for the examples given in Sect. 4, in which the development of the network model is discussed. We describe how methods commonly advocated for network construction may fail in some situations. Techniques that have been developed to effectively deal with these problems. The paper is rounded off with some conclusions and a description of our future work in Sect. 5.

2 Decision-Theoretic Networks

A *decision-theoretic network*, or *influence diagram*, is a concise representation of a decision problem. It comprises a qualitative and a quantitative part. The qualitative part of a decision-theoretic network encodes in a *directed acyclic graph* all variables that are relevant to the decision problem at hand. In the graph, three types of node are distinguished. A *decision node* represents viable decisions or actions that can be taken by the decision maker, a *probabilistic variable* represents an uncertain entity, the outcome of which cannot be selected by the decision maker, and the *value node* models the desirability of the various decisions and their consequences. The arcs in the digraph bear different meanings, depending on the types of their incident vertices. For example, the set of all arcs between probabilistic vertices captures the (conditional) independency relation between these variables; informally speaking, these arcs may be interpreted as directed 'influential' or 'causal' relationships between the linked variables. Associated with the qualitative part of the network is a quantitative part. This part consists of a numerical assessment of the strengths of the represented probabilistic relationships and of the desirabilities of the various decisions and their consequences. For the purpose of computing best decisions from a decision-theoretic network, several algorithms have been developed (e.g. [17]). *Belief networks* may be taken as decision-theoretic networks without decision and value nodes. In the design of a decision-theoretic network, a belief network can act as a convenient basis. In this paper, we restrict ourselves to the construction of belief networks.

Decision-theoretic networks may be abstracted to *qualitative networks* by replacing their numerical assessments with signs ('+', '−' or '?'), expressing qualitative influences and synergies [20]. Although qualitative networks are not as expressive as fully quantified networks, they bring several advantages. Qualitative networks may replace decision-theoretic networks where numerical assessments are either not available or not necessary for solving the decision problem at hand, or they may be used in addition to quantified networks for explaining reasoning in qualitative terms [10]. Also, qualitative networks may serve as an intermediate representation in the knowledge-acquisition process [3]. In this paper, we address this last application of qualitative probabilistic networks.

3 The Problem Domain: Ventricular Septal Defects

A significant problem for the paediatric cardiologist in the management of patients with a cardiac anomaly is to decide if and when a patient has to be submitted to surgical treatment. In the management of these patients, there is always a trade-off between the benefits gained by waiting before surgical intervention in the hope that the patient's condition will improve, and the risks caused by the poor natural history of these disorders [14]. The number of factors involved in this decision-making process is large and their interplay is subtle. Therefore, it is extremely difficult for the clinician to determine which timing of medical and surgical treatment will be optimal for a given patient. In general terms, this problem may be characterised as planning under uncertainty with time constraints. Although the need for decision support in this problem domain is recognised by paediatric cardiologists, no system currently exists to support this decision-making process.

Ventricular septum defect (VSD) is a relatively well-understood disorder with many clinical features that are characteristic for congenital heart disease in general. It was therefore chosen as the first problem domain to be examined in the Tetrade project. VSD is a defect in the ventricular septum, the fibromuscular wall that separates the left and the right ventricle. An immediate consequence of this defect is blood flow ("shunt") from the left to the right ventricle due to ventricular pressure differences. The shunt size, *i.e.*, the amount of blood flowing through the defect, depends primarily on the size of the defect and the relation of pulmonary and systemic vascular resistances. During the foetal stage, the muscular pulmonary arteries are small in diameter with a thick smooth muscular wall, thus preventing massive shunting by their high resistance. Following birth, the arteries change to thin-walled structures with increased internal diameter. These changes are accompanied by a decline in pulmonary vascular resistance, resulting in an increased shunt size.

Left-to-right shunting causes oxygenous blood to be pumped into the lungs again. As a result, the pulmonary pressure will rise, and systemic cardiac output will decrease. The latter effect usually causes the patient to be pale and easily sweating. With large defects, the high pulmonary pressure (*pulmonary hypertension*) may lead to left heart failure, and also, in the long run, to right heart failure. Left heart failure is typically accompanied by shortness of breath, feeding problems, and a complex of symptoms that is usually termed 'failure to thrive'. Furthermore, abnormal breath sounds can be heard on auscultation (*pulmonary crepitations*). Signs of right heart failure are *cardiomegaly* (enlarged heart), *hepatomegaly* (enlarged liver), and *oedema*.

With small defects, the clinical course is favourable throughout infancy and childhood [11]. About 75 to 80% of the defects close spontaneously, with the majority closing in the first two years of life. Patients with moderate-sized defects may develop large left-to-right shunts and associated complications in infancy, but the majority of this group can be managed medically without surgical intervention. Patients with large defects are more difficult to manage, because of the risks of mortality in the first year of life due to heart failure and associated pulmonary infections. Elevated pulmonary vascular resistance may also develop as a response to continuous pulmonary overflow and hypertension [7]; this is termed *Eisenmenger's complex*. It may result in severe, irreversible damage to the pulmonary arteries (*arteriopathy*). Early surgical intervention is therefore strongly recommended for these patients. The majority of patients with repair of uncomplicated VSD in infancy or early childhood have an excellent result with no clinical signs or symptoms and apparently normal long-term survival.

4 Building the Network Model

Building a decision-theoretic network for a domain of application involves various tasks. The first of these is to identify the *variables* that are of importance in the domain at hand, along with their possible values. Once the important variables have been identified, the construction of the qualitative part of the network can start: the second task is to identify the *probabilistic relationships* among the variables discerned and to express these relationships in an acyclic digraph. The last task in building a decision-theoretic network is to estimate the (conditional) probabilities that are required to constitute its quantitative part.

Here, we focus on the second task in the building of a network model: the construction of the qualitative part of the network, *i.e.*, the topology of the digraph. Formally, this task comprises identification of the independence relation of the joint probability distribution on the variables discerned. In practice, however, the digraph typically is constructed directly without explicitly identifying the independence relation. For most application domains, the qualitative part of a network model has to be *hand-crafted* with the help of one or more domain experts. For eliciting the topology of the digraph of the network, often the concept of *causality* is used as a heuristic guiding rule during the interview with a domain expert; typical questions asked are "What could cause this effect?", "What manifestations could this cause have?" [9]. The thus elicited causal relations among the variables discerned are easily expressed in graphical terms by taking the direction of causality for directing the arcs between related variables; this graphical representation can then be taken as a basis for feedback to the domain expert for further refinement. Building on the concept of causality has the advantage that domain experts are allowed to express their knowledge in either the *causal* or *diagnostic* direction. Since they are allowed to express their knowledge in a form they feel comfortable with, the experts' statements tend to be quite robust. This especially holds in medical domains, where the various factors involved in the clinical description of a disorder are often characterised in terms of cause-effect relations.

Yet, not every influential relationship among variables can be interpreted causally. If a non-causal influential relationship comes to the fore, a more elaborate analysis of the independences involved is required before it can be expressed in graphical terms. In the sequel, we discuss three situations where using causality as a principle modelling guideline may be confusing or even lead to incorrect results. For each of these situations, we provide a method to circumvent or solve the problem.

First, causality is not a well-understood concept and therefore may leave room for multiple interpretations. In particular, there may be substantial differences in the amount of time it takes for 'causes' to render their 'effects'. Sometimes the relations described by directed graph found in medical textbooks are better understood in terms of state transitions over time than in terms of causality. This was one of the reasons that we decided to make a separate description of the clinical course of VSD in terms of major pathophysiological development stages. This description complements the static description provided by the network model; a full account is given in Subsect. 4.1. A second situation in which causality may hamper instead of help the construction of the digraph is the presence of feedback loops. To avoid directed cycles in the topology of the digraph, alternative modelling techniques are then required. In Subsect. 4.2, we discuss two example feedback loops in the VSD domain, and the way we decided to model them. Finally, it is not uncommon to find many qualitative abstractions in the vocabulary of a clinician. Such abstractions cannot be understood in terms of cause-effect relations, and therefore have to dealt with differently. The modelling of abstractions is discussed in Subsect. 4.3.

4.1 Modelling Development Stages of a Disorder

One of the problems we encountered during model building was the fact that there are several stages in the pathophysiological development of a VSD, and each stage has its own characteristics. Although it was possible to construct a single, static model that accounted for each of the stages and its characteristics, the resulting model did not seem to suit the clinician's intuition very well. For instance, this model (to which we will refer as the *general network model*) includes a variable SHUNT, taking a value from the domain {*no_shunting*, *small_left-to-right_shunt*, *large_left-to-right_shunt*, *right-to-left_shunt*}. Among the successors in the digraph of this variable are included both typical signs of left-to-right shunting, such as paleness and sweating, as typical signs of right-to-left shunting, such as cyanosis. Simultaneous occurrence of these signs, however, is excluded.

As the domain expert pointed out, it is therefore not very natural to see these signs co-occurring in a single network model.

Our solution to this problem consisted of the following steps. First, the pathophysiological stages of the disease development were identified. Then, we explored which reductions to the general network model were possible in each stage. The models resulting from applying these reductions are called *stage models*. They are reduced versions of the general model, and contain only the parts that are relevant for the associated pathophysiological development stage. Reductions of the model consist of (possibly partial) value assignments to variables and removing variables and relations where possible.

The stages in the pathophysiological development of a VSD were distinguished by the domain expert. First, there is an initial stage (six to thirteen weeks after birth) during which the pulmonary vascular resistance decreases and the left-to-right shunt increases. In the second stage the left-to-right shunt has reached its maximum, causing heart failure with its associated signs. Subsequently, in the third stage, (a) either the defect size gradually decreases or (b) the Eisenmenger's complex may follow. In both cases left-to-right shunting will diminish, rendering a significant improvement in the condition of the patient. However, whereas decreasing defect size will lead to defect closure and vanishing clinical signs (fourth stage, a), increased pulmonary vascular resistance due to Eisenmenger's complex will eventually cause shunt reversal and cyanosis (fourth stage, b).

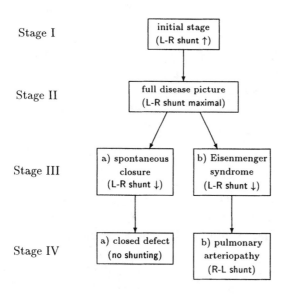

Fig. 1. Stages in the pathophysiological development of a VSD.

Central to model reduction was the variable SHUNT. Recall that right-to-left shunting is excluded in the first three stages of development. We can therefore remove the value *right-to-left_shunt* from the variable's domain in the associated stage models. Consequently, a number of variables representing characteristic effects of right-to-left shunting (e.g., CYANOSIS) can be removed from the stage models. On the other hand, left-to-right shunting cannot occur in the fourth stage. So, the values *small_left-to-right_shunt* and *large_left-to-right_shunt* can be excluded from the SHUNT domain in the stage model for stage IV. In this case, the variables representing characteristic effects of left-to-right shunting (e.g. HEART FAILURE and PULMONARY FLOW-HYPERTENSION) can be removed.

Node removal is valid in these cases because some of the relations between the variable SHUNT and its successors are not probabilistic but *deterministic* in nature. Deterministic relations can often be detected in the vocabulary and reasoning of the clinician. In the present example, it was detected that the domain expert often equated 'right-to-left shunting' and 'cyanosis' in his explanations. Detecting deterministic relations is useful in several respects: it reduces the number of probabilities that have to be assessed, and can be used to infer strong conditional independency statements that facilitate efficient computations [19].

4.2 Coping With Feedback Loops

The main physiological component in the domain of congenital heart disease is a closed-loop haemodynamic system. It is not very surprising, then, that one of the problems we were confronted with during model development was the occurrence of *feedback loops*. In the case of a VSD, the size of the left-to-right shunt depends on the interventricular pressure gradient, which in turn depends on the relative pulmonary pressure (compared to systemic pressure). On the other hand, the relative pulmonary pressure is increased by the shunting of blood through the defect. When we try to model these dependences in causal fashion, a (directed) cycle occurs in the network (see Fig. 2a).

Another example feedback process is Eisenmenger's complex. Continued left-to-right shunting through the VSD will increase the pulmonary arterial pressure. In time, this results in damage to the pulmonary arterioles, and increasing pulmonary vascular resistance. Although the pulmonary pressure will remain high, the pulmonary blood volume (*i.e.*, the shunt size) will decrease. This is depicted in Fig. 2b.

We note that a cyclic digraph representing a feedback process can be viewed as a compact representation of an infinite acyclic digraph containing each variable indexed by time [18]. A possible solution to the problem of directed cycles is therefore to reject the compact representation and to explicitly model the feedback process in a *dynamic network model* [2]. Dynamic network models extend the belief-network formalism by allowing temporal reasoning over a series of (structurally identical) static networks ("slices") indexed by time.

Although dynamic network models provide an elegant and mathematically sound way to represent feedback processes, their usefulness in practical circumstances is limited. Not only the size of the network model and computational complexity increase drastically, dynamic representation of the feedback process is

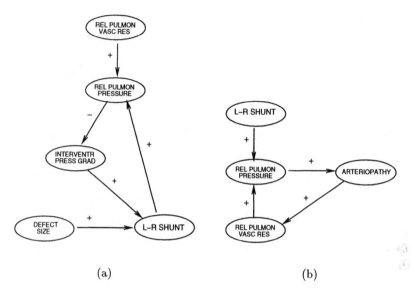

Fig. 2. (a) haemodynamic feedback loop, and (b) Eisenmenger's complex.

also very fine-grained, and a regression model of the feedback process is needed. Therefore, we think that dynamic network models only should be used when the time spanned by the feedback process is large and multiple observations on the variables involved may be performed within that time span. This applies to the feedback process due to Eisenmenger's complex: this process may take several years, and usually many observations on the clinical state of patient are made during this period. The dynamic part of the network model for Eisenmenger's complex is shown in Fig. 3b (see below for an explanation of the variable PRESSURE RATIOS).

For short-term feedback processes, a solution within the static domain model is favourable. Then, an alternative representation without directed cycle has to be found, for which various options exist. These include adding and removing arcs, reversing one or more arcs, adding one or more variables to the digraph, and clustering multiple variables in a single network node. We do not believe there is a single, best option; the solution that is chosen should, however, yield a satisfactory model and be supported by domain-specific arguments. An example of solution of 'cutting' cycles by adding and removing arcs supported by domain-specific arguments can be found in [12]. We have chosen to cluster the variables RELATIVE PULMONARY PRESSURE and INTERVENTRICULAR PRESSURE GRADIENT into one super node PRESSURE RATIOS. The argument is that in under normal circumstances, the values of the two aforementioned variables are equal; the clinician considers both variables to be known with certainty once either of both has been observed. Subsequently, a topology for the network containing the super node was designed in collaboration with the domain expert. The relevant part of the resulting network is shown in Fig. 3a.

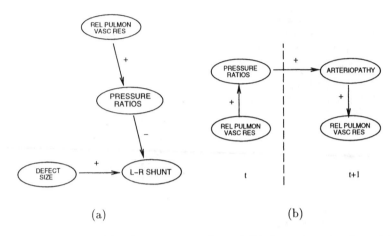

Fig. 3. Solutions: (a) using a super node, and (b) dynamic network model.

4.3 Modelling Qualitative Abstractions

In many medical domains, the vocabulary that is used by clinicians contains qualitative abstractions of biochemical and physiological states or processes involved. Typically, a specific term is introduced to indicate that some quantity has reached some (critical) value, or that a typical combination of values is at stake. For instance, in the domain of cardiac anomalies, when the oxygen saturation of the systemic blood drops below 92%, this is classified as *cyanosis*. Similarly, when the systolic pulmonary pressure exceeds 1/4 of the systolic systemic pressure due to large left-to-right shunting, one speaks of *pulmonary flow-hypertension* (see Fig. 4).

It is useful to recognise such abstractions during the model building for several reasons. First, there is usually a "hard" condition involved in the classification step; We have indicated this in Fig. 4 by the label 'c: > 1/4' on the arc between REL-ATIVE PULMONARY PRESSURE and PUL-MONARY FLOW-HYPERTENSION. As was noted in Subsect. 4.1, recognition of such deterministic relations reduces the num-

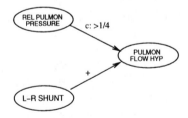

Fig. 4. Abstraction variable.

ber of probabilities to be assessed. Second, if an abstraction variable has successors in the digraph, this will usually indicate an undesired loss of precision. It will be favourable to re-evaluate the relation between these nodes and the predecessors of the abstraction variable; In many circumstances, a direct, influential relation can then be found. Returning to the aforementioned example, our domain expert initially stated that pulmonary flow-hypertension causes arteriopathy in the long run. While this is not untrue, it is more precise to state that continuous elevated pulmonary vascular pressure causes arteriopathy. As the pulmonary vascular pressure is modelled in quantitative terms, modelling the latter relation instead of the former yields more precision. We remark that the introduction of an abstraction variable has no effect on the complexity of the network model if the classification variable has no successors in the digraph. This is due to the fact that the variable itself will not be instantiated. Therefore, no dependencies between its predecessors in the graph are introduced.

Figure 5 shows the network model for VSD in stage III. We have made a distinction between primary and secondary determinants of the patient's clinical state, and variables whose values only result from this state, but do not have effect on others. In the case of VSD, the clinical state of the patient depends primarily on the size of the defect and the relative pulmonary vascular resistance. These variables are grouped by the dashed box with label A in the figure; They determine the state of variables like the relative pulmonary pressure, ventricular pressure gradient, direction and size of the shunt and the degree of heart failure. Dashed box B contains these secondary determinants. These variables in turn affect the state of many observable variables representing signs and symptoms. Finally, we have distinguished to variables that represent critical developments in the clinical state of the disorder. These are spontaneous closure of the defect, and Eisenmenger's complex; They are contained in dashed boxes with label C.

5   Conclusions and Future Work

The framework of decision-theoretic networks is becoming increasingly popular as a basis for medical decision-theoretic expert systems. The framework has proven its usefulness in a number of real-world applications. However, detailed methodologies for building decision-theoretic networks are still lacking.

In this paper, we have described the manual construction of network model for ventricular septal defect with the help of a paediatric cardiologist. We followed the often advocated heuristic of using 'causality' as a guideline in the modelling process. Although this heuristic proved to be useful in large part, it was found that in some situations its applicability falls short, or even may hamper efficient model construction. These include the situation that several stages of development are discerned in the clinical state of the patient, that feedback processes may exist in the domain, and that qualitative abstractions are used. To deal with each of these situations, specific techniques have been developed.

We have described a simplified version of the VSD model that will be used as a basis for a decision-theoretic expert system. We are currently implementing the model, which counts up to 38 nodes and 52 arcs, as a qualitative probabilistic network. The resulting preliminary system will be used as feedback to the domain expert for possible refinement. Subsequently, the numerical prob-

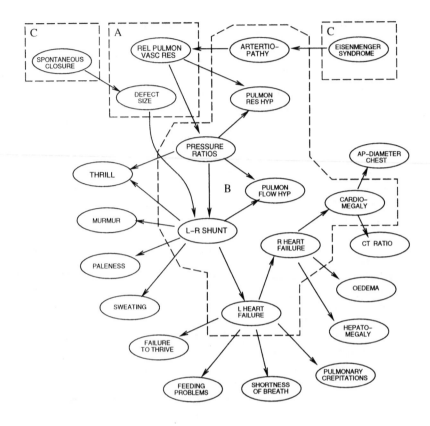

Fig. 5. VSD model for stage III.

abilities forming the quantitative part of the network model will be assessed. For this task, the framework described in [3] will be used to combine numerical information from various sources. Finally, the model will be embedded in a decision-support architecture.

Acknowledgements. The authors wish to thank Linda van der Gaag and Peter Lucas for many useful comments on earlier drafts of this paper.

References

1. Andreassen, S., Hovorka, R., Benn, J., Olesen, K. and Carson, E.: A model-based approach to insulin adjustment, In: M. Stefanelli et al., *Proc 3rd Conf on Artificial Intelligence in Medicine*, Berlin: Springer Verlag (1991) 239–248
2. Dagum, P. and Galper, A.: Forecasting sleep apnea with dynamic network models. *Proc 9th Conf on Uncertainty in Artificial Intelligence* (1993) 41–48

3. Druzdzel, M. and Van der Gaag, L.: Eliciation of probabilities for belief networks: combining qualitative and quantitative information. *Proc 11th Conf on Uncertainty in Artificial Intelligence* (1995) 141–148
4. Druzdzel, M., Van der Gaag, L., Henrion, M. and Jensen, F. (*eds.*): *Building Probabilistic Networks: Where Do the Numbers Come From?* IJCAI-95 Workshop, Montreal, Quebec, Canada (1995)
5. Egar, J., Puerta, A. and Musen, M.: Graph-grammar assistance for modeling of decisions, In: B.R. Gaines et al., *Proc 7th AAAI Knowledge Acquisition for KB Systems WS*, Banff: SRDG Publications (1992)
6. Goldman, R. and Charniak, E.: A language for the construction of belief networks. *IEEE Trans on Pattern Analysis and Machine Intelligence*, **15(3)** (1993) 196–208
7. Graham, T., and Gutgesell, H.: Ventricular septal defekts. In: A.J. Moss, F.H. Adams et al., *Heart Disease in Infants, Children, and Adolescents*, Baltimore: Williams & Wilkins (1995) 724–746
8. Heckerman, D., Horvitz, E. and Nathwani, B.: Toward normative expert systems: part II – probability-based representations for efficient knowledge acquisition and inference, *Methods of Information in Medicine* **31** (1992) 106–116
9. Henrion, M.: Some practical issues in constructing belief networks. In: L.N. Kanal et al., *Uncertainty in Artificial Intelligence 3*, Amsterdam: Elsevier (1989) 161–173
10. Henrion, M. and Druzdzel, M.: Qualitative propagation and scenario-based approaches to explanation of probabilistic reasoning. In: L.N. Kanal and J.F. Lemmer, *Uncertainty in Artificial Intelligence 6*, Amsterdam: Elsevier (1991) 17–32
11. Kidd, L., Driscoll, D. and Gersony, W.: Second natural history study of congenital heart defects: results of treatment of patients with ventricular septal defects. *Circulation* **87** (1993) 138-151
12. Korver, M. and Lucas, P.: Converting a rule-based system into a belief network. *Medical Informatics* **18(3)** (1993) 219–241
13. Lucas, P.: Knowledge acquisition for decision-theoretic expert systems. *AISB Quarterly* **94** (1996) 23–33
14. Macartney, F., Spiegelhalter, D. and Rigby, M.: Medical management, in: R.H. Anderson et al., *Paediatric Cardiology*, Vol. 1, Edinburgh: Churchill Livingstone (1987) 421–442
15. Pearl, J.: *Probabilistic Reasoning in Intelligent Systems: Networks of Plausible Inference*, Morgan Kaufmann Publishers, Palo Alto, 1998
16. Schreiber, A., Wielinga, B., De Hoog, R., Akkermans, H. and Van de Velde, W.: CommonKADS: a comprehensive methodology for KBS development. *IEEE Expert*, **9(6)** (1994) 28–37
17. Shachter, R.: Evaluating influence diagrams. *Operations Research* **34** (1996) 79–90
18. Spirtes, P.: Directed cyclic graphical representations of feedback models. *Proc 11th Conf on Uncertainty in Artificial Intelligence* (1995) 491–498
19. Van der Gaag, L. and Meyer, J.-J.: Characterising normal forms for informational independence. *Proc 6th Int Conf on Information Processing and Management of Uncertainty in Knowledge-Based Systems* (1996) 973–978
20. Wellman, M.: Fundamental concepts of qualitative probabilistic networks. *Artificial Intelligence* **44(3)** (1990) 257–303

A Theory of Medical Diagnosis as Hypothesis Refinement

Peter Lucas

Utrecht University, Department of Computer Science,
Padualaan 14, 3584 CH Utrecht, The Netherlands
E-mail: lucas@cs.ruu.nl

Abstract. In this paper, medical diagnosis is viewed as a two-stage process: medical knowledge is first interpreted in a diagnostic sense; next, observed findings are interpreted with respect to this interpreted knowledge and a given hypothesis, yielding a diagnosis. A new set-theoretical framework is introduced that captures this view of diagnosis; it is used to formalize various notions of diagnosis, those proposed in the literature included. Next, a new theory of flexible diagnosis, called refinement diagnosis, is proposed and defined in terms of this framework. Relationships with notions of diagnosis known from the literature are investigated.

1 Introduction

In recent years, several theories of diagnosis have been proposed, providing different foundations for diagnostic problem solving in intelligent systems. Much of this work focuses on techniques for diagnosing hardware faults in technical equipment; relatively little of this work has been applied to the medical field. Nevertheless, much of this research is also relevant for medical diagnosis.

In the literature on diagnosis, diagnostic problem solving is variously described in terms of *abductive reasoning* (cf. [4, 9, 10]), as a specific form of *consistency-based reasoning* (cf. [12, 5, 7]), or as *deductive reasoning* (cf. [1]). In the context of diagnosis, one usually speaks of *abductive diagnosis, consistency-based diagnosis*, and *heuristic classification* [3], respectively. Abductive diagnosis is used in medical expert systems incorporating causal disease models. Such systems have been developed by Tuhrim et al., [13], and by Punch et al., [11], among others. Consistency-based diagnosis was shown to be suitable for diagnosing problems using models of normal structure and functional behaviour, such as models of electronic equipment [12]. K.L. Downing, however, has investigated the application of consistency-based diagnosis to medical physiology [6]. Abductive and consistency-based diagnosis are often classified as *model-based* approaches to diagnosis. Heuristic classification is used in systems based on empirical knowledge, typically, but not always, rule-based expert systems [1].

The diagnostic frameworks mentioned above differ in several respects, but in all of them diagnostic problem solving can be viewed as a special instance of *hypothetical* reasoning [10]. In solving a diagnostic problem, a hypothesis is first generated and next tested with respect to diagnostic knowledge and observed findings. If it passes the tests, it is accepted and called a diagnosis; when it fails to pass the tests, it is rejected. Although this view of diagnosis seems quite general, it is still unnecessarily restrictive, certainly when considering diagnosis in the medical field. Instead of simply rejecting a hypothesis that does not comply with all requirements, it seems more natural to adjust or refine it, when possible. Since medical knowledge bases are, almost without exception, incomplete, e.g. knowledge of certain interactions among disorders may be missing, and certain patient findings may be unknown, e.g. due to restricting to non-invasive diagnostic tests, or unreliable, e.g. the findings may be obtained by telephone, rigorous notions of diagnosis may be too strong. In medicine, it is usually better to arrive at a diagnosis that does not account for all observed findings, or that suggests findings that have not been observed, than to establish no diagnosis at all. The formalization of this as *refinement diagnosis* is the subject of this paper.

The structure of this paper is as follows. In Section 2, a brief summary of a set-theoretical framework of diagnosis, which may be viewed as a much generalized version of set-covering theory [9], is presented. In our description of diagnosis, we focus on the *structure* of diagnosis, not on the handling of uncertainty, which aspect is also central to diagnosis. The framework is employed to investigate notions of refinement diagnosis in Section 3.

2   A Framework of Diagnosis

In this section, we provide a brief overview of a set-theoretical framework of diagnosis that is used in the remainder of the paper (cf. [8]).

2.1   The Representation of Interactions

Consider the following piece of medical knowledge: "Influenza causes fever and infection of the trachea and bronchial tree, which causes a sore throat; if the patient suffers from asthma, dyspnoea will occur as well." In Fig. 1(a), the directed-graph representation of the causal knowledge embodied in this medical description is depicted, where an arc denotes a cause-effect relationship. The medical meaning ascribed to the elements in the causal graph is indicated in Fig. 1(b). Elements d_i represent disorders; elements f_i are observable findings. Note that in the graph the disorders d_1 and d_2 are causally related to each other.

Interactions among disorders, such as in the example above, can be captured more precisely by means of a mapping of sets of disorders to sets of observable findings, yielding a diagnostic interpretation of this knowledge. Such a mapping will be called an evidence function. More formally, let $\Sigma = (\Delta, \Phi, e)$ be a *diagnostic specification*, where Δ denotes a set of disorders, and Φ denotes a set of findings. Positive disorders d (findings f) and negative disorders $\neg d$ (findings $\neg f$) denote *present* disorders (findings) and *absent* disorders (findings), respectively. If a disorder d or a finding f is not included in a set, it is assumed to be unknown. Let a set X_P denote a set of positive elements, and let X_N denote a set of negative elements, such that X_P and X_N are disjoint. It is assumed that

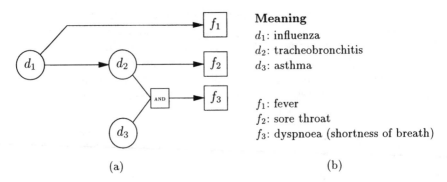

Meaning

d_1: influenza
d_2: tracheobronchitis
d_3: asthma

f_1: fever
f_2: sore throat
f_3: dyspnoea (shortness of breath)

(a)   (b)

Fig. 1. Causal net.

$\Delta = \Delta_P \cup \Delta_N$ and $\Phi = \Phi_P \cup \Phi_N$. The power set of a set S is denoted by $\wp(S)$. Now, an *evidence function* e is a mapping

$$e : \wp(\Delta) \to \wp(\Phi) \cup \{\bot\}$$

such that: (1) for each $f \in \Phi$ there exists a set $D \subseteq \Delta$ with $f \in e(D)$ or $\neg f \in e(D)$ (and possibly both, which simply means that these findings may alternatively occur); (2) if $d, \neg d \in D$ then $e(D) = \bot$; (3) if $e(D) \neq \bot$ and $D' \subseteq D$ then $e(D') \neq \bot$. If $e(D) \neq \bot$, it is said that $e(D)$ is the set of *observable findings* for D (D is *consistent*); otherwise, it is said that D is *inconsistent*.

For the medical knowledge depicted in Fig. 1, it holds, among others, that:

$$
\begin{aligned}
e(\{d_1\}) &= \{f_1, f_2\} & e(\{d_3\}) &= \varnothing \\
e(\{d_2\}) &= \{f_2\} & e(\{d_2, d_3\}) &= \{f_2, f_3\} \\
e(\{d_1, d_2\}) &= e(\{d_1\}) & e(\{d_1, d_2, d_3\}) &= e(\{d_1, d_3\}) = \{f_1, f_2, f_3\}
\end{aligned}
$$

The property $e(\{d_i\}) \subseteq e(\{d_1, d_2\})$, $i = 1, 2$, formally expresses that the interaction between d_1 and d_2 is monotonic; the evidence function e is monotonically increasing. An evidence function may also be monotonically decreasing (an example of such a function, describing physiological knowledge, is given below), or nonmonotonic. Nonmonotonic interactions may be due to masking of observable findings due to the presence of more than one disorder in a patient at the same time, e.g. fever is masked in a patient with an infectious disease and Cushing's disease at the same time.

Local as well as global interactions between disorders can be expressed readily in terms of evidence functions. A typical global property of evidence functions encountered in the literature is interaction freeness (cf. [9, 14]). A set of disorders Δ is called *interaction free* iff $e(D) = \bigcup_{d \in D} e(\{d\})$ for each consistent $D \subseteq \Delta$. This shows that an evidence function can be partially specified, which may be exploited for computational purposes (cf. [2, 9, 14]).

2.2 Notions of Diagnosis

An evidence function provides a semantic interpretation of a knowledge base in terms of expected evidence for the combined occurrence of (present or absent) disorders; yet, it does not yield a diagnosis. To employ an evidence function for the purpose of diagnosis, it must be interpreted with respect to actually observed findings. Such interpretations will be called notions of diagnosis.

More formally, let $\mathcal{P} = (\Sigma, E)$ be a *diagnostic problem*, where $E \subseteq \Phi$ is a set of *observed (patient) findings*; it is assumed that if $f \in E$ then $\neg f \notin E$, i.e. contradictory observed findings are not allowed. Let R_Σ denote a *notion of diagnosis* R applied to Σ, then a mapping

$$R_{\Sigma,e_{|H}} : \wp(\Phi) \to \wp(\Delta) \cup \{u\}$$

will either provide a diagnostic solution for a diagnostic problem $\mathcal{P}$, or indicate that no solution exists, denoted by u (undefined). Here, H denotes a *hypothesis*, which is taken to be a set of disorders ($H \subseteq \Delta$), and $e_{|H}$, called the *restricted evidence function* of e, is a restriction of e with respect to the power set $\wp(H)$:

$$e_{|H} : \wp(H) \to \wp(\Phi) \cup \{\bot\}$$

where for each $D \subseteq H$: $e_{|H}(D) = e(D)$. A restricted evidence function $e_{|H}$ can be thought of as the relevant part of a knowledge base with respect to a hypothesis H. An *R-diagnostic solution*, or *R-diagnosis* for short, with respect to a hypothesis $H \subseteq \Delta$, is now defined as the set $R_{\Sigma,e_{|H}}(E)$, where $R_{\Sigma,e_{|H}}(E) \subseteq H$ if a solution exists. In Fig. 2, the idea underlying the definition of a notion

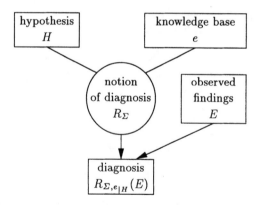

Fig. 2. Schema of notion of diagnosis, diagnostic problem and solution.

of diagnosis R and diagnostic solution to a diagnostic problem is illustrated schematically.

A notion of diagnosis R provides the possibility to express interactions among disorders and observed findings at the level of diagnosis, which we call dependencies. We may also have that $R_{\Sigma,e_{|H \cup H'}}(E) = R_{\Sigma,e_{|H}}(E) \cup R_{\Sigma,e_{|H'}}(E)$, with $R_{\Sigma,e_{|H \cup H'}}(E) \neq u$, which means that the diagnostic solution with respect to the hypothesis $H \cup H'$ is obtained as the union of the solutions for the two separately examined hypotheses H and H'. This is called the *independence (or compositionality) assumption*. For many notions of diagnosis described in the literature, in particular for abductive diagnosis and consistency-based diagnosis, the independence assumption fails to hold.

To demonstrate how the definitions above can be employed, we consider a notion of diagnosis US (Unique Subset), such that $US_{\Sigma,e_{|H}}(E) = H'$ if it holds that H' is the only nonempty subset of H such that $e_{|H}(H') \subseteq E$; otherwise, $H' = u$. This notion of diagnosis expresses that a diagnosis consists of a set of disorders which, on the one hand, can account for at least part of all observed findings, and, on the other hand, every finding associated with the set of disorders that is taken as a diagnosis has been observed. Furthermore, there is only one such subset of the given hypothesis H. Some interesting diagnostic conclusions for the medical example from Fig. 1 are: $US_{\Sigma,e_{|\{d2,d3\}}}(\{f_2\}) = \{d_2\}$, i.e. a patient with sore throat may have tracheobronchitis, $US_{\Sigma,e_{|\{d_2,d_3\}}}(\{f_2,f_3\}) = u$, i.e. there exists no *unique* subset of H accounting for both sore throat and dyspnoea as signs, and finally, $US_{\Sigma,e_{|\{d_2\}}}(\{f_2\}) = \{d_2\}$. In the first case, it is said that the hypotheses has been *adjusted*, in the second case, that the hypothesis is *rejected*, and in the last case, that the hypothesis has been *accepted*. This example demonstrates the flexibility of the approach.

It is also straightforward to define notions of diagnosis proposed in the literature. For example, consider the following typical instances of notions of diagnosis:

- *Abductive diagnosis using 'may' relations (weak-causality diagnosis)* [4, 9]:

$$WC_{\Sigma,e_{|H}}(E) = \begin{cases} H \text{ if } e_{|H}(H) \supseteq E \\ u \text{ otherwise} \end{cases}$$

  i.e. all observed findings must be observable. A notion of *strong-causality diagnosis*, SC, is obtained by replacing $\supseteq$ by equality. This expresses that all observable findings must be observed, and vice versa.
- *Consistency-based diagnosis* [7, 12]:

$$CB_{\Sigma,e_{|H}}(E) = \begin{cases} H \text{ if } \forall f \in E : f \in e_{|H}(H) \vee \neg f \notin e_{|H}(H) \\ u \text{ otherwise} \end{cases}$$

  i.e. observed findings may not contradict with observable findings.

These notions of diagnoses will be used below as reference points for notions of refinement diagnosis. When we apply these notions of diagnosis to the example depicted in Fig. 1, the following results are obtained: $SC_{\Sigma,e_{|\{d_2,d_3\}}}(\{f_2\}) = u$, $WC_{\Sigma,e_{|\{d_2,d_3\}}}(\{f_2\}) = \{d_2,d_3\}$, and $CB_{\Sigma,e_{|\{d_2,d_3\}}}(\{f_2\}) = \{d_2,d_3\}$. Hence, SC is stronger than the notion of diagnosis US defined above, whereas WC and CB are weaker, potentially producing superfluous disorders as part of a diagnosis. The notion of heuristic classification can also be expressed in terms of the framework; here, an evidence function stands for the empirical associations between disorders and findings (see below).

It is informative to relate these notions of diagnosis to each other in terms of a restriction relation $\sqsubseteq$; it holds that $R \sqsubseteq R'$ iff the diagnoses resulting from the notion of diagnosis R are a subset of those resulting from R' (for any legal diagnostic specification Σ). It is easily seen that: $SC \sqsubseteq WC \sqsubseteq CB$; which reveals that consistency-based diagnosis is a very weak form of diagnosis, a well-known fact in the diagnosis community.

3   Refinement Diagnosis

What can be taken as a basis for notions of diagnosis which incorporate certain principles of refinement? Obviously, there exists a wide range of possibilities. Which of the possible choices yields the most natural result depends, to a large extent, on the nature of the problem domain, which is partially expressed by the characteristics of the evidence functions e. Dependencies between an interpretation of observed findings (notion of diagnosis) given an interpretation of a knowledge base (evidence function) are important in this respect.

Two classes of refinement diagnosis will be studied here. Firstly, the class of notions of refinement diagnosis, called *most general diagnosis*, is examined, where the least upper bound of accepted hypotheses (with respect to set inclusion) is taken as a diagnostic solution. Secondly, the class of notions of refinement diagnosis, called *most specific diagnosis*, based on taking the greatest lower bound of accepted hypotheses is studied. In most general diagnosis, the smallest set of disorders that includes every accepted subhypothesis is considered most plausible; in contrast, in most specific diagnosis, the largest set of disorders that is included in every accepted subhypothesis is considered most plausible.

3.1   Most General Diagnosis

Notions of most general diagnosis capture the idea that if a specific diagnostic hypothesis is not accepted, then the 'nearest' subhypothesis should be taken instead. The least upper bound with respect to set inclusion of the set of accepted subhypotheses is an example of such a 'nearest' subhypothesis. The notions of most general diagnosis enforce independence or compositionality of diagnostic components in the sense of the previous section.

The notion of *most general subset diagnosis*, denoted by GS, is defined as follows:

$$
\mathrm{GS}_{\Sigma,e_{|H}}(E) = \begin{cases} \bigcup_{\substack{H' \subseteq H \\ e_{|H}(H') \subseteq E}} H' & \text{if } H \text{ is consistent, and} \\ & \exists H' \subseteq H : e_{|H}(H') \subseteq E \\ u & \text{otherwise} \end{cases}
$$

Intuitively, a most general subset diagnosis is the smallest set of disorders that includes all accepted subhypotheses of a given hypothesis, where an accepted subhypothesis concerns observable findings that all have been observed.

For the example in Fig. 1 with $E = \{f_1, f_2\}$, we have that $\mathrm{GS}_{\Sigma,e_{|\{d_1,d_2\}}}(E) = \{d_1, d_2\}$, which is also an abductive diagnosis, because $\mathrm{SC}_{\Sigma,e_{|\{d_1,d_2\}}}(E) = \{d_1, d_2\}$. However, it holds that $\mathrm{GS}_{\Sigma,e_{|\{d_1,d_2\}}}(\{f_2\}) = \{d_2\}$, whereas $\mathrm{SC}_{\Sigma,e_{|\{d_1,d_2\}}}(\{f_2\}) = u$. Hence, $e(\{d_1, d_2\})$ predicts a finding that cannot be accounted for, causing the disorder d_1 to be ignored. This may be a suitable approach to medical prob-

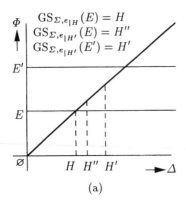
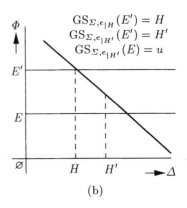

(a)   (b)

Fig. 3. Monotonically increasing (a) and decreasing (b) evidence functions.

lems in which neglecting a particular disorder may be dangerous, such as in life-threatening situations. If the evidence function represents empirical associations, GS may be viewed as a special form of heuristic classification.

In Fig. 3, the relationship between a diagnostic hypothesis H, a set of observed findings E and the resulting diagnosis $GS_{\Sigma,e_{|H}}(E)$ is summarized by schematically depicting these sets as if they were real numbers and by taking set inclusion as the $\leq$ total order on the real numbers. If most general subset diagnosis is applied to a monotonically decreasing evidence function, the resulting diagnosis is either undefined or equal to the given hypothesis H. This contrasts with GS applied to a monotonically increasing evidence function, which may also yield subsets of the hypothesis as a diagnosis. The case $GS_{\Sigma,e_{|H'}}(E) = H''$ in Fig. 3(a) illustrates that $e(H'')$ may even be a superset of E.

Where most general subset diagnosis can be viewed as a more flexible version of strong-causality diagnosis SC, which for certain evidence functions is as little restrictive as consistency-based diagnosis, a similar, flexible notion of diagnosis can be designed for weak-causality diagnosis. This suggests replacing the subset relation in most general subset diagnosis by the superset relation, yielding the notion of most general superset ('cOntains') diagnosis GO.

The notion of *most general superset diagnosis*, denoted by GO, is defined as follows:

$$
GO_{\Sigma,e_{|H}}(E) = \begin{cases} \bigcup_{\substack{H' \subseteq H \\ e_{|H}(H') \supseteq E}} H' & \text{if } H \text{ is consistent, and} \\ & \exists H' \subseteq H : e_{|H}(H') \supseteq E \\ u & \text{otherwise} \end{cases}
$$

Most general superset diagnosis has much in common with weak-causality diagnosis WC defined in the previous section. If the notion of most general superset diagnosis is applied to evidence functions that are monotonically decreasing, or nonmonotonic, for the resulting diagnosis $GO_{\Sigma,e_{|H}}(E) = H'$ it may even hold that $e(H') \subset E$, although for each of the diagnostic hypotheses $H'' \subseteq H$ that contribute to the diagnosis it holds that $e_{|H}(H'') \supseteq E$. Hence, the situation is the reverse of that for most general subset diagnosis discussed above, as might be expected from their respective definitions. A similar figure can be constructed for GO as for GS in Fig. 3.

As is true for weak-causality diagnosis WC, most general superset diagnosis restricted to monotonically increasing evidence functions is very unrestrictive, which is revealed by the fact that $GO_{\Sigma,e_{|H}}(\varnothing) = H$ if $e(H) \neq \bot$, meaning that all disorders constituting the hypothesis may have occurred, even if none of the associated findings have been observed. Note that the same diagnosis would have been produced by weak-causality diagnosis WC in this case. By adopting some criterion for the selection of relevant diagnoses, such as minimality according to set inclusion – such criteria are known as parsimony criteria – the unrestrictiveness is alleviated; the empty diagnosis $\varnothing$ would then be produced.

An alternative to the definition of subset diagnosis is to consider all sets of disorders D that have at least one finding f in common with the findings E observed. This leads to the notion of *most general intersection diagnosis*, denoted by GI:

$$GI_{\Sigma,e_{|H}}(E) = \begin{cases} \bigcup_{\substack{H' \subseteq H \\ (E = \varnothing \lor e_{|H}(H') = \varnothing \lor \\ e_{|H}(H') \cap E \neq \varnothing)}} H' & \begin{array}{l} \text{if } H \text{ is consistent, and } (E = \varnothing \text{ or} \\ \exists H' \subseteq H : e_{|H}(H') = \varnothing \text{ or} \\ e_{|H}(H') \cap E \neq \varnothing) \end{array} \\ u & \text{otherwise} \end{cases}$$

If the sets of observed and observable findings are nonempty, intersection diagnosis with respect to H stands for the least upper bound of subsets H' of H, where for each H' admitted to the most general intersection diagnosis $GI_{\Sigma,e_{|H}}(E)$, the associated set of observable findings $e_{|H}(H')$ is empty or has at least one finding in common with the set of observed findings E.

The advantage of most general intersection diagnosis over most general subset and superset diagnosis is that only disorders that have at least one associated observable finding that has actually been observed, are included in a diagnosis. This will be an acceptable assumption in medical domains where not all findings associated with a set of disorders need be observed and not all observed findings need be accounted for. In representing a domain, however, it may be required to restrict to those observable findings that are in some way 'typical'.

3.2 Comparison

Most general subset, superset and intersection diagnosis are three refinement approaches to diagnosis. The restriction relationships between these notions of diagnosis are shown in Fig. 4. Notions of diagnosis can also be classified in terms of elements included in individual diagnoses using set inclusion; the subdiagnostic relation $\trianglelefteq$ does exactly this. The three notions of diagnosis discussed above stand in a subdiagnostic relation to each other: GS $\trianglelefteq$ GI and GO $\trianglelefteq$ GI, i.e., a most general intersection diagnosis will always contain at least as many elements as the corresponding most general subset and superset diagnoses.

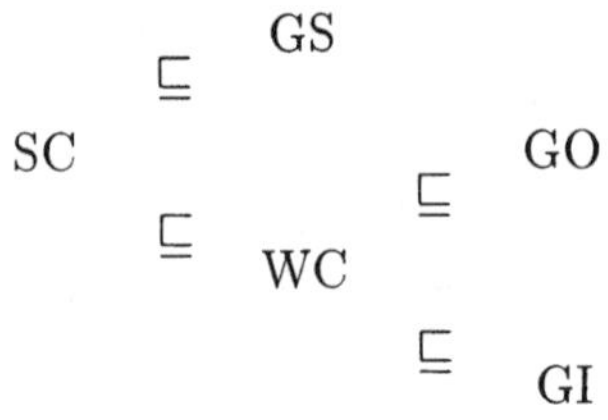

$$GS$$
$$\sqsubseteq$$

$$SC \qquad\qquad GO$$

$$\sqsubseteq \qquad\qquad \sqsubseteq$$

$$WC$$

$$\sqsubseteq$$
$$GI$$

Fig. 4. Restriction taxonomy of notions of diagnosis.

3.3 Most Specific Diagnosis

Rather than taking the least upper bound of a set of accepted subhypotheses of a given hypothesis, taking the greatest lower bound provides another approach to refinement diagnosis. We shall refer to notions of diagnosis based on taking the greatest lower bound as notions of *most specific diagnosis*. Where the concept of 'most general diagnosis' formalizes notions of diagnosis that yield diagnoses that include *every* accepted subhypothesis, most specific diagnosis formalizes notions of diagnosis that yield diagnoses that are *common* to every accepted subhypothesis. In general it holds for a notion of most specific diagnosis S that if $S_{\Sigma,e_{|H}}(E) = \varnothing$ and $S_{\Sigma,e_{|H'}}(E) = H''$, then, by definition, $S_{\Sigma,e_{|H \cup H'}}(E) = \varnothing$. Hence, notions of most specific diagnosis are very restrictive.

As with the notion of most general subset diagnosis, in the notion of most specific subset diagnosis, subhypotheses are admitted to a diagnosis if their associated sets of findings are included in the set of observed findings of a diagnostic problem. However, of these accepted subhypotheses, only the disorders the subhypotheses have in common constitute a diagnosis. Hence, the notion of *most specific subset diagnosis*, denoted by SS, is defined as follows:

$$
SS_{\Sigma,e_{|H}}(E) = \begin{cases} \bigcap_{\substack{H' \subseteq H \\ e_{|H}(H') \subseteq E}} H' & \text{if } H \text{ is consistent, and} \\ & \exists H' \subseteq H : e_{|H}(H') \subseteq E \\ u & \text{otherwise} \end{cases}
$$

This notion of diagnosis is extremely restrictive. For example, if an evidence function is interaction free, then the most specific subset diagnosis will almost always (with the exception when only one subhypothesis is accepted) be equal to the empty set, or undefined.

If the evidence function is monotonically decreasing, then most specific subset diagnosis tries to construct the smallest diagnosis possible. It may be viewed as a flexible form of consistency-based kernel diagnosis in the sense of [7] (a kernel diagnosis is a diagnosis that is a common part of certain diagnoses). The reason for the similarity between kernel diagnosis and most specific subset diagnosis is that any hypothesis H' for which $e_{|H}(H') \subseteq E$ is also consistent with E.

The correspondence between kernel diagnosis and most specific subset diagnosis is illustrated by means of an example of the diagnosis of blood-vessel pathology. Consider Fig. 5, which shows a schematic picture of five connected

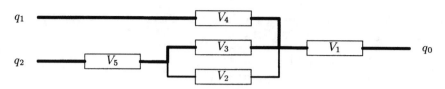

Fig. 5. Schematic picture of an arterial net.

arteries, referred to as V_1 = aortic arc, V_2 = collateral circulation (consisting of the internal thoracic, posterior intercostal, and inferior epigastric arteries) V_3 = descending aorta, V_4 = subclavian artery, and V_5 = femoral artery.

Normally, blood flows from the aortic arc to the arms via the subclavian arteries, and to the legs through the descending aorta and femoral arteries. If there exists an obstruction to blood flow at the level of the descending aorta (V_3), e.g. due to aortic coarctation, the blood may still flow to the legs through other vessels, collectively denoted by V_2, establishing what is called a collateral circulation. The flow in the femoral arteries, however, is then significantly reduced. Of course, the blood flow in any artery may be obstructed, e.g. due to atherosclerosis. The blood flow in an artery, denoted by Q, is defined by $Q = \frac{\delta P}{R}$, where δP is the pressure gradient, and R is the resistance of the vessel. Let $\Sigma = (\Delta, \Phi, e)$ be a diagnostic specification representing the arterial net. Obstruction of an artery V_i to blood flow will be denoted by v_i; patency of an artery V_i is indicated by $\neg v_i$. It is convenient to assume that the input blood flow to the arterial net is fixed, as indicated in Fig. 5 by q_0. The normal output blood flow of the arterial net is denoted by q_1 (blood flow to the arms) and q_2 (blood flow to the legs); reduced or absent blood flow due to obstruction is denoted by $\neg q_j$, $j = 1, 2$.

The following values of the evidence function e are among those that correspond to the arterial net's (normal) physiological behaviour:

$$e(\{\neg v_1, \neg v_2, \neg v_3, \neg v_4, \neg v_5\}) = \{q_1, q_2\}$$
$$e(\{\neg v_1, \neg v_2, v_3, \neg v_4, \neg v_5\}) = \{q_1\}$$
$$e(\{\neg v_1, v_2, v_3, \neg v_4, \neg v_5\}) = \{q_1\}$$
$$e(\{\neg v_1, v_3, \neg v_4, \neg v_5\}) = \{q_1\}$$
$$e(\{v_3\}) = \{q_1\}$$
$$e(\{\neg v_1, \neg v_2, \neg v_4\}) = \{q_1, q_2\}$$
$$\vdots$$
$$e(\varnothing) = \{q_1, q_2\}$$

($e(\varnothing) = \{q_1, q_2\}$ indicates that if it is unknown whether occlusions are present or absent, all normal findings may be observed.) Note that we have refrained from specifying information about abnormal behaviour (e.g. when V_3 is occluded, we might add $\neg q_2$ to the set of observable findings, which we have not done above), since it is assumed that the model used for diagnosis is a physiological model, not a *patho*physiological model. The most specific subset diagnosis with respect to the hypothesis $H = \{v_3\}$ is equal to

$$SS_{\Sigma, e_{|\{v_3\}}}(\{q_1, \neg q_2\}) = \{v_3\}$$

which is indeed a kernel diagnosis for the diagnostic problem $\mathcal{P} = (\Sigma, E)$ using consistency-based diagnosis. Note that

$$SS_{\Sigma, e_{|H}}(\{q_1, \neg q_2\}) = \{v_3\}$$

if $\{\neg v_1, v_3, \neg v_5\} \subseteq H$, for consistent $H \subseteq \Delta$.

The notion of *most specific superset diagnosis*, denoted by SO, is defined as follows:

$$SO_{\Sigma, e_{|H}}(E) = \begin{cases} \bigcap_{\substack{H' \subseteq H \\ e_{|H}(H') \supseteq E}} H' & \text{if } H \text{ is consistent, and} \\ & \exists H' \subseteq H : e_{|H}(H') \supseteq E \\ u & \text{otherwise} \end{cases}$$

If the evidence function to which most specific superset diagnosis is applied, is monotonically increasing, the result may be intuitively attractive. The basic idea of most specific superset diagnosis is that the observed findings that are common to the accepted subhypotheses are due to the common disorders of accepted subhypotheses.

Reconsider Fig. 1. For $E = \{f_2, f_3\}$ (i.e. the patient has a sore throat and dyspnoea), the most specific superset diagnosis is equal to

$$SO_{\Sigma, e_{|\{d_1, d_2, d_3\}}}(E) = \{d_3\}$$

because, it holds that $e_{|H}(D) \supseteq E$, for $D = \{d_1, d_3\}, \{d_2, d_3\}, \{d_1, d_2, d_3\}$, where $H = \{d_1, d_2, d_3\}$. All other subsets of H have associated sets of findings that are no supersets of E. The disorder d_3 stands for asthma. While both d_1 and d_2 participate in subhypotheses that also account for E, only the disorder d_3 occurs in all accepted subhypotheses, i.e. it turns out to be essential. It seems therefore intuitively right to accept d_3 as the most plausible diagnosis.

As the example above indicates, a most specific superset diagnosis need not account for all observed findings on the basis of the given evidence function. If an evidence function is interaction free, then most specific superset diagnosis is likely to produce a singleton set diagnosis for a given hypothesis that is very plausible if the associated sets of observed findings $e(\{d\})$ are mutually disjoint.

As discussed above, the notion of most general intersection diagnosis is very unrestrictive. All disorders that, either individually or in combination with other disorders, have findings in common with the set of observed findings, are included in a diagnosis. The notion of *most specific intersection diagnosis*, denoted by SI, obtained by replacing union by intersection in the definition of GI, is much more restrictive than most general intersection diagnosis. If the evidence function e is monotonically increasing, the resulting diagnosis will be equal to the empty set if the function values $e(\{d\})$ have many observable findings in common.

3.4 Comparison

Although the notions of most specific diagnosis are very restrictive, they do not stand in a simple restriction relation to the other notions of diagnosis. However, it is easy to see that $SS_{\Sigma, e_{|H}}(E) \subseteq GS_{\Sigma, e_{|H}}(E)$ holds for each consistent $H \subseteq \Delta$. Obviously, similar set inclusion relations hold for the other notions of diagnosis, i.e. SS $\trianglelefteq$ GS, SO $\trianglelefteq$ GO, and SI $\trianglelefteq$ GI.

4 Discussion

In this paper, we introduced a general set-theoretical framework as a tool for the formalization of notions of diagnosis. As was shown, the particular properties of evidence functions to which a notion of diagnosis is applied, are important with respect to the suitability of a notion of diagnosis. Several new notions of diagnosis have been proposed that are more flexible in dealing with observed findings and domain knowledge than common notions of diagnosis. We expect that these flexible notions of diagnosis are particularly valuable for use in the field of medicine, because both medical knowledge and patient data are often incomplete and inaccurate. Of course, it is desirable to gather experimental evidence for the usefulness of refinement diagnosis as a basis for medical diagnostic applications, which may also result in particular extensions.

References

1. B.G. Buchanan and E.H. Shortliffe (1984). *Rule-based Expert Systems: the MYCIN Experiments of the Stanford Heuristic Programming Project.* Reading: Addison-Wesley.
2. T. Bylander, D. Allemang, M.C. Tanner and J.R. Josephson (1992). The computational complexity of abduction. *Artificial Intelligence,* **49**, 25–60.
3. W.J. Clancey (1985). Heuristic classification. *Artificial Intelligence,* **27**, 289–350.
4. L. Console, D. Theseider Dupré and P. Torasso (1989). A theory of diagnosis for incomplete causal models. In *Proceedings of the 10th International Joint Conference on Artificial Intelligence,* pp. 1311–1317.
5. L. Console and P. Torasso (1990). Integrating models of correct behaviour into abductive diagnosis. In *Proceedings of ECAI'90,* pp. 160–166.
6. K.L. Downing (1993). Physiological applications of consistency-based diagnosis. *Artificial Intelligence in Medicine,* **5**, 9–30.
7. J. de Kleer, A.K. Mackworth and R. Reiter (1992). Characterizing diagnoses and systems. *Artificial Intelligence,* **52**, 197–222.
8. P.J.F. Lucas (1996). Modelling interactions for diagnosis. In *Proceedings of CESA'96 IMACS Multiconference: Modelling, Analysis and Simulation,* **1**, pp. 541–546, Lille, France.
9. Y. Peng and J.A. Reggia (1990). *Abductive inference models for diagnostic problem solving.* New York: Springer-Verlag.
10. D. Poole (1990). A methodology for using a default and abductive reasoning system. *International Journal of Intelligent Systems,* **5**(5), 521–548.
11. W.F. Punch III, M.C. Tanner, J.R. Josephson and J.W. Smith (1990). PEIRCE: a tool for experimenting with abduction. *IEEE Expert,* **5**(5), 34–44.
12. R. Reiter (1987). A theory of diagnosis from first principles. *Artificial Intelligence,* **32**, 57–95.
13. S. Tuhrim, J. Reggia and S. Goodall (1991). An experimental study of criteria for hypothesis plausibility. *Journal of Experimental and Theoretical Artificial Intelligence,* **3**, 129–144.
14. T.D. Wu (1991). A problem decomposition method for efficient diagnosis and interpretation of multiple disorders. *Computer Methods and Programs in Biomedicine,* **35**, 239–250.

A New Approach to Feature Selection

Matthias Scherf

GSF - National Research Center for Environment and Health, medis Institute
85754 Neuherberg
e-mail: scherf@gsf.de

Abstract. The design of classifiers for medical decision tasks is often based on a small set of high dimensional feature vectors [1]. Therefore we have to curtail the effect of the curse of dimensionality phenomenon on the complexity of the classifier by the application of data pre-processing techniques [Dev82].
One possible way to reduce the dimensionality of the input space is to select a subset of features which give the best characterisation of the class membership of the given feature vectors. This technique, which is called "feature selection" is also very interesting for knowledge acquisition because the calculated feature subset can be examined by the medical expert to improve the decision process and the data acquisition technique.
The main drawback of the feature selection techniques known so far is, that their search procedures for optimal feature subsets are very time consuming when the dimension of the feature vectors is high.
We present a new feature selection technique which leads to a high reduction of computation time by determining the feature subset through "learning" according to neural network techniques.

1 Introduction

The design of classifiers for medical decision tasks is often based on a lot of features, which are determined in expensive, protracted examinations, e.g. perimetry or computer tomography. Since the design of classifiers for medical tasks is mostly based on a small set of preclassified samples, data pre-processing techniques must be applied to reduce the dimensionality of the input space to circumvent the curse of dimensionality. The general way to reduce dimensionality is to project the samples of the input space in a lower dimensional space by an arbitrary function.
The advantage of orthonormal projections, which means the selection of a feature subset, against non-orthonormal projection techniques is, that the result can be interpreted. The medical expert is therefore able to improve on the one hand the decision process and on the other hand the data acquisition technique.

---

[1] If we talk about feature vectors we mean real valued vectors.

2 Feature Selection

Given a set $Y = \{y_1, y_2, ..., y_Q\}$ of Q features, the goal of feature selection is to determine an optimal feature subset $X = \{x_1, x_2, ...x_q | x_i \neq x_j, x_i \in Y, q \leq Q\}$, which is given by

$$J(X) \leq J(\tilde{X}), \forall \tilde{X} \in \aleph,$$

where $J(.)$ is an arbitrary criterion function and $\aleph$ is the set of all 2^Q feature subsets.

Since we are interested in data pre-processing for classifiers, the criterion function should give a measure for class separability. From a theoretical point of view the optimal criterion function is therefore the probability of correct classification which is very difficult to evaluate [Dev82]. Consequently criterion functions are mostly based on criteria like the inter- and intraclass-distances which can easily be calculated without any assumptions about the class conditional probability density functions.

Given a criterion function $J(.)$ an optimal feature subset is determined through the application of search procedures. Most of them, as for example introduced in [Dev82] and [Fuk90] suffer from the fact, that they are very time consuming when dealing with high dimensional input spaces or that they only take advantage of a small subset of possible solutions. The reason is, that all known search procedures find a solution through iteratively comparing the results of the criterion function with different feature subsets as arguments. Even there exist a lot of optimised techniques as for example the branch and bound technique [Fuk90], there is no guarantee, that not all 2^Q subsets have to be compared during the search process which will lead to unacceptable computation time if the input space is of high dimensionality [Bis96].

3 Learning an Optimal Feature Set

To circumvent the drawbacks of the subset selection strategies we developed a feature selection technique which searches for the optimal subset by optimising a criterion function via gradient descent. For reasons mentioned above we base our criterion function on the inter- and intraclass-distances.

To calculate the distance d_{ij} between feature vectors V^i and V^j of dimension Q we use the Euclidean distance, modified by introducing weights $w_q \in [0, 1]$, weighting the quadratic distances between the features y_q^i and y_q^j respectively:

$$d_{ij} = \sqrt{\sum_{q=1}^{Q} w_q (y_q^i - y_q^j)^2}$$

We define

$$\delta^s(i, j) = \begin{cases} 1 \text{ if } V_i \text{ and } V_j \text{ are feature-vectors of the same class} \\ 0 \text{ otherwise} \end{cases}$$

and

$$\delta^d(i,j) = \begin{cases} 1 \text{ if } V_i \text{ and } V_j \text{ are feature-vectors of different classes} \\ 0 \text{ otherwise} \end{cases}$$

Let N be the number of available feature vectors, $N_s = \sum_{i=1}^{N} \sum_{j=i+1}^{N} \delta^s(i,j)$ and $N_d = \sum_{i=1}^{N} \sum_{j=i+1}^{N} \delta^d(i,j)$. We choose a criterion function which measures the relation between the inter- and intraclass distances:

$$J = \frac{1}{N_s} \sum_{i=1}^{N} \sum_{j=i+1}^{N} \delta^s(i,j) d_{ij} - \frac{1}{N_d} \sum_{i=1}^{N} \sum_{j=i+1}^{N} \delta^d(i,j) d_{ij}.$$

To find a set of weights which minimises $J(.)$ we initialise the weights with random values in a suitable range [2] and modify them iteratively through gradient descent. The gradient of weight w_q is calculated by

$$\frac{\partial J}{\partial w_q} = \frac{1}{N_s} \sum_{i=1}^{N} \sum_{j=i+1}^{N} \frac{\delta^s(i,j)(y_q^i - y_q^j)^2}{2\sqrt{\sum_{t=1}^{Q} w_t(y_t^i - y_t^j)^2}} - \frac{1}{N_d} \sum_{i=1}^{N} \sum_{j=i+1}^{N} \frac{\delta^d(i,j)(y_q^i - y_q^j)^2}{2\sqrt{\sum_{t=1}^{Q} w_t(y_q^i - y_q^j)^2}}.$$

The weights are adapted through

$$w_q(t+1) = w_q(t) + \lambda \frac{\partial J}{\partial w_q}$$

where $w_q(t)$ is the q'th weight at iteration step t and λ is a suitable chosen learning constant. The search space for the weights is restricted through $[0,1]$.

We applied the feature selection method to a wide range of artificial and real world datasets and got the very promising result, that in most of the cases every weight is set exactly to one or zero after the optimisation process has terminated. In all these cases the optimal feature subset is given by the features y_q, with $w_q = 1$.

Since the criterion function is nonlinear it is very difficult to give an analytic statement about conditions, when the feature selection technique can be successfully applied to a given set of feature vectors, meaning that after the termination of the optimisation process every weight is clearly set to one or zero. Nevertheless we had only a few cases where we did not get a clear decision and by introducing a threshold function $\Phi(.)$ with

$$\Phi(x_q) = \begin{cases} 1 \text{ if } x_q \geq 0.5 \\ 0 \text{ if } x_q < 0.5 \end{cases}$$

we even got acceptable results.

Like in neural network tasks the solution gained by the introduced method depends on the initialisation values of the weights and therefore it might be advisable to run the optimisation process with different initialisations and to compare the results.

---

[2] In most of our experiments we used an initialisation range of $[0.4, 0.6]$

4 Application and Results

We applied the feature selection method to perimetry data which show glaucomatous and pathologic but not glaucomatous defects. The data set contained 983 samples, preclassified by a medical expert. Every perimetry is characterised through a 59 dimensional vector of real values, whereas every value (feature) gives the relative sensitivity loss in a location of the visual field. We applied our method for feature selection with different weight initialisations and got the same subset of 30 features respectively. The computation time was about 35 min on a Sparc10 Station, whereas the branch and bound algorithm [Dev82] needed weeks, giving the same result. Using a RBF neural network classifier we got an improvement of 20% in specificity and equal sensitivity when using the reduced feature set for the classifier design instead of all features available.

5 Discussion

We presented a new method for determining an optimal subset of features according to a criterion function which is much faster in the presence of high dimensional measurement spaces than all search procedures known so far.
The method is similar to neural network methods, meaning that the solution is determined by optimising a nonlinear energy function with respect to some weights. Like in training neural networks there is no guarantee, that the optimisation process will find the global optimum of the energy function but since all known search procedures suffer from the fact, that they need unacceptable computation time it seems to be a very promising solution for high dimensional input spaces.

References

[Bis96] Bishop, C.M.
Neural Networks for Pattern Recognition
Clarendon Press Oxford

[Dev82] Devijever P., Kittler J.
Pattern Recognition: A Statistical Approach
Prentice/Hall, 1982

[Fuk90] Fukunaga K.
Introduction to Statistical Pattern Recognition
ACADEMIC PRESS INC, Harcourt Brace Jovanovich, Publishers
Boston San Diego New York London Sydney Tokyo Toronto, 1990

A Heuristic Approach to the Multiple Diagnoses Problem

Randolph A. Miller, M.D., Division of Biomedical Informatics, Vanderbilt University
Medical Center, Nashville, TN USA

Abstract

A new heuristic model for the diagnosis of multiple related disorders in a patient case is presented. The model constructs differential diagnoses of single and related disorders, based on a medical knowledge base containing disease descriptions and linkages among diseases in the knowledge base.

1. Introduction

The problem of computer-assisted diagnosis in medicine has been the subject of research for nearly a half-century [1-11]. While much progress has been made, there remain both conceptual and pragmatic obstacles to the creation of general, broad-based programs for medical diagnosis. One such conceptual obstacle is the problem of multiple diagnoses [7]. There have been few workable or efficient algorithms for solving cases in which multiple concurrent disorders are present. Existing approaches have emphasized theory over pragmatics, resulting in computationally intensive, medical knowledge-poor algorithms unlikely to be useful in clinical practice.

Approaches to general medical diagnosis (as opposed to focused, device-associated diagnostic problems, such as EKG interpretation or automated cytology analysis) fall on a spectrum [25] from formal mathematical models (for example, simple Bayesian approaches [3-4, 10],Set Covering approaches [12], and Bayesian Belief networks [13-16]) to heuristic methods (for example, INTERNIST-I/QMR [17-18], ABEL [19], ILIIAD [20], MEDITEL [21]), and neural network systems [22-24]). A daunting problem is that formal mathematical models often require unrealistic assumptions to make them computationally tractable [25] – such as the well-known independence assumption adopted by simple Bayesian approaches [3-4, 10]. Conversely, most computationally tractable heuristic models of diagnosis suffer from lack of formal grounding [25]. Both approaches suffer from lack of high-quality, accurate, large medical knowledge bases [26-28].

Given that all approaches to medical diagnosis are flawed in one way or another, the ultimate measure of success for a diagnostic decision support system should be whether objective evidence demonstrates that (a) use of the system causes no harm, and/or (b) the system improves the performance of its users on specified tasks when compared to the users' baseline performance (without the system) on similar tasks at an acceptable level of risk to patients and at an acceptable cost in time and money [29-31].

This paper presents a novel heuristic approach to the multiple diagnoses problem. It is based on the author's experience over the past two decades as both a co-developer of the INTERNIST-I/QMR knowledge base and diagnostic programs [17-18, 26-29], and as a practicing clinician. The approach described is general, and could be applied to any diagnostic system in which the knowledge base contains both descriptions of diseases (with the strengths of association between a disease and each finding of the disease) and descriptions of the causal and epidemiological associations among disorders (including frequency of association or similar measures).

2. Background and Description of the Problem

Most medical computer programs approach diagnosis by combining and resolving the individual differential diagnoses of findings present (or absent) in a patient case [11, 17]. Unfortunately, the medical literature, which is the existing "gold standard" for medical expert system knowledge base construction, is disease-centric, rather than finding-centric. Case reports or case series that appear in the literature are clustered by diagnoses rather than by presenting findings. As a result, medical diagnostic systems' knowledge bases are primarily disease-centric. By compiling lists of the findings reported to occur in patients with each given disease, it is possible to construct differential diagnoses for each finding through inversion of the disease descriptions. This limits system's diagnoses to those diseases described in the system.

Individual findings in a given case may represent either (1) findings caused by a single active disease process; (2) findings present in the patient unrelated to any active disease process ("red herring" findings) that represent false indicators of active disease, including (a) residual findings from past, currently inactive disease, (b) congenital or acquired pseudo-abnormalities, such as congenital clubbing of the fingers or macroamylasemia, and, (c) "false positive" findings, based on faulty interpretations during the clinical examination or erroneous measurement or reporting of laboratory results; (3) findings caused by multiple independent disorders present in the patient (such as co-occurring osteoarthritis, essential hypertension, and emphysema in an elderly patient); and, (4) findings caused by concurrent presence of multiple diagnoses that are interrelated causally or predispositionally (for example, essential hypertension, stroke, and hypertensive heart disease). The "multiple diagnoses" problem occurs whenever a confirmed, single disorder does not explain all of the findings present in a patient case. A "true" multiple diagnoses problem is encountered when a patient's findings are due to any combinations of (2) through (4) above; and an apparent ("false") multiple diagnoses situation is encountered when a patient presents with a combination of (1) and (2) above.

Several computational approaches have been proposed for the multiple diagnoses problem in the past. In 1968, G. Anthony Gorry wrote a visionary paper on heuristic methods for medical diagnosis [7]. Gorry proposed a formal definition of the diagnostic problem. He enumerated appropriate roles for system components, including a pattern-sorting function to determine whether competing diagnoses are members of the same "problem area" -- i.e., whether diagnostic hypotheses should be considered together because they are related to pathology in the same organ system, or separately, as potential complementary multiple diagnoses. The latter constituted Gorry's proposed solution to the multiple diagnoses problem.

In the 1970s, Ben-Bassat [32] and colleagues developed a method to allow multiple diagnoses in Bayesian systems by considering diagnosis as a task that first establishes either the presence or absence of each disease in the system's knowledge base, and which then ranks and resolves surviving hypotheses. This approach subsequently evolved as part of the MEDAS system during the 1980s and 1990s [33].

INTERNIST-I, an experimental system for diagnosis in general internal medicine, was developed by Myers, Pople, and Miller from 1973-1984 [17-18]. The program could diagnose multiple disorders in the same patient (whether the diagnoses were related or not) by serially solving the problem, "identify and conclude the best single diagnosis consistent with the currently unexplained set of patient findings". In developing the INTERNIST-I diagnostic algorithm, Pople employed a partitioning heuristic to determine whether a given diagnosis was a competitor or an alternative to the current top-most ranked single diagnosis [17-18]. Stated simply, the heuristic was, "if two diagnoses taken together explain no more of the significant findings of the case than either of the diagnoses individually, then they are competitors; otherwise, they are alternatives". Competitor diagnoses to the topmost diagnosis were assumed to be mutually exclusive, with only one of the set present in the given patient case. Alternative diagnoses were assumed to represent potentially complementary diagnoses to the topmost diagnosis that could be present concurrently with the topmost diagnosis. After conclusion of a diagnosis from a set of competitors, INTERNIST-I would mark all findings of the concluded diagnosis as "explained" and recycle, attempting to find diagnostic causes for any remaining unexplained findings in the case. INTERNIST-I gave bonus weight to any hypotheses that were causally (or predispositionally) related to previously concluded diagnoses.

The multiple related diagnoses problem is a component of the multiple diagnoses problem, as noted previously. In general, the INTERNIST-I system displayed an uncanny ability to solve cases with multiple diagnoses sequentially, but on a number of cases, the system suffered from its inability to take a broad overview of a case in which related diseases were present in multiple organ systems [17-18, 40], especially when overwhelming evidence was lacking for the cause in any of the involved organ systems. To solve the multiple diagnoses problem sequentially, the INTERNIST-I approach relied on the ability of the program to identify a problem area (set of competitor diagnoses) in which the program could correctly conclude a diagnosis. The program's ability to solve the multiple related diagnoses problem depends on first concluding a diagnosis that is related to the other (yet undiagnosed) conditions in the patient. The program's approach of assuming that all findings potentially caused by a diagnosis were explained by the diagnosis upon its conclusion presented a problem for the system. Findings are often multifactorial in nature, with more than one cause present in the patient concurrently. Marking a finding as explained by the first concluded hypothesis consistent with the finding potentially eliminates consideration of better explanations for the finding among subsequently hypothesized diagnoses. Even worse, upon explanation, the finding is not available to evoke any hypotheses directly itself, nor does it contribute to the scoring of hypotheses that potentially explain the finding better than the previously concluded diagnosis. The new multiple-related diagnoses algorithm presented in this paper represents an attempt to overcome these known shortcomings in the INTERNIST-I program.

Patil developed ABEL in the late 1970s and early 1980s as an approach to multiple diagnoses employing pathophysiological reasoning about acid-base and electrolyte disorders [19]. The approach depended heavily on a deep model of domain knowledge. ABEL used semi-quantitative reasoning, based on its deep pathophysilogical knowledge, to predict when additional disorders should be hypothesized. When the degree of change represented by the patient's abnormal test results could not be accounted for by existing hypotheses, ABEL generated additional hypotheses to explain the "unaccounted-for" portion of the patient's abnormalities. While ABEL represented a tour-de-force in diagnostic reasoning, its knowledge base requirements made it an impractical model for general diagnosis, and its computational complexity made it cumbersome for real-time applications. The applicability of the ABEL approach is limited in that deep knowledge representations can be constructed in the areas of acid-base physiology or cardiovascular physiology, but not for most other areas of medicine (such as dermatology, rheumatology, or psychiatry).

During the 1980s, Reggia and Peng [12] developed parsimonious set covering theory as a formal approach to the multiple diagnoses problem. The formalism led to a decrease in computational tractability compared to earlier heuristic approaches. The set covering approach viewed the individual differential diagnoses of findings present in a patient case as creating a domain from which subsets of diagnoses could be selected that individually explain subsets of the findings present   They defined a minimal cover set as the smallest number of diagnoses required to explain concurrently all findings in the case, and an irreducible cover set as one where the removal of any individual diagnosis from the set would cause some findings to become "unexplained".   Ultimately, Peng and Reggia proposed an INTERNIST-I-like Bayesian overlay for set covering that would be capable of ranking various cover sets against one another [34-35]. This approach in many ways represented a more formal mathematical codification of the heuristic approaches used by Pople in INTERNIST-I [17-18].   However, the approach suffered from lack of ability to conclude any particular diagnosis conclusively. The most parsimonious set covering is not always the correct diagnosis for the patient, and in fact, sometimes it a portion of the multiple diagnoses problem is solved easily in a patient (e.g., the patient is presenting with AIDS but the problem is to diagnose which complications of that disease are also present).

Several problems exist with the cover set model.   First, its computational tractability was questionable (eventually heuristic methods were introduced to help with this problem [12]).   Second, the model did not take into account interrelationships among diseases -- i.e., the presence of disease A (such as hypertension) may cause or predispose to disease B (such as stroke or end-stage renal disease). Clinicians use such relationships regularly in solving complex multi-system diagnostic problems. In contrast, the Bayesian version of the cover set model Peng and Reggia proposed in 1987 required the independence of diseases [34-35]. The sequential INTERNIST-I approach allowed the system (when possible) to correctly conclude an "anchor point" diagnosis and then all of its potentially related diagnoses would receive extra consideration, improving the chances that related diagnoses would be concluded when appropriate, but allowing appropriate consideration of "independent" alternatives as well.

Beginning in the early 1980s, Pearl [13], Cooper and colleagues at Stanford [14-16], and a number of other groups have developed Bayesian Belief Networks as a method for handing multiple concurrent diagnoses. This approach also suffers from computational intractability for large medical knowledge bases, as well as the lack of reliable probabilistic and causal data. When three numbers with confidence bounds of plus or minus ten percent are multiplied together as a product, the resulting product has error bounds of plus or minus 30%. Few medical decisions can be made under such uncertainty. These systems require large numbers of multiplications of "fuzzy numbers" (estimates of prior probabilities of disease; estimates of sensitivities of findings for diseases; similar estimates for pathophysiological states that have not been carefully studied epidemiologically), making any result subject to considerable question. In general, such systems require a number of medically unrealistic assumptions to be made to make the approach computationally tractable. The great clinician-philosopher Alvin Feinstein of Yale University had a remarkably insightful comment on computationally difficult, mathematically-oriented systems two decades ago:

"Iatromathematical enthusiasts could make substantial contributions to clinical medicine if the efforts now being expended on Bayesian and decision-analytic fantasies were directed to the major challenges of algorithmically dissecting clinical judgment, based on the way the judgments are actually performed. Instead, however, the enthusiasts usually become infatuated with the mathematical processes and with the associated potential for computer manipulations, so that the basic clinical challenges become neglected or evaded ... " [18, 37].

Miller and Masarie developed and refined the QMR relationships function during the late 1980s, and described the algorithm in detail in a 1992 MEDINFO paper [38]. The goal of the relationships function is to quickly and efficiently identify all plausible single- and multi- (up to a limit of four) diagnosis hypotheses that could completely explain the presence of a small number of (less than 10) input findings. The algorithm answers the question, "If I could explain all of the following small number of critical findings in the patient case, I believe I would have a correct diagnostic solution. What are the sets of single or multiple interrelated diagnoses that explain each and every one of the following findings?" The efficiency of the QMR relationships function results from recognition that physicians can summarize the salient features of cases in order to provide brief computer input, and acknowledgment that the program's output needs only to mention relevant diagnostic considerations, since the physician-user can determine which ones are relevant to the actual patient case (QMR also provided other tools to assist in this process). The use of pre-compiled knowledge base structures in the form of bitmaps stored in disk files greatly improved the computational efficiency of what would otherwise be difficult combinatorial calculations. Constraints were that all multiple diagnosis hypotheses had to be causally or predispositionally interrelated, and the insistence that all input findings be explained. The algorithm was not useful for cases with multiple independent (unrelated) disorders concurrently present, and would not suggest correct diagnoses if one of the input findings was a misleading "false positive" finding. The INTERNIST-I diagnostic algorithm (which also is an independent component of the QMR tool set), because of its quasi-probabilistic nature, and its partitioning heuristic, was less susceptible to false positive findings.

Wu, from 1988-1991, developed a symptom-clustering approach to the multiple diagnoses problem [39]. While heuristic in nature, the approach was computationally intensive. Like the model proposed by Eddy and Clanton [36] for human reasoning in complex cases, Wu's approach relied on the identification of pivotal, or focal, findings, whose differential diagnoses (in Wu's model) did not subsume the differential diagnoses of any other finding present in the patient case. Wu's algorithm constructed symptom clusters whose differential diagnoses included a common set of disorders that could explain all findings within the cluster. Wu noted that the multiple diagnoses problem could be solved by taking the Cartesian product of the sets of diagnoses associated with each symptom cluster.

3. Description of Method
3.1. Assumptions underlying the new algorithm for multiple diagnoses
The new method for multiple diagnoses relies on the following assumptions:

3.1.1 A medical diagnostic knowledge base (MDKB) exists describing the findings (Mi) associated with each disorder (Dj). The MDKB must provide the equivalent of positive predictive values (PPVij) of findings (Mi) for disorders (Dj), as well as the sensitivity (Sij) of each finding for each disorder in which it occurs. As an aside, based on decades of literature review of hundreds of articles regarding each of 600+ diagnoses, the author believes that the medical literature supports such information (PPV and sensitivity) to approximately one part in five (i.e., plus or minus 10 percent) [26-27]. In the INTERNIST-I and QMR knowledge bases, "evoking strength" scores on a scale of 0 to 5, with 0 being non-specific and 5 "pathognomic", are used for PPVij; and, scores on a scale of 1 to 5 are used for Sij, with 1 indicating "very rare but reported by at least two groups independently" and 5 meaning "essentially all - a sine qua non for the diagnosis".

3.1.2 A table or list exists for each disorder (Dj) in the MDKB which specifies:
(a) the other disorders Dk in the knowledge base that the given disease Dj either causes or is caused-by, with a frequency (sensitivity) of causation Cjk and a frequency of being caused-by Bjk;
(b) the other disorders Dm in the knowledge base with which the given disease Dj co-occurs (empirically verified association based on epidemiological evidence) with a forward associational frequency Fjm and a reverse associational frequency Rjm. Refer to these relationships collectively as R(Dj -> Dn), where Dn represents the union of Dk and Dm.

Note that in the INTERNIST-I and QMR MDKBs, the Cjk, Bjk, and Fjm are given on the same 1 to 5 scale as the Sij.

3.1.3 A metric G(Mi) exists which gives the global significance of each diagnostic finding Mi in isolation (i.e., a measure of how strongly a clinician should be compelled to explain the presence of the finding in a patient by making a diagnosis related to the finding). In the INTERNIST-I and QMR MDKBs, this G(Mi) "import" is given on a 1 to 5 scale, with 1 indicating a finding that rarely merits diagnostic explanation, and 5 indicating a finding which must always be explained diagnostically [17]. A second metric, H(Di, Dj) calculates the percent homology of two disorders by computing the intersection of the modified disease profiles, Di' and Dj' (after removing from each disease description any laboratory tests classified as "moderately or extremely expensive or invasive"), and using the function G(M) to weight the significance of the remaining findings from the intersection (obtaining $G(I)$). The $G()$ function then is used to weight the modified disease descriptions Di' and Dj', and the homology score is calculated as

$H(Di,Dj) = 100 \times G(I) / ((min (G(Di'), G(Dj')) + 0.1*max (G(Di'),G(Dj')))$ [40]

The derivation and utility of homologies is discussed by Berman in reference [40].

3.1.4 The goal of the multiple-related diagnoses algorithm is to identify the best-supported set of related (causally or epidemiologically) disorders that are consistent with the observed patient findings (but which do not necessarily explain all observed findings).

3.1.5 The basis for the algorithm is several observations about clinical diagnosis.

(a) It is unusual in a patient case for "hidden diagnoses" or "hidden states" to be present when multiple diagnoses are concurrently present. Usually, there will be clinical evidence, in the form of observable or measurable findings, to support each diagnosis that applies to the patient. The algorithm hypothesizes that in a causal chain (e.g., disorder A causing disorder B causing disorder C causing disorder D), there will at most be one disorder where there may not be much direct clinical evidence to support the hypothesis.

(b) The underlying assumption is that clinicians recognize interrelated disorders by the "company they keep". Not only do patient findings support diagnostic hypotheses that directly explain them, but they also provide indirect support for diagnoses causally or otherwise related to the diagnoses that directly explain them. In the causal chain listed in 3.1.5(a) above, evidence directly supporting disorder B and disorder D indirectly gives credence to disorder C, which is causally related to both B and D. A medical knowledge base can be "compiled" in a manner to take advantage of indirect evidence of this sort.

3.2. The algorithm for knowledge base construction for multiple diagnosis

The new method for multiple diagnoses requires construction of the following knowledge base components (from other pre-existing KB structures):

3.2.1 For each disorder (disease or high-level pathophysiological state, such as chronic congestive left heart failure) Dj in the medical knowledge base, construct a list Dn of all causally or predispostionally related disorders (causes of Dj, complications of Dj, and disorders that co-occur with Dj with more than chance frequency). This list is constructed from the relationships R(Dj->Dn) described above. Dj is called the "focal disorder" below.

3.2.2 For each Dn related to the focal disorder, take the list of all findings Mn of Dn and merge them into a union of all findings for all Dn. From this merged list of findings U(Mn), subtract out the findings that are the direct findings of the focal disorder Dj: the result is U(Mn)-Mj = Rj, the related findings of focal disorder Dj.

3.2.3 Construct a new knowledge base structure Rj for each disorder Dj in the knowledge base. For each finding Mr in Rj, compute a "strength of relationship" score that represents the maximum (across all Dn related to Dj) of either (a) the frequency with which Dn occurs given Dj multiplied by the frequency of the current Mr in the disorder Dn; plus (b) the frequency with which Dn explains Mr (as opposed to other causes of Mr) multiplied by the frequency with which Dj occurs given Dn.

3.2.4 Invert the data structures created in step 3.2.3. This will give, for any finding Mx, the list of disorders Dz for which Mx provides indirect associational evidence: call this list A(Mx->Dz). Maintain with this list the associational strengths calculated as part of step 3.2.3.

3.3 The algorithm for diagnosis of multiple interrelated conditions
The diagnostic algorithm that uses the knowledge structures outlined in Section 3.2 follows:

3.3.1 Assume that a case is described by a series of findings present in the patient, M+, and a set of "pertinent negative" findings sought for but found to be absent in the case, M-.

3.3.2 Construct a list of scored, directly evoked set of "single best diagnoses" using the INTERNIST-I (or similar) algorithm [17], using M+, M-, and the available knowledge base.

3.3.3 For each finding Mi of M+, retrieve the list of indirectly associated disorders A(Mi->Dz). Construct a list of "indirectly supported diagnoses" from these lists for all Mi in M+. Weight each of these diagnoses Dz by both the "strength of relationship" score calculated as part of the supporting knowledge structures, and by the combined importance of the findings explained by Dz, given by G(Mi).

3.3.4 Review the 15 top-most single diagnoses generated by the "best single diagnosis" (INTERNIST-I/QMR) scoring algorithm. Using the topmost diagnosis as a seed, determine its problem area cohorts from the list using the homology function H(), described above, with a cutoff threshold for "similarity" at 35% (i.e., diseases belong to the same problem area if their homology score is >34%). Repeat passes through the same list of 15 diagnoses, using the highest ranked disease hypothesis not yet part of a problem area as the seed for the next problem area. Repeat the same process for the 15 top-ranked indirectly evoked disorders generated by step 4.3.3.

3.3.5 Create aggregate hypotheses. Call the list of directly evoked single hypotheses "List D" and the list of indirectly evoked hypotheses "List I". Create aggregate hypotheses using the problem areas from List I. For each problem area in List I, determine if 1-step linkages exist to any of the 15 diseases on List D. If such links exist, add related diseases from List I and List D to the new aggregate. Continue to grow the aggregate by determining if there are additional links from new members of the aggregate to other members of List I or List D. Limit aggregates to size of 5 or fewer related problem areas.

3.3.6 Use the other available tools in the diagnostic decision support system to investigate the plausibility (concludability) of members of the aggregate hypotheses.

4. Results
The algorithm described above was implemented in Turbo Pascal as an extension

---

Figure 1: Global Overview: NEJM 1991, Volume 324, Page 547
Please refer to published case report [44] for findings and "correct" diagnoses

UNIFYING HYPOTHESIS #1: 212
   512 Takayasus Arteritis
   With one or more CONSEQUENT diseases including:
      One Disease from the following list:
         57 Myocardial Infarction Acute
         67 Angina Pectoris
         8 Cardiomyopathy Secondary
      Plus One Disease from the following list:
         45 Aortic Dissection

UNIFYING HYPOTHESIS #2: 165
   459 Renal Artery Stenosis
   [Rest of hypothesis similar to CONSEQUENT list above]

UNIFYING HYPOTHESIS #3: 162
   372 Mitral Stenosis
   One ANTECEDENT from the following:
      25 Aortic Valvular Stenosis
   With one or more CONSEQUENT diseases including:
      One Disease from the following list:
         48 Angina Pectoris
      Plus One Disease from the following list:
         16 Aortic Regurgitation Chronic

UNIFYING HYPOTHESIS #4: 124
   370 Arteriolar Nephrosclerosis Benign <ESSENTIAL HYPERTENSION>
   With one or more CONSEQUENT diseases including:
      One Disease from the following list:
         33 Aortic Dissection
      Plus One Disease from the following list:
         37 Arteriosclerotic Heart Disease
         27 Hypertensive Heart Disease
      Plus One Disease from the following list:
         10 Cerebral Artery Thrombosis Or Dissection With Encephalomalacia

---

of the final non-commercial version of the QMR program (1990 version). No formal evaluation of its performance has yet been conducted. Anecdotally, the algorithm is capable of suggesting correct sets of diagnoses on several difficult NEJM CPC [17, 38] type cases (with several dozen positive and negative findings); Figure 1 illustrates the output from the new algorithm in analyzing such a case [44]. The anatomically proven correct diagnosis for the case was aortic dissection. The timing performance (global overview produced in 2 to 20 seconds on an Intel pentium-class CPU) is substantially better than the speed of earlier algorithms for multiple diagnoses, with the exception of the QMR relationships function (which is limited to a maximum of 10 input findings).

5. Discussion

The new multiple-diagnoses algorithm was developed as a part of the QMR program [17,26-29,38,40-43]. The general approach taken in developing QMR was to abandon the model of a monolithic expert system which could solve any challenging diagnostic case while the physician-user watched passively in awe [29]. Instead, the philosophy of QMR is to present a number of "expert" tools, to be selectively and sequentially applied by the clinician-user. The tools that comprise QMR provide useful perspectives on various individual components of diagnostic problem-solving. A human diagnostician, when faced with a challenging problem, will often seek the advice of expert colleagues, review portions of the medical literature, compare the case to similar ones, and re-examine the patient more carefully in the light of any new information received. The result of these activities is that the clinician synthesizes aspects of multiple divergent approaches to the case. It is unusual for multiple consultants and information sources to produce a single, integrated, and uniformly correct answer for a complex case. The QMR tool set contains a variety of approaches to solving diagnostic problems, ranging from the program's ability, at the textbook level, to display the differential diagnosis of any of 4500 findings in general internal medicine [41-42]; at the integrative level, to quickly provide suggestions for multiple diagnoses explaining a small set of critical input findings, through the QMR relationships function [38], and, at the expert consultant level, through a modified version of the original INTERNIST-I algorithm [17], to provide a list of "single best hypotheses" that can be manipulated by the user to generate questions for the user to answer selectively. What was missing from the QMR tool set was an algorithm that could take into consideration all of the input findings in a complex case, and which could suggest clinically plausible "unifying hypotheses" – sets of interrelated diagnoses that taken together that explain most of the clinically important findings presented in the case. This viewpoint would be a particularly valuable complement to the QMR/INTERNIST-I "find the best single diagnosis" algorithm [17]. The new multiple related diagnoses algorithm fills this niche.

The method for constructing complex inter-related multi-disease differential diagnoses is intended to serve as a complement to previous algorithms designed to identify the best single-disease hypothesis [17] and the QMR relationships function, which provides a quick approach to multiple diagnoses [38]. The new algorithm does not work well in cases with a single diagnosis or when only multiple unrelated diagnoses are present, since these conditions violate its underlying assumptions. A more formal evaluation of this promising approach is warranted.

References

1. Nash FA. Differential diagnosis: an apparatus to assist the logical faculties. Lancet 1954; 1:874.
2. Lipkin M and Hardy JD. Differential diagnosis of hematological diseases aided by mechanical correlation of data. Science. 1957; 125:551-552.
3. Ledley RS and Lusted LB. Reasoning Foundations of Medical Diagnosis. Science 1959; 130:9-21.

4. Warner HR, Toronto AF, Veasey LG, Stephenson RA. Mathematical Approach to Medical Diagnosis. J. Am Med Assoc (JAMA). 1961; 177:75-81.

5. Reichertz P: Diagnosis and automation Medizinische Monatsschrift. 1965; 19:344-7.

6. Gremy F. Joly H: Problem of the application of electronic computers to diagnosis Revue Francaise D Etudes Cliniques Et Biologiques. 1967; 12(4):322-9.

7. Gorry A. Strategies for Computer-Aided Diagnosis. Mathematical Biosciences 1968; 2:293-318.

8. Gorry GA. Barnett GO: Experience with a model of sequential diagnosis. Computers & Biomedical Research. 1968; 1(5):490-507.

9 Bleich HL. Computer evaluation of acid-base disorders. Journal of Clinical Investigation. 1969; 48(9):1689-96.

10 de Dombal FT. Hartley JR. Sleeman DH: A computer-assisted system for learning clinical diagnosis. Lancet. 1969; 1(586):145-8.

11. Miller RA. Medical diagnostic decision support systems - past, present, and future. J. Am. Med. Informatics.Assoc (JAMIA). 1994; 1:8-27.

12. Reggia JA, Nau DS, Wang PY. Diagnostic expert systems based on a set covering model. Internat J Man-Machine Stud. 1983; 19:437-460.

13. Pearl J. Evidential reasoning using stochastic simulation of causal models. Artificial Intelligence. 1987; 32(2):245-252.

14 Cooper GF. NESTOR. Doctoral dissertation thesis, Medical Information Science Program, Stanford University. 1984.

15 1991.47. Shwe MA Middleton B Heckerman DE Henrion M Horvitz EJ Lehmann HP Cooper GF: Probabilistic diagnosis using a reformulation of the INTERNIST-1/QMR knowledge base. I. The probabilistic model and inference algorithms. Methods Inf Med. 1991; 30:241-55.

16. Middleton B, Shwe MA, Heckerman DE, et al. Probabilistic diagnosis using a reformulation of the INTERNIST-I/QMR knowledge base. II: Evaluation of diagnostic performance. Methods Inf Med. 1991; 30:256-67.

17. Miller RA, Pople HE Jr, Myers JD. INTERNIST-1, An Experimental Computer-based Diagnostic Consultant for General Internal Medicine. N Engl J Med. 1982; 307:468-76.

18.. Pople HE Jr. Heuristic methods for imposing structure on ill-structured problems: the structuring of medical diagnostics. In: Szolovits P (ed). Artificial Intelligence in Medicine. AAAS Selected Symposium Series. Westview Press:Boulder, CO. 1982. pp 119-190.

19. Patil RS, Szolovits P, Schwartz WB. Modeling knowledge of the patient in acid-base and electrolyte disorders. In: Szolovits P (ed). Artificial Intelligence in Medicine. AAAS Selected Symposium Series. Westview Press:Boulder, CO. 1982. pp 190-226.

20. Warner HR Jr. ILIIAD: Moving medical decision-making to new frontiers. Meth Inform Med. 1989; 28:370-2.

21. Waxman HS, Worley WE. Computer-assisted adult medical diagnosis: subject review and evaluation of a new microcomputer-based system. Medicine (Baltimore) 1990; 69:125-36.

22. Rumelhart DE McClelland JL et al. Parallel Distributed Processing, Volumes I and II. MIT Press: Cambridge, MA. 1988.

23. Hart A Wyatt J: Evaluating black-boxes as medical decision aids: issues arising from a study of neural networks. Med Inf (Lond), 15:229-36, 1990 Jul-Sep.

24 Baxt WG: Use of an artificial neural network for the diagnosis of myocardial infarction. Ann Intern Med, 1991; 115:843-8.

25 Aliferis CF, Miller RA. On the Heuristic Nature of Medical Decision Support Systems. Meth Inform Med. 1995; 34:5-14.

26 Miller RA. Internist-1/CADUCEUS: Problems Facing Expert Consultant Programs. Meth Inform Med. 1984; 23:9-14.

27. Giuse DA, Giuse NB, Miller RA. Towards Computer Assisted Maintenance of Medical Knowledge Bases. Artificial Intelligence in Medicine. 1990; 2:21-33.

28. Miller RA, Giuse NB. The Medicine in Medical Informatics: Medical Knowledge Bases.Academic Medicine. 1991; 66:15-17.

29. Miller RA. (Editorial) The Demise of the "Greek Oracle" Model for Medical Diagnostic Systems. Meth Inform Med. 1990; 29:1-2.

30. Miller RA, Schaffner KF, Meisel A. Ethical and Legal Issues Related to the Use of Computer Programs in Clinical Medicine. Ann Intern Med. 1985; 102:529-36.

31. Miller RA. Evaluating Evaluations of Medical Diagnostic Systems (Editorial). J. Am. Med. Informatics Association (JAMIA). 1996; 3:429-31.

32. Ben-Bassat M, Carlson RW, Puri VK, et al. Pattern-based interactive diagnosis of multiple disorders: the MEDAS system. IEEE transactions on Pattern Analysis and Machine Intelligence. PAMI-1,2 1980a, pp. 148-60.

33.Ben-Bassat M, Campbell D, McNeil A, Weil MH. Evaluating multimembership classifiers: a methodology and application to the MEDAS system. IEEE transactions on Pattern Analysis and Machine Intelligence. PAMI-5, 2 March 1983, pp. 225-9.

34. Peng Y and Reggia JA. A Probabilistic Causal Model for Diagnostic Problem Solving -- Part I: Integrating Symbolic Causal Inference with Numerica Probabilistic Inference. IEEE Transactions on Systems, Man, and Cybernetics 1987; SMC-17:146-162.

35. Peng Y and Reggia JA. A Probabilistic Causal Model for Diagnostic Problem Solving -- Part II: Diagnostic Strategy. IEEE Transactions on Systems, Man, and Cybernetics 1987; SMC-17:395-406.

36. Eddy DM, Clanton CH. The art of diagnosis: solving the clinicopathological conference. N Engl J Med. 1982; 306:1263-1269.

37. Feinstein AR. Clinical Biostatistics XXXIX. The haze of Bayes, the aerial palaces of decision analysis, and the computerized Ouija board. Clin Pharm Therapeutics. 1977; 21:482-496, p. 495.

38. Miller RA, Masarie FE. The Quick Medical Reference (QMR) Relationships Function: Description and Evaluation of a Simple, Efficient "Multiple Diagnoses" Algorithm. In: Lun et al (eds), Proceedings of MEDINFO 92, Geneva, Switzerland, September 1992. pp. 512-8.

39. Wu TD. A problem decomposition method for efficient diagnosis and interpretation of multiple disorders. In Miller RA (ed). Proc 14th Ann Sympos Comput Applic Med Care (SCAMC). IEEE Press: New York. 1990. pp. 86-92.

40. Berman L, Miller RA. Problem area formation as an element of computer-aided diagnosis: a comparison of two strategies with Quick Medical Reference (QMR). Meth Inform Med. 1991; 30:90-95.

41. Miller RA, Masarie FE, Myers JD. "Quick Medical Reference" for diagnostic assistance. MD Computing. 1986; 3:34-48.

42. Miller RA, McNeil MA, Challinor S, Masarie FE, Myers JD. Status Report: The INTERNIST-1 / Quick Medical Reference Project. West J Med. 1986; 145:816-22.

43. Bankowitz RA, McNeil MA, Challinor SM, Parker RC, Kapoor WN, Miller RA. A computer-assisted medical diagnostic consultation service: implementation and prospective evaluation of a prototype. Ann Intern Med. 1989; 110:824-32.

44. Case records of the Massachusetts General Hospital. A 69-year-old man with abdominal pain six weeks after a coronary revascularization procedure. N Engl J Med. 1991; 324:547-55.

Intelligent Assistance for Coronary Heart Disease Diagnosis: A Comparison Study

Guido Bologna, Ahmed Rida, Christian Pellegrini

Artificial intelligence group, Computing Science Center, University of Geneva
24 rue General Dufour, CH-1211 Geneva 4, Switzerland

Abstract. Using only non invasive medical information, we propose inductive decision trees exploiting C4.5 algorithm, artificial neural networks with three MLP models, and linear discriminant analysis to diagnose coronary heart disease. The first neural network model is a constructive MLP called OIL (Orthogonal Incrementing Learning) that builds its hidden neurons during the training phase. The second one is a fixed MLP architecture with the same number of hidden neurons obtained from the first network building methodology. The last one is a special "interpretable" MLP model with a fixed architecture (IMLP), which is interpretable through symbolic rule extraction. In general, explanation of connectionist model responses are difficult to obtain, especially when input examples have continuous variables. This is not acceptable for real world diagnosis applications. The novelty in our study consists in the interpretability of the IMLP model we have developed. For this diagnosis application, all neural networks globally obtain better predictive accuracies than C4.5 and the linear discriminant analysis. Results obtained with the OIL method are slightly better than those obtained by IMLP, but they lack interpretability.

1   Introduction

Classification problems are among the most promising fields for neural network applications; problems which are hardly solved by classical deterministic algorithms or by conventional expert systems may be handled efficiently by well-trained neural networks.

In the context of coronary heart disease, using only non invasive medical information, we propose to compare the diagnosis performed by inductive decision trees, artificial neural networks, and linear discriminant analysis. The MLP (Multi Layer Perceptron) model [1] is widely used in the connectionist community. However, justifications of network responses are difficult to obtain, especially when input examples have continuous variables. This is not acceptable for real world diagnosis applications. In fact especially for critical diseases, the physician using a diagnosis help system strictly needs to understand the decision making mechanism.

In general, several rule extraction techniques from neural networks are carried out from binary input variables (as an example see [2] [3]). The rule extraction becomes particularly difficult when input observations contain continuous variables [4]. Andrews and Jeva introduced the Rulex model that is close to a dynamic RBF model in which rules are extracted in a natural manner even with continuous input neurons [5].

Many authors have presented comparisons between MLPs and inductive decision trees [6] [7] [8] [9] [10] [11]. We propose to perform diagnosis with C4.5 [12], a standard algorithm which produces interpretable inductive decision trees, three MLP models, and linear discriminant analysis. The first MLP model is a constructive network where hidden neurons are generated during the learning phase, the second one is a fixed architecture MLP, and the last one we have developed is a special interpretable MLP (IMLP[1]) through symbolic rule extraction. In this last model, rules are extracted in a natural manner even when the datasets include continuous variables. The novelty in our approach resides in the architecture of the model. Neither explicit transformation of the datasets, nor clustering algorithms applied both to model and datasets are needed. To our knowledge, applying in all cases the so-called exact rule extraction method, IMLP is the sole model able to provide zero order categorical rules from continuous attributes which exactly mimic the neural network classification.

2 Application Description

The Coronary Heart Disease application data was supplied by the Institute of Cardiology of the University of Pisa (Italy) [13]. The total number of patients, symptomatic of CHD (Coronary Heart Disease) included in the study is 884; each patient had a complete angiographic study of the coronary tree. The results of angiography are considered the "gold standard" for correct classification. The patients were thus classified as not having (314 cases) or having (570 cases) CHD. A subject was included in the CHD group when his coronary angiography showed the presence of at least one stenosis greater than 75% of the lumen. For each patient the following 16 variables were recorded: age, sex, height, weight, smoking habits (yes/no, where yes denotes smokers or ex-smokers with less than 10 years of abstinence), family history (yes/no, where yes denotes the presence of CHD in at least one relative), presence of diabetes (according to blood glucose level values and the use of anti-diabetic drugs), arterial systolic and diastolic pressures measured at the admission, serum cholesterol level, total High Density Lipoprotein, α-High Density Lipoprotein, triglycerides, β/α ratio (defined as the ratio between the β-High Density Lipoprotein and the α-High Density Lipoprotein), low density lipoprotein, and fibrinogen.

3 Inductive Decision Trees

Inductive decision tree algorithms recursively build a descending tree by selecting at each step the variable with the highest splitting power. Then a training set with known classes (having CHD, non-having CHD) is split according to some

---

[1] For simplicity IMLP will denote Interpretable Multi Layer Perceptron

determined threshold for the value of a given variable. The leaves are made up of images belonging to the same class. The variables determined at the nodes on the path between the root and a leaf form a class description. Later, newly analyzed patients may be associated with one of the classes by descending the tree along the path on which the successive variable values match. We experimented with inductive decision trees using Quinlan's C4.5 implementation [12].

4 Feed-Forward Neural Networks

In this section we describe the approach we adopt to solve this classification problem using feedforward neural networks. To use them, we consider our problem as a regression problem which consists in approximating a true real function f from a compact sub-domain $\Omega \subset \Re^m$ into $\Re^p$ (for our problem $m = 16$ $p = 1$ and $\Omega = [0, 1]^{16}$), according to the L^2 norm:

$$\|f - g\|_{L^2}^2 = \int_\Omega \|f(x) - g(x)\|^2 dx; \tag{1}$$

where $\|.\|$ is the euclidean norm in $\Re^p$. But, since the available information about the problem is a sample (a set of variable's measures, target diagnosis class) $(x_1, f(x_1)), ..., (x_N, f(x_N))$, the feed-forward network will be trained by minimizing the mean square error function:

$$E = \frac{1}{2N} \sum_{i=1}^{N} \|g(x_i) - f(x_i)\|^2 . \tag{2}$$

After preprocessing of the data (feature selection, normalization), the most difficult tasks are:

1. neural network topology determination;
2. training the neural network (optimization according to the available data).

For the first task, the methodology we choose is described by the following two steps:

1. determine the topology by an incremental self configuring algorithm;
2. train the obtained different network architectures given by this algorithm.

For the first phase of the topology determination, we had a choice among several algorithms: Cascade-Correlation [14] Internal Representation Optimization (IRO) [15] and Orthogonal Incremental Learning(OIL) [16]. After preliminary trials, we chose the OIL algorithm as it gave the most promising results on our coronary heart disease application[2]. This algorithm consists in incrementally building-up a sequence of n-dimensional one-hidden-layer feedforward neural networks $(g_n)_{n \geq 1}$ which converge to the true function f. The characteristic of this algorithm is that the hidden neurons are orthogonal from functional point of view(see [16] for details). .

---

[2] this assumption concerns only the CHD application

The second task pertains to optimization techniques. In the case of feedforward neural networks, the optimization problem induced by the learning task is highly non-convex. In large spaces, such optimization is NP-hard because of the existence of many local optima and the optimization schemata used are not able to deal with them efficiently. The second related problem is the parameter optimization procedure set, the tuning of which depends on given application and topology. So, for this task when the error (2) is a differentiable function of the weights,[3] we decided to use a gradient based optimization schema which allows a self-tuning parameter set. After preliminary results obtained with Scaled Conjugate Gradient (SCG) [17] and Rprop [18], the latter has given better results on the CHD application. When the error function (2) is not differentiable we use the Simulated Annealing algorithm [19] (see sect. 5).

4.1 Learning with a fixed architecture

For this phase, we use Rprop [18] to train the network architectures produced by OIL. Moreover, in order to follow the general architecture model given by OIL we used:

- the sigmoidal activation function without bias $h(x) = (1 + e^{-x})^{-1}$ for the hidden units;
- the identity with bias for the output units $act(x) = x + b$

5 An interpretable MLP

In this section we propose a method related to the rule extraction hybrid learning paradigm. For this purpose, we translate a particular trained MLP architecture into a rulebase [20]. Hence, if such an MLP is used in a diagnosis help system, physicians could have justification of its responses.

5.1 The MLP architecture and learning

The architecture: We define an MLP with an input layer, one or two hidden layers and an output layer (cf. fig. 1). In this model, each neuron of the first hidden layer is connected to only one input neuron and to the bias virtual unit. All the other layers are fully connected. The output value h_j of the jth hidden unit of the first hidden layer is given by the threshold function:

$$h_j = \begin{cases} 1 \text{ if } \sum_k w_{jk}.x_k > 0 \\ 0 \text{ otherwise} \end{cases} \tag{3}$$

---

[3] the bias is considered as a weight from a virtual unit with constant activity set to 1

When the model has two hidden layers, the second hidden layer responses are not given by the threshold function but rather by the sigmoid function. The output value o_i of the ith output unit is given by the sigmoid function :

$$o_i = \sigma(\sum_j v_{ij} \cdot h_j) = 1/(1 + exp(-\sum_j v_{ij} \cdot h_j)) \qquad (4)$$

where v_{ij} represents the weight associated with the connection from hidden neuron j to output neuron i.

Hence, this MLP architecture differs from the previous architectures used in section 4 on three main points:

1. each hidden node in the first hidden layer is connected to only one input node;
2. the activation function used for the first hidden layer units is the threshold function instead of the sigmoid function. Therefore the mean sum square criterion (2) is not differentiable.
3. The first hidden layer size is determined experimentally from multiples of the input layer size.

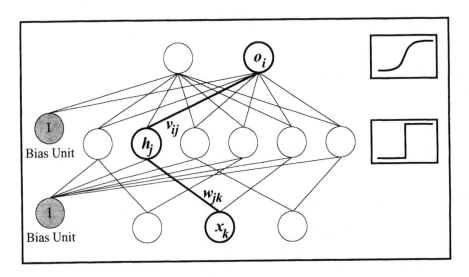

Fig. 1. a MLP network with one hidden layer of threshold units. Symbols x, h, and o represent respectively input units, hidden units, and output units. Weights going from the first to the second layer are denoted by symbol w, and weights going from the second to the third layer by symbol v. Each hidden unit is connected to only one input neuron and to the first bias unit.

Units of the first hidden layer define thresholds on input variables. These are represented in the conditions of extracted rules (cf. 5.2). The maximum number of thresholds is determined by the number of hidden neurons in the first hidden layer. In other terms, if an extracted rule from IMLP contains the condition $LDL > 0.445$ this does not imply that all the conditions including the LDL variable will have the same threshold. For instance, assuming that the first hidden layer size is at least twice the input layer size, we can also find the condition $LDL > 0.333$. Thus, the "expressive power" of the model can be enhanced by increasing the number of hidden neurons.

Learning algorithm: Since the error function (2) is not differentiable, the training algorithm used in this phase is Simulated Annealing [19] controlled by two parameters: the initial temperature and the maximum weight variation.

Weights changes are selected randomly from a uniform distribution. Each weight is modified individually according to the error variation ΔE. When ΔE is positive, the probability $P(accept)$ of accepting the weight change is given by

$$P(accept) = e^{-\frac{\Delta E}{T}} \tag{5}$$

where T represents the current temperature. If ΔE is negative the weight change is always accepted.

5.2 Rule extraction

The aim of our rule extraction techniques is to explain the IMLP decision making process by decoding its internal state into a *if..then* zero order set of conjunctive rules. We describe two methods for deriving such rules. *Exact rule extraction* which results represents the exact IMLP network classification and *Approximate rule extraction* wich represents an approximation of the former.

Exact rule extraction: Rules are extracted in the following way. We define a domain as a region split by at least one hyper-plane defined by the relation (eq.3). Because each hidden unit receives a connection from only one input neuron, all hyper-planes are parallel to the axes defined by input variables. If a hyper-plane separates two domains of different classes, the associated hidden unit is a discriminator. The values of all the connections between the first hidden layer and the output layer determine whether a hidden unit is a discriminator in each region of the input space.

Figure 2 illustrates the process of rule extraction for a two-dimensional example. This process follows three main steps:

1. All the output values of the first hidden layer are determined with training examples. This produces the set of all domains associated with the training set. Each domain is represented by a binary vector. As an example: $h_1=1$, $h_2=1$, describes domain D_4 in figure 2.

2. With an algorithm equivalent to boolean expression simplification, the set of domains determined in the first step is reduced to the set of fundamental domains. This corresponds to the elimination of all hyper-segments that are not discriminators. In figure 2 all domain descriptions (D_1, D_2, D_3, D_4) are simplified by fundamental domains F_1, F_2, and F_3.

3. Any fundamental domain binary description in the hidden unit space is replaced by hyper-segment inequalities in the input space. In figure 2 the domain F_2 defined by $h_2=1$ verifies rule R_2 in the input space. Rule R_2 is defined as $w_{20}+w_{22}x_2 > 0$ (or $x_2 > -w_{20}/w_{22}$), where w_{20} is the weight associated with the connection going from the first bias unit to the second hidden neuron, and w_{22} is the weight associated with the connection going from the second input neuron to the second hidden neuron.

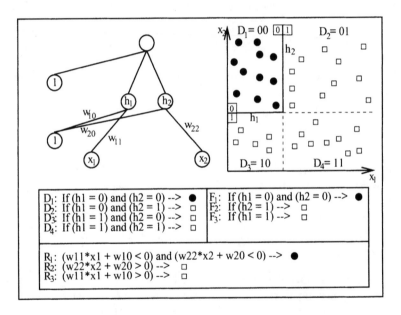

Fig. 2. Input space partition of a two class problem by a MLP network using threshold units in the hidden layer. Each domain is represented by hidden unit outputs. Each hidden neuron represents a potential discriminator (h_1 h_2 are partial discriminators). Using boolean expression simplification, domains D_1, D_2, D_3, and D_4 are replaced by fundamental domains F_1, F_2, and F_3. Finally, their reformulation in the input space gives rules R_1, R_2, and R_3.

Approximate rule extraction: For the approximate rule extraction method the only difference with respect to the exact rule extraction algorithm resides in the second step. In this case, the C4.5 algorithm is applied directly on all binary domains descriptions rather than performing boolean expression simplification. As a consequence, the obtained symbolic rules generally reflect the hidden units' approximate classification.[4] After step 3 of the exact rule extraction method, these rules are transcribed in the input space.

6   Results and Discussion

6.1   Description of experiments

The dataset contains 12 continuous and 4 binary variables. Therefore all the MLP models have 16 input neurons. The continuous variables are normalized into $[0, 1]$. The binary variables are encoded with values 0 or 1. Class CHD or non-CHD are respectively converted into binary values 0 or 1. Thus, all the MLP architectures used have one output neuron.

For the experiments we used a Stratified Cross Validation protocol (SCV). Half of the examples of each class are randomly selected to form the training sets. The remaining examples are not considered during the training phase. In fact, they are fed into the models to estimate their predictive accuracy (i.e. the global ratio of correct classifications to unknown examples). The operation is repeated 10 times and for each partition we perform a learning process 10 times.

Architectures obtained from the OIL constructive algorithm have given rise to a number of hidden neurons comprised between 1 and 5. Thus, fixed MLP architectures with 1 to 5 hidden neurons have been trained according to the SCV protocol. The interpretable MLP contains in its first and second hidden layer 256 and 10 neurons, respectively. This architecture has been tried empirically, because the OIL constructive algorithm is only relevant to those MLP networks fully connected between two successive layers.

For C4.5, we tried 360 parameter configurations. For each configuration we performed 100 trials obtained by SCV sampling method. For comparisons, we considered the best parameter configuration.

Finaly as a standard classification method we perform a linear discriminant analysis performed over 100 SCV trials.

6.2   Results

Results summarized in figure 3 show that all MLP networks globally obtain better predictive accuracies than C4.5 and discriminant linear analysis. The obtained predictive accuracies of the interpretable MLP are close to those obtained by the fixed architecture MLPs. The OIL algorithm has given slightly better results but its predictions are not interpretable into simple symbolic rules which could be understood by physicians.

---

[4] In fact the algorithm achieves a compromise between accuracy and number of generated rules.

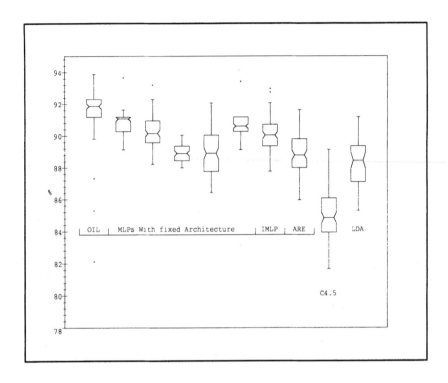

Fig. 3. Predictive accuracy distributions of different paradigms. From the left; first:OIL; following five boxplots: fixed architecture (resp. 1,2,3,4 and 5 hidden neurons); seventh: IMLP using exact rule extraction; eighth: IMLP using approximate rule extraction (ARE); nineth: linear discriminant analysis (LDA); on the extreme right: C4.5. Vertical axis represents the percentage of predictive accuracy.

Rule Extraction: We compare obtained rules from IMLP and C4.5 along three dimensions: mean predictive accuracy, mean number of rules, and mean number of conditions per rule. As shown by figure 4 the mean number of rules obtained with the exact rule extraction method is larger than that obtained by C4.5. However, using the approximate rule extraction method we obtain better mean predictive accuracy than C4.5 with close mean number of rules and mean number conditions per rule.

About rule examples: For all IMLP networks we obtained between 46 to 78 rules. Below we give an example of two rules extracted from a particular network. The two rules, referred to as R_1 and R_2, are used in 13.1% and 13.2% of the whole dataset, respectively. Moreover their respective accuracies on the testing set are 100% and 96.6%.

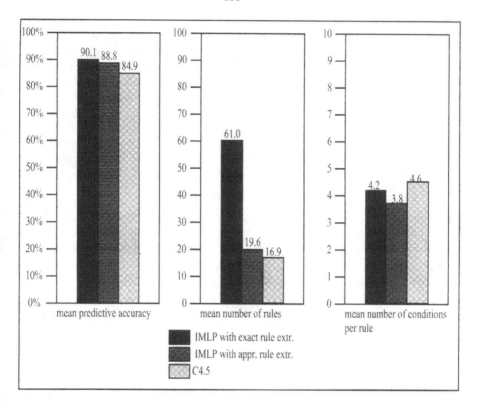

Fig. 4. From left to right barcharts represent: average accuracy performance, average number of rules and average number of conditions by rule.

R₁: If (*Woman*) and (Not *Family_History*) and ($\beta/\alpha < 0.146$) and (*Fibrinogen* < 0.307) then *Non_CHD*

R₂: If (*Man*) and (*Weight* < 0.657) and (*LDL* ≥ 0.445) then *CHD*

6.3 Discussion

Qualitative comparison between IMLP and C4.5: During the training phase of the IMLP model the error function (cf. 2) is minimized by the global working of all weights. Thus, during the training phase, all the attributes (via input neurons) intervene simultaneously to minimize the error criterion. On the other hand, during the tree construction C4.5 selects for each node only one attribute (according to the entropy criterion)[11]. Thus, at each node of the generated tree all attributes are not globally involved into the learning process. Consequently, if the classification process requires complex combinations between attributes C4.5 may obtain worse predictive accuracy than IMLP. Reciprocally, if just simple cutting up of attributes is sufficient to solve the problem C4.5 may obtain better predictive accuracy than IMLP [11].

Generally, a neural network with a fixed architecture builds a redundant internal representation of the problem. Thus, when rules are extracted from IMLP using the exact rule extraction method the generated rulebase contains some redundant information. Therefore, for the same classification problem more rules will be extracted from the IMLP model than those obtained from C4.5. However, using approximate rule extraction the number of previously generated rules is reduced (cf. fig.4) without reducing significantly the related performances.

Utilization in real life: For a non-expert in learning techniques, C4.5 is obviously simpler to use than any neural based technique. In fact, default C4.5 parameters work fine for many applications [12], whereas building up and training a neural network requires quite good knowledge of such techniques. To use C4.5 more optimaly than the default configuration a physician should aware about inductive decision tree manipulation. Such a user would not try to build up a classifier by fine tuning parameters related to an inductive decision tree construction or related to a neural network configuration and training, but would use directly the classifier (rulebase, trained neural network with interpretation...) *previously generated for his specific problem* by an expert in machine learning techniques.

7 Conclusion

Using only non invasive information, we presented a coronary heart disease diagnosis application realized by linear discriminant analysis, C4.5, and MLP neural networks. We showed that in this particular task MLP models are globally more accurate than C4.5 and linear discriminant analysis. Finally, the IMLP neural network classification mechanism has been transcribed into simple symbolic rules. This model, compared to fixed architecture MLPs has given similar predictive accuracies. On the other hand, the network building methodology OIL obtained slightly better results; but IMLP has an explanation capability through rule extraction, whereas OIL is not interpretable. Moreover, at first sight with the same observable attributes, IMLP (accuracy $\approx 90\%$) seems to reach better accuracies than those met in the typical clinical practice (accuracy $\approx 70\%$) [21]. Therefore, larger statistical analysis of IMLP results should be done. After that, comparisons between physicians with and without the IMLP diagnosis assistance may be carried out.

Acknowledgments

The authors are deeply in debt to U. Bottigli for having provided us with the Coronary Heart Disease dataset.

References

1. White H. Connectionist non-parametric regression. multi-layer feedforward networks can learn arbitrary mappings. Neural Networks 1990: 3 (3); 535–551.

2. Towell G.G, Shawlik J.W. Extracting Refined Rules from Knowledge-Based Neural Networks, Machine Learning, 13 (1), 1993.

3. Setiono R, Liu H. Understanding Neural Networks via Rule Extraction. IJCAI 1995: 1; 480–485.

4. Gorman R.P, Sejnowski T.J. Analysis of Hidden Unites in a Layered Network Trained to Classify Sonar Targets. Neural Networks 1988: 1(1); 75–88.

5. Andrews R, Geva S. Extracting Rules From a Constrained Error Backpropagation Network, Proc of the 5th Australian Conference on Neural Networks, Brisbane, 1994.

6. Mooney R, Shavlik J, Towell G, Gove A. An experimental Comparison of Symbolic and Connectionist Learning Algorithms, Proc. IJCAI-89 Morgan Kaufmann Los Altos, CA 775–780, 1989.

7. Atlas L, Cole R, Connor J, El-Sharkawi M, Marks R.J, Muthusumi Y, Barnard E. Performance Comparison Between Backpropagation Networks and Classification Trees on Three Real-World Applications, Touretzky (ed) Advances in Neural Information Processing 2, Morgan Kaufmann, San Mateo, CA, 622–629, 1990.

8. Tsoi A.C, Pearson R.A. Comparison of Three Classification Techniques, CART, C4.5 and MLP, Lippman R.P. et Al (eds) Advances in Neural Information Processing 3, Morgan Kaufmann, San Mateo CA 963–969.

9. Mitchell T.M, Thsun S.B. Explanation Based Learning. A comparison of symbolic and connectionist Learning Algorithms, Proc 10th Int. Conf. on Machine Learning, Morgan Kaufmann San Mateo CA 197–204, 1993

10. Feng G, Sutherland A, King R, Muggleton S, Henery R. Comparison of Machine Learning Classifiers to Statistics and Neural Networks, Proc. 4th Int. Workshop on Artificial Intelligence and Statistics, Florida 1993.

11. Quinlan J.R. Comparing Connectionist and Symbolic Learning Methods, Hanson et al, 445–456, 1994.

12. Quinlan JR. C4.5: Programs for Machine Learning. Morgan Kaufmann 1993.

13. Amendolia S.R, Bertolucci E, Biadi O, Bottigli U, Caravelli P, Fantacci M.E, Fidecaro E, Mariani M, Messineo A, Rosso V, Stefanini A. Neural Network Expert System for Screening Coronary Heart Disease. Physica Medica 1993: IX (1); 13–17.

14. Fahlman S. E, Lebiere C. The Cascade-Correlation Learning Architecture TechReport 1990: CMU-CS-90-100 *Carnegie Mellon University*;

15. Lengellé R, Denoeux T, Training MLPs Layer by Layer Using an Objective Function for Internal Representations. Neural Networks 1996 vol:9 Nbr: 1; 83–98.

16. Vysniauskas V, Groen F.C, Krose J.A. Orthogonal Incremental Learning of a feedforward Network. ICANN'95, Paris; vol:1; p311.

17. Møllerr M. A Scaled Conjugate Gradient Algorithm for Fast Supervised Learning. Neural Networks 1993 vol: 6 nbr: 4; 525–533

18. Riedmiller M. Rprop—Description and Implementation Details. TechReport riedmiller-94a. 1994

19. Huang HH, Zhang C, Lee S. Implementation and Comparison of Neural Network Learning Paradigms: Back Propagation, Simulated Annealing and Tabu Search. Artificial Neural Networks in Engineering 1991: ASME Press, New York; 95–100.

20. Bologna G, Pellegrini C. Three Medical Examples in Neural Network Rule Extraction (Submitted on 1996) to Physica Medica, ed. Giardini Editori e Stampatori in Pisa.

21. Delogu P. Uso di Reti Neurali per Diagnosi Cliniche Automatiche. Master Thesis, University of Pisa (Italy), 1996.

Diagnosis and Monitoring of Ulnar Nerve Lesions

Jürgen Rahmel, Christian Blum

University of Kaiserslautern

Centre for Learning Systems and Applications

PO Box 3049, 67653 Kaiserslautern, Germany

e-mail:*rahmel@informatik.uni-kl.de*

Peter Hahn, Björn Krapohl

Neustadt Hand Centre

Salzburger Leite 1

97616 Bad Neustadt, Germany

e-mail:*hahn@hand.franken.de*

Abstract

In this paper we introduce a novel approach for diagnosis and monitoring of ulnar nerve lesions, affecting the coordination of movement of the ring and little finger of the human hand. Based on data generated by ultrasound measurements, we developed suitable preprocessing methods for automatic extraction of relevant features from the movement pattern to be examined. The partial absence of class information even for the pattern in the training set requires the use of unsupervised methods for the learning and class assignment procedures. For that reason, we use a new dynamic and hierarchic neural network for the analysis of the generated pattern vectors. The dynamically structured architecture of the network satisfies the special needs of this medical task, such as providing variable levels of generalization and efficient retrieval of similar cases.

1 Introduction

Periphal nerve injuries are common and frequently disabling. Functional recovery following nerve repair in upper extremity or hand injuries is often the rate-limiting factor in determining ultimate hand function. Besides external injuries, all nerves can be damaged by entrapment neuropathies, whereby nerves are injured due to compression in anatomical bottlenecks.

The human hand is provided with the radial, median and ulnar nerve. The ulnar nerve provides sensory function for the small and ring finger and innervates the intrinsic muscles of the hand. These muscles are crucial in balancing and coordinating the flexor and extensor muscles, rendering possible fine movement such as grip and pinch. While assessing sensory function is feasible, objective analysis of motor function is quite difficult. Clinical investigation includes grip force measurement and recording of active and passive range of motion. Besides these factors, ulnar nerve dysfunction causes changes in coordination of the movement which cannot be measured by instruments. In contrast to a normal, physiological movement pattern (Fig. 1(a)), the dynamic disorder 'rolling' describes the pathological flexion of the finger. This movement resembles the rolling of a carpet (Fig. 1(b)). As an effect, patients are not able to grasp an object because their fingers push it out of the palm. The dynamic disorder 'clawing' describes the hyperextension of the MP joint with flexion of the PIP and DIP joint[1] while the finger is in resting position (Fig. 1(c)). These descriptions are based on the experience of the examiner. Changes in quality and especially improvement of fine motor activities after nerve repair are difficult to detect and to quantify. If nerve repair fails, there are different operations to rebuild the movement pattern. In these cases, the outcome of surgery also cannot be quantified. Until now, there was no convenient measurement system to distinguish finger movement patterns.

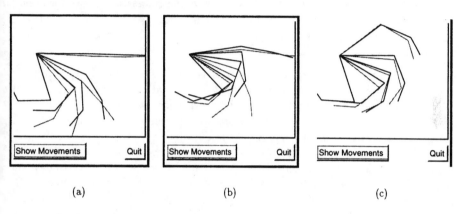

(a)   (b)   (c)

Figure 1: Different forms of finger movement pattern: (a) normal, physiological movement, (b) rolling and (c) clawing (see text). Each picture shows nine steps of finger movement during one cycle of closing (black lines) and opening (gray lines) the fist.

Based on kinematic research we established a measurement system to get real-time data of human finger movement. Trials to analyze these data with classical mathematical methods like discriminant analysis failed to distinguish between normal and pathological movement. Statistical clustering provides a good first insight in the structuring of the data but is not able to support the specific needs in this application (cf. Sec. 2). Other decision methods like CART [BFOS84] or decision trees [Qui93] have some desired diagnostical properties, but are not applicable because of missing class information in the data records of our domain. Another crucial point is the fact that the prospected diagnosis system should efficiently support the medical experts in decision making. Thus, for any given data vector, the system has to be able to retrieve a number (which is possibly not known exactly in advance) of similar stored vectors. This group of similar vectors may then provide a basis for a decision for the current data vector.

In Sec. 2, we will outline certain domain specific problems that determine some of the required properties of a suitable analysis method. Section 3 describes some commonly used methods in the field of ulnar nerve examination and previously used diagnosis approaches. The approach proposed in this paper is described in Sec. 4 and results as well as a comparison to a conventional statistical analysis follow in Sec. 5.

---

[1]The MP, PIP and DIP joints are the three finger joints ordered from the base joint between hand and finger to the tip.

2 Domain-specific Medical Requirements

In this section, we will describe some of the characteristic problems in our domain of ulnar nerve diagnosis and outline the main medical goals to be aimed at with current and future research.

The first problem for data analysis in this domain is the visualization and explanation of data structure to the human observer. We found a hierarchical organization to be both computationally tractable and easily providing access to useful information on data structure and various levels of abstraction. A comparison of a conventional hierarchical method and our approach with a new hierarchical neural network is given later in the paper.

A particular characteristic of our domain is the (at least) partial absence of class information. From the patient records we only know if a patient has had a nerve lesion or not, but this knowledge is not necessarily relevant for diagnosis. Fully recovered finger motion should be considered to be healthy, regardless of the former presence of a lesion. Such diagnostic information has to be supplied by the experienced medical expert. Since visual inspection of finger movement can reveal strongly developed symptoms only and provides merely a subjective judgement, we first had to develop measurement and preprocessing methods for objective quantification of movement pattern. Section 4.1 gives details on this approach. Generated pattern vectors always have to be related to similar cases in order to be interpretable by the medical expert. The analysis method therefore has to support the retrieval of similar cases, at best in an incremental way, because the number of pattern needed for comparison is usually not known a priori and depends on the particular situation. Thus, one of the crucial points for application development is the generation of appropriate memory and indexing structures.

Such an indexing structure can also be the basis of a method that is able to detect less severe forms of motion dysfunctions. Only very strong changes in static and especially dynamic anomalities are accessible by visual inspection of finger motion. Lighter forms (e.g. caused by slowly progressing entrapment neuropathies) as well as possibly not yet discovered kinds of motion disturbances should be detectable and quantifiable. A similar problem arises for the task of monitoring motion recovery success after healing of the nerve or surgical reconstruction of motoric function of the finger. Recovery after nerve repair depends on several factors, e.g. age of the patient, level of injury, and delay of repair. Besides these predictable factors, individual biology plays an important role especially in motoric recovery. Thus the results are not exactly predictable, but should be made comparable.

3 Conventional Approaches

This section outlines the need for a new approach to ulnar nerve diagnostics and summarizes one of the well known methods for pattern analysis that usually is applicable for related tasks.

3.1 Previous Attempts to Ulnar Nerve Examination

Traditionally, monitoring of finger motion served two different aims. Global hand function can be assessed by measurement of grip and pinch strength, active (AROM) and passive (PROM) range of motion and description of individual tendon function. In contrast to this, specific lack of hand or finger function is described by different clinical signs. These signs give a pictorial description of disturbed function as e.g. rolling or clawing. They strongly depend on subjective impressions of the examiner, so they cannot be used for objective quantification. [Sri83] for the first time tried to establish a system for assessing motor function using a grapical representation of defined finger positions. This system more or less defines a working space, but it is not able to evaluate fine changes in dynamic finger function. Electrophysiological investigations as neurography and myography describe the degree of nerve or muscle recovery, but they do not correlate with functional outcome [BH93]. Patients with anomalous innervation pattern as Martin-Gruber communication can present normal movement pattern even if ulnar nerve is damaged.

3.2 Related Methods for Structuring Data

In this section, we give a brief summary of a basic method that usually is applicable in a pattern analysis task. Since we are interested in an unsupervised method for structuring the data set, we have to focus our discussion on the hierarchical cluster analysis. A short review on neural networks related to our approach concludes this section.

Hierarchical Cluster Analysis. For the hierarchical cluster analysis, divisive and agglomerative variants exist, based on the direction of construction of the hierarchy. In agglomerative methods, the clustering starts with as many clusters as samples are available, and successively groups of one or more samples are merged to form new clusters of a higher level. Divisive methods start with the whole population as one big cluster and iteratively divide larger sample sets into parts. In the following, we restrict ourselves to agglomerative methods.

The *closeness* of clusters decides which two clusters are merged. Several choices exist for the definition of this closeness. One chooses the minimal distance of members of two clusters for their distance, another selects clusters according to the maximal distance between cluster members. For the comparison of the results in Sect. 5 we chose still another method, viz. the centroid-algorithm, which looks for the minimum distance of cluster means and thus is a kind of compromise of the before-mentioned variants. For details of these methods, we refer to e.g. [DH73] or any textbook on cluster analysis. The result of the hierarchical clustering can be visualized as a dendrogram, which is a two-dimensional tree structure that shows the order of linkage (for the agglomerative case) and the distance or similarity at which this linkage of clusters was performed. Thus, this method is able to display the clustering of data but it is not possible to reason about the real spatial relationship of the observed pattern. There is no similarity information other than the one for linked clusters. Similar statements are true of course for divisive methods. So the hierarchical clustering methods are useful tools for a preliminary analysis of the data, but they do not provide additional ways for explaining the classification result or reason on alternative solutions based on neighborhood observations.

Tree Networks. There exist a number of neural network models that are called to be tree-structured and which, considering the network topology of nodes and propagating links, are indeed trees. The construction of these neural trees however is not done in a hierarchical way by a neural training mechanism.

Tree-structured MLP networks like the Perceptron Trees [Utg88] are quite comparable to decision trees, because they use an attribute test at each decision node. But unlike decision trees, now the terminal nodes are not class assignment nodes, but Linear Treshold Units (LTU), which divide the current subspace by a hyperplane. Thus, the terminal nodes require an additional test and then provide a class assignment. Since class information is not fully available in our data sets, we are restricted to unsupervised or competitive methods.

A model based on a competitive tree-structured network is proposed in [FJW+91], [LFJ92]. Those binary Neural Trees have a predefined size and structure and may be trained with variants of the competitive learning scheme. Input data is forwarded through the tree and at each level takes the path with the winning neuron. The weight adaptation affects the complete subtree of the first winning neuron. Thus, we again have a subsequential division of the data space by hyperplanes, but for the Neural Trees, the orientation of the planes may change during weight adaptation. The classification structure is more flexible than e.g. for the Perceptron Trees, but the need to predefine the network structure is a drawback.

4 A New Approach to Ulnar Nerve Diagnostics

In this chapter, we briefly introduce the methods we use for the task of analyzing finger movement pattern. Details on patient data and interprtation of training results follow in section 5.

4.1 Data Generation and Preprocessing

We used a real time motion analysis system based on ultrasound (CMS50, Zebris, Germany). Principles of this system are described in [GK87]. By fixing eight markers, paired by two, on the dorsum of the metacarpal bones and on each phalanx we obtained the 3-dimensional coordinates of each marker. Each marker emits 25 pulses per second. From the coordinates, we calculated the angles in the two-dimensional plane of movement during opening and closing of the fist. Details of the measurement are described in [HKHL95]. The plots of the data obtained by the measurements resemble three time-dependent, sometimes phase-shifted, sinus-like curves. Preprocessing of these data was difficult, because two different problems had to be solved.

First of all, selected sets of data should represent the same view of the original data. Simple methods failed, because patients moved their fingers with different velocities in different cycles of opening and closing the fist. Thus these original sets were not comparable directly. Second, selected sets and the results of training should include interpretability for medical experts. As a result, we implemented a tool to automatically select feature vectors from the measurement data by observing predefined positions of finger movement during the closure and opening of the fist. This set of data containes the three angles of the respective finger joints for each selected finger position. Using these angles and the lengths of the phalangeal segments as described by [LT87], who defined a length of 2 for the distal, 3 for the middle, and 5 for the proximal phalanx, we could reconstruct an image of the individual movement pattern (see Fig. 1 for examples). For the reason of retransformability of training results into interpretable pictures (see Fig. 3), we used no further dimension reducing preprocessing methods like, e.g., principal component analysis.

4.2 The SplitNet Model: Hierarchical Structuring of Data

Existing approaches to hierarchical clustering and classification neglect the spatial relations of clusters or partial solution spaces. A particular class of neural network models has the potential to overcome this problem. Regarding the mapping from the input space onto the space spanned by the neighborhood relations of the neurons in the network, the property of certain neural network models to keep track of neighborhood relationships of clusters of data even in cases of reduction of dimensionality is called *topology preservation*. The degree of topology preservation can be determined by the observation, how well neighborhood relationships in one space are preserved by the mapping onto the other space. Thus, one question is: for two input vectors that are close in input space, are their best matching units close[2] in the network topology? The other question is: for two neurons that are neighbors in the network topology, are their associated weight vectors close in the input space? These questions led to the development of the topographic function [VDHM96], that effectively quantifies the topology preservation in topographic maps. Topology preserving models are, among others, the Growing Cell Structures [Fri93] and the Topology Representing Network [MS94]. But all the existing models lack the ability of hierarchically structuring the training set.

SplitNet is a topology preserving, dynamically growing model for unsupervised learning and hierarchical structuring of data [Rah96b]. Starting with a single, small Kohonen chain [Koh90], localized insertion and deletion criteria enable an efficient quantization of the data space. The hierarchy in the architecture develops, when one of the following splitting criteria is satisfied: (i) detection of topological defects, (ii) deletion of neurons by an aging mechanism, (iii) significant local variances in quantization errors and (iv) significant local variances in edge lengths. Those criteria are checked several times during the training progress. If a criterion is satisfied, the affected chain is split into two or more subchains that are added to the network at one level lower in the hierarchy. The node in the hierarchy representing the formerly

---

[2]As different input vectors may be mapped onto the same neuron, in this informal explanation, the *closeness* of neurons includes also the identity of those neurons.

unsplit chain now serves as a generalized description and access structure for the new son nodes. Figure 2 illustrates this basic mechanism. If a topological defect is found (e.g. between neurons 1 and 7, which are close in input space but distant in the chain of neurons), the chain is split and nodes representing the fragments are added as descendants to the tree. Path decisions in the so constructed hierarchy will be drawn according to the mean of the weight vectors of the neurons in the chain, thus the mean is also indicated in the figure. The topology preserving construction of the network structure provides local neighborhood information that is necessary for incremental retrieval of nearest neighbor to a given input vector. The dashed lines in

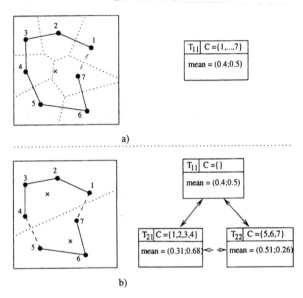

Figure 2: Example of splitting a chain because of a topological defect

Fig. 2 indicate this type of knowledge. The neighborhood relations are kept as lateral connections defining the topology of the network space. They are responsible for the high degree of topology preservation in SplitNet and enable a fast and incremental search for a set of nearest neighbors. A more rigorous and exhaustive treatment of these aspects and retrieval results can be found in [RV96].

Since unsupervised learning methods provide no direct classification, the training result has to be interpreted in the context given by the training data. For the SplitNet model, we observe three containers of knowledge that can be used for the tasks in diagnosis applications like the one described in this paper:

Neuron distribution: The insertion criterion determines the error function to be minimized. Quantization of the data set allows local estimation of density and probability of class occurrences.

Topology: The connections between neighboring neurons provide information on where to find similar cases. Measuring topological defects yields the search depth for incremental retrieval of nearest neighbors to a given query [Rah96a].

Hierarchy: The hierarchical structure of the network contains different levels of generalization and abstraction. It allows a fast tree search for best matches and insightful visualization of the data structure for the domain expert.

In the current domain of ulnar nerve diagnosis, the latter two points are of greater interest. The task of comparing a given data vector of a new patient to similar vectors in the pretrained network is fully accomplished by the topology-based retrieval algorithms described in [RV96]. The result is an effective diagnosis support based on the well established k-nearest-neighbor rule. The utility of the constructed hierarchy is explained in detail in the following section.

5 Application Results and their Interpretation

5.1 Patients, data sets and network training

So far, a total of 55 measurements of 45 subjects were obtained. These patients suffered from different types of ulnar nerve lesion. 14 patients had posttraumatic lesion of the ulnar nerve at different levels. 17 patients suffered from nerve compression at the level of the elbow. For the sake of explainability and readability of the tree representations in this paper, we will present the results of a smaller sample set consisting of 22 measurements of ring finger of 14 patients suffering from traumatic lacerations of the ulnar nerve. Further conclusions to be drawn from the network trained with all vectors will be mentioned where appropriate.

One patient (**gru**) was measured before and two times after release of the ulnar nerve at the elbow level. Two patients (**wei, rap**) were measured before and four patients (**wei2, rap2, mic, hof**) after reconstruction of motoric function by Zancolli lasso plasty. These data were compared to the data of ten fingers of six healthy persons.

Training data sets were generated by the methods decribed in Sec. 4.1. We currently have more than 550 data vectors available for the analysis. However, for the results reported here, we used 93 data vectors of the above mentioned subjects. Figure 3 shows the hierarchical representation of the data as it was generated by SplitNet. The training was automatically stopped, when a good diversification of the pattern was reached. Current research is concerned on defining automated stopping criteria based on characteristics of this domain. A framework for this decision is given by the following medical interpretation of training results.

5.2 Medical Interpretation of Tree Content

The division of the tree into branch #2 and #3 at the early beginning already divides the data into physiological movement depending on branch #3 and mainly pathological ones in the leaf nodes of branch #2. Further examination of branch #2 has to interpret 6 leaves, four of which are of special interest. Leaf #6 contains movements where, in full extension of the finger, MP joints are hyperextended whereas PIP and

219

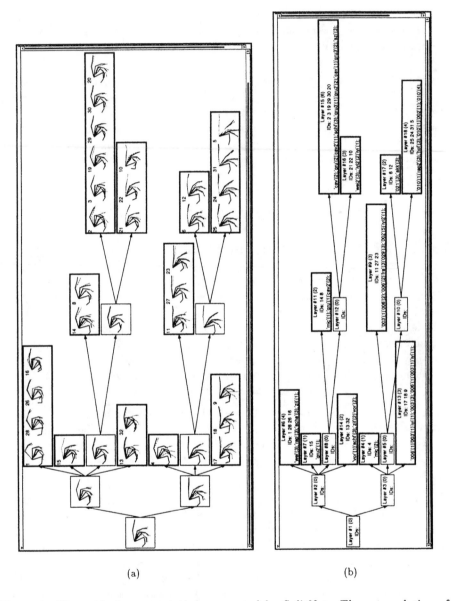

(a)   (b)

Figure 3: Hierarchical representations generated by SplitNet. The retranslation of
neuron weights allows the display of interpretable finger movements in the learned
hierarchical arrangement (a). The same tree is shown with a text output (b) for naming nodes by their box number (first line in each box) and mapping training vectors
onto neurons. The three-letter acronyms denote the subjects, names for neighboring
neurons are separated by a semicolon.

DIP joints never reach full extension. This type of dysfunction was termed *clawing* above. In contrast to this, leaf #14 represents mainly dynamic dysfunction. PIP and DIP joint flexion precedes MP joint flexion, resembling the *rolling* of a carpet. Thus the medically wellknown phenomena of clawing and rolling could be recognized. Leaves #11 and #15 present different forms of combined clawing and rolling. From a clinical point of view, all patients suffering from ulnar nerve palsy can be found in leaves #6, 11, 14 and 15. In our case, the degree of handicap decreases from left to right in SplitNet, a fact that can be deduced by a physician from the graphical representations of the individual neurons.

The leaves of branch #3 mainly contain physiological movement data. Among these data are only a few data of patients with ulnar nerve lesion, e.g. data of (iyi), a patient with partial lesion of the ulnar nerve and only minor changes in movement leading to a distribution of the movement vectors over layer # 16, 9, 13. Leaves #4 and #18 are of special interest. They contain neurons representing patients after Zancolli-plasty. This is an operation to prevent clawing by transposition of a flexor tendon. Respective neurons show that clawing, as e.g. preoperatively demonstrated by **rap** in leaf #6 is changed to exclusive MP-flexion initiating the flexion curve and late PIP and DIP during fist closure (#18). In contrast to this, leaf #4 **mic** shows still clawing and rolling although operated by Zancolli-plasty. This is an effect of tendon adhesions which have to be reoperated since physiotherapy will gain no effect. The separation of this patient's data is thus supported by medical evidence. Six patients who underwent Zancolli-plasty were monitored until now and were analysed with the larger data set available up to now. That analysis revealed that preoperative movement pattern is changed to an extra leaf depending on the branch of normal movement. This leaf presented patterns with exclusive MP-flexion initating the flexion curve as already described above for **rap**. Interpretation of the results thus support the fact that movement pattern is changed to a less disturbed one, but movement characteristics still differ from normal ones. So by means of SplitNet, other techniques for prevention of clawing can be investigated.

Monitoring recovery of one patient (**gru**) after neurolysis of the damaged nerve at the level of the elbow showed a shift of movement pattern from layer #11 to 15. Again, by observation of the images for the individual neurons in Layer #15, a change in finger movement from worse to better can be recognized. Clawing and rolling reduces from left to right. In the network generated with the larger sample set, this shift can be seen more clearly. This is interesting because the patients feels better after the operation but classical clinical investigation failed to determine the degree of improvement. From a clinical point of view, SplitNet provides a method to evaluate ulnar nerve lesion by movement pattern. Compared to neurophysiological methods, SplitNet provides extended diagnostic facilities, because functional changes do not exclusively depend on the neurophysiological state, but in addition on laxity of ligaments, skin and joints as well as other factors. Thus diagnosis and monitoring can be done based on function. In addition we could get more insight in the biomechanics changes caused by nerve regeneration or tendon transfer.

A comparison of the results obtained by SplitNet with those of a hierarchical cluster analysis clarifies the strength of the neural model. We performed a run of the clustering process and examined a subgraph of the dendrogram with about as many terminal nodes as the SplitNet tree described above. The result was not surprising. The clustering produced nearly the same groups of data represented by leaf nodes, thus supporting the clustering abilities of the SplitNet model. However, despite of the distance information that is available for the merging level of two clusters, interpretation of the dendrogram from a medical point of view was possible only in a very limited way. Whereas the neuron chains representing the terminal nodes in SplitNet arrange themselves in a direction that best reflects the largest variation in the associated movement pattern (an intrinsic property of the underlying Kohonen model), such information is not available in the cluster analysis. Moreover, the dendrogram provides information on the order of the cluster merges, yet it does not contain explicit or implicit information on the spatial relationships of clusters. This is a crucial property for a reliable diagnosis of new cases which are not contained in the center of existing clusters. In order to compare those with nearest neighbors, reliable information on cluster connectivity is necessary. The lateral connections between neurons in the SplitNet model facilitate reasoning for class assignment based on neighborhood considerations.

6 Conclusion

Our system for the first time applies a neural pattern recognition approach to human finger movement. As evident from the results, SplitNet is able to distinguish between normal and pathological movements. From a statistical point of view, part of its function resembles a cluster analysis. But in addition to that, it allows further examination of the learning results. Thus, interpretation of the images (which are retranslations of neuron weights into the semantics of training vectors) enhances our knowledge of the movement pattern. For example, we recognized that most of the data for Zancolli-lasso-plasty are separated, because they represent a special type of movement pattern that resembles intrinsic-plus movement. In similar way, other types of dynamic or static reconstructions can be tested in the future. At the moment we still do not know if we portray the whole spectrum of ulnar nerve dysfunction by the available data. More measurements have to be recorded in order to decide which and how many different types of changes in movement pattern exist. Data from nontraumatic lesions as compressions neuropathies have to be gathered. Our general aim is to build up a neural net containing all types of normal and pathological movement, labeled with verified diagnostic class information. Then we are able to classify ulnar nerve lesions by recording finger movement measurements and observing the mapping of the movement pattern by the neural net onto a certain location in the tree, for which clinical diagnosis is already accessible.

The aim of gaining more data for the different pathological forms of the ulnar nerve dysfunctions also yields a need for incremental learning of new pattern without relearning the old ones. This is part of current research, where we try to use a structured case memory for training. Each training vector can be associated with its best matching neuron in the network. Newly generated pattern are trained together with the topologically adjacent located older pattern, a form of training that is enabled by the construction of a network topology as it is achieved by the SplitNet model.

References

[BFOS84] L. Breiman, J.H. Friedman, R.A. Olsen, and C.J. Stone. *Classification and Regression Trees.* Belmont, CA, Wadsworth, 1984.

[BH93] P.W. Brandt and A. Hollister. *Clinical Mechanics of the Hand.* Mosby Year Book, 1993.

[DH73] R.O. Duda and P.E. Hart. *Pattern Classification and Scene Analysis.* Wiley, 1973.

[FJW+91] L. Fang, A. Jennings, W. X. Wen, K. Li, and T. Li. Unsupervised learning for neural trees. In *Proceedings of the IJCNN*, 1991.

[Fri93] B. Fritzke. Growing cell structures - a self-organizing network for unsupervised and supervised learning. Technical Report TR-93-026, ICSI, 1993.

[GK87] U. Guggenbühl and H. Krüger. Bewegungsanalyse an verschiedenen industriellen Arbeitsplätzen. *Sozial- und Präventivmedizin*, 32:266–268, 1987.

[HKHL95] P. Hahn, H. Krimmer, A. Hradetzky, and U. Lanz. Quantitative analysis of the linkage between the interphalangeal joints of the index finger. in vivo study. *Journal of Hand Surgery*, 20B:696–699, 1995.

[Koh90] T. Kohonen. The self-organizing map. *Proceedings of the IEEE*, 78(9):1464–1480, 1990.

[LFJ92] T. Li, L. Fang, and A. Jennings. Structurally adaptive self-organizing neural trees. In *Proc. of the ICNN*, 1992.

[LT87] J. W. Littler and J. S. Thompson. Surgical and functional anatomy. In W.H. Bowers, editor, *The interphalangeal joints*, pages 14–20. Churchill Livingstone, Edinburgh, 1987.

[MS94] Thomas Martinetz and Klaus Schulten. Topology representing networks. *Neural Networks*, 7(2), 1994.

[Qui93] J.R. Quinlan. *C4.5: Programs for Machine Learning.* Morgan Kaufman, 1993.

[Rah96a] J. Rahmel. On the Role of Topology for Neural Network Interpretation. In W. Wahlster, editor, *Proc. of the ECAI*, 1996.

[Rah96b] J. Rahmel. SplitNet: Learning of Hierarchical Kohonen Chains. In *Proc. of the ICNN '96*, Washington, 1996.

[RV96] J. Rahmel and T. Villmann. Interpreting Topology Preserving Networks. Technical Report LSA-96-01E, University of Kaiserslautern, 1996.

[Sri83] H. Srinivasan. Universe of finger postures and finger dynamography. *Handchir. Mikrochir. Plastische Chirugie*, 15:3–6, 1983.

[Utg88] P. Utgoff. Perceptron trees: A case study in hybrid concept representations. In *Proc. of the Nat. Conf. on AI*, pages 601–606, St. Paul, MN, 1988.

[VDHM96] Th. Villmann, R. Der, M. Herrmann, and Th. Martinetz. Topology preservation in self-organizing feature maps: Exact definition and measurement. *IEEE Transactions on Neural Networks*, 1996. To appear.

Hypothesist: A Development Environment for Intelligent Diagnostic Systems

David McSherry

School of Information and Software Engineering,
University of Ulster, Coleraine BT52 1SA,
Northern Ireland, UK

A model of diagnostic reasoning based on the hypothetico-deductive reasoning strategies used by doctors is presented. The model includes strategies for confirming a likely diagnostic hypothesis, eliminating alternative hypotheses, and discriminating between competing hypotheses. There is also a mechanism for recognising when there is sufficient evidence to support a firm diagnosis. An implementation of the model in an environment providing integrated support for knowledge acquisition, diagnostic reasoning and explanation is described.

1 Introduction

Early Bayesian programs for computer-assisted diagnosis were criticised for failing to explain their reasoning in terms that were meaningful to doctors and for assumptions of mutually exclusive disease hypotheses and conditional independence of symptoms (Fox et al. 1980, Shortliffe et al. 1979, Szolovits 1980, Szolovits & Pauker 1978). However, programs based on the independence Bayesian framework often perform well in practice. A well-documented example is the Leeds program which offers a differential diagnosis of the nine most common causes of acute abdominal pain based on the observed values of about 30 patient attributes (e.g. de Dombal et al. 1972). Multi-centre trials in the UK have shown that the program significantly increases accuracy in diagnosis (Adams et al. 1986).

The development of AI techniques to enable such programs to emulate the reasoning strategies used by doctors may increase their chances of more widespread acceptance and use (Shortliffe et al. 1979). Some Bayesian programs (e.g. Gorry et al. 1973) use the method of minimum entropy to guide test selection in sequential diagnosis. A similar strategy is the basis of the theory of measurements developed by de Kleer and Williams (1987) in their General Diagnostic Engine, which combines model-based reasoning with sequential diagnosis to localise faults in digital circuits. However, the absence of a specific diagnostic hypothesis in the entropy approach can lead to the selection of tests which seem irrelevant to human diagnosticians (Pearl 1988, Spiegelhalter & Knill-Jones 1984).

This paper presents a model of diagnostic reasoning based on the hypothetico-deductive reasoning (HDR) strategies used by doctors (Elstein et al. 1978, Kassirer & Kopelman 1991, Shortliffe & Barnett 1990) and its implementation in HYPOTHESIST, an environment providing integrated support for knowledge acquisition, diagnostic reasoning and explanation. Modified and extended from previous work (McSherry 1986, McSherry 1992, McSherry & McClean 1995), the model includes strategies for confirming a likely diagnostic hypothesis, eliminating alternative hypotheses, and discriminating between competing hypotheses. There is also a mechanism for recognising when there is sufficient evidence to support a firm diagnosis.

The HDR strategies used in HYPOTHESIST are described in the following section. Section 3 describes the tools provided in the environment to support the reasoning process and the explanations available to the user. Examples based on data from the Leeds acute abdomen program and a well-known data set from the machine learning literature are used to illustrate the approach.

2 HDR Strategies

Defined within the independence Bayesian framework, the HDR model can be applied to any diagnostic task for which the following are available: the hypotheses to be discriminated and their prior probabilities, relevant tests, and the conditional probabilities of their results in each hypothesis. The hypotheses are assumed to be mutually exclusive and exhaustive and the results of the tests are assumed to be independent in each hypothesis.

HYPOTHESIST repeats a diagnostic cycle of identifying a target hypothesis, choosing an appropriate diagnostic strategy, selecting the most useful test to support the chosen strategy, obtaining the result of the selected test, and updating the probabilities of all the competing hypotheses. Unless otherwise specified by the user, the target hypothesis is the one that is currently most likely, and is continuously revised as new evidence is obtained. The diagnostic strategy used at each stage of the reasoning process is selected from the following HDR strategies, in order of priority:

HDR-1   confirm the target hypothesis
HDR-2   eliminate the likeliest alternative hypothesis but not the target hypothesis
HDR-3   increase the probability of the target hypothesis
HDR-4   decrease the probability of the likeliest alternative hypothesis
HDR-5   increase the probability of the target hypothesis relative to the likeliest alternative hypothesis
HDR-6   eliminate, or decrease the probability of, any alternative hypothesis

First priority is given to test results that confirm outright the target hypothesis. Such findings, though unfortunately rare in medicine, are said to be *pathognomonic*. For example, a Pap smear with grossly abnormal cells is essentially never seen unless there is cancer of the cervix or uterus (Shortliffe & Barnett, 1990). Second priority is given to test results that eliminate the likeliest alternative hypothesis. For example, a male patient cannot have a pregnancy-related illness, however strongly other evidence may support that hypothesis.

The usual absence of tests that confirm outright or eliminate any hypothesis means that doctors must look for findings that will increase the probability of a target hypothesis (HDR-3), decrease the probability of an alternative hypothesis (HDR-4) or discriminate between two competing hypotheses (HDR-5).

Table 1. Conditional probabilities for one of the patient attributes from the Leeds acute abdomen program (e.g. de Dombal et al. 1972).

Disease	Type of pain		
	INTERMITTENT	STEADY	COLICKY
Acute appendicitis	0.11	0.59	0.30
Diverticular disease	0.24	0.47	0.29
Perforated peptic ulcer	0.07	0.76	0.18
Non-specific abdominal pain	0.24	0.45	0.31
Acute cholecystitis	0.11	0.53	0.37
Small bowel obstruction	0.15	0.23	0.63
Acute pancreatitis	0.07	0.70	0.24
Renal colic	0.15	0.34	0.51
Dyspepsia	0.20	0.54	0.25

2.1 Identifying Useful Tests

HYPOTHESIST's choice of diagnostic strategy is determined by the availability of relevant tests (or patient attributes). A test is relevant in the context of a given diagnostic strategy if at least one of its results supports the strategy (e.g. confirms the target hypothesis). However, a test is selected to support HDR-3 only if one of its results *always* increases the probability of the target hypothesis. The reason for this is to enable the reasoning process to be explained in general rather than case-specific terms. Similarly, a test is selected to support HDR-4 only if one of its results always decreases the probability of the likeliest alternative hypothesis.

To illustrate how tests are selected in HYPOTHESIST, Table 1 shows the conditional probabilities for different types of pain in the common causes of acute abdominal pain. Although the most likely type of pain in acute appendicitis is STEADY, this does not mean that STEADY pain will necessarily increase the probability of acute appendicitis. In fact, it may either increase or decrease the probability of acute appendicitis depending on the current probabilities of the other diseases. Because it occurs more often in acute appendicitis than in non-specific abdominal pain, STEADY pain will always increase the probability of the former *relative* to the latter. Thus if the target hypothesis is acute appendicitis and the likeliest alternative hypothesis is non-specific abdominal pain, TYPE OF PAIN will support HDR-5 but not HDR-3.

As the following theorem shows, a test result always increases the probability of a target hypothesis if it occurs more often in the target hypothesis than in any other hypothesis. Attributes that support HDR-3 can easily be identified, therefore, from the conditional probabilities of their values. The theorem also shows how attributes that support the other HDR strategies are identified in HYPOTHESIST. For example, an attribute will support HDR-1 if one of its values occurs only in the target hypothesis.

Theorem 1. In the independence Bayesian framework, given a target hypothesis H_t and alternative hypothesis H_a such that $0 < p(H_t) < 1$ and $0 < p(H_a) < 1$, a finding E will:

(a) confirm H_t if and only if it occurs only in H_t

(b) eliminate H_a but not H_t if and only if it occurs in H_t but not in H_a

(c) always increase the probability of H_t if it occurs more often in H_t than in any other hypothesis

(d) always decrease the probability of H_a if it occurs less often in H_a than in any other hypothesis

(e) increase the probability of H_t relative to H_a if it occurs more often in H_t than in H_a.

Proof. (a) and (b) follow easily from Bayes' theorem.

(c) This is a specific case of a more general result that a finding will increase the probability of a given hypothesis provided it occurs more often in that hypothesis than in any other hypothesis (McSherry 1986).

(d) Let H_1, H_2, ... H_n be the hypotheses to be discriminated and suppose that $p(E|H_a) < p(E|H_i)$ for all $i \neq a$. Then by Bayes' theorem,

$$p(H_a|E) = p(H_a)\,p(E|H_a) \, / \, (\sum_{i=1}^{n} p(H_i)\,p(E|H_i))$$

$$< p(H_a)\,p(E|H_a) \, / \, (\sum_{i=1}^{n} p(H_i)\,p(E|H_a))$$

$$= p(H_a)\,p(E|H_a) \, / \, p(E|H_a)$$

$$= p(H_a).$$

(e) If $p(E|H_t) > p(E|H_a)$ then by Bayes' theorem,

$$p(H_t|E)/p(H_a|E) = (p(E|H_t)/p(E|H_a))\,(p(H_t)/p(H_a)) > p(H_t)/p(H_a).$$

According to Theorem 1, INTERMITTENT pain always increases[1] the probabilities of diverticular disease and non-specific abdominal pain and decreases the probabilities of perforated peptic ulcer and acute pancreatitis. STEADY pain always increases the probability of perforated peptic ulcer and decreases the probability of small bowel obstruction. Finally, COLICKY pain always makes small bowel obstruction more likely while providing evidence against perforated peptic ulcer.

TYPE OF PAIN will therefore support HDR-3 whenever the target hypothesis is diverticular disease, non-specific abdominal pain, perforated peptic ulcer, or small bowel obstruction. With another hypothesis as the target hypothesis, it will support HDR-4 if the likeliest alternative hypothesis is perforated peptic ulcer, acute pancreatitis, or small bowel obstruction. No value of TYPE OF PAIN, however, can confirm or eliminate any hypothesis. In fact, none of the attributes from the acute abdomen program will support HDR-1 or HDR-2.

---

[1] As condition (c) of Theorem 1 is not strictly satisfied, it would be more correct to say *never decreases*.

Table 2. Conditional probabilities for two attributes in the contact lens data (Cendrowska 1987).

	TEAR PRODUCTION RATE		ASTIGMATISM	
Contact lens type	reduced	normal	present	absent
NO contact lenses	0.80	0.20	0.53	0.47
Soft contact lenses	0.00	1.00	0.00	1.00
Hard contact lenses	0.00	1.00	1.00	0.00

Cendrowska's (1987) contact lens data is based on a simplified version of the optician's real-world problem of selecting a suitable type of contact lenses, if any, for an adult spectacle wearer. The hypotheses to be discriminated are NO contact lenses, soft contact lenses and hard contact lenses. Table 2 shows the conditional probabilities for two attributes in the data set. One of the attributes, TEAR PRODUCTION RATE, has a value (reduced) that occurs only in NO contact lenses and will therefore support HDR-1 when NO contact lenses is the target hypothesis. The other attribute, ASTIGMATISM, has one value that never occurs in soft contact lenses and another that never occurs in hard contact lenses. It will therefore support HDR-2 whenever the likeliest alternative hypothesis is soft contact lenses or hard contact lenses.

2.2 Selecting the Most Useful Test
When two or more attributes will support the same HDR strategy, some measure of their usefulness is required to enable HYPOTHESIST to select the most useful attribute. Different measures are used depending on the strategy supported. For attributes that support HDR-3, HDR-4 or HDR-5, the measure is based on the concept of weights of evidence (e.g. Spiegelhalter & Knill-Jones 1984).

Definition 1. The weight of evidence of a finding E in favour of a given hypothesis H_1, relative to an alternative hypothesis H_2, is:

$$w(E, H_1, H_2) = p(E|H_1) / p(E|H_2).$$

An overall measure of the usefulness of an attribute is provided by its *expected* weight of evidence in favour of the target hypothesis, relative to the likeliest alternative hypothesis.

Definition 2. The expected weight of evidence of an attribute A with values $V_1, V_2, ... V_m$ in favour of a given hypothesis H_1, relative to an alternative hypothesis H_2, is:

$$\psi(A, H_1, H_2) = \sum_{i=1}^{m} p(A = V_i \mid H_1) \, w(A = V_i, H_1, H_2).$$

If the strategy of highest priority which can be supported in HYPOTHESIST is HDR-3, HDR-4 or HDR-5, and two or more attributes will support it, then the attribute selected is the one for which $\psi(A, H_t, H_a)$ is greatest, where H_t is the target hypothesis and H_a is the likeliest alternative hypothesis.

In the diagnosis of acute abdominal pain, for example, TYPE OF PAIN will support HDR-3 when the target hypothesis is perforated peptic ulcer. Its usefulness, however, depends on the likeliest alternative hypothesis. For example, its expected weight of evidence relative to a likeliest alternative hypothesis of non-specific abdominal pain is:

$$\psi(\text{TYPE OF PAIN, perforated peptic ulcer, non-specific abdominal pain})$$
$$= 0.07^2/0.24 + 0.76^2/0.45 + 0.18^2/0.31 = 1.41.$$

With acute pancreatitis instead as the likeliest alternative hypothesis, its expected weight of evidence (again in favour of perforated peptic ulcer) is only 1.03.

McSherry (1995) has shown that $\psi(A, H_1, H_2) \geq 1$ for any attribute A and hypotheses H_1, H_2. However, the expected weight of evidence of an attribute is infinite if any value occurs in H_1 but not in H_2. Expected weights of evidence cannot therefore discriminate between attributes that support HDR-1 or HDR-2. The solution to this problem is to use a different quantitative measure for these attributes.

Definition 3. The eliminating power of a finding E, denoted el(E), is the sum of the probabilities of the hypotheses eliminated by E, or zero if none is eliminated. The expected eliminating power of an attribute A with values $V_1, V_2, ... V_m$, in favour of a given hypothesis H, is :

$$\gamma(A, H) = \sum_{i=1}^{m} p(A = V_i \mid H) \, el(A = V_i).$$

If the strategy of highest priority which can be supported in HYPOTHESIST is HDR-1 or HDR-2, and two or more attributes will support it, then the attribute selected is the one for which $\gamma(A, H_t)$ is greatest, where H_t is the target hypothesis.

Unlike its expected weight of evidence, an attribute's expected eliminating power depends on the current probabilities of the hypotheses to be discriminated. In the contact lens data, the prior probabilities of NO contact lenses, soft contact lenses and hard contact lenses are 0.63, 0.21 and 0.17. At the start of the reasoning process, the expected eliminating power of TEAR PRODUCTION RATE in favour of a target hypothesis of NO contact lenses is therefore:

$$\gamma(\text{TEAR PRODUCTION RATE, NO contact lenses})$$
$$= 0.80 \times (0.21 + 0.17) + 0.20 \times 0 = 0.30.$$

Similarly, the expected eliminating power of ASTIGMATISM in favour of a (user-selected) target hypothesis of soft contact lenses is initially:

$$\gamma(\text{ASTIGMATISM, soft contact lenses}) = 0 \times 0.21 + 1 \times 0.17 = 0.17.$$

2.3 Recognising Sufficient Evidence for a Firm Diagnosis

An important aspect of diagnostic reasoning is the ability to recognise when there is sufficient evidence to support a firm diagnosis and thus avoid the unnecessary cost of further tests. Another reason to discontinue testing is when further evidence can have only a limited impact on the probability of the target hypothesis. A strategy often used in programs for sequential diagnosis (Gorry et al. 1973, de Kleer & Williams 1987) is to terminate the reasoning process when the probability of any hypothesis reaches a predetermined threshold. The following theorem, adapted from (McSherry & McClean 1995), provides a basis for a more reliable and flexible strategy in which upper and lower bounds for the probability of the target hypothesis are computed as the result of each test is obtained.

Theorem 2. In the independence Bayesian framework, let H be any hypothesis which cannot be confirmed or eliminated. If one of the results of a binary test occurs more often in H than in any alternative hypothesis, then any combination of test results which maximises the probability of H must include that test result. Any combination of test results which minimises the probability of H must include the other result of the binary test.

To compute, for example, a lower bound for the probability of a hypothesis without the advantage of this theorem, it would be necessary to compute the posterior probabilities corresponding to every possible combination of results of the remaining tests[2]. As each qualifying test reduces the number of combinations of test results by a factor of two, the net result may be a dramatic reduction in the computational effort required. However, the search for upper and lower bounds remains a significant computational overhead and is undertaken only when the probability of the target hypothesis is high and a reasonable response time is possible given the number of combinations of test results still to be evaluated.

3 The HYPOTHESIST Environment

Written in Prolog for the Apple Macintosh, HYPOTHESIST incorporates tools for eliciting all the domain knowledge necessary to apply the HDR model, namely the hypotheses to be discriminated and their prior probabilities, relevant tests, and the conditional probabilities of their results in each hypothesis. A knowledge base editor provides tools for editing or extending the knowledge base and checking its completeness.

3.1 Mixed-Initiative Dialogue

At the beginning of a consultation, the user can volunteer as much information as she wishes. A graphics window (Fig.1) is updated to show the impact of each new piece of evidence. On receiving the initiative, HYPOTHESIST seeks further evidence, selecting tests in order of their usefulness to support the current diagnostic strategy

---

2   Szolovits (1980) reports experiments in which a lower bound was approximated by assuming the result of each test that was least favourable on a sequential basis.

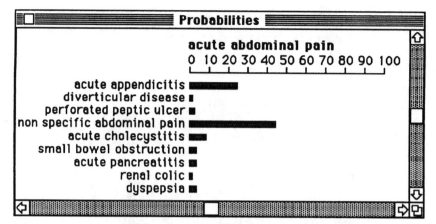

Fig. 1. Prior probabilities of disease hypotheses based on data from the Leeds acute abdomen program (e.g. de Dombal et al. 1972).

(Fig. 2). Initially the target hypothesis, if chosen by HYPOTHESIST, is the one that is most likely given any evidence already reported. Alternatively, the user can nominate any hypothesis as the target hypothesis. Before answering any question, the user can ask why it is relevant, review the evidence in favour of the target hypothesis, initiate sensitivity analysis, select a new target hypothesis, or update findings previously reported.

3.2 Explanation of Reasoning

The explanation provided when the user asks why a question is relevant is automatically generated by HYPOTHESIST and depends on the current diagnostic strategy. In HDR-4, for example, the user is told which result (or results) of the selected test can always be guaranteed to decrease the probability of the likeliest alternative hypothesis. HYPOTHESIST also provides on request a summary of the evidence in favour of the target hypothesis. The findings listed are those which can always be guaranteed to increase its probability. Similarly, the user can review the evidence against the target hypothesis.

3.3 Sensitivity Analysis

At any stage of the consultation, the user can examine the potential effects of any tests whose results are unknown (or not yet reported) on the probability of the target hypothesis. By Theorem 2, some of the test results that minimise the probability of the target hypothesis may be predictable in advance. If a reasonable response time is not possible, the user is requested to select fewer tests. The analysis may reveal evidence that could drastically reduce the probability of the target hypothesis, or may show that a firm diagnosis is possible even in the absence of missing information. Provided the current probability of the target hypothesis is at least 80% and a reasonable response time is possible, HYPOTHESIST computes upper and lower bounds for the probability of the target hypothesis as each new piece of evidence is reported. However, the decision to end the consultation is left to the user.

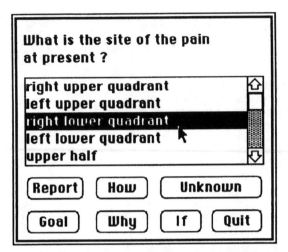

Fig. 2. Tests are selected in order of their usefulness
to support the current diagnostic strategy.

3.4 Example Consultations

The first example is based on data from the Leeds acute abdomen program (e.g. de Dombal 1972). Because of the limitations of space, the dialogue presented is text based. At the start of the consultation, the user has selected acute appendicitis as the target hypothesis, but chosen not to volunteer any information.

TARGET HYPOTHESIS: acute appendicitis
Is there rebound tenderness? WHY
> *The presence of rebound tenderness always increases the probability
> of acute appendicitis*

Is there rebound tenderness? YES
What is the site of tenderness? RIGHT LOWER QUADRANT
What is the site of the pain at present? RIGHT LOWER QUADRANT
What is the site of rectal tenderness? NONE
Is there aggravation by movement? YES
What is the site of the pain at onset? WHY
> *Because if the site of pain at onset is central or right lower quadrant, this
> always increases the probability of acute appendicitis*

What is the site of the pain at onset? CENTRAL
What is the appetite of the patient? DECREASED
What is the duration of the pain? HOW

The following findings always increase the probability of acute appendicitis:
- rebound tenderness is present
- the site of tenderness is right lower quadrant
- the site of the pain at present is right lower quadrant
- aggravation by movement is present
- the site of the pain at onset is central
- the appetite of the patient is decreased

What is the duration of the pain? UNKNOWN

At this stage of the consultation, the probability of acute appendicitis is over 90% and HYPOTHESIST is still pursuing its HDR-3 strategy, having not yet exhausted attributes with values that always increase the probability of the target hypothesis. The findings considered most relevant by HYPOTHESIST are reasonably consistent with textbook guidelines for the diagnosis of acute appendicitis. Findings that favour acute appendicitis are listed by de Dombal (1991) in the following order: site of pain moving from the centre of the abdomen to the right lower quadrant; pain aggravated by movement and coughing; nausea, vomiting and loss of appetite; flushed colour; tenderness in the right lower quadrant; rebound tenderness and guarding; and rectal tenderness on the right side.

The second example is based on the contact lens data (Cendrowska 1987). In contrast to Cendrowska's rule-based approach, only NO contact lenses can be established with certainty in the independence Bayesian framework. Starting with NO contact lenses as the target hypothesis, HYPOTHESIST uses a combination of its HDR-1, HDR-2 and HDR-3 strategies.

TARGET HYPOTHESIS: NO contact lenses
What is the tear production rate? WHY
> *Because if the tear production rate is reduced, this will confirm NO contact lenses*

What is the tear production rate? NORMAL
TARGET HYPOTHESIS: soft contact lenses
Is there astigmatism? WHY
> *Because if astigmatism is absent, this will eliminate hard contact lenses*

Is there astigmatism? NO
What is the age of the patient? WHY
> *Because if the age of the patient is pre-presbyopic, this always increases the probability of soft contact lenses*

What is the age of the patient? PRE-PRESBYOPIC
> *The likeliest hypothesis, with a probability of 81%, is soft contact lenses. Its probability cannot be less than 79% or more than 83%.*

What is the spectacle prescription? QUIT

Given the strength of evidence in favour of soft contact lenses, and limited possible impact of further evidence, the user decides to end the consultation.

4 Conclusions

HYPOTHESIST's diagnostic strategies are essentially heuristic and cannot be guaranteed to minimise the number of tests required to reach a firm diagnosis. In this respect, a test selection strategy based on the method of minimum entropy is likely to perform better on average. However, the ability to explain the reasoning process may be an important advantage not only from the point of view of acceptability to users but also for educational purposes (Klemenz & McSherry 1995). Although the absence of intermediate hypotheses means that HYPOTHESIST cannot provide multiple levels of explanation like a rule-based expert system, its explanation of the reasoning process in terms of the diagnostic strategy it is currently pursuing may resemble more closely the kind of explanation a human expert would be expected to provide.

By selecting the tear production rate as the most useful test in the contact lens data, HYPOTHESIST reveals a limitation it shares with any system lacking an awareness of the relative costs of tests. The tear production rate requires a lengthy and expensive examination which can be avoided in practice if other tests show the patient is unsuitable for contact lenses (Cendrowska 1987). Research on extending the HDR model to take account of the relative costs and risks of tests is currently in progress.

Some of HYPOTHESIST's reasoning strategies resemble those of INTERNIST (Pople 1982), which can also formulate an initial set of hypotheses to be differentiated, an aspect of diagnostic reasoning that HYPOTHESIST does not address. Although the HDR model could be extended to include a similar mechanism, obtaining reliable probability estimates seems likely to remain a limiting factor for the application of probabilistic reasoning in medical diagnosis. Nevertheless, probabilistic reasoning can play a complementary role once the problem has been constrained (e.g. by model-based reasoning) to a narrow differential diagnosis (de Kleer & Williams 1987, Spiegelhalter & Knill-Jones 1984, Szolovits 1980, Szolovits & Pauker 1978). The model of HDR presented here may enhance the reasoning capabilities, and acceptability to users, of programs based on such an integrated approach.

Acknowledgement.
The author is grateful to the anonymous referees for their comments.

References

ADAMS, I. D., CHAN, M., CLIFFORD, P. C. et al. (1986). Computer aided diagnosis of acute abdominal pain: a multicentre study. *British Medical Journal*, 293, 800-804.

CENDROWSKA, J. (1987). PRISM: An Algorithm for Inducing Modular Rules, *International Journal of Man-Machine Studies*, 27, 349-370.

de DOMBAL, F. T. (1991). *Diagnosis of acute abdominal pain.* Churchill Livingstone.

de DOMBAL, F. T., LEAPER, D., STANILAND, J. et al. (1972). Computer-aided diagnosis of acute abdominal pain. *British Medical Journal*, 2, 9-13.

de KLEER, J. and WILLIAMS, B. C. (1987). Diagnosing multiple faults. *Artificial Intelligence*, 32, 97-130.

ELSTEIN, A. S., SCHULMAN, L. A., and SPRAFKA, S. A. (1978). *Medical problem solving: an analysis of clinical reasoning.* Harvard University Press.

FOX, J., BARBER, K. D. and BARDHAN, K. D. (1980). Alternatives to Bayes? *Methods of Information in Medicine,* 19, 210-214.

GORRY, G. A., KASSIRER, J. P., ESSIG, A. and SCHWARTZ, W. B. (1973). Decision analysis as the basis for computer-aided management of acute renal failure. *American Journal of Medicine,* 55, 473-484.

KASSIRER, J. P. and KOPELMAN, R. I. (1991). *Learning clinical reasoning.* Williams & Wilkins.

KLEMENZ, B. and McSHERRY, D. (1995) Computer-assisted learning through interaction with a model of diagnostic reasoning. *International Conference on Initiatives for Change in Medical Education in Europe (MedEd-21),* Vaals, The Netherlands.

McSHERRY, D. (1986). Intelligent dialogue based on statistical models of clinical decision making. *Statistics in Medicine,* 5, 497-502.

McSHERRY, D. (1992). A domain independent theory for testing fault hypotheses. *IEE Colloquium on Intelligent Fault Diagnosis,* London.

McSHERRY, D. (1995) Hypothetico-deductive data mining. *Proceedings of the Seventh International Symposium on Applied Stochastic Models and Data Analysis,* Dublin, 398-407.

McSHERRY, D and McCLEAN, S. (1995) Intelligent techniques for analysis of inconsistent and missing data in a distributed database environment. *Proceedings of Intelligent Data Analysis 95,* Baden-Baden, 119-123.

PEARL, J. (1988). *Probabilistic reasoning in intelligent systems.* Morgan Kaufman.

POPLE, H. E. (1982). Heuristic methods for imposing structure on ill-structured problems: the structuring of medical diagnostics. In Szolovits, P. (ed.) *Artificial Intelligence in Medicine,* 119-190. Westview Press.

SHORTLIFFE, E. H. and BARNETT, G. O. (1990). Medical data: their acquisition, storage and use. In Shortliffe, E.H. et al. (eds.) *Medical informatics: Computer Applications in Health care,* 37-69. Addison-Wesley.

SHORTLIFFE, E. H., BUCHANAN, B. G. and FEIGENBAUM, E. A. (1979). Knowledge engineering for medical decision-making: a review of computer-based clinical decision aids. *Proceedings of the IEEE,* 67, 1207-1224.

SPIEGELHALTER, D. and KNILL-JONES, R. (1984). Statistical and knowledge-based approaches to clinical decision-support systems, with an application in gastroenterology. *Journal of the Royal Statistical Society Series A,* 147, 35-77.

SZOLOVITS, P. and PAUKER, S. G. (1978). Categorical and probabilistic reasoning in medical diagnosis. *Artificial Intelligence,* 11, 115-144.

SZOLOVITS, P. (1980). The lure of numbers: how to live with and without them in medical diagnosis. In Statland, B.E and Bauer, S. (eds.) *Computer-assisted decision making using clinical and paraclinical (laboratory) data,* 65-75. Mediad Inc.

The Clinical Spectrum of Decision-Support in Oncology with a Case Report of a Real World System

Antoine Geissbühler, MD, Randolph A. Miller, MD, William W. Stead, MD
Division of Biomedical Informatics, Vanderbilt University Medical Center

Abstract

Clinical decision-support opportunities in oncology are numerous. Application programs may assist the diagnostic process, help define the proper therapy and adjust it to the patient's characteristics, streamline the delivery and follow-up of the treatments, provide tools for patient tracking and outcome measurements, and support patient care in the community. The authors and their colleagues have extended a novel general-purpose direct care-provider order entry system to take into account the particular aspects of chemotherapy ordering and decision-support. This new approach takes advantage of the infrastructure and functions of the integrated medical information system.

Introduction

Various computer-based tools have been developed to assist clinicians in the task of caring for oncology patients, and include broad-based [6] and specialized [1] diagnostic support systems, information resources on prognosis and treatment [5], and therapy management tools [2,4].

Ideally, these functions could be integrated around an electronic medical record: clinical information could be used to assist in the diagnostic process and in the detection of complications; treatment protocols could intelligently generate medical orders which would then be translated into dispensing and administration information, thus minimizing transcription errors and allowing for various checks to be performed. Results from laboratory tests and other sources, including textual reports processed by natural language processing techniques, could be monitored and trigger alerts or reminders to adapt the therapy, watch for complications and detect deviations from optimal protocols. The same data could be used to document research protocols, to look for similar cases, or to automatically retrieve relevant patient-specific information from various resources, such as literature reference databases or patient information databases. Interfaces to the Internet could facilitate the decentralization of care and would help community care-providers [8] and patients to access information and knowledge available in specialized facilities.

This paper describes how a general-purpose care-provider order entry system, as a part of an integrated advanced information management system (IAIMS), has been extended to provide decision-support and safety functions for the treatment of oncology patients in a tertiary-care hospital.

WizOrder and the IAIMS Project at Vanderbilt University

VUMC has adopted a fast track approach to IAIMS [7], based on the following objectives: demonstrate that an environment can be established that redirects and coordinates individual initiatives so they come together into an IAIMS, demonstrate models of the core resources that are required as a foundation to the IAIMS, and evaluate the effectiveness of strategies to overcome the obstacles to IAIMS implementation, by measuring progress against predefined milestones.

As part of this effort, the WizOrder project provides a user-friendly interface at the point of care for both the capture of medical orders and the intelligent integration of information resources and clinical decision-support tools [3]. The rationale of focusing on the time when orders are entered as a central point for data integration and decision-support is based on the hypothesis that this represents the precise moment where medical decisions, based on the care-provider's knowledge and data from the patient care information system, are formalized and ready to be communicated to the hospital personnel. Medical decisions are mature enough to be critiqued, but not processed yet, so that they can easily be altered by the person who conceived them, when given appropriate advice; they are captured at the source and represent the closest approximation of what is really intended. Within the Vanderbilt system, once orders are captured and validated, they are passed to a commercial order processing (transaction) system and then dispatched to the appropriate ancillary departments (e.g., pharmacy, laboratory, radiology, dietary services) through a custom-built interface engine.

Based on a modular and distributed architecture, WizOrder's capabilities evolve with the development of the patient care information system and of techniques for accessing remote information resources. As of December 1996, it is routinely used in the medicine and surgery services of the hospital (400 out of 660 total beds), including oncology and bone marrow transplant units. 60 to 70% of the 3000 daily orders are entered directly by physicians and the system generates more than 100 warnings every day. The WizOrder interface encompasses features such as an intelligent completer that translates users' orders from free text to structured records using a relational dictionary which defines the nomenclature and syntax of what can be ordered in the medical center (7000 items); the simultaneous display of active orders, patient demographics, allergies and current alerts detected by the program; and, single-key access to the integrated information resources. These resources include an extensive drug information database, developed and maintained by the hospital pharmacy, which contains drug dosing information, monographs, general drug-drug interactions, infusion compatibility tables and institution-specific information for research protocols. A laboratory reference manual is available on-line. Laboratory results and other reports can be queried, either interactively or by WizOrder from the MARS data repository [9]. Along with demographic information, these results are used to perform drug dose checking (by taking into account the age, weight, body surface area, renal function of the patient and pharmacokinetic models) and generate alerts. Other tools available during the order entry process include an ICD9 completer for diagnoses and procedures and automated link to literature references related to the patients diagnoses and treatments that make use of the UMLS Metathesaurus for translation across different nomenclatures.

WizOrder incorporates a protocol-generation facility that enables end-users to create complex, logic-based protocols for therapy of specified diseases or conditions. More than 600 diagnostic- and procedure-based order sets have been created. They are maintained directly by clinicians.

WizOrder also generates integrated reports such as the nurses worksheet which combines demographics information and medical orders, the physicians rounds report which integrates alerts, demographic data, diagnoses, medications, recent laboratory results and textual reports, and the sign-out sheet which contains summarized patient information in order to facilitate overnight coverage.

WizOrder Extensions for Oncology Patient Care

In oncology, more than in any other medical specialty, therapy depends on a critical balance between achieving therapeutic benefit, and avoiding potentially serious side-effects. It is therefore essential to take into consideration several safety issues.

Capturing the orders at the source of medical expertise and avoiding errors due to their transcription by transmitting them electronically should improve data quality for the enterprise. However, the users might not be familiar with the computer encoding schemes, and it is unacceptable to leave room for divergent interpretations. WizOrder contains heuristic rules that limit how chemotherapeutic agents can be ordered and the system unambiguously spells out how the program understood the order.

Rule-based and knowledge-based drug dosing checks take into account the age, weight, body surface area and renal function of the patient, for single doses, daily doses, doses per chemotherapy cycle and cumulative doses. Other checks performed when orders are captured include drug-drug interactions, allergy checks, and the exclusion of certain medications from research protocols. The necessary information is contained in the drug information databases developed and maintained by the pharmacists at our institution, in the computerized pharmacy dispensing system. Processes have been implemented so that these database can be regularly and automatically transferred into the WizOrder database to be used at the front-end, but their maintenance remains the responsibility of the pharmacy.

Computerized protocols help standardize patient care, control costs while maintaining quality, and reduce ambiguities and prescription errors. We extended the functionalities of protocols in WizOrder so that complex calculations, temporal information and questionnaires could be represented. The translation to computerized protocols is performed directly by senior clinicians who not only know appropriate dosages but also understand the logistical implications of the orders, so that the actions generated by the use of these protocols really match what is intended. Protocols can contain recommendations and can be embedded in other protocols. Simple, standard sets of orders, such as anti-emetic treatments, nursing instructions for neutropenic patients or blood transfusion recommendations, can be built separately then embedded into larger protocols which ensures a greater level of consistency and simplify the maintenance. Questionnaires can be used to dynamically present the part of the protocol that is relevant based on the answers of the user. WizOrder currently provides access to more than 80 chemotherapy protocols.

Once generated, medication orders are automatically sent to pharmacists who are responsible for translating medical orders into dispensing and administration information. To avoid a transcription step, WizOrder reformats chemotherapy, pre-medications and post-medication orders and sorts them for each day of the chemotherapy. The document can then be annotated by pharmacists who will add information such as drug concentration, infusion rate and other specific recommendations. The result is the chemotherapy medication administration record (MAR) which will be used by the nurses as a worksheet.

Patients are often seen in the outpatient oncology clinic before they are hospitalized to receive chemotherapy. Orders generated during the visit are validated and stored until the patient is admitted. When a treatment needs to be delayed, for example when the recovery from the previous treatment is longer than expected, sets of orders can be rescheduled.

Conclusion

The capture of accurate data and the ability to interact directly with the care-providers are pre-requisites to efficient clinical decision-support applications. The same is true for the maintenance of knowledge bases, which must be the responsibility of the relevant experts, the role of information technologists being to provide tools for their manipulation and consistency checking.

WizOrder has been developed to fulfill these roles and its architecture was designed to enable the seamless integration of decision-support tools. The implementation of functions specific to oncology patients, including safety issues as well as decision-support capabilities, has shown that this model is viable.

As a part of an IAIMS project, WizOrder benefits from institution-wide information resources and technologies to provide relevant information during the order entry process, and to streamline the information communication process. As standard protocols and nomenclatures are developed, information and knowledge sharing across the Internet will increase, extending the institutional capabilities and facilitating the outreach of patient care.

References

1. Baak JP. Artificial intelligence systems (expert systems) as diagnostic consultants for the cytologic and histologic diagnosis of cancer. Report from the Second International Conference, March 13-15, 1988, Chicago, Illinois. Journal of Cancer Research & Clinical Oncology. 1988; 114(3):325-34.
2. Enterline JP, Lenhard RE Jr., Blum BI, et al.. OCIS: 15 years' experience with patient-centered computing. MD Computing. 1994; 11(2):83-91.
3. Geissbuhler A, Miller RA. WizOrder, a user-friendly interface for order entry and clinical decision support tools. Proceedings of the SCAMC; 1995:1002.
4. Hickam DH, Shortliffe EH, et al. The treatment advice of a computer-based cancer chemotherapy protocol advisor. Annals of Internal Medicine. 1985; 103:928-36.
5. Hubbard SM, Marin NB, Thurn AL. NCI's cancer information systems--bringing medical knowledge to clinicians. Oncology. 1995; 9(4):302-6
6. Miller RA. Medical diagnostic decision support systems - past, present and future: a threaded bibliography and brief commentary. JAMIA. 1994; 1:8-27.
7. Stead WW, Borden R, Bourne J, Giuse D, et al. The Vanderbilt University fast track to IAIMS: transition from planning to implementation. JAMIA. 1996;3:308-17.
8. Wirtschafter D, Carpenter JT, Mesel E. A consultant-extender system for breast cancer adjuvant chemotherapy. Annals of Internal Medicine. 1979; 90(3):396-401.
9. Yount RJ, Vries JK, Councill CD. The Medical Archival System: an information retrieval system based on distributed parallel processing. Information Processing & Management, 1991; 27(4):379-389.

A Case-Based Reasoning Method for Computer-Assisted Diagnosis in Histopathology

Marie-Christine Jaulent*, Christel Le Bozec**,
Eric Zapletal* and Patrice Degoulet*

* Service d'Informatique Médicale - Hôpital Broussais - 96 rue Didot - 75014 Paris, France
** IGR - rue Camille Desmoulins - 94800 Villejuif, France

Abstract

This article addresses the issue of exploiting knowledge acquired from experience in the diagnosis process in histopathology. We present the functional architecture of a Case-Based-Reasoning system in this domain. The main procedure, the selection of similar previous cases, has been implemented. The selection procedure is based on an original similarity measure that takes into account both semantic and structural resemblances and differences between the cases. A first evaluation of the system was performed on a base of 35 pathological cases of specimen of breast palpable tumours.

1. Introduction

The identification of the various histologic tumour types requires the integration of various and complex data. In front of the abundance of histologic patterns, the physician faces several diagnostic problems and the expert uses heuristics and his/her own experience to adapt old solutions to new situations.

In histopathology, diagnosis and prognosis decision support systems rely on a wide variety of methods. Many of them are based on a bayesian network approach like Pathfinder [1] and others [2][3]. Expert systems like CancerStage [4], using Artificial Intelligence methods, are the usual alternative to the probabilistic approach. The decisive advance brought by the most recent knowledge-based systems is the ability to process symbolic information and to provide "intelligent" retrieval of diagnostic clues from a reference set. These systems work in situations where optimal solutions to problems can be logically proved.

Histopathologic imagery can hardly be modelised in the format of logical knowledge representation. The lack of data and the enormous effort which would be necessary to assert such data impedes the relationships between morphological features to be expressed in terms of logical conditions. Besides, a part of medical reasoning is associative, intuitive and based on raw cases. This is especially the case in histopathology where experts use heuristics rather than logically formulated rules. They are in particular good at recognizing a new problem as analogous to a certain kind of problem that they already know how to solve. We address the issue of considering that the previous experience is rich enough to help decision making in this domain. The case based reasoning approach seems to be a good framework for studying and exploiting the knowledge sources and the reasoning attitude of experts in histopathology.

In this paper, we present the conception of a computer system using a case-based reasoning approach to modelise the expert diagnosis process in histopathology. The main contention of this work is that the case and the collection of cases include the necessary and sufficient information (e.g. morphological features and implicit mutual correlation between features) to solve new problems.

2. Method

Case Base Reasoning is an approach to problem-solving that uses the specific knowledge of previously experienced concrete situations (cases). A new problem is solved by finding a similar case and reusing it in the new problem situation [5]. At the highest level of generality, a general CBR cycle is composed by the four following steps [5] (figure 1):

- *RETRIEVE* the most similar case (or cases). Firstly, the *extraction* of interesting cases allows to restrict the searching base. Secondly, the *selection* phase allows to retrieve the most similar cases. The retrieval capacity stems from the definition of a similarity measure between the case and the new problem that encompasses the notion of distance. Gentner in [6] discusses a general classification of similarity measures depending on whether the similarity is based on structural information (architectural aspects of the case) or surface information (semantic description).

• *REUSE* the information and knowledge present in the most similar case to solve the new problem. This phase is often called the *adaptation* step.
• *REVISE* the proposed solution. This phase consists in comparing the solution provided by the system to the reality.
• *RETAIN* the parts of this experience likely to be useful for future problem solving.

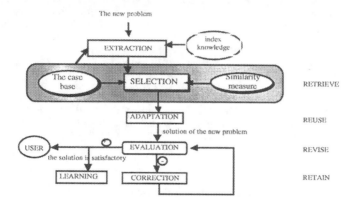

Figure 1 : Functional architecture of a CBR system

The restriction of the domain to breast tumour specimen determines the nature of the cases present in the base and the context in which a new problem occurs.
    In figure 1, the grey area corresponds to what has been realized in the current state of the system. In the context of our application, we have focused on the selection process.The two main aspects that are presented concern - the representation of a case and - the definition of a similarity algorithm.

3. A CBR System in Histopathology
3.1. Representation of a case

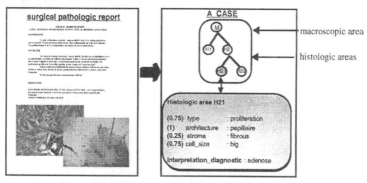

Figure 2 : The representation of a case

    The usual description of a case is written in natural language by the physician in a more or less standardized report [7]. From the analysis of several reports, a model has been developed in which a case is described as a collection of macroscopic areas, each of them associated to a collection of histologic areas. An histologic area can contain several histologic areas as well as a cytological description. Each type of macroscopic area, each type of histologic area is defined by a set of specific features. For instance, (stroma fibrous) and (architecture papillary) are two features, among others, of a histologic area of a type proliferation (figure 2). Inside a case, some features are descriptive (semiological features) and others are conclusive (goal features). In order to express to what extent a descriptive feature is responsible for a conclusive feature, a degree of importance is assigned to each semiological feature (figure 2). The set of degrees is heuristically given by the expert.

3.2. The Selection Procedure

The selection procedure computes a similarity measure between a new problem n (a case without goal features) and a well known case c. The entities to compare are composite and their descriptions include structural and semantic characteristics. The semantic characteristics are given by the set of features. The structural characteristics correspond to the tree structure of the global entity. The global measure is computed as the arithmetic mean of a surface similarity and a structure similarity.

Surface similarity expresses the semantic resemblance between two macroscopic areas or two histologic areas. The surface similarity relies on the similarity of each corresponding feature of n and c. For each feature, a similarity table has been defined in order to compare the different possible values of the feature. For instance, the table 1 corresponds to the feature "consistency". The similarity is rated between 0 and 1. The rate can be given by an expert (for instance $s(5,2) = 0.5$) or calculated by the following formula: let p be the number of possible values for a given feature,

$$\forall i, j \in [1,p] \qquad sim = s(i, j) = max\left(0, k \cdot \frac{|i - j|}{p}\right) \text{ where } k = \frac{3}{2} \qquad (1)$$

Table 1: Example of a similarity table

consistency	soft	supple	hard	very hard	heterogeneous
soft	1	s(1,2)	s(1,3)	s(1,4)	s(1,5) = 0.5
supple	s(2,1)	1	s(2,3)	s(2,4)	s(2,5) = 0.5
hard	s(3,1)	s(3,2)	1	s(3,4)	s(3,5) = 0.5
very hard	s(4,1)	s(4,2)	s(4,3)	1	s(4,5) = 0.5
heterogeneous	s(5,1) = 0.5	s(5,2) = 0.5	s(5,3) = 0.5	s(5,4) = 0.5	1

Moreover, let n and c be described as an ordered set of features: $n = (n_1, n_2, ..., n_i, ..., n_T)$ and $c = (c_1, c_2, ..., c_i, ..., c_T)$. Let a_i be the importance given to the ith descriptive feature, the *surface similarity* is then given by the weighted aggregation of the similarities established inside the areas between each common feature. The aggregation is based on the minimum operator.

$$S_{surface}(n, c) = min_{i \in \{1...T\}}\{max(sim(n_i, c_i), 1 - a_i)\} \qquad (2)$$

where a_i = weight of attribute i , $n = \{n_i\}, i \in \{1...T\}$ and $c = \{c_i\}, i \in \{1...T\}$

Structure similarity is based on a tree matching algorithm. The procedure consists in finding the best matching between the tree structure of the new problem and the tree structure of the known case.

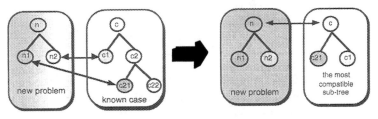

Figure 3 : Structure matching

A flexibility has been introduced in the matching process in order to take into account the fact that the histologic areas are not necessarily described at the same level of hierarchy by the experts. Indeed, an histologic area of the new problem will match the histologic area of the known case for which the surface similarity is the best one.

4. Results and Conclusion

Thirty-five pathological specimen were selected to constitute the case base. These cases correspond to confirmed reference cases in an histopathology department. In order to test the retrieve phase, a first prototype has been implemented in C++. Once the most similar case has been selected, the system presents to the user the semiology, the associated images and the diagnostic for this closest case. It gives also the value of the computed similarity as well as the computed partial similarity.

In this article, we presented a case-based reasoning method for diagnostic decision making in histopathology. The main advantage of this method is the fact that the knowledge is expressed in a natural way. The expert does not need to express his/her knowledge through production rules or decision trees. The first purpose of the system that has been realized is to help the non expert pathologist in his/her diagnostic process by providing similar, solved expert cases.

The first prototype of the system demonstrates clearly the interest of this method in the sense that a meaningful resemblance rate between cases is obtained. The system is efficient in the sense that it can find similar examples even when the hierarchical organisation of the areas is not strictly identical. Indeed, the definition of the similarity measure takes into account the variability of the case description, in particular in the structure similarity. Nowadays, the system is not yet formally evaluated. Moreover, the fact to provide partial degrees of similarities allows the expert to analyse the causes of a potential failure. It is then possible to modify the different parameters of the measure in order to improve the performances.

From this preliminary study, it appears that this approach is adapted and robust to missing information and provides important clues to the pathologist.

Besides the completion of the CBR cycle (reuse, revise, retain), the perspectives of this work are both methodological and applicative. At the methodological level, an important point concerns the representation of the imprecision inherent of the information contained in the case through the use of the fuzzy set theory. Another point concerns the representation of the case, in particular the necessity to improve the description of images by introducing morphometric attributes. At the applicative level, the perspectives are broad. For instance, the domain can be extended to the whole breast pathology and other domains of pathology. Furthermore, the possibility to access, through a network, large multi-experts bases of anonymous cases could be useful in the daily practice for both medical and educational purposes.

Bibliographie

[1]   Heckerman DE, Natathwani BN.An evaluation of the diagnostic accuracy of Pathfinder.1992.Comput Biomed Res.1992;25(1): 56-74.

[2]   Bartels PH, Thompson D, Bibbo M, Weber JE. Bayesian belief networks in quantitative histopathology. Analyt Quant Cytol Histol 1992;14:459-473.

[3]   Montironi R, Bartels PH, Thompson D, Scapelli M, Hamilton P. Prostatic Intraepithelial Neoplasia, development of a Baysian belief network for diagnosis and grading. Analyt Quant Cytol Histol 1994;16:101-112.

[4]   Marchevsky AN, Coons G.Expert systems as Aid for the Pathologist's role of clinical consultant: Cancer-Stage. 1993;6(3):265-269.

[5]   Aamodt A. Case-Based Reasoning: Foundational Issues, Mathodological Variations, and System Approaches. AICOM 1994; 7:39-59.

[6]   Gentner D. Analogical inference and analogical access. Analogica : Proceedings of the first workshop on analogical reasoning 1987;

[7]   Rosai J. Standardized Reporting of Surgical Pathology Diagnoses for the Major Tumor Types. A proposal. Am J Clin Pathol 1993;100: 240-255.

The Validation of an Expert System for Diagnosis of Acute Myocardial Infarction

A.Rabelo Jr.[1] A.R.Rocha[2] A.Souza[1] A.Araujo[1] A.Ximenes[1] C.Andrade[1]
D.Onnis[1] I.Olivaes[1] K.Oliveira[1,2] N.Lobo[1] N.Ferreira[1] S.Lopes[1] V.Werneck[1,2]

[1] Cardiology and Cardiovascular Surgery Unit (UCCV), Federal University of Bahia
Fundação Bahiana de Cardiologia (FBC)
Rua Augusto Viana s/n, 40140-060 Salvador,Brazil
e-mail: arabelo@ufba.br

[2] COPPE, Computer Science Department, Federal University of Rio de Janeiro
Caixa Postal 68511, 21945-970 Rio de Janeiro, Brazil
e-mail:darocha@cos.ufrj.br

Abstract. This paper describes the validation of an expert system for diagnosis of acute myocardial infarction developed to support doctors without cardiology specialization. The conception of this expert system took into account the characteristics and problems of Brazilian Health Care System. However since similar features are found in the Health Care Systems of other countries, the usefulness of this system is not restricted to the Brazilian context.

1 Introduction

The diagnosis of acute myocardial infarction is based on the patient's history, the physical examination and on the electrocardiogram (ECG) interpretation. However due to the deficiencies of many countries' health care systems, many primary and secondary hospitals and primary emergency units lack cardiologists on call. This situation, is responsible for delays in therapeutic actions, preventing patients to receive adequate treatment and often leading to unnecessary deaths.

Considering the incidence of acute myocardial infarction and the health care situation of Brazil and many other countries we decided to develop an expert system to support doctors non specialized in cardiology for diagnosis of acute myocardial infarction. The system, named SEC, arrives to a diagnostic conclusion taking into consideration symptoms, previous events, risk factors, the physical examination and an automatic interpretation of the ECG.

The final result should be in one of the ranges as follows:

Range 1: There is a low probability of an acute myocardial infarction and the patient may be discharged.

Range 2: There is a moderate probability of an acute myocardial infarction and the patient should be referred to a Cardiology Service.

Range 3: There is a high probability of an acute myocardial infarction and the patient should be immediately referred to a Coronary Care Unit.

The project started in April, 1994 with the definition of the software development process made by the software engineering team. We decided to have an evolutionary development process and to work first on aspects related to the patient's clinical information. In June, we began the knowledge acquisition process. The construction of version 1.0 finished in September, 1994. Following the approval of this version, the system was submitted to a process of refinement until December. These refinements produced versions 1.1, 1.2 and 1.3. In January, 1995 we began version 2.0. During 1995, version 2.0 was refined producing versions 2.1, 2.2 and 2.3. On all these versions the ECG was interpreted by the physician who was responsible for entering the result of this interpretation into the system. With the results of the validation of version 2.3 we considered that SEC achieved our goals for the analysis of clinical information. Thus we began to work on knowledge acquisition for ECGs interpretation. This process led to version 3.0 which integrates clinical information and ECG interpretation.

2 Software Quality Assurance Procedures

It is well known that software cannot be made reliable only by means of testing. Software quality cannot be added to a product after its development. It must be built in. This was the approach used in this project for software quality assurance. The chosen technique for software evaluation during development was phased inspection [1]. The criteria considered in each evaluation were defined based on a set of attributes we have identified as desirable for an expert system [2].

Differences between conventional software and expert systems determine validation peculiarities for these systems. As no method alone can assure program reliability, we decided to use a combination of testing methods [3], [4], [5]. The system validation was first made using face validity [6] where the project team compared the system performance to human expert performance. The next step in validation was to perform sensitivity analysis [5] where the experts systematically changed the expert system input variable values observing the effect upon the system performance. These two validation methods were supported by operational prototyping [7] and were used for testing versions 1.0 to 1.3.

Another validation method used was to perform comparative tests. This method was used for validating version 2.0. Sixty three test cases were used to compare the judgment of the expert system with that of specialists in cardiology, cardiology fellows and residents in order to classify the performance of our system among physicians with different levels of expertise. As the correct diagnosis was not known, we decided to use the most cited solution for theses cases, the right answer being the one upon which the majority of experts agree [8]. Each case was accompanied by a form demanding a reply according to the three levels of diagnostic conclusion made by the system. Seven test cases were eliminated as they were considered not sufficiently clear by the cardiologists or because it was not possible to decide for the right answer. The error rate among experts range from 12.5% to 41%, among the cardiology fellows from 23.2% to 60.7% and among residents from 32.1% to 41%. With 30.3% errors the SEC system began to behave as an expert.

The tendency of SEC in this version was, in a case of a diagnostic error, to overprotect the patient, as we had already observed with test results of versions 1.0, 1.1, 1.2 and 1.3. This may be considered as a factor that increases its reliability. Insufficient diagnosis is a major reason for patient mortality and one of the motivations for the development of SEC, even though we decided to refine this version to obtain a more specific system without losing the achieved sensibility. This process has led to versions 2.1, 2.2 and 2.3.

Version 2.3 was validated with 320 real cases collected in the emergency room of UCCV/FBC. All these cases have the record of a physician's diagnosis and the outcome (whether or not the patient had an acute myocardial infarction). With the validation of version 2.3 we have obtained the following results. In range 1, the system judged 168 patients, 167 of whom effectively did not have an acute myocardial infarction. This result means that when SEC classified a patient in range 1 this judgment was correct in 99.4 % of cases. In range 3, SEC judged 72 patients, 58 of whom effectively had an acute myocardial infarction. This result means that when SEC judged a patient in range 3 the patient was suffering from a myocardial infarction in 80.5% of these cases. Only 14 in 320 patients (4.3%) without myocardial infarction were referred to a Coronary Care Unit. Eighty patients were judged to be in range 2 (25% of a total of 320 patients). Among those, 12 patients were suffering from a myocardial infarction. These results made us confident about SEC's evaluation of clinical data as we achieved specificity without losing sensibility. Thus, we began to work on ECGs interpretation which led to version 3.0.

At present we are validating version 3.0 which integrates the analysis of clinical data with the interpretation of the ECG. This version is also being validated with real cases from our emergency room. Version 3.0 is being validated with only 67 cases. For all these cases we have recorded the outcome and the ECG. We have obtained the following results, which should be considered already partial. In range 1, the system judged 21 patients, 20 of whom effectively did not have an acute myocardial infarction. This result means that when SEC classified a patient in range 1 this judgment was correct in 95.2% of cases. In the only one case where SEC judge the patient in range 1 and he had an acute myocardial infarction, this was also the cardiologist diagnosis in the emergency room. In range 3, SEC judged 23 patients, 20 of whom effectively had an acute myocardial infarction. This result means that when SEC judged a patient in range 3 the patient was suffering from a myocardial infarction in 86.9% of these cases. Only 3 of those 67 patients (4.4%) were referred to a Coronary Care Unit without myocardial infarction. 23 patients were judged to be in range 2 (34.3% of a total of 67 patients). Among those, 10 patients were suffering from a myocardial infarction.

The next step on the validation of SEC will be to conduct field tests in one State Public Hospital, where it will be possible to compare the performance of a physician assisted by SEC with those not assisted.

3 Conclusion

This paper describes an expert system developed to support doctors without cardiology specialization for diagnosis of acute myocardial infarction. One important feature of this project is the validation process it was submitted all over its development. Inspections were performed since the initial phases allowing errors to be detected in the same phase they occur, and thus avoiding their propagation, increasing the productivity and reducing project costs. The validation using real cases is another important feature of the process and it was possible because the whole cardiovascular unit was involved in the project.

Acknowledgment

This project has been partly sponsored by grants from FINEP, CNPq and IBM-Brazil, the financial support of which the authors acknowledge.

References

1. J.Knight and E.A.Myers. Improved inspection technique. Communications of the ACM, 36:51- 61, 1993.
2. A.Rabelo Jr. et al. An expert system for diagnosis of acute myocardial infarction: software quality assurance procedures. In Proc. European Symposium on the Validation and Verification of Knowledge Based-Systems pages 117-128, 1995.
3. P.Meseguer and E. Plaza. Validation of KBS: the VALID project. In L.Steels and B. Lepape, editors, Enhancing the Knowledge Engineering Process, pages 55-78. Elsevier, 1992.
4. P.Meseguer. Conventional software and expert systems: some comparative aspects regarding validation. In J.Cuena, editor, Knowledge Oriented Software Design, pages 193-204. Elsevier, 1993.
5. R.O'Keefe, O. Balci and E.P. Smith. Validating expert systems performance. IEEE Expert 4:81-87, 1987.
6. T.J.O'Leary, M.G.Goul, K.E.Hoffitt and A.E.Radwan. Validating expert systems. IEEE Expert 7:51-58, 1990.
7. A.M.Davis. Operational prototyping: a new development approach. IEEE Software 9:70-78, 1992.
8. P.François et al. Comparative study of human expertise and an expert system: application to the diagnosis of child's meningitis. Computers and Biomedical Research 26:383-392, 1993.

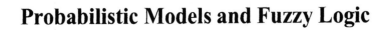

Probabilistic Models and Fuzzy Logic

A Causal-Functional Model Applied to EMG Diagnosis

Jorge Cruz and Pedro Barahona

Departamento de Informática, Universidade Nova Lisboa, 2825 Monte da Caparica, Portugal

Abstract. This paper presents an EMG diagnostic Knowledge Based System, that is the first application of our methodology for reasoning with causal-functional (meta-)models. Despite past difficulties, diagnosis is still an important application of KBSs, if considered in an appropriate context of medical practice. We argue that this is the case with neurophisiology, which lends to deep modelling of the domain and associated reasoning. The results obtained with our prototype system, and the clinical context where the system may be used make it a quite promising application, not only to experiment advanced artificial intelligence techniques but also to provide an useful decision support system for medical practice.

Keywords: Knowledge representation, reasoning under uncertain, diagnostic KBS.

1. Introduction

Although one of the first focus of artificial intelligence applications in Medicine, diagnosis has more recently lost some of its appeal, and it is arguable that health care professionals are more interested in more global patient management [1,2]. Diagnosis is nevertheless quite important, if considered in an appropriate context of medical practice. For example, the diagnosis of acute abdominal pain [3] and the automatic interpretation of ECGs [4], are possibly the most successful applications of artificial intelligence (as well as other) in the medical field. A main reason for this success, namely in ECG, is the appropriate interface with medical devices, which makes it possible to analyse in real time the data obtained from them.

Other medical domains exhibit the same potential for diagnosis, namely the diagnosis of disorders of the peripheral nervous system (PNS) from electromyography studies (EMG). Early diagnostic systems [5,6,7] have already addressed this domain, but their widespread use has been hampered, by lack of agreement in common terminology (for representation of data, disorders, etc.) and adequate interfaces. These problems were addressed in project ESTEEM, where a multinational team agreed on a number of common data sets for EMG findings (raw data), their symbolic interpretation and the set of disorders to be diagnosed. A telematics platform has been built around these data sets, and one EMG manufacturer has even produced a prototypical connection to this platform, thus allowing the automatic collection of EMG data, which could thus support the diagnostic task [8,14].

EMG diagnosis is particularly interesting, since it involves the application of a number of artificial intelligence techniques. Firstly, EMG disorders are not syndromatic, and hence do not require mere pattern-matching between sets of findings and possible diagnosis. On the contrary, EMG diagnosis require a more complex reasoning strategy, involving gathering of information from where working hypotheses can be abduced from a domain model, and further verified by deduction in the model (a typical methodology to model medical reasoning in AI [9, 10]).

Secondly, the peripheral nervous system is sufficiently well understood so as to enable the specification of deep models, that represent knowledge at a more detailed level than findings and disorders. Anatomic and physiologic knowledge may be represented in such deep models, together with causal relationships between the state of the model components.

Thirdly, deep models can be regarded at a number of abstraction/refinement levels. Quantitative data (such as EMG raw data) might be abstracted into qualitative symbolic data. Conversely, refinement into more detailed knowledge levels is required to obtain more accurate deductions from the refined models.

Fourthly, relationships in the model are usually not deterministic. Although at a sufficient deep level one may argue that causal relations are deterministic, such levels are usually not workable (either not observable, or involving untractable computations). More abstract models must thus consider uncertainty in their relations.

In this paper we present the first realistic application of a methodology we developed for reasoning with causal-functional (meta-)models [11], well suited for the EMG domain. Section 2 briefly outlines the basic knowledge regarding the EMG domain. Section 3 describes the causal-functional model adopted for this domain, including the representation of uncertainty. Section 4 addresses the reasoning process at the various abstraction levels, by means of an example. Section 5 discusses some preliminary results, and section 6 presents the concluding remarks.

2. Medical Domain

The Peripheral Neuro-Muscular System (PNS) is deeply involved in two main body functions, namely, motion and sensation. Sensations are triggered by specialised cells (receptors) able to react to particular forms of stimuli by producing nervous impulses which, when properly propagated through sensory fibres, reach a specific Central Nervous System (CNS) sensory area. Motion is the result of muscle contraction in response to the arrival of nervous impulses originated in particular CNS motor areas and propagated through the motor fibres that enervate the involved muscles.

The nervous sensory and motor fibres are the basic units for the transmission of nervous impulses. A nervous fibre is an extension of a nervous cell (axon) surrounded by specialised cells (Schwann cells) forming an involving sheath which sometimes enclose a conductive substance called myelin. The nervous fibres connect directly the sensory receptors and muscles to the CNS, grouping themselves in their course into a complex network of nerves composed of fibre bundles enclosed in connective tissue. The fibres that constitute the nerves are countless and it is thus impossible to differentiate their individual paths.

Neuromuscular disorders are responsible for the anatomical problems concerning the PNS. Local neuropathies directly affect a restricted nerve area, polyneuropathies are diffuse problems affecting the nervous fibres in all their extent, and myopathies affect muscles. All these problems induce some damage in the involved nerve or muscle fibres which, in case of axonal loss, is propagated distally (away from the CNS) to other fibre areas not directly affected by the disorder.

In order to obtain data from patients, several electrophysiological studies can be performed. In nerve studies, nervous impulses are induced by stimulation of a particular nerve point (stimulation site) and the electrical waveforms produced are recorded in another point of the nerve or attached muscle (recording site). The characteristics of these recorded electrical signs such as amplitude and velocity are used to assess the state of the fibre bundles involved in the impulse propagation. In muscular studies, the electrical waveforms produced by the muscles are recorded using electrodes giving direct information about muscle condition.

3. Qualitative and Quantitative Model

The knowledge about this medical domain spreads through different abstraction levels, explicitly represented in our system by a causal-functional model. The model explicitly represents structural, functional and causal knowledge through various abstraction levels. Moreover it supports consistent abstraction and refinement mechanisms that enable an efficient diagnostic reasoning.

3.1. Structural and Functional Knowledge

Two major structural concepts are considered in our model to represent transmission structures: the nervous fibre and the nervous bundle, defined as a set of nervous fibres sharing a common path. Other anatomical concepts (muscular fibres, muscles, receptor cells, sensory regions) are represented in a similar way.

The structural attributes associated with a nerve fibre characterise the state of its most important components: the myelin sheath and the axon. These components are not independent, showing a gradual degradation with structural damage. Hence the state of a nerve fibre is represented by a single attribute with values ranging from normal to complete axonal loss (Table I). The structural attributes related to a nerve bundle abstract the structural states of their fibres by their relative proportions.

Longitudinal composition/decomposition relate nerve fibres and bundles with their longitudinal components (points and segments). Transversal composition and decomposition relate sets of fibres that share a parallel path in some stages of their length, with each of its possible subsets. Abstraction and refinement operations relating the state of a structure with the state of its substructures can then be defined. The structural state of a nerve fibre is related with the worst damage suffered by its longitudinal components. The structural state of nerve bundles is abstracted from their transversal components by their relative proportions.

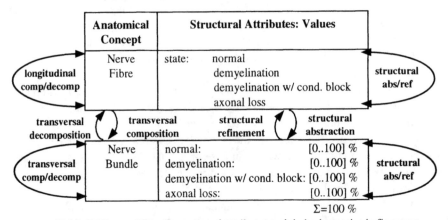

Table I-Fibre and Bundle structural attributes and their abstraction/refinement.

In addition to structural attributes, the model considers functional states, which represent particular views about the functioning of structures and support the representation of causal knowledge.

Functional attributes of nerve fibres specify the state of propagation of nervous impulses. For example, a functional attribute characterises the structure conduction properties in terms of delay or blocking. Functional attributes of nerve bundles can be directly associated with the interpretation of raw data from electrophysiological studies.

Anatomical Concept	Functional Attributes: Values	
Nerve Fibre	conduction:	normal, delayed, blocked
Nerve Bundle	cond. velocity:	decreased, decreased border, normal
	amplitude:	decreased, decreased border, normal

Table II - Fibre and Bundle functional attributes.

The physiological knowledge about nerve fibres allows the definition of abstraction and refinement operations relating the structural state of a fibre component with its functional conduction attribute. For example, if the structural state denotes demyelination without conduction block then a conduction delay is expected, while demyelination with conduction block or axonal loss obstruct impulse propagation.

Due to its higher degree of abstraction, the structural-functional abstraction and refinement operations for nerve bundles and muscles is typically uncertain. In practice, there is no way to compute precisely the value of the functional attributes from the structural states (e.g. the conduction velocity from the structural state of a nerve bundle), although it is known that demyelination and axonal loss are the structural parameters responsible for a possible delay and demyelination is more important than axonal loss to conduction delay. Such non-deterministic knowledge leads to a probabilistic definition of these structural-functional abstraction and refinement operations: a conditional probability function represents the likelihood of a functional attribute value given the possible structural states (Table III).

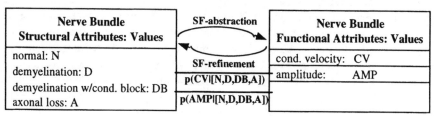

Nerve Bundle Structural Attributes: Values	SF-abstraction	Nerve Bundle Functional Attributes: Values
normal: N	SF-refinement	cond. velocity: CV
demyelination: D	p(CV|[N,D,DB,A])	amplitude: AMP
demyelination w/cond. block: DB	p(AMP|[N,D,DB,A])	
axonal loss: A		

Table III - Nerve Bundle structural-functional abstraction and refinement operations for conduction velocity and amplitude attributes.

The conditional probability function considers the relative importance of each structural attribute effect combining them into an overall composite effect, used as a deviation of the normal probability distribution for the functional value. For example, in case of a completely normal structural state for the nervous bundle, the normal distribution is assumed and the probability of the functional values is given by the correspondent areas (figure 1 for the decreased border value).

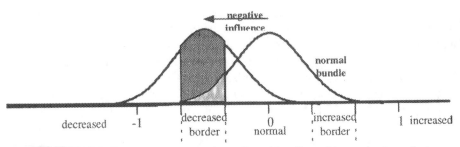

Fig. 1- The relation between normal and demyelinated bundles and its conduction velocity.

If there are demyelinated fibres then a negative influence is identified by a negative deviation of the normal distribution proportional to the percentage of the affected fibres, and the probability of the functional values is now given by the new correspondent areas (in figure 1 the shift caused by the negative influence clearly increased the decreased border value by comparison with the normal case). If a structural state presents both demyelination and axonal loss, the overall influence is obtained by aggregating both contributions, taking into account their relevance.

3.2. Causal Knowledge

In the causal-functional model, changes caused by normal or abnormal functioning of structures, as well as those caused by external agents, are modelled by means of processes, expressed at the appropriate level of abstraction.

The diagnostic hypotheses, i.e. the anatomical problems (local neuropathies, polyneuropathies and myopathies) that induce the deep pathological processes, are described in our system as causes of processes at the abstraction level of nerve bundles and muscles.

A local neuropathy is a lesion in a nerve point that causes deep pathologic processes of local demyelination and axonal loss. Only nerve fibres passing in the lesion point are affected. Two aspects are of major importance to characterise a neuropathy. First, the proportion of fibres involved in each of the deep pathological processes, that is, the proportion of fibres that suffer axonal loss and demyelination with or without conduction block. Second, the extension of the damage along the nerve fibres, since a neuropathy induces pathological processes in the affected fibres not only in the lesion point but also, in neighbouring points. The model includes transversal and longitudinal dispersion functions for the lesion severity. The causal processes that describe neuropathy effects have two arguments, the lesion nerve point and the lesion severity, and are constrained by the transversal and longitudinal dispersion functions.

process: local neuropathy   **effects:** $segment_{kl}$ of fibre $bundle_{FB}$:
     causes: neuropathy   normal=N
           ($point_i$ of $nerve_N$,Severity)   demyelination=D
    constraints: transversal dispersion   demyelination w/ cond. block=DB
                  longitudinal dispersion   axonal loss=A

The transversal dispersion function captures the gradual increase of structural damage caused by the severity of the lesion. In our model this dependency is based

on a binomial distribution of the structural damage caused by a lesion severity [12].
(Table IV).

	Lesion Severity		
	Mild	**Moderate**	**Severe**
normal (N):	42%	13%	2%
demyelination (D):	42%	37%	14%
demyelination w/ cond. block (DB):	14%	37%	42%
axonal loss (Ax):	2%	13%	42%

Table IV- Proportions of the deep pathological processes induced by the lesion severity

The longitudinal dispersion function captures the decrease of structural damage with
the distance from the directly affected nerve point. A Normal distribution is used to
characterise this dispersion around the lesion nerve point (figure 2). In this case,
whereas the directly lesioned nerve point A presents 42% demyelinated fibres, a
neighbouring point B situated at a distance Δ presents only 20% of demyelination
and a distant point C is considered unaffected [12].

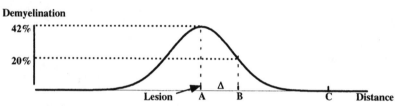

Fig. 2- Longitudinal demyelination caused by a mild lesion of nerve point A.

Equally important for the longitudinal dispersion of axonal loss is the contribution of
the deep pathological processes of axonal degeneration, implying a complete axonal
damage of the involved fibres (defined by transversal dispersion) for any distal point.

The process of local neuropathy relates a lesion in a nerve point with the
induced structural state of the affected fibre bundles, assuming that it is the only
anatomical problem in presence. However several problems can occur
simultaneously and their individual contributions for the fibre bundles structural state
should be considered. To compute the global structural state, we assume the effects
of two problems to be independent, and that the severest subsumes the weaker. Table
V shows an example of such computation.

P1 \ P2	N: 60%	D: 0%	DB: 10%	Ax: 30%
N: 40%	N: 24%	D: 0%	DB: 4%	Ax: 12%
D: 30%	D: 18%	D: 0%	DB: 3%	Ax: 9%
DB: 0%	DB: 12%	DB: 0%	DB: 2%	Ax: 6%
Ax: 10%	Ax: 6%	Ax: 0%	Ax: 1%	Ax: 3%

N: 24%
D: 18%
DB: 21%
Ax: 37%

Table V- Combination of two structural effects

To improve efficiency, the model is able to further abstract the above causal
processes (still at the nerve bundle and muscle level), by simply linking a lesioned
structure, abstracting away the lesion's severity, with possible problems that caused it.

4. Reasoning

The diagnostic reasoning of the system has two phases. In the first, it explores basic anatomical properties of the problem, in a superficial abductive search to elicit abstract hypotheses offering reasonable explanations for the observations. Anatomical relations, defined explicitly in the model, are used in order to restrict the huge number of initial possibilities, and only the abstracted processes referred in section 3 are used. In a second phase, each of these hypotheses is refined and the structural and corresponding functional states of the examined structures are deduced from the non abstracted processes. The evaluation of the suggested hypotheses is thus made taking into account the physiological knowledge added by context refinement. A comparison between predicted functional states and observations is then used to evaluate the plausibility of each hypothesis.

The system's diagnostic reasoning is explained by means of a simple example, which example only requires knowledge about anatomical structures of a single arm, namely two nerves (median and ulnar nerves), five sensory regions (the hand digits) and two hand muscles (abductor pollicis brevis/apb and abductor digiti minimi/adm) (see figure 3). The anatomical problems are restricted to local neuropathies in some typical points and the conduction velocity of five electrophysiological tests is the only information available.

Three sensory nerve studies were made (A, B and C) by stimulation of a sensory region (digits 1, 3 and 5 respectively) and recording of the induced electrical waveform in a proximal nerve point (wrist). The time elapsed between these two events (stimulation and recording) defines the conduction velocity of the nervous segment involved in the propagation (A was decreased border, B was decreased and C was normal). Two motor nerve studies were made (D and E) by stimulation of a nerve (median and ulnar) in two different points (elbow and wrist, distal sulcus and wrist) and recording of the induced electrical waveform in a muscle enervated by that nerve (apb and adm). The difference between the propagation times of the two stimulation's characterise the conduction velocity between the two stimulated points (D was decreased, E was normal).

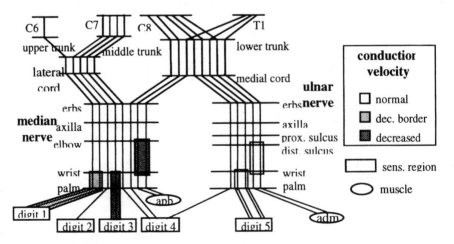

Fig. 3- Interpretation of electrophysiological data into conduction velocity of nerve bundles.

Even in this reduced and discrete subset of possible diagnoses (local neuropathies at discrete points) and given the number of nerve points (19) and the nervous segments that enervate the sensory regions and muscles (5+2), there is a huge number of possible diagnoses, (26 sites each with 4 severity values -absent, mild, moderate or severe: 4^{26}= 4.5×10^{15}). By only considering abstracted processes, the system only searches the localisation of neuropathies, postponing the evaluation of severity, but the number of possibilities remains very high (2^{26}=6.7×10^7).

In searching possible causes of abnormal findings, the system uses structural-functional refinement (Table III) to determine which of the analysed anatomical structures are necessarily in an abnormal structural state. As shown in figure 1, normal structures are only compatible with normal or (less likely) with decreased border conduction velocities. Consequently, a decreased value observed for the conduction velocity necessarily implies an abnormal structure. So, in our example, structures B and D are abnormal and diagnosis should identify local neuropathies responsible for this. Abduction made with the abstracted local neuropathy processes (with effects over B and D) identified the nerve areas shown in figure 4:

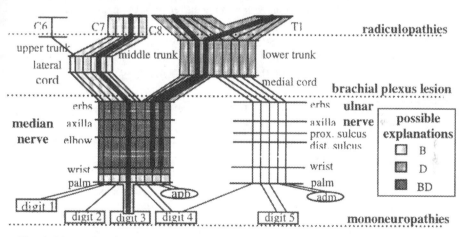

Fig. 4 - Nerve areas for local neuropathies capable of explaining the observed abnormalities

4 possible nerve points (median nerve: wrist, elbow, axilla and erbs) explain both abnormalities, 5 nerve points (median nerve: digit 3 and palm; lateral cord, middle trunk and C7) explain abnormality B alone, and 4 nerve points (medial cord, lower trunk, C8 and T1) explain abnormality D alone.

To restrict the set of raised hypotheses the system applies a parsimony criteria (which reflects empirical knowledge). Even if it is not the purpose of the system (at this stage) to suggest etiologic causes of the problems, it is reasonable to look for structural hypotheses that minimise the number of diseases. The system considers several etiologic groups (radiculopathies, plexus lesions and mononeuropathies, cf. figure 4) and takes into account that they can be responsible for several simultaneous local neuropathies.

A secondary parsimony criteria is used, that minimises the structural involvement within each etiology, aiming at reproducing the characteristic involvement of these groups of diseases.

The huge number of all possible diagnoses is now restricted to a few abstracted local neuropathies:

i) mononeuropathy on the median nerve (between the wrist and the erbs);
ii) brachial plexus lesion with two foci: one in lateral cord or middle trunk and the other in the medial cord or lower trunk;
iii) radiculopathy involving C7 and, C8 or T1.

The next reasoning step evaluates each hypothesis by considering the refined causal processes for the local neuropathy where the lesion severity and the dispersion functions are explicitly represented. For each lesion severity the structural state of every observed nervous segment is determined (see Table IV).

Once obtained the structural state of the observed structures, the system evaluates, for each observation, the explanation quality of each hypothesis, based on conditional probability functions p(CV [N,D,DB,Ax]) defined for the corresponding structural-functional abstractions (Table III).

Assuming the independence of the different observed functional attributes, the result of the multiplication of all these conditional probability values is the probability of the set of observations given the occurrence of the hypothesis.

$$p(\text{observations} \mid \text{hypothesis}) = \Pi_i\, p(CV_i \mid [N,D,DB,Ax]) \quad i \in \{A,B,C,D,E\}.$$

This value is used by the system as a plausibility value to rank the possible hypotheses, and eventually to guide the choice between alternatives (Table VI).

refined hypotheses		A Dec. bord	B Dec	C Normal	D Dec	E Normal	Π
median:	mild	0.41	0.49	0.82	0.49	0.82	6.62×10^{-2}
wrist	mod	0.26	0.71	0.82	0.71	0.82	8.81×10^{-2}
	sev	0.30	0.66	0.82	0.66	0.82	8.79×10^{-2}
median:	mild	0.09	0.00	0.82	0.49	0.82	-
elbow	mod	0.13	0.01	0.82	0.71	0.82	6.21×10^{-4}
	sev	0.28	0.03	0.82	0.66	0.82	3.73×10^{-3}
median:	mild	0.09	0.00	0.82	0.00	0.82	-
axilla or erbs	mod	0.13	0.01	0.82	0.01	0.82	8.74×10^{-6}
	sev	0.28	0.03	0.82	0.03	0.82	1.69×10^{-4}
lat. crd and	mild	0.09	0.00	0.82	0.00	0.82	-
(med. crd or	mod	0.13	0.01	0.80	0.01	0.80	8.32×10^{-6}
low. trk)	sev	0.28	0.03	0.67	0.03	0.67	1.13×10^{-4}
mid. trk and	mild	0.09	0.00	0.82	0.00	0.82	-
(med. crd or	mod	0.11	0.01	0.80	0.01	0.80	7.04×10^{-6}
low. trk)	sev	0.17	0.03	0.67	0.03	0.67	6.87×10^{-5}
C7 and	mild	0.09	0.00	0.82	0.00	0.82	-
(C8 or T1)	mod	0.11	0.01	0.81	0.01	0.81	7.22×10^{-6}
	sev	0.17	0.03	0.71	0.01	0.71	2.57×10^{-5}

Table VI - Conditional probability of functional values given hypothesis

Some of the alternatives are immediately excluded because their plausibility is null. For instance, although a local neuropathy in a median nerve point proximal w.r.t. the wrist (e.g. at the elbow) is possible and is thus present as a working hypotheses, its refinement into a mild severity is excluded. The reason is that the system assumes that a mild lesion causes only 2% of axonal damage (see Table IV) and all distal segments of the median nerve should be almost normal being impossible to justify the decreased conduction velocities (cf. figure 1).

From the remaining hypotheses, the system must decide which should be presented as potential diagnoses. The diagnoses are a set of alternatives, sorted by the belief of each hypothesis qualified symbolically as conclusive, probable or possible. The decision process thus involves the elimination of some of the alternatives based on their plausibility values.

A diagnosis may arguably be excluded in the presence of an alternative and comparable diagnosis with better plausibility. The criteria assumes the adoption of some thresholds to guide this elimination: if the ratio between the plausibility of two diagnoses exceeds these thresholds, the least plausible diagnosis is eliminated. The threshold defined for two alternatives belonging to the same etiologic group is smaller (i.e. it favours allowing more exclusions), than that for two alternatives from different etiologic groups. This difference is justified on the grounds that in general, the relative evaluation of the two hypotheses belonging to different etiologic groups is subject to more uncertainty and hence the system is more cautious in eliminating alternatives. By using thresholds 100 (for the same etiology) and 1000 (otherwise), the system produced in this example the following diagnosis:

- Probable local neuropathy of median nerve at wrist (moderate, severe or mild);
- Possible severe local neuropathy of median nerve at elbow;
- Possible severe local neuropathy of lateral cord and medial cord or lower trunk;

5. Preliminary Evaluation

In order to make a preliminary evaluation of the system's performance, 60 clinical cases were collected from the ESTEEM database of real cases and input to the system. Each of them had been previously analysed by a group of medical experts that reached consensus diagnoses. Consensus diagnoses thus provided the reference with which the system diagnoses were compared to.

This comparison is not trivial because diagnoses can disagree in several aspects making it difficult to quantify the quality of diagnoses. A diagnosis is a set of possible hypotheses with an associated belief value. Two different diagnoses can disagree in the set of suggested hypotheses, in the belief of each hypothesis, or in the hypotheses parameters. Hence, we adopted comparison criteria that classifies the similarity between two diagnoses in the following similarity levels:

3. The best hypotheses of both diagnoses strongly match. A strong match means a total identity or some small difference in qualifiers (e.g. mild severity and moderate severity).

3'. The best hypotheses of both diagnoses match weakly. A weak match means an identity of the hypotheses type with some more significant difference in the qualifiers (e.g. mild severity and severe severity).

2. The best hypothesis of one of the two diagnoses match with a secondary hypothesis of the other.

1. The best hypotheses of both diagnoses do not match with any alternative but some secondary hypotheses match with each other. In this group were included

cases where the system could not find any electrophysiological problem whilst the consensus diagnosis suggests a mild anatomical lesion.

0. Complete discrepancy between both diagnoses.

Table VII shows the results obtained by applying this methodology to the 60 collected cases.

Similarity Level	3	3⁻	2	1	0
Number of Cases	33	12	6	4	5

Table VII - Results for 60 collected cases.

Observing each individual case it is possible to conclude that most of the diagnostic discrepancies are the result, on the one hand, of the need to restrict the context of the hypotheses search, and on the other hand, of the system ignorance about the real clinical context in which the examination were performed.

The strategy adopted to reduce the huge number of initial hypotheses relies on several assumptions and criteria that are adequate in the majority of cases but not quite so in others. For instance, the assumption than only anatomical structures that are certainly lesioned require an explanation explains why, in such cases, the system did not produce any hypothesis whilst the consensus diagnosis was some mild disorder. Another example is the application of a minimal etiology criteria, where hypotheses with less associated etiologies are preferred to hypotheses with a higher number of etiologies. In some cases, the consensus diagnoses were produced in the context of a previously known disease and the results involved multiple etiologies that were ignored by the system.

6. Conclusion

This paper presented an instantiation of the causal-functional (meta-)model to the neurophysiology domain, and in particular to EMG diagnosis. As such it briefly described ways in which this instantiation handled the abductive and deductive phases of the reasoning, taking into account the complexity and uncertainty underlying the various abstraction levels at which medical knowledge is considered.

Some of the steps in this instantiation might be further improved in the future, namely the abstraction/refinement between qualitative and quantitative representations, as well as the uncertainty involved in the model relationships. At present, the uncertainty in the relationship between two abstracted representations is obtained by aggregation of the corresponding refined representations, but the underlying mathematical models have weak justification. In the future, we intend to develop such relationships based on constraints on both qualitative and quantitative data, and to evaluate the likelihood of potential hypothesis by some measurement on the constraints of the model that ought to be defeated (as outlined in [13] for the finite and discrete data sets).

Nevertheless, the results obtained so far are quite encouraging with respect to their accuracy. Moreover, a prototype of our diagnostic system is being installed, together with a modification of an EMG machine, in the University Hospital of Lille, as part of project ISAR[14]. Results from this instalation, together with further evaluation from the clinical group of ESTEEM (whose work has extended beyond the end of this project), will provide us with valuable information to improve the system.

References

[1] P. Barahona et al, *Knowledge Processing for Decision Support in the Health Sector - A Perspective for the Next Decade*, in Knowledge and Decisions in Health Telematics, P. Barahona and J.P.Christensen (Eds.), IOS Press, pp. 3-58, 1994.

[2] J. Wyatt, *Promoting Routine Use of Medical Knowledge Systems: the Lessons from Computerised ECG Interpreters*, in Knowledge and Decisions in Health Telematics, P. Barahona and J.P.Christensen (Eds.), IOS Press, pp. 73-80, 1994.

[3] I.D. Adams et al, *Computer Aided Diagnosis of Acute Abdominal Pain: a Multicentre Study*, British Medical Journal, no. 293 , pp.800--804, 1986.

[4] J.L Willems et al, *The Diagnostic Performance of Computer Programs for the Interpretation of Electrocardiograms*, New England Journal of Medicine, no. 325, pp. 1767-1773, 1991.

[5] A. Fuglsang-Frederiksen, J. Rønagar and S. Vingtoft, *PC-KANDID: An expert system for electromyography*, Artificial Intelligence in Medicine, pp. 117-124, 1989.

[6] A. Vila, D. Ziebelin and F. Reymond, *Experimental EMG expert system as an aid in diagnosis*, Electroenceph. Clin. Neurophysiol., no. 61, 1985.

[7] S. Andreassen, B. Falck and K.G. Olesen, *Diagnostic Function of the Microhuman Prototype of the Expert System MUNIN*, Electroencephalography in Clinical Neurology, 1992.

[8] M. Veloso et al, *ESTEEM: European Standardised Telematics Tool to Evaluate EMG Knowledge Based Systems and Methods*, in Health in the New Communication Age, M.F. Laires, M.J. Ladeira and J.P.Christensen (Eds.), IOS Press, pp. 348-356, 1995.

[9] M. O'Neil, A. Glowinski and J. Fox, *A Symbolic Theory of Decision Making Applied to Several Medical Tasks*, in Lecture Notes in Medical Informatics, Springer-Verlag, no. 38, pp.62-71, 1989.

[10] G. Lanzola and M. Stefanelli, *A Specialized Framework for Medical Diagnostic Knowledge Based Systems*, Computers and Biomedical Research, no. 25, pp. 351-365, 1992.

[11] P. Barahona, *A Causal - Functional Model for Medical Knowledge Representation*, in Deep Models for Medical Knowledge Engineering, E. Keravnou (Ed.), Elsevier, pp. 101-127, 1992.

[12] J. Cruz, *A Causal-Functional Model for the Diagnosis of Neuromuscular Disorders* (in Portuguese), M.Sc Thesis, Dep. of Computer Science, New University of Lisbon, 1995.

[13] F. Menezes and P. Barahona, *Defeasible Constraint Solving*, Lecture Notes in Computer Science, Springer-Verlag, no. 1106, pp.151-170, 1996.

[14] R. Beuscart, B. Modjeddi and M. DeMeester, *ISAR: Integration System Architecture*, in Health in the New Communication Age, M.F. Laires, M.J. Ladeira and J.P.Christensen (Eds.), IOS Press, pp. 392-403, 1995.

Learning Bayesian Networks by Genetic Algorithms: A Case Study in the Prediction of Survival in Malignant Skin Melanoma

Pedro Larrañaga[1], Basilio Sierra[1], Miren J. Gallego[1], Maria J. Michelena[2], and Juan M. Picaza[3]

[1] Department of Computer Science and Artificial Intelligence, University of the Basque Country, Spain.
[2] Oncological Institute of Gipuzkoa, Spain.
[3] Department of Computer Languages and Systems, University of the Basque Country, Spain.

Abstract. In this work we introduce a methodology based on Genetic Algorithms for the automatic induction of Bayesian Networks from a file containing cases and variables related to the problem. The methodology is applied to the problem of predicting survival of people after one, three and five years of being diagnosed as having malignant skin melanoma. The accuracy of the obtained model, measured in terms of the percentage of well-classified subjects, is compared to that obtained by the so-called Naive-Bayes. In both cases, the estimation of the model accuracy is obtained from the 10-fold cross-validation method.

1 Introduction

Expert systems, one of the most developed areas in the field of Artificial Intelligence, are computer programs designed to help or replace humans beings in tasks in which the human experience and human knowledge are scarce and unreliable. Although, there are domains in which the tasks can be specifed by logic rules, other domains are characterized by an uncertainty inherent in them. Probability was not taken into account, for some time, as a reasoning method for expert systems trying to model uncertain domains, because the specifications and computer cost it requires are too expensive. At the end of the 80s, Lauritzen and Spiegelhalter [14] showed that these difficulties can be overcome by exploiting the modular character of the graphical models associated with the so-called probabilistic expert systems, that we in this work call Bayesian Networks.

Bayesian Networks (BNs) [9], [13], [15] constitute a probabilistic framework for

* We thank Gregory F. Cooper for providing his simulation of the ALARM Network. We also thank the referees for their work and comments. This work was supported by the Diputación Foral de Gipuzkoa, under grant OF 92/1996, by the grant UPV 140.226-EA186/96 from the University of the Basque Country, and by the grant PI 95/52 from the Gobierno Vasco - Departamento de Educación, Universidades e Investigación.

reasoning under uncertainty. From an informal perspective, BNs are directed acyclic graphs (DAGs), where the nodes are random variables and the arcs specify the independence assumptions that must be held between the random variables. BNs are based upon the concept of conditional independence among variables. This concept makes possible a factorization of the probability distribution of the n-dimensional random variable $(X_1, ..., X_n)$ in the following way:

$$P(x_1, ..., x_n) = \prod_{i=1}^{n} P(x_i | pa(x_i))$$

where x_i represents the value of the random variable X_i, and $pa(x_i)$ represents the value of the random variables parents of X_i.

Thus, in order to specify the probability distribution of a BN, one must give prior probabilities for all root nodes (nodes with no predecessors) and conditional probabilities for all other nodes, given all possible combinations of their direct predecessors. These numbers in conjunction with the DAG, specify the BN completely. Once the network is constructed it constitutes an efficient device to perform probabilistic inference. This probabilistic reasoning inside the net can be carried out by exact methods, as well as by approximated methods. Nevertheless, the problem of building such a network remains. The structure and conditional probabilities necessary for characterising the network can be either provided externally by experts or obtained from an algorithm which automatically induces them.

In this paper, a methodology for inducing automatically Bayesian Networks is introduced. This methodology is based on Genetic Algorithms and tries to obtain from the file of cases the most probable structure of the Bayesian Network. The work is organized as follows, in Sect. 2 some structure learning methods are reviewed, taking an special interest in the method proposed by Cooper and Herskovits [5]. Section 3 introduces Genetic Algorithms, while Sect. 4 presents the structure learning methodology integrating both, the metric proposed by Cooper and Herskovits and the adaptative searching process characteristic of the Genetic Algorithms. In Sect. 5 we present the results obtained from applying the previous methodology to a file of cases, which contains information about 311 patients diagnosed as having malignant skin melanoma. The induced Bayesian network is used for classifying patients according to their prognosis of survival after one, three and five years of being diagnosed. These results are compared to those obtained by the called Naive-Bayes paradigm. Section 6 gathers the conclusions.

2 Structure Learning in Bayesian Networks

2.1 Introduction

During the last five years a good number of algorithms whose aim is to induce the structure of the Bayesian Network that better represents the conditional independence relationships underlying in the file of cases have been developed. In our opinion, the main reason for continuing the research in the structure learning problem is that modeling the expert knowledge has become an expensive, unreliable and time-consuming job.

The different approaches to the structure learning mentioned here are related with multiple connected networks, and have been grouped according to the necessity or not of imposing order on the variables. See Heckerman et al. [7] for a good review.

Assuming order among variables means that a variable X_i can have the variable X_j as parent only if, in the established order among the variables, X_j precedes X_i. With this restriction, the cardinality of the space that contains all the structures is given by $2^{\binom{n}{2}}$, where n is the number of variables in the system. Some methods under this restriction are those developed by Cooper and Herskovits [5], and Bouckaert [4].

If we do not assume ordering between the nodes the cardinality of the search space is bigger, and it is given by the Robinson's formula [17]:

$$f(n) = \sum_{i=1}^{n} (-1)^{i+1} \binom{n}{i} 2^{i(n-i)} f(n-i); f(0) = 1; f(1) = 1.$$

Several authors have been working under these general assumptions. Among them, Bouckaert [3], and Provan and Singh [16].

2.2 The K2 Algorithm

As it will be seen in Sect. 4, the proposed approach - based on Genetic Algorithms - use the CH metric proposed by Cooper and Herskovits [5] for evaluating the goodnes of a Bayesian Network structure, as well as the K2 algorithm developed by the previously mentioned authors. K2 is an algorithm that creates and evaluates a BN from a database of cases once an ordering between the system variables is given. The CH metric is used for the evaluation of the network that it constructs. K2 searches, given a database D for the BN structure B_{S^*} with maximal $P(B_S, D)$, where $P(B_S, D)$ is as described in the following theorem proved in [5].

Theorem Let Z be a set of n discrete variables, where a variable x_i in Z has r_i possible value assignments: $(v_{i1}, \ldots, v_{ir_i})$. Let D be a database of cases of m cases, where each case contains a value assignment for each variable in Z. Let B_S denote a BN structure containing just the variables in Z. Each variable x_i in B_S has a set of parents, which are represented with a list of variables π_i. Let w_{ij} denote the jth unique instantiation of π_i relative to D. Suppose there are q_i such unique instantiations of π_i. Define N_{ijk} to be the number of cases in D in which variable x_i has the value v_{ik} and π_i is instantiated as w_{ij}. Let $N_{ij} = \sum_{k=1}^{r_i} N_{ijk}$. If given a BN model, the cases occur independently, there are not cases that have variables with missing values and the density function $f(B_P|B_S)$ is uniform, then it follows that

$P(B_S|D) = P(B_S) \prod_{i=1}^{n} g(i, \pi_i)$, where $g(i, \pi_i) = \prod_{j=1}^{q_i} \frac{(r_i-1)!}{(N_{ij}+r_i-1)!} \prod_{k=1}^{r_i} N_{ijk}!$

The K2 algorithm assumes that an ordering on the variables is available and that, a priori, all structures are equally likely. It searches, for every node, the set of parent nodes that maximizes $g(i, \pi_i)$ - CH metric-. K2 is a *greedy* heuristic. It starts by assuming that a node does not have parents, after which in every step it adds incrementally that parent whose addition most increases the probability of the resulting structure. K2 stops adding parents to the nodes when the addition of a single parent cannot increase the probability. Obviously, this approach does not guarantee the selection of a structure with the highest probability.

3   Genetic Algorithms

The computing complexity inherent in a great number of real problems of combinatorial optimization has carried, as a consequence, the development of heuristic methods that try to tackle these problems successfully. An heuristic is a procedure which will give a good solution - not necessarily the optimal - to problems which can be catalogued as difficult, if you try to solve them obtaining the exact solution. Although there are heuristics developed for specific problems, in the past years there have been an explosion in the applications of what we could call metaheuristics, because its formulation is independent of the problem to solve. Among the most studied metaheuristics we quote Simulated Annealing, Tabu Search and Genetic Algorithms.

Genetic Algorithms [6] are adaptive methods that can be used for solving problems of search and optimization. They are based on the genetic process of living organisms. Through generations the populations evolve in nature according to the principles of natural selection and survival of the fittest postulated by Darwin. Imitating this process, the Genetic Algorithms are capable of creating solutions for real world problems.

Genetic Algorithms use a direct analogy with the natural behaviour. They work with a population of individuals, each individual representing a feasible solution to a given problem. To each individual we assign a value or score according to the goodness of that solution. The better the adaptation of the individual to the problem, the more probable is that the individual will be selected for reproduction, crossing its genetic material with another individual selected in the same way. This cross will produce new individual - offspring of the previous - which share some of the features of their parents. In this way a new population of feasible solutions is produced, replacing the previous one and verifing the interesting property of having greater proportion of good features than the previous population. Thus, through generations good features are propagated through the population. Favouring the cross of the fittest individuals, the most promising areas of the search space are being explored. If the Genetic Algorithms have been well designed, the population will converge to an optimal solution of the problem.

Figure 1 summarizes the pseudocode for the so-called Abstract Genetic Algorithm. In it the parent selection doesn't need to be made by asigning to each individual a value proportional to its objetive function, as is usual in the so-called Simple Genetic Algorithm. This selection can be carried out by any function that selects parents in a natural way. It is worth notice that descendants are not necessarily the next generation of individuals, but that this generation is made by the union of parents and descendents. That is why we need the operations of extension and reduction in the cycle.

```
begin AGA
      Make initial population at random
      WHILE NOT stop DO
        BEGIN
        Select parents from the population.
        Produce children from the selected parents.
        Mutate the individuals.
        Extend the population by adding the children to it.
        Reduce the extended population.
        END
      Output the best individual found.
end AGA
```

Fig. 1. The pseudo-code of the Abstract Genetic Algorithm.

4   Genetic Algorithms in the Induction of Bayesian Networks

In this approach, each individual in the Genetic Algorithm will be a Bayesian Network structure.

4.1   Notation and Representation

Denoting with D the set of BN structures for a fixed domain with n variables, and the alphabet S being $\{0,1\}$, a Bayesian Network structure can be represented by an $n \times n$ connectivity matrix C, where its elements, c_{ij}, verify:

$$c_{ij} = \begin{cases} 1 \text{ if } j \text{ is a parent of } i, \\ 0 \text{ otherwise.} \end{cases}$$

4.2   Assuming an ordering between the nodes

In this case, the connectivity matrices of the network structures are triangulated and therefore the genetic operators are closed operators with respect to the DAG conditions. We represent an individual of the population by the string:

$$c_{21}c_{31}c_{41}\ldots c_{n1},\ldots c_{32}c_{42}\ldots c_{n2},\ldots c_{n-2n-1}, c_{n-2n}, c_{n-1n}.$$

With this representation in mind, we show how the crossover and mutation operators work by using simple examples.

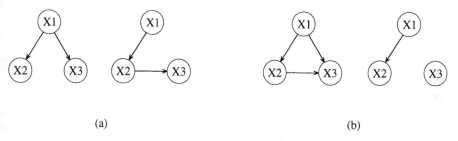

(a)   (b)

Fig. 2. With order assumption: Crossing over two BN structures.

Example 1. Consider a domain of 3 variables on which the two BN structures of Fig. 2(a) are defined. Using the above described representation, the networks are represented by the strings : 110 and 101. Suppose now that the two network structures are crossed over and that the crossover point is chosen between the second and the third bit. This gives the offspring strings 111 and 100. Hence, the created offspring structures are the ones presented in Fig. 2(b).

Example 2. Consider the DAG of Fig. 3(a). It is represented by the string 100.

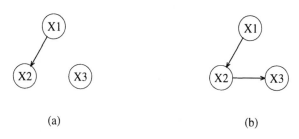

(a)   (b)

Fig. 3. With order assumption: Mutating a BN structure.

Suppose that the third bit is altered by mutation. This gives the string 101, which corresponds with the graph of Fig. 3(b).

4.3 Without assuming an ordering between the nodes

If no ordering assumption on the variables is made, we represent an individual of the population by the string:

$$c_{11}c_{21}\ldots c_{n1}c_{12}c_{22}\ldots c_{n2}\ldots c_{1n}c_{2n}\ldots c_{nn}.$$

As can be seen in the following examples, the genetic operators are not closed operators with respect to the DAG conditions.

Example 3. Consider a domain of 3 variables on which the two BN structures of Fig. 4(a) are defined. Using the above described representation, the networks are represented by the strings : 001001000 and 000000110. Suppose now that the two network structures are crossed over and that the crossover point is chosen between the sixth and the seventh bit. This gives the offspring strings 001001110 and 000000000. Hence, the created offspring structures are the ones presented in Fig. 4(b). We see that the first offspring structure is not a DAG.

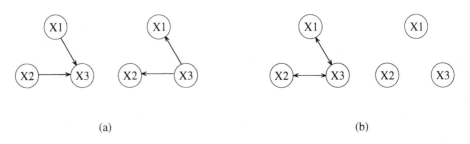

(a)   (b)

Fig. 4. Without order assumption: The crossover operator is not a closed operator.

Example 4. Consider the DAG of Fig. 5(a). It is represented by the string 010001000. Suppose that the seventh bit is altered by mutation. This gives the string 010001100, which corresponds with the cyclic graph of Fig. 5(b).

To assure the closeness of the genetic operators we introduce a *repair operator*, which transforms the child structures that do not verify the DAG conditions into DAGs, by randomly eliminating the edges that invalidate the DAG conditions.

This approach has been evaluated empirically with a simulation of the ALARM network [2]. For details see Larrañaga et al. [10], [11].

Another different approach, in which the individuals of the population are orderings, has been proposed by Larrañaga et al. [12].

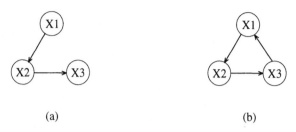

(a)   (b)

Fig. 5. Without order assumption: The mutation operator is not a closed operator.

5   Predicting Survival in Malignant Skin Melanoma

5.1   The malignant skin melanoma

In spite of the advances achieved in last years in the treatment of cancer, the prognosis of patients having developed skin melanoma has changed very little. The incidence of the disease has grown without stopping in the last decade. Annual incidence has increased and the progressive reduction of the ozone layer, if not stopped, will expand it even more.

Experimental data and the results of epidemiological studies suggest two main risk factors: sun exposure along with phenotype characteristics of the individual. Thus, for example, the continuous sun exposure represents an odds ratio of 9, while the acute intermitent exposition has got associated an odds ratio of 5.7.

Malignant skin melanoma is a rather uncommon tumour in our country. It entails between the 8% and the 10% of the total malignant tumours that affect the skin. According to the Cancer Register of the Basque Country [8], in 1990 the rate of incidence was 2.2 for every 100,000 people for males and 3 for every 100,000 for females.

The database contains 311 cases - diagnosed at the Oncological Institute of Gipuzkoa in the period between the first of January, 1988, and the 31 of December, 1995 - and for each case we have information about eight variables. The five predictor variables are: sex (2 categories), age (5 categories), stage (4 categories), thickness (4 categories) and number of positive nodes (2 categories). The variable to predict has two categories taking into account if the person survives or not one, three or five years after being diagnosed as malignant skin melanoma.

5.2   The Models

Two models have been taken into account. First, we have induced a BN structure using GAs, as explained in Sect. 4. In order to get it, we have searched in the space of all structures without imposing any order restriction among the variables. Therefore we have tried to find, given a file with cases, the a posteriori most probable structure. The second model used is the so-called Naive-Bayes.

This model assumes independence among predictor variables. In both models the estimations of the rate of well-classified individuals have been obtained using 10-fold cross-validation[18]. The propagation of the evidence has been done using the software HUGIN [1].

Model I. The a posteriori most probable structure. CH-GA. Figures 6, 7 and 8

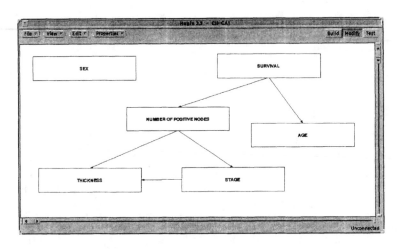

Fig. 6. The a posteriori most probably structure for the one year case.

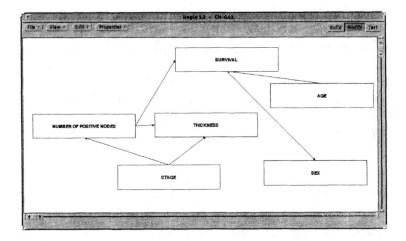

Fig. 7. The a posteriori most probably structure for the thee year case.

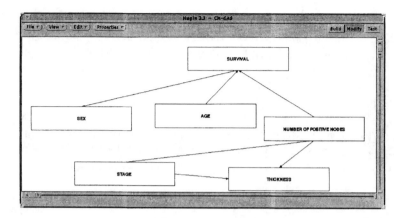

Fig. 8. The a posteriori most probably structure for the five year case.

show the structures of the Bayesian Networks induced by the Genetic Algorithm. They correspond to the predictions of survival after one, three and five years of being diagnosed. In Table 1, estimations of the probability of succes in classification obtained by each of the previous models can be seen.

Model II. Naive - Bayes classifier. N-B. In spite of the strong assumptions of inde-

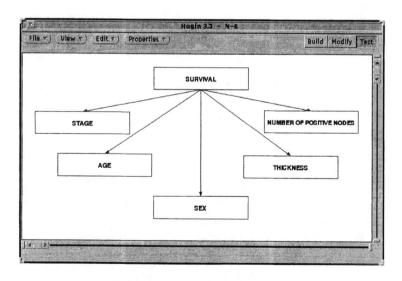

Fig. 9. The Naive-Bayes classifier.

pendence upon which the model is built, Naive - Bayes classifier has proved itself competitive against other more refined classifiers. It is assumed that all variables are conditionally independent given the value of the variable to predict. Therefore, the model ignores the correlations among variables which can prejudice its predictive capacity. In Fig. 9 it can be seen the structure of the Bayesian Network corresponding to the Naive-Bayes. This structure is common to the three classification problems. Table 1 shows that the estimations obtained by two of the Naive-Bayes models are inferior to those obtained by the previous approach. The bad result obtained by the CH-GA approach for the 5 years problem can be explained by the scarce number of cases - 161 of the 311 - diagnosted five or more years before 31 of December of 1995, that has been used to induce the structure.

Table 1. Accuracy of the different approaches for the prediction of survival one-year, thee-years and five-years after be diagnosed

Survival of Malignant Skin Melanoma		
1 year 3 years	5 years
CH-GA 93.06% 81.95%	69.57%
N-B 91.43% 79.02%	71.43%

6   Conclusions and Futher Research

A method of induction of Bayesian Networks has been introduced. This method is based on intelligent search made by Genetic Algortihms. The method uses the CH metric and tries to find the a posteriori most probable Bayesian Network structure given the file of cases.

The Bayesian Network structures induced by this method have been empirically compared to the Naive-Bayes structures in one classification problem consisting on the prediction of survival of individuals after one, three or five years of being diagnosed as having malignant skin melanoma. Although in the inductive method does not exist an especial treatment for the variable to classify, the estimations of the 10-fold croos-validation for the probability of survival are better in two of the three examples than those obtained by the Naive-Bayes paradigm.

In the future, we plan to combine the previous two techniques for finding the a posteriori most probable structure that contains, at least, the Naive-Bayes. Besides, it would be interesting to develop a method of intelligent search based on Genetic Algorithms, Simulated Annealing or Tabu Search that take into account the purpose the induced Bayesian Network will be use for - in our case supervised classification -.

References

1. Andersen, S.K., Olesen, K.G., Jensen, F.V. and Jensen, F.: "HUGIN - a shell for building Bayesian belief universes for expert systems". In *Eleventh International Joint Conference on Artificial Intelligence* (1989) 1128-1133
2. Beinlinch, I.A., Suermondt, H.J., R.M. Chavez R. M. and Cooper G.F.: "The ALARM monitoring system: A case study with two probabilistic inference techniques for belief networks". In *Proceedings of the Second European Conference on Artificial Intelligence in Medicine* (1989) 247-256
3. Bouckaert, R.R.: "Optimizing causal orderings for generating DAGs from data". In *Uncertainty in Artificial Intelligence. Proceedings of the Eighth Conference* (1992) 9-16
4. Bouckaert, R.R.: "Properties of Bayesian belief networks learning algorithms". In *Uncertainty in Artificial Intelligence. Tenth Annual Conference*, (1994) 102-109
5. Cooper, G.F., and Herskovits, E.A.: "A Bayesian method for the induction of probabilistic networks from data". *Machine Learning* 9 (1992) 309-347
6. Goldberg, D.E.: *"Genetic Algorithms in Search, Optimization and Machine Learning"*. Addison-Wesley, Reading, MA (1989)
7. Heckerman, D., Geiger, D. and Chickering, D.M.: "Learning Bayesian networks: The combination of knowledge and statistical data". *Technical Report MSR-TR-94-09*, Microsoft (1994)
8. Izarzugaza, M.I.: "Informe del registro de Cáncer de Euskadi 1990". *Osasunkaria* (1994) 8-11
9. Jensen, F. V.: *"Introduction to Bayesian networks"*. University College of London (1996)
10. Larrañaga, P., Poza, M., Yurramendi, Y., Murga, R., and Kuijpers, C.: "Structure Learning of Bayesian Networks by Genetic Algorithms: A Performance Analysis of Control Parameters". *IEEE Transactions on Pattern Analysis and Machine Intelligence.* 18 (1996) 912-926
11. Larrañaga, P., Murga, R., Poza, M., and Kuijpers, C.: "Structure Learning of Bayesian Networks by Hybrid Genetic Algorithms". In *Learning from Data: AI and Statistics V, Lecture Notes in Statistics 112*. D. Fisher, H.-J. Lenz (eds.), New York, NY: Spriger-Verlag, (1996) 165-174.
12. Larrañaga, P., Kuijpers, C., Murga, R., and Yurramendi, Y.: "Learning Bayesian Network Structures by searching for the best ordering with genetic algorithms". *IEEE Transactions on System, Man and Cybernetics* 26 (1996) 487-493
13. Lauritzen, S.L.: *"Graphical Models"*. Oxford University Press (1996)
14. Lauritzen, S.L., and Spiegelhalter, D.J.: "Local computations with probabilities on graphical structures and their application on expert systems". *Journal Royal of Statistical Society B* 50 (1988) 157-224
15. Pearl, J.: *"Probabilistic Reasoning in Intelligent Systems: Networks of Plausible Inference"*. Morgan Kaufmann, San Mateo (1988)
16. Provan, G.M., and Singh, M.: "Learning Bayesian Networks Using Feature Selection". In *Learning from Data: AI and Statistics V, Lecture Notes in Statistics 112*. D. Fisher, H.-J. Lenz (eds.), New York, NY: Spriger-Verlag (1996) 291-300
17. Robinson, R. W.: "Counting unlabeled acyclic digraphs". In C. H. C. Little (ed.) *Lectures Notes in Mathematics 622: Combinatorial Mathematics V*, Springer-Verlag, New York, (1977) 28-43.
18. Stone, M.: "Cross-validation choice and assessment of statistical procedures". *Journal Royal of Statistical Society* 36 (1974) 111-147

A Neuro-Fuzzy-Classifier for a Knowledge-Based Glaucoma Monitor

Gudrun Zahlmann[1]), Matthias Scherf[1]), Aharon Wegner[2])

[1])GSF, National Research Center for Environment and Health, Institute of Medical Informatics
and Health Services Research, Ingolstädter Landstr. 1, 85764 Neuherberg,
[2])Department of Ophthalmology, Clinic rechts der Isar, Technical University of Munich,
Ismaninger Str. 22, 81675 Munich

Abstract: A knowledge-based glaucoma monitor is developed to detect
critical or suspicious situations in patient's ophthalmic data sets. The decision, which
type of situation occurs is made by a neuro-fuzzy classifier. The neural net part is
based on a special developed feature selection algorithm and a RBF network. Fuzzy
classification is realised by a fuzzy rule set combining all patient data with the
classification results of the neural net classifier to the final decision.

1 Introduction

Glaucoma is one of the most severe eye diseases according to the number of
blindness cases in the western industrial countries [1]. Besides new developments in
clinical research environments [2], investigating new and more sensitive methods for
an early glaucoma detection the main focus should be given to the primary care
facilities and their available information and data (intraocular pressure, perimetry,
description of the papilla).
Therefore this knowledge-based glaucoma monitor is designed to detect early
changes in a patient's data set in a primary care environment, which can be related to
known glaucomatous changes [3].
The structure overview is shown in Figure 1.

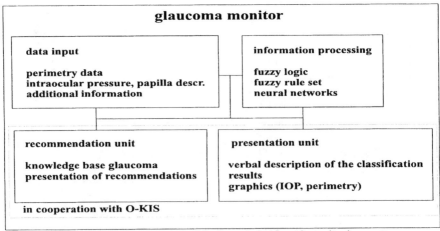

Figure 1:   Structure of the knowledge-based monitoring system

The main function of this system is to react as a 'watch dog', 'barking' if critical or suspicious situations are detected, otherwise to rely in a 'sleeping' condition. Both cases require the assessment and classification of new data sets. This classification into 'situation classes' has to be done in two different ways, as a differential diagnosis decision and an evaluation of time-dependent changes. The reaction of the monitoring system is to generate messages about the found situation and give the possibility to get more information using a special query technique in co-operation with the ophthalmic knowledge-based information system (O-KIS).

This paper describes the classification methods leading to a differential diagnosis decision.

2 Input data

The decision of medical experts about glaucomatous changes of a patient's eye rely on the following data sets:

- direct measurable data
- parameter estimations
- more or less unstructured verbal descriptions

To the *direct measurable data* belong the intraocular pressure (IOP) given as a real number in a pressure unit (or as data set of several IOP values as a diurnal profile) and perimetry data sets.

The latter data describe the status of the visual field of the patient measured by special devices (perimeters), which detect the loss in light sensitivity at different stimulus points of the retina (number and locations depend on the applied perimeter type and measuring regimen). These locations are stimulated by flash light of different intensities at different locations within a hemisphere with a background illumination while the patient is fixating to the center. The 'answer' whether or not a stimulus could be seen is given pressing a response button by the patient. Therefore, perimetry is a subjective measuring method in general. Additionally the perimetry method has different measuring regimes (static, dynamic) and different error handling procedures implemented by the perimeter companies like stimulating the same point different times within a measuring procedure to detect changes over time and verify previous findings [4-6]. An example of the output of an OCTOPUS perimeter (static perimetry) processed by Peridata software package [7] is shown in Figure 2.

At the lower right side the age-corrected sensitivity loss values are plotted. The upper left side shows a grey-scale 'image' based on these values. Upper right is shown the Bebie-curve [8] which shows the cumulative defect values. All other parameters are calculated from the sensitivity loss values under special consideration of the measurement regimen.

Perimetry is therefore a time consuming method. Considering that the patients normally suffering from glaucoma are of higher ages, it is understandable, that the results are not only subjective but also insecure. Nevertheless it is the best available method today.

Another problem related to the perimetry data is, that there exists no gold standard, meaning that the data can not be verified by an objective reference method. Therefore we asked four medical experts (1 clinician, 3 private ophthalmologists) to classify the same data set of 244 perimetries independently. The variability of the classification decision is used as a measure of uncertainty of the neural net decision. This work is in progress and will be published later on. For the purpose of this paper we will compare

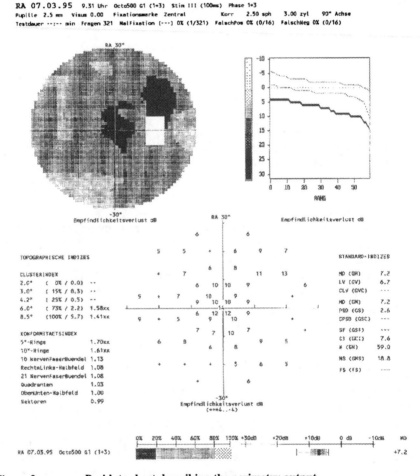

Figure 2:   **Peridata sheet describing the perimetry output**

the classification results of two medical experts to illustrate the problems inherent of the perimetry classification and give a motivation for our neural net investigations. The decision was given at different hierarchy levels (for details see chapter about neural net).

Perimetry data, as used for our investigations, is described through a 59-dimensional vector of real values. To determine the relation between the distribution of the perimetry data in the feature space and the classification agreements/disagreements of the experts we visualised the perimetry-samples by the non-linear projection technique introduced by Sammon [9]. Sammon's mapping directly tries to approximate local geometric relations of samples in a two dimensional graphic plot: Given a set of samples in a high dimensional feature space, Sammon's mapping

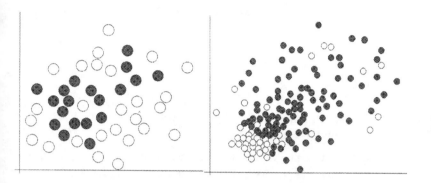

Figure 3:   **Sammon's mapping of perimetries, which are classified as normal (left) / pathologic(right) by at least one expert[1].**

places every sample on a two dimensional plane, such that the Euclidean distances between them are as closely as possible to their Euclidean distances in the high dimensional feature space.

The results are shown in Figure 3 and 4. The grey circles represent perimetries where the experts agreed in their diagnosis, the white circles represent those where the experts gave a different diagnosis.

The results comparing the 'normal' and 'pathological' decision tasks are shown in Figure 3. In this case the measurement space seems to be separable in two clustered regions containing the 'normal' and 'pathological' perimetries which were classified in agreement. The perimetries where the experts disagreed in their diagnoses build a broad boundary, surrounding the regions of agreement. This result implies, that the perimetries, classified in agreement and disagreement are similar according to their Euclidean distances.

Figure 4 shows Sammon's mapping for all perimetry samples, which were classified as glaucomatous by at least one expert. Here the white circles represent the perimetry-samples which were classified both 'glaucomatous' as well as 'pathological but not glaucomatous'. In contrast to Figure 3 the cases of disagreement are uniformly distributed and no boundary is detectable. Even if we take into account, that Sammon's mapping does not guarantee the correct geometric relations of the samples

---

[1] Grey points: agreement in diagnosis, white points: disagreement.

it seems, that the similarity between glaucomatous perimetries which were classified in agreement is very weak according to their Euclidean distances.

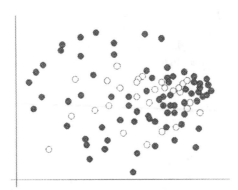

Figure 4:   **Sammon's mapping of perimetries, which are classified as glaucomatous by at least one expert[2]**

The results make clear, that the diagnosis of perimetry data is a very difficult task with a great degree of uncertainty. As a consequence the results of a neural network classifier which is based on the decision-behaviour of one expert should be seen in this context when using the results as input values to fuzzy-rules.

Another input to the decision process are papilla descriptions. These are mainly made by watching the papilla on-line during the eye examination and *estimating several parameters* like the cup-disc-ratio (CDR), the location of the excavation or a comparison of the CDR's of the right and left eyes. The CDR and the right-left-difference are given as real numbers (estimated), the location is given in linguistic terms like 'central, inferior, superior'. The CDRs and the differences are transformed by the medical experts into a meta level of classification, evaluating them as 'normal, increased' etc.

The third information source are the patient's own reports which are mainly given *verbally* and *unstructured* but contain valuable information about the status at the time point of visiting the ophthalmologist and about changes in this status.

Based on these data the ophthalmologist has to decide, whether or not these data and the related findings (transformation to the decision level - situation description at the knowledge level [14]) belong to glaucomatous findings or not and additionally what type of reaction is required. Reactions here can be the decision about a shorter or longer interval to the next examination, a medication or a decision about a type of eye surgery (depending on the glaucoma type, like open angle glaucoma etc.).

Our goal is to model this decision process giving finally a decision support to the ophthalmologist. The final decision maker remains the physician.

Several approaches have been tested in the past trying to realize this decision support functionality. One approach is to use a rule-based diagnostic system like CASENET [10] or in an advanced approach [11]. This expert system approach is not suitable for

---

[2] Grey points: agreement in diagnosis, white points: disagreement.

the working regimen at a physician's working place in a primary care setting with its examination interval per patient of about 3 minutes.

Several working groups use neural net approaches to classify perimetry data (for a detailed literature overview see [3]). Others [12] try to classify perimetric data with statistical approaches like cluster analysis.

The last two approaches give only support in the classification of perimetry data , which are only one parameter of the required triple data set IOP, papilla findings and perimetry data to detect early changes in the human eye related to glaucoma.

A fuzzy set approach is described [13] with the main focus of testing defuzzification methods based on ERG-data, which are not available in primary care settings.

These experiences, the available data sources and types of our application area - primary care settings (private ophthalmologists, optometrist, small eye hospitals) have led us to a combination of fuzzy rules and neural networks as classification methods.

3 Neural Networks

Due to the fact that it is very difficult to give a formal description about how to classify perimetry data we use artificial neural networks (ANN) to learn the classification task on the basis of pre-classified perimetry data samples.

One general problem in designing ANNs with valid generalisation properties is the curse of dimensionality, which means, that the number of examples needed for training increases exponentially with the input dimension [15]. To weaken the curse of dimensionality we developed a method for feature selection which was applied as a pre-processing step to the perimetry data.

In the following we describe our approach for the ANN classifier design and introduce briefly our method for feature selection.

3.1 Classification hierarchy

The design of the ANN classifier is based on the classification tree which is shown in Figure 5 (left side). The motivation in modelling the classification tree is to introduce several decision stages, ranging from rather crude decisions like the 'normal'/'pathological' classification up to refined decisions, like the 'questionable'/'probably' glaucomatous classification. Our approach in modelling the ANN-perimetry-classifier is to design an ANN for every decision level from the root to the leaves of the classification tree respectively (see Figure 5 right).

The development of each ANN is consequently based on different data sets. As an example, the training, test and evaluation sets of the ANN1 contain all available perimetry data, whereas the training, test and evaluation sets of the ANN6 only contain perimetry data, pre-classified as probably glaucomatous or questionable glaucomatous.

In the application a perimetry data sample is classified by ANN1 through ANN6 respectively. Their output values are interpreted top down according to the classification hierarchy. If for example the ANN 2 classifier gives the result that the perimetry data is more 'normal' than 'pathological', we will give more attention to the results of the ANN 3 classifier than to the results of the ANN 4, ANN 5 and ANN 6 classifiers. This kind of interpretation is taken into consideration when using the ANN outputs as inputs to the fuzzy system and is possible due to the fact that we use RBF networks [16], which do an interpolation between samples of a certain feature space region.

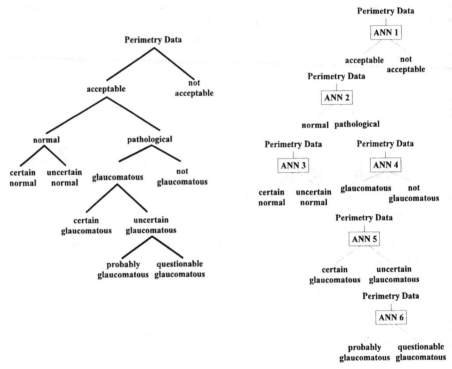

Figure 5: Classification tree, introducing several decision stages (left) and the ANN classifier approach (right), where an ANN is introduced for every decision stage.

3.2 Data pre-processing

Our goal in data pre-processing is to reduce the dimension of the perimetry data while improving the classification results of the applied ANNs. To receive interpretable results we developed a feature selection technique. The goal of feature selection techniques is the determination of a combination of d features which optimise an arbitrary criterion function. We apply the data pre-processing step on the training-database of the six ANNs respectively to get an idea which features of the perimetry data have good discrimination properties according to the special classification task.

In a classification task, feature vectors which belong to the same class should be as similar as possible in contrast to feature vectors, which belong to different classes. The similarity of two feature-vectors is generally determined by their distance in measurement space, which can be calculated by different metrics. To select a feature subset, which gives the best results according to the similarities/dissimilarities of the resulting feature vectors we developed a criterion function which has its global optimum when the distances between feature vectors of the same class (intra-class distances) are zero and the distances of feature vectors, belonging to different classes (inter-class distances) are maximal according to the bounds of the underlying measurement space:

Let $D^a = \{d_1^a, d_2^a, ..., d_{N_a}^a\}$ be the set of the N_a intra-class distances and $D^e = \{d_1^e, d_2^e, ..., d_{N_e}^e\}$ the set of the N_e inter-class distances. We define the criteria-function by:

$$J = \frac{1}{N_a}\sum_{i=1}^{N_a} d_i^a - \frac{1}{N_e}\sum_{i=1}^{N_e} d_i^e \tag{1}$$

Let Q be the dimensionality of the feature vectors and p_q^i the q'th feature of the i'th feature vector. We calculate the inter- and intra-class distances by the Euclidean metric, modified by the introduction of real valued weights w_q, $q = 1,2,...,Q$.

$$d_{ij} = \sqrt{\sum_{q=1}^{Q} w_q \left(p_q^i - p_q^j\right)^2} \tag{2}$$

and determine the minimum of (1) by iteratively modifying the weights via gradient descent: $w_q(t+1) = w_q(t) - \lambda \frac{\partial J}{\partial w_q}$, (3)

where λ is an arbitrary chosen learning constant and $w_q(t+1)$ is the q'th weight at the modification step t+1. The gradient is calculated by:

$$\frac{\partial J}{\partial w_q} = \frac{1}{N_a}\sum_{i=1}^{N_a} \frac{\left(p_q^{g_1^a(i)} - p_q^{g_2^a(i)}\right)^2}{2\sqrt{\sum_{t=1}^{Q} w_t \left(p_t^{g_1^a(i)} - p_t^{g_2^a(i)}\right)^2}} - \frac{1}{N_e}\sum_{i=1}^{N_e} \frac{\left(p_q^{g_1^e(i)} - p_q^{g_2^e(i)}\right)^2}{2\sqrt{\sum_{t=1}^{Q} w_t \left(p_t^{g_1^e(i)} - p_t^{g_2^e(i)}\right)^2}} \tag{4}$$

$g_1^a(i), g_2^a(i), g_1^e(i), g_2^e(i)$ are functions which give the indices of the two feature vectors, from which the i'th inter/intra-class distances are calculated.

The search space for the weights w_q is restricted to [0,1] respectively. Even there is no guarantee, that every weight will be clearly set to zero or one after the optimisation process terminates by reaching a local minimum, it could be shown experimentally, that there are only a few special cases with no clear decisions.

3.3 Results

ANN1 through ANN6 were trained by 2/3 and tested/evaluated by 1/3 of their perimetry- sample sets. The feature selection method which was applied respectively to the training set gave clear results in every case, that is the weights were unequally set to one or zero after the optimisation process terminated. Table 1 gives an overview of the sensitivity/specificity results of the ANN classifiers with and without data pre-processing.

Hierarchy	All Features Sens/Spec	Reduced Features Sens/Spec	Number of neglected Features
ANN 1	85 % / 76 %	83 % / 81 %	5
ANN 2	82 % / 93 %	85 % / 93 %	2
ANN 3	91 % / 91 %	91 % / 92 %	1
ANN 4	71 % / 51 %	72 % / 81 %	30
ANN 5	71 % / 52 %	79 % / 56 %	16
ANN 6	69 % / 61 %	62 % / 74 %	36

Table 1: Results of the specialised ANN, comparing the results of ANNs which were trained with all features and of a features subset, determined by the feature selection technique.

Applying the feature selection technique as an data pre-processing step we got the very promising result, that all ANNs gave equal or better results compared to the ANNs which were trained with all features. Consequently it seems, that there are some locations in the visual field which are most significant according to a special classification task.

4 Fuzzy rule sets

The overall decision about the differential diagnosis is given by a fuzzy rule set. The main structure is shown in Figure 6.

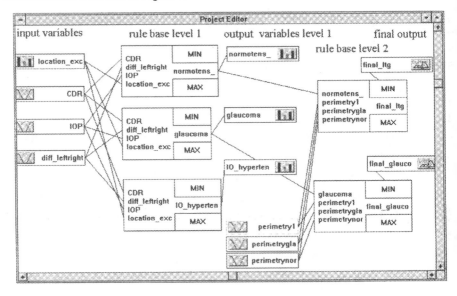

Figure 6:   **Main structure fuzzy rule set**

CDR (cup-disc-ratio of the disc), IOP and the left-right-difference values are input directly as real numbers which will be fuzzified by membership functions (MBF[3]) defined by the medical expert in co-operation with the knowledge engineer.

The first rule level combines these values using min-max decision rules to get output values of the first level : These are intraocular hypertension, normotensive glaucoma and all other glaucoma types (glaucoma).

The result is given as a membership value to the variable terms 'yes' and 'no'.

These provisional results are used as an output and input to the next rule level, respectively.

The second rule level gets additional input from the classification of perimetry data. As shown in Figure 6 this pre-classification step can be done by the medical expert or automatically by the neural network classifier.

The classification of the perimetry data is input at all three hierarchical levels. Starting with the highest one (normal-pathological-not acceptable) down to the deeper classification of normal and pathological/glaucomatous classes.

Input fuzzification can take place at different levels. As illustrated above we use fuzzy input data for each class using 'yes' and 'no' decision for each class.

The decision given for test purposes by the medical expert then were always deterministic: This perimetry data set belongs to classes 'pathological' , 'questionable_glaucomatous'. This can be modelled using the neural network classifiers with dual output values. The 'fuzzy' decision level is then only implemented in the definition of classes. Neural networking implies the advantage to make the classification output 'fuzzy' using real numbers as direct input either to a fuzzy class or as direct input to a membership function fuzzifying the input additionally.

The final decision will be made in the second rule set with the output 'final_low_tension_glaucoma' and 'final_glaucoma'. We use these fuzzy outputs without defuzzification to produce messages based on a situation classification (comparable to perimetry classes, but based on the overall decision of the neuro-fuzzy-classifier) of the monitoring system, because the information contents dealing with suspicious situations is higher then that using a defuzzification algorithm and getting a winner class.

These ideas are realised using the software package fuzzyTech (inform GmbH).

The interesting point is now to investigate the influence of the input from perimetry data classification on the final output decision depending on the different input types. Table 2 shows a comparison of the 'preclassification' of perimetry data given by the physician or implementing the ANN hierarchy, interpreting the real output values of each ANN as a fuzzy membership function value input to second level fuzzy rules.

---

[3] The graphical representation of these two different input fuzzification levels are colored columns (location of the excavation) or functional graphs (IOP).

283

Class	physician		neural nets	
	A	**B**	**A**	**B**
perimetry_normal	0	0	0	.1
_pathological	1	1	1	.97
_glaucomatous	1	0	.7	.45
_probably_glauc.	0	0	.1	.51
_question._glauc.	0	1	.35	.5

Table 2: Perimetry-classification by a physician or using the ANN's

A and B respectively illustrate two different cases describing the situation classes A - 'glaucomatous' and B - 'questionable glaucomatous'. Whereas the 'glaucomatous' class is equivalently classified by both decision ways, the ANN classifiers give a different answer to the 'questionable-glaucomatous' situation class. The insecurity, vagueness or fuzziness in the decision is shown in a 'may-be' decision given by output values around .5. To detect the appropriate final decision outcome an additional fuzzy rule level (level 2) is necessary.

5 First results and discussion

The final classification method is a combination of automatic classification by hierarchical ordered neural nets and fuzzy rule sets at different levels.

'situation class'	physician		neural nets	
	final_glaucoma		**final_glaucoma**	
	no	**yes**	**no**	**yes**
'pathoplogical'	0	.25	.09	.4
'glaucomatous'	0	1	0	.7
'questionable_glau comatous'	0	.35	.1	.4

Table 3: Final decision output of the neuro-fuzzy-classifier for different situation classes

Testing the complex classifier with first patient data sets for different situation classes and using the classification of perimetry data given by the physician and the ANN's (Table 3) it seems to give acceptable results to the medical user because of the fuzzy strategy and a trend to 'summarise' even small membership values for each single perimetry class in connection with the degree of support of the rules. It is very difficult to separate pathological (not glaucomatous) from early glaucomatous (questionable_glaucomatous) changes within the visual field, when all other input parameter (papilla. IOP) give no additional information. Testing with additional patient data sets from an eye clinic and 6 private ophthalmologists is in progress.
The interpretation of the final decision outcome in form of messages to the user is under development. In parallel the time dependencies are investigated.

284

Acknowledgements
This work is part of the OPHTEL project funded by the European Commission within the
'Telematics Application Programme'.

Literature

[1]   S.E. Spenceley, D.B. Henson, D.R. Bull, Visual field analysis using artificial
        neural networks, *Ophthal. Physiol. Opt.* **14** (1994) 239-248
[2]   R.A. Hitchings,Perimetry-back to the future, *British J. of Ohthalmol.* **78**
        (1994), 805-806.
[3]   G. Zahlmann, M. Obermaier, C. Ritzke, M. Scherf, Knowledge-Based
        Monitoring of Glaucoma Patients - a Connectionist's Approach, in
        *J. Brender, J.P. Christensen, J.R. Scherrer, P. McNair (Eds.) Medical
        Informatics '96, Technology and Informatics 34 IOS-Press, 1996, S.555-559*
[4]   H. Bebie, Computer-assisted evaluation of visual fields, *Graefe's Arch Clin
        Exp Ophthalmol (1990) 228, 242-245*
[5]   B. Lachenmayr, O.-E. Lund; 15 Jahre automatisierte Perimetrie - Wohin
        führt der Weg?, *Klin Monatsbl Augenheilkd (1994) 205, 325-328*
[6]   J. Flammer, The concept of visual Field indices, , *Graefe's Arch Clin Exp
        Ophthalmol (1986) 224, 389-392*
[7]   H. Bebie, J. Flammer, Th. Bebie, The cumulative defect curve: separation of
        local and diffuse components of visual field damage, *Graefe's Arch Clin Exp
        Ophthalmol (1989)227, 9-12*
[8]   J. Weber, Perimetrische Äquivalente der Glaukomprogression,
        Ophthalmologe (1992) 89, 175-189
[9]   J.W. Sammon Jr., A nonlinear mapping for data structure analysis, *IEEE
        Trans. Comp. C- 18, (1969), 401*
[10]   S.M. Weiss,C.A. Kulikowski,A.S. Safir, A model-based method for
        computer-aided medical decision-making, *Artificial Intelligence II,* North-
        Holland publ. Co 1978
[11]   C.E.T. Krakau, Artificial Intelligence in computerized perimetry, *Doc.
        Ophthalmol. / Proc. of the Int. Visual Field Symp.,* 1986 Amsterdam
        49(1987), 169-174
[12]   B.C. Chauhan et all., Cluster analysis in visual field quantification, *Doc.
        Ophthalmol.* **69** (1988), 25-39
[13]   B. Losch, Application of fuzzy sets to the diagnosis of glaucoma, *Proc.
        IEEE-EMBS* 1996
[14]   A. Newell, The Knowledge level, *Artificial Intelligence* **18**(1982), 87-127
[15]   E.B. Baum, D. Haussler: What size net gives valid generalisation ?, *Neural
        Computation 1(1989), 151-160*
[16]   J. Moody and C. Darken, Learning with localized receptive fields, *in
        Proceedings of the 1988 Connectionist Models Summer School, G. Hinton,
        T.Sejnowski, and D. Touretzsky, eds, 133-134*

A Method for Diagnosing in Large Medical Expert Systems Based on Causal Probabilistic Networks

Marko Suojanen, Kristian G. Olesen and Steen Andreassen
Department of Medical Informatics and Image Analysis,
Institute of Electronic Systems, Aalborg University,
Fredrik Bajersvej 7 D, DK-9220 Aalborg, Denmark
Phone   +45 9815 8522, Fax: +45 9815 4008,
Email: ms@miba.auc.dk, kgo@miba.auc.dk and sa@miba.auc.dk

Abstract: Diagnosis of multiple diseases in large medical expert systems based on causal probabilistic networks may require resources that are not available on common computers. We propose a method that is able to diagnose multiple diseases by systematic investigation of subsets of diseases. The method is illustrated in the MUNIN expert system for diagnosis of muscle and nerve diseases. In MUNIN the requirements for memory space and calculation time were reduced by about 5 orders of magnitude, which is sufficient to make the method practical. We conclude that the method is viable under reasonable assumptions.

1 Introduction

MUNIN is a decision support system designed to assist in the diagnosis of muscle and nerve diseases in the peripheral nervous system (Andreassen et al. 1989; 1992; 1996; Olesen et al. 1989). The current prototype of the system covers most common general muscle and nerve disorders, that is, disorders that affect multiple muscles and/or nerves, and a range of local nerve lesions that affect only single nerves. The anatomy of the prototype covers a sensory nerve, a motor nerve and two mixed nerves on each side of the body. This anatomy is adequate to describe all principal features of the diagnostic process, but is, of course, too limited for practical purposes. This is why we call it the microhuman prototype. MUNIN is modelled as a Causal

Probabilistic Network (CPN), also known as a Bayesian Network (Pearl 1988; Andreassen et al. 1991; Jensen 1996), and consists of about 1100 discrete random variables linked together in a graphical structure that describes dependencies among the variables. One of the virtues of CPNs is that they offer a complete coherent updating of all variables based on probability theory. In order to obtain this, a representation of the joint probability table of all variables has to be maintained. The size of such a table grows exponentially with the number of variables, which means it is impossible to construct and store even moderate-sized CPNs. Fortunately methods have been developed to factorise the state space into a number of smaller tables (Lauritzen and Spiegelhalter 1988, Jensen et al. 1990a; 1990b). This is done by grouping the variables in cliques, that is, (small) sets of variables. Each clique has an attached table that holds the joint probability distribution for the nodes in the clique. The cliques are organised in a tree structure, a junction tree. All computations are performed in the junction tree by *propagation* and the correct marginal belief in all variables can be calculated, conditioned on available evidence. The construction of the junction tree is known as a *compilation* of the original CPN specification and the size of the junction tree also determines the calculation time, since this is roughly proportional to the sum of the sizes of all clique tables. The compilation includes a *triangulation* of the CPN, that is a manipulation of the graph in order to identify the cliques. The problem of finding the best triangulation is NP-hard, and although several heuristics for this procedure exist, the resulting junction tree most often includes large cliques. It turns out that large clique tables are usually quite sparse and we are able to reduce the space requirements by techniques for representation of sparse matrices. We call this transformation of representation *compression*. The table sizes can be further reduced by *approximation* (Jensen and Andersen 1990), simply by eliminating rare states. Empirical studies have shown that elimination of configurations with a probability less than 0.0001 yields acceptable results. For such states we simply set the probability to zero and thus the tables can be compressed further.

Although we have exploited these and other tricks in MUNIN the size of the resulting junction tree is still measured in terabytes. This means that other methods, such as conditioning (Pearl 1986), have to be considered. Conditioning eliminates a set of nodes from the CPN, resulting in a reduced space demand for the junction tree. The cost is an increase in computation time, because a propagation has to be done for each possible combination of the states of the eliminated nodes. If the size of MUNIN is reduced to a manageable size by conditioning, we get a resulting computation time that is measured in the order of years. The problem is that we consider all possible diseases simultaneously because we wish to be able to diagnose multiple diseases. Multiple diseases are not a problem if the diseases do not have overlapping findings, but this is not the case in general. In practise, patients with two diseases with overlapping findings are seen occationally, whereas patients with three diseases with overlapping findings are extremely rare. We are therefore faced with the practical problem of developing a method for diagnosis under the assumption that at most two diseases with common findings are present.

2 Method

The method we propose systematically considers subsets of the diseases (Olesen and Andreassen 1996). Conceptually we first consider single diseases, then pairs of diseases, triplets of diseases, etc.

1) We generate all single disease nets from the original CPN with all diseases represented. A single disease net is a CPN consisting of a single disease and all variables affected by that disease. Findings are inserted and propagated in those nets, and that leaves us with a list of diseases, where the a posteriori probability of the disease is larger than the a priori probability. We assume that the list contains the patient's actual diseases, along with a number of false positive diseases, essentially the diseases that share findings with the actual diseases.

2) Next, we generate all double disease nets. A double disease net is a CPN consisting of two diseases and the union of all variables affected by those diseases. We insert and propagate findings in all double disease nets, provided the diseases belong to the list of diseases generated by propagation in the single disease nets. If the patient only has a single disease, then we assume that propagation in the double disease nets eliminates all false positive diseases. In that case the diagnostic procedure can be terminated. If the patient has more than one disease, the list of diseases with a posteriori probabilities larger than their a priori probability may still contain false positive diseases.

3) In that case all triple disease nets must be generated. A triple disease net is a CPN consisting of three diseases and the union of all variables affected by those diseases. We insert and propagate findings in all triple disease nets, provided the diseases belong to the list of diseases generated by propagation in the double disease nets. If the patient only has two diseases, then the assumption is that this will eliminate all false positive diseases. If the patient has more than two diseases, the list of diseases with a posteriori probabilities larger than their a priori probabilities may still contain false positive diseases. If desired this can be dealt with by considering quadruple disease nets, etc.

Before demonstrating this procedure on MUNIN the concept of anatomical units will be introduced. A set of variables in the original CPN that is d-separated (Jensen 1996) from the rest of the CPN by the disease nodes is called an anatomical unit. In MUNIN the variables in an anatomical unit all relate to a given anatomical structure, hence the name anatomical unit. Without going into the detailed arguments, we will postulate that two things can be gained by introducing the concept of anatomical units. The first advantage is that we can modularise the nets. We let a single disease net consist of only the disease and one anatomical unit, and the double and triple disease nets contain only the diseases and the intersection of the affected nodes, instead of the union of the affected nodes. Then, for example, in the double disease nets, the influence of the variables in the union, but not in the intersection, can be taken into account by using appropriate results, available from the propagations in the single disease nets.

The second advantage that we postulate is that an n-tuple disease net can be used to diagnose patients with more than n diseases, provided that the patient only has n-1 diseases affecting the same anatomical unit.

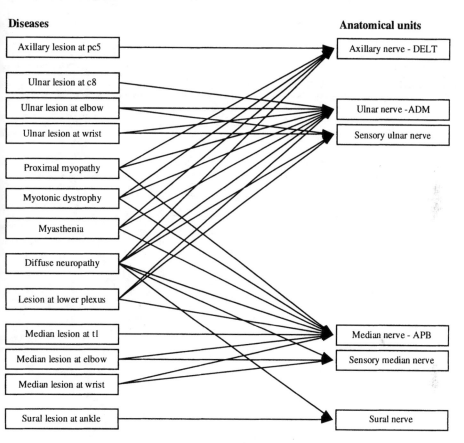

Figure 1. The structure of the MUNIN microhuman network for one side of the body. The left column lists the 13 included diseases that each is described by 1-5 variables and the right column shows the 6 included anatomical units, consisting of between 20 and 150 variables. The arrows show that between 2 and 8 diseases affect each anatomical unit.

To illustrate the method Figure 1 shows the principal structure of the MUNIN microhuman network for one side of the body. In the left column all diseases affecting one side of the body are shown, and the right column displays the anatomical units. Each entity consists of several variables. Diseases are described by between one and five variables of which one specifies the severity of the disease. This variable determines whether the disease should be considered relevant and if this is the case, a further description of the nature of the disease is detailed by other variables that comprise e.g. pathology or time course. The anatomical units describe either a sensory nerve or a motor nerve together with a muscle it innervates and consist of between 20 and 150 variables. These variables describe how the diseases affect the anatomical units through expected pathophysiological effects and findings. The links in the figure show the anatomical units that are affected by a given disease.

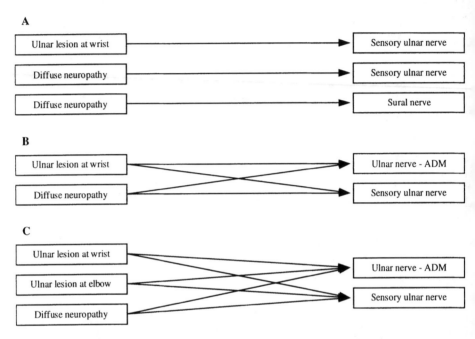

Figure 2. A: Three single disease nets, where an ulnar lesion at wrist affects the sensory ulnar nerve, diffuse neuropathy affects the sensory ulnar nerve and diffuse neuropathy affects the sural nerve. **B:** A double disease net, where an ulnar lesion at wrist and diffuse neuropathy both affect the sensory ulnar nerve and the ulnar motor nerve together with the ADM muscle. **C:** A triple disease net, where ulnar lesion at elbow is present together with the two diseases in part B.

Figure 2A shows examples of single disease nets for an ulnar lesion at wrist affecting the sensory ulnar nerve, and for diffuse neuropathy affecting respectively the sensory ulnar nerve and the sural nerve. Similar nets exist for the other anatomical units affected by the diseases including e.g. the ulnar motor nerve together with the abductor digiti minimi muscle (ADM). In figure 2B the double disease net describing both an ulnar lesion at wrist and diffuse neuropathy is shown. This net only includes common anatomical units, in this case the sensory ulnar nerve and the ulnar motor nerve together with ADM. As stated above partial results on for example the influence of the sural nerve on diffuse neuropathy can be transferred from the corresponding single disease net. In figure 2C an example of a triple disease net is shown. In this net an ulnar lesion at elbow has been added. This disease affects the same anatomical units as the ulnar lesion at wrist and diffuse neuropathy. Altogether the method results in 60 single disease nets, 96 double disease nets and 212 triple disease nets (left and right side). With these 368 nets we are able to diagnose patients with at most two diseases affecting the same anatomical unit. The question is whether we are able to provide the computational resources required to handle this collection of nets. To investigate this we have compiled the nets using the HUGIN system (Andersen et al. 1989).

3 Results

3.1 Single Disease Nets

We compiled all the single disease nets using the default triangulation heuristic (fill-in weight) provided by HUGIN. After this we compressed the single disease nets. We also approximated the single disease nets and subsequently compressed them again. The results of these operations are presented in Table 1. To make the specification of the required memory independent of the actual computer's representation of numbers, all sizes are given as the number of elements in the clique tables. For example, in our computer one number corresponds to four bytes. The percentages in parentheses give the size relative to the initial size.

Single disease net	Size [kilonumbers]	Compressed size [kilonumbers]	Size after approx. [kilonumbers]
Smallest	1.7	0.4 (22%)	0.3 (16%)
Largest	76.6	8.5 (11%)	4.9 (6%)
Average	26.4	8.0 (30%)	4.5 (17%)
Total	1581.4	477.4 (30%)	269.4 (17%)

Table 1. Sizes of the 60 single disease nets after compilation, compression and approximation.

The total memory requirement of the single disease nets after compilation is about 1.6 Meganumbers, which is readily available on our computer. We can further reduce the memory requirement by compressing and approximating the single disease nets. We achieve a factor 3.3 saving in memory requirement after compression and a factor 5.9 saving after approximation and a following compression. The conclusion is that our computer can handle the single disease nets without problems.

3.2 Double Disease Nets

MUNIN has altogether 96 double disease nets. We compiled all these double disease nets using again the fill-in weight triangulation heuristic. Since the total size of the compiled double disease nets was almost 110 Meganumbers (Table 3), we wanted to investigate, whether other triangulation heuristics would give better results. To do this, we selected the 40 largest double disease nets, since their total size was almost 95 % of the total size of the 96 double disease nets. These 40 double disease nets were then compiled using all the built-in triangulation heuristics provided by HUGIN. The results are presented in Table 2.

Triangulation heuristic	Total size [Meganumbers]	Total compressed size [Meganumbers]	Total size after approx. [Meganumbers]
fill-in weight	103	23 (23%)	6 (6%)
clique weight	97	34 (35%)	5 (5%)
fill-in size	184	n.a.	7 (4%)
clique size	151	n.a.	6 (4%)

Table 2. Total sizes of the 40 largest double disease nets after compilation, compression and approximation using different triangulation heuristics.

The total sizes of the 40 largest double disease nets after compilation with fill-in weight and clique weight heuristics were somewhat smaller than after fill-in size and clique size heuristics. We went on to investigate, whether this would also hold after compression and approximation. With the current version of HUGIN we were not able to compress all the double disease nets after compilation with fill-in size and clique size heuristics. We were however able to compress all the double disease nets after approximation. After approximation and a subsequent compression all the built-in triangulation heuristics gave very similar results. We conclude that other triangulation heuristics do not give essentially better results than the fill-in weight heuristic. We went on to investigate the 96 double disease nets further. The results are shown in Table 3.

Double disease net	Size [kilonumbers]	Compressed size [kilonumbers]	Size after approx. [kilonumbers]
Smallest	8	7 (85%)	4 (48%)
Largest	5152	831 (16%)	143 (3%)
Average	1141	272 (24%)	71 (6%)
Total	109548	26157 (24%)	6831 (6%)

Table 3. Sizes of the 96 double disease nets after compilation, compression and approximation.

The total memory requirement of the double disease nets was almost 110 Meganumbers. This is more than available on our computer. After compression the total size of the double disease nets was 26 Meganumbers, which is smaller than the original size by a factor of 4.2. Still, 26 Meganumbers is quite a large memory requirement. After approximation and a following compression we achieved a factor 16 reduction in size, and the memory requirement was under 7 Meganumbers. This can be handled conveniently. Our conclusion is that we should always approximate and subsequently compress the double disease nets. Otherwise we have too large memory requirements. Note that we gain more with compression and approximation in the double disease nets than in the single disease nets. The reason for this is that the double disease nets have larger clique tables than the single disease nets, and large clique tables are usually quite sparse.

3.3 Triple Disease Nets

MUNIN contains 212 triple disease nets. Most of these nets have very large memory requirements after compilation. We consider as an example the net with two local nerve lesions, an ulnar lesion at elbow and an ulnar lesion at wrist and diffuse neuropathy. An attempt to compile this triple disease net provides the information that the size of the compiled net would be 160 Meganumbers. This is more than is available on our computer and the compilation therefore failed. A possible solution is to reduce the size of the net by conditioning. A straight forward choice is to use the variables representing the diseases for the conditioning. In that case we can produce a triple disease net by taking any of the double disease nets with two of the diseases and adding the third disease as conditioned. The size of this net is only marginally larger than the size of the original double disease net. The three possible choices of conditioned disease are considered in Table 4. From the column giving the size of the compiled nets it can be seen that the conditioned nets are much smaller than the unconditioned triple disease net by a factor of 20 to 40. However, in the conditioned nets, several propagations have to be carried out. Therefore we multiply the size of the conditioned net by the necessary number of propagations, which is equal to the size of the state space in the conditioned nodes. This measure is then used to compare calculation times. We give the calculation times in numbers rather than in seconds in order to make them independent of the actual computer. For example, in our computer we can process approximately one Meganumber per second. It can be seen that the calculation time in the conditioned nets is 2.6 to 4 times longer than in the net without conditioning. This increase in calculation time must be balanced against the large reduction in the size of the nets and thereby in the memory requirements.

Conditioned disease	Size [Meganumbers]	Calc. time [Meganumbers]	Calc. time after compr. [Meganumbers]	Calc. time after approx. [Meganumbers]
None	160 (100%)	160 (100%)	n.a.	n.a.
Ulnar lesion at elbow	4.1 (2.6%)	418 (261%)	193 (120%)	23 (14%)
Ulnar lesion at wrist	4.2 (2.6%)	419 (261%)	130 (81%)	21 (13%)
Diffuse neuropathy	7.9 (4.9%)	635 (396%)	208 (130%)	24 (15%)

Table 4. Sizes and calculation times of the triple disease net with the diseases "ulnar lesion at elbow", "ulnar lesion at wrist" and "diffuse neuropathy". Sizes and calculation times are shown following conditioning on each of the three diseases and after compression and approximation of the compiled nets.

The requirements for calculation time and memory can be reduced by compression and approximation. It is interesting to note that after approximation, the differences between the calculation times for the three conditioned nets are quite similar. This indicates that the choice of disease to be conditioned in the triple disease nets may not be important. However, even for the best of the three conditioned nets the propagation time is equivalent to propagation in a net with a size of 21.4 Meganumbers. This exceeds the sum of the propagation times for all double disease nets, which was equivalent to 6.8 Meganumbers (Table 3). Assuming that one Meganumber can be processed per second, propagation in this triple disease net can be done in 21 seconds. This is not in itself prohibitive, but enough to make it necessary to consider in how many of the triple disease nets it will be necessary to propagate.

The first observation to make is that it will only rarely be necessary to make any propagation in triple disease nets. The assumption is that propagation in the double disease nets eliminates all false positive diseases if the patient only has one disease. If this assumption holds true, then propagation in triple disease nets will only be necessary in patients that actually have two diseases, affecting the same anatomical unit. This implies that the most frequent example of patients with two nerve lesions, a median nerve lesion at the wrist (carpal tunnel syndrome) in both sides will not make it necessary to do propagations in triple nets, since the two lesions affect different anatomical units. A typical example of a patient with two lesions affecting the same anatomical unit may be a patient with a diffuse neuropathy and a local nerve lesion. Analysis of this situation shows that a typical number of triple nets in which propagation is necessary will be 4 - 6. The number does depend on the order in which the disease triplets are considered and an unfortunate choice of order may give a worst case number of 21 propagations in triple disease nets. This does not seem prohibitive either, but it does rest on the assumption that propagation in triple nets eliminates all false positive diseases, if the patient has only two diseases. Although this seems to agree with previous experience (Andreassen et al. 1996), an experimental verification of the assumption will be necessary.

4 Conclusion

A method has been proposed for diagnosing multiple diseases in large medical domains. The initial problem was that compilation of a CPN, containing all diseases yielded junction trees with large cliques, measured in teranumbers. In the proposed method, diagnosis was done by first considering single diseases and all findings affected by that disease. In the MUNIN CPN, the sum of the sizes of all the 60 single disease nets was quite modest, about 1.6 Meganumbers, which could be reduced to 269 kilonumbers by compression and approximation.

In the subsequent step of the proposed method, the double disease nets were considered. In MUNIN the sum of the sizes of all the 96 double disease nets was about 110 Meganumbers. With current computer technology this may be inconvenient, but compression and approximation reduced the size to 6.8 Meganumbers.

The final step was to consider the 212 triple disease nets. Compilation of one of these nets was attempted, but failed because the net had a size of 160 Meganumbers. As an alternative, conditioning on one of the three diseases was attempted. This reduced the size of the net to 4.1 Meganumbers, but increased the calculation time by a factor of 2.6. After compression and approximation the calculation time was about 21 sec., assuming that one Meganumber can be processed per second. Based on combinatorial considerations it was estimated that about 6 propagations in triple disease nets typically will be necessary. This is within acceptable limits, and we thus conclude that a practical method for diagnosing multiple diseases in large CPNs has been proposed. This conclusion rests on the assumptions that propagation in double disease nets eliminates all false positive diseases, provided that the patient only has one disease, and that propagation in triple disease nets eliminates all false positive diseases, provided that the patient only has two diseases. This assumption is supported by past experience (Andreassen et al. 1996), but must be verified experimentally on cases with multiple diseases.

References

Andersen, S.K., Olesen, K.G., Jensen, F.V. and Jensen, F. (1989). HUGIN - A shell for building Bayesian belief universes for expert systems. Proceedings of the 11th International Joint Conference on Artificial Intelligence, 1080-1085. Morgan Kaufman. Reprinted in: Shafer, G. and Pearl, J. (Eds.): Readings in Uncertain Reasoning, Morgan Kaufman, 1990.

Andreassen, S., Jensen, F.V., Andersen, S.K., Falck, B., Kjærulff, U., Woldbye, M., Sørensen, A.R., Rosenfalck, A. and Jensen, F. (1989). MUNIN - An expert EMG assistant. In: Desmedt, J.E. (Ed.): Computer-Aided Electromyography and Expert Systems. Elsevier.

Andreassen, S., Jensen, F.V. and Olesen, K.G. (1991). Medical expert systems based on causal probabilistic networks. *International Journal of Biomedical Computing* **28**, 1-30.

Andreassen, S., Falck, B. and Olesen, K.G. (1992). Diagnostic function of the Microhuman prototype of the expert system MUNIN. *Electroencephalography and Clinical Neurophysiology* **85**, 143-157.

Andreassen, S., Rosenfalck, A., Falck, B., Olesen, K.G. and Andersen, S.K. (1996). Evaluation of the diagnostic performance of the expert EMG assistant MUNIN. *Electroencephalography and Clinical Neurophysiology*, **101**, 129-144.

Jensen, F. and Andersen S.K. (1990). Approximations in Bayesian belief universes for knowledge-based systems. Proceedings of the sixth conference on uncertainty in artificial intelligence, Cambridge, Massachusetts, U.S.A., 162-169, 1990.

Jensen, F.V. (1996). An introduction to Bayesian networks. UCL Press.

Jensen, F.V., Lauritzen, S.L., and Olesen, K.G. (1990a). Bayesian updating in causal probabilistic networks by local computations. *Computational Statistics Quarterly* **4**, 269-282.

Jensen, F.V., Olesen, K.G., and Andersen, S.K. (1990b). An algebra of Bayesian belief universes for knowledge-based systems. *Networks* **20**, 637-659.

Lauritzen, S.L. and Spiegelhalter, D.J. (1988). Local computations with probabilities on graphical structures and their application to expert systems. *Journal of the Royal Statistical Society Series B* **50**, 157-224.

Olesen, K.G. and Andreassen, S. (1996). A heuristic method for diagnosing multiple diseases in complex medical domains modelled by causal probabilistic networks. In: Brender, J. et al. (Eds.). Medical Informatics Europe '96, IOS Press.

Olesen, K.G., Kjærulff, U., Jensen, F., Jensen, F.V., Falck, B., Andreassen, S. and Andersen, S.K. (1989). A MUNIN network for the median nerve - A case study on loops. *Applied Artificial Intelligence* **3**, 385-403.

Pearl, J. (1986). A constraint-propagation approach to probabilistic reasoning. In: Kanal, L.N. and Lemmer, J.F. (Eds.). Uncertainty in artificial intelligence, North-Holland.

Pearl, J. (1988). Probabilistic reasoning in intelligent systems. Morgan Kaufmann.

Dynamic Decision Making in Stochastic Partially Observable Medical Domains: Ischemic Heart Disease Example

Milos Hauskrecht

MIT Lab for Computer Science, NE43-421, 545 Technology Square, Cambridge, MA 02139

E-mail: *milos@medg.lcs.mit.edu*

Abstract

The focus of this paper is the framework of partially observable Markov decision processes (POMDPs) and its role in modeling and solving complex dynamic decision problems in stochastic and partially observable medical domains. The paper summarizes some of the basic features of the POMDP framework and explores its potential in solving the problem of the management of the patient with chronic ischemic heart disease.

Introduction

Dynamic decision problems in medicine usually deal with two sources of uncertainty. First is due to the action outcome uncertainty, the second is due to imperfect observability of the underlying process state. While most of the work on dynamic decision making addresses the issue of action outcome uncertainty, the feature of partial observability is often considered irrelevant or is abstracted out. Research work falling into this category includes the management of diabetes [5] or chronic heart disease [6]. The assumption of perfect observability may not work well for problems in which observations are imprecise indicators of the patient state and when investigative actions have significant cost (invasiveness, economic cost). In such cases careful evaluation of costs and benefits associated with both treatment and investigative actions with regard to the global objectives is necessary.

A framework that allows one to model both sources of uncertainty is the partially observable Markov decision process [1] [9] [7] [2] [3]. In the following I will summarize the POMDP framework and illustrate its potential on the problem of the management of patients with chronic ischemic heart disease.

Partially Observable Markov Decision Process

A *partially observable Markov decision process (POMDP)* describes the stochastic control process with partially observable states and formally corresponds to a 6-tuple (S, A, Θ, T, O, C) where S is a set of states, A is a set of actions, Θ is a set of observations, T is a set of transition probabilities between states that describe the dynamic behavior of the modeled environment under different actions, O stands for a set of observation probabilities that describe the relationship among observations, states and actions, and C denotes a cost model that assigns costs to state transitions and models payoffs associated with such transitions (alternative formulations can include rewards). Note that the basic model does not impose any restrictions on details of the actual representation and one can use a factored representation of states, observations and probabilistic relations with explicitly represented independencies.

The *decision (or planning) problem* in the context of POMDP requires one to find an action or a sequence of actions that minimizes the objective cost function. An *information state* represents all the information available to the agent at the decision time that is relevant to the selection of the optimal action. The information state consists of either a complete history of actions and observations or corresponding sufficient statistics ensuring the Markov property of the information process. An *objective function* represents (quantifies) control objectives by combining costs incurred over time using various kinds of models. Typically, the objective function is additive over time and based on expectations, e.g. the cost function often uses a finite horizon model $\min E(\sum_{t=0}^{n} c_t)$, that minimizes expected costs for the next n steps or an infinite discounted horizon $\min E(\sum_{t=0}^{\infty} \gamma^t c_t)$, with $0 \leq \gamma < 1$ being a discount factor. In the following we will focus on these two models.

Solving the POMDP Problem

For the n step-to-go problem the optimal value of the objective function, so called *value function*, and the optimal control can be computed using the Markov property of the information state process and Bellman's principle of optimality via standard recursive formulas [3]:

$$V_n^*(I_n) = \min_{a \in A} \rho(I_n, a) + \gamma \sum_{o \in \Theta_{next}} P(o|I_n, a) V_{n-1}^*(\tau(I_n, o, a))$$

$$\mu_n^*(I_n) = \mathrm{argmin}_{a \in A} \rho(I_n, a) + \gamma \sum_{o \in \Theta_{next}} P(o|I_n, a) V_{n-1}^*(\tau(I_n, o, a))$$

where $V^*(.)$ and $\mu^*(.)$ are optimal value and control functions, I_n denotes the current information state; $\rho(I_n, a)$ is the expected transition cost from state I_n under action a and can be computed as $\rho(I_n, a) = \sum_{s \in S} \sum_{s' \in S} P(s'|s, a) P(s|I_n) C(s, a, s')$; Θ_{next} is a set of observations that are available in the next step; τ is a transition function that maps the information state, new action and observation to the next step information state; and γ is the possible discount factor. Identical formulas (less the index denoting the number of steps to go) can be derived for the infinite discounted horizon problem.

The problem of finding optimal actions or policies can be computationally very expensive. It has been shown to be PSPACE-hard even for a single initial state and finite horizon cost function [8]. This is because the number of information states one potentially needs to visit grows exponentially with the number of steps to be explored. An even worse situation may emerge when one is required to find the solution for all initial information states — the so called policy problem. Although exact methods for solving both decision and policy problems are available for standard POMDP models [9] [2] [3], the computational complexity of such methods naturally leads to the exploration of various approximations that allow good solutions with less computation. Efficient approximation methods are mostly based on the idea of approximate dynamic programming (for the finite horizon case) and approximate value iteration (for the infinite discounted horizon). Methods can be based on sampling schemes combined with function approximation and fitting strategies, or based on reducing the complexity of the information vector space in various ways, e.g. through feature extraction mappings. Description of the exact and approximate solution methods is outside the scope of this paper (see [7] [2] [3]).

Management of Ischemic Heart Disease

The POMDP framework can be exploited in representing various complex problems of patient management, e.g. the management of chronic ischemic heart disease (IHD) [10] [6] [4]. The objective is to determine the optimal plan for managing the patient's chronic disease relative to cost criteria, including, e.g., invasiveness of the treatment, risk of death etc.

Basic components of the POMDP model include state, action and observation variables (see figure 1) describing the state of the patient, possible actions, and available observations.

State variables	Actions	Observation variables

status
    / \\
dead   alive
    coronary artery disease
    ischemia level
    history of MI
    history of PTCA
    history of CABG
	no action
	angiogram investigation
	stress test
	medication treatment
	angioplasty (PTCA)
	coronary artery bypass
	surgery (CABG)
		death
		angiogram result
		stress test result
		resting EKG
		chest pain
		acute MI symptoms

Fig. 1. Ischemic heart disease: basic model components

The dependencies between components of the model are captured in figure 2. The dynamics is represented by a controlled stochastic transition model with states and actions. States (circles) describe the underlying coronary artery disease (status of artery occlusion), severity of ischemia and other information influencing the transition, e.g. past MI or past angioplasty. Actions (rectangle) decribe possible decision choices, e.g. no action (wait), medication treatment, angiogram investigation, or coronary artery bypass surgery.

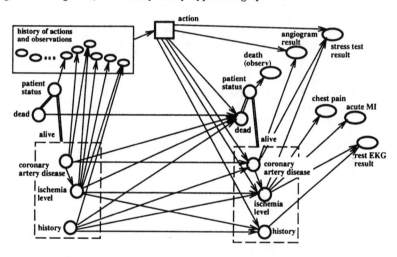

Fig. 2. Dynamic model of the ischemic heart disease

Observations (represented by ovals) are probabilistically dependend on the underlying patient state and can be conditioned on actions, e.g. angiogram result is conditioned on the choice of angiogram investigation. The conditioning is suitable when one wants to stress the presence of the test and its possible transition and cost effects. For example the angiogram investigation increases the incidence of MI or death and is also associated with higher invasiveness and economic cost. On the other hand many observations can be assumed "costless" and always available, e.g. EKG results.

The cost model describes payoffs associated with possible transitions, e.g. maximum cost is associated with the transition to the dead state, smaller but still substantial cost is associated with severe ischemia or occurrence of an MI. The decision criteria that try to reduce the expected cost then try to avoid these highly negative states.

Given the model, the objective of the problem solver is to find an action or a sequence of actions that minimizes the expected cost of management. Decision horizons applicable in the IHD case include both the finite horizon in which one optimizes the treatment for the next n time steps and infinite discounted horizon in which an infinite number of steps is considered, with more distant steps discounted.

Conclusion

Although the basic methodology for modeling dynamic decision processes via POMDPs has been available for some time, its potential has not been exploited in medical applications. In the paper I have described the basics of the POMDP framework and its solution methods. More detailed description of various exact and approximation methods can be found in [3]. The usefulness of the framework in medical settings is being examined with the example of the management of ischemic heart disease. Challenging problems in building and using the model include reliably estimating the many parameters and choosing appropriate approximation methods that yield timely and useful solutions.

This research was supported by the grant 1T15LM07092 from the National Library of Medicine. Peter Szolovits and William Long have provided valuable feedback on early versions of the paper and Hamish Fraser has helped with the ischemic heart disease example.

References

1. K.J. Astrom. Optimal control of Markov decision processes with incomplete state estimation. Journal of Mathematical Analysis and Applications, 10, pp. 174-205, 1965
2. A.R. Cassandra. Optimal policies for partially observable Markov decision processes. Brown University, Technical report CS-94-14, 1994.
3. M. Hauskrecht. Planning and control in stochastic domains with imperfect information. MIT EECS PhD thesis proposal, August 1996, 133 pages.
4. M. Hauskrecht. Dynamic decision making in stochastic partially observable medical domains. AAAI Spring symposium, pp. 69- 72, 1996.
5. R. Hovorka et.al. Causal probabilistic network modelling - An illustration of its role in the management of chronic diseases. IBM Systems Journal, 31:4, pp.635-648, 1992.
6. T.-Y. Leong. An integrated approach to dynamic decision making under uncertainty. MIT/LCS/TR-631, 1994.
7. W.S. Lovejoy. A survey of algorithmic methods for partially observed Markov decision processes. Annals of Operations Research, 28, pp. 47-66, 1991.
8. C.H. Papadimitriou, J.N. Tsitsiklis. The complexity of Markov decision processes. Mathematics of Operations Research, 12:3, pp. 441-450, 1987.
9. R.D. Smallwood, E.J. Sondik. The optimal control of partially observable processes over a finite horizon. Operations Research, 21, pp. 1071-1088.
10. J.B. Wong et.al. Myocardial revascularization for chronic stable angina. Annals of Internal Medicine, 113 (1), pp. 852-871, 1990.

Self-Learning Fuzzy Logic Control in Medicine

D.G. Mason*, D.A. Linkens*, N.D. Edwards[#]

Depts Automatic Control & Systems Engineering*,

Surgical & Anaesthetic Sciences, Northern General Hospital [#]

University of Sheffield, Sheffield, United Kingdom S1 3JD

(e-mail: D.Mason@Sheffield.ac.uk)

Abstract

Self-learning fuzzy logic control has the important property of accommodating uncertain, non-linear and time-varying process characteristics. This intelligent control scheme starts with no fuzzy control rules and learns how to control each process presented to it in real-time without the need for detailed process modelling. Medicine abounds with suitable applications for this technique. Following an outline of the methodology we demonstrate its clinical effectiveness for application in anaesthesia. We have investigated its application to atracurium-induced neuromuscular block during surgery and have observed improved control over complex numerical techniques. This self-learning fuzzy control technique shows much promise for other medical applications such as post-operative blood pressure management, intra-operative control of anaesthetic depth, and multivariable circulatory management of intensive care patients.

Keywords : Fuzzy logic, Intelligent control, Medicine, Anaesthesia

Introduction

It appears a common misconception that fuzzy logic endows a control system with 'intelligence'. Many fuzzy control systems operate with a fixed fuzzy rule base derived using heuristics and are not really 'intelligent'. The fuzzy logic merely provides a means of processing linguistic data. This does bring considerable benefits in the design of control systems for uncertain and complex systems [1]. It provides a simple way to construct a non-linear controller. It also enables a small collection of fuzzy control rules to be used rather than seeking a general control law expressed in complex mathematical terms. The derivation of these fuzzy control rules is a common problem in the development of fuzzy control systems. A simple way to overcome this problem is the on-line learning of fuzzy control rules. This gives the controller a form of 'intelligence' because it   then exhibits the ability to adapt to changeable characteristics of each individual process. Of course, in the case of medicine, the process we are talking about is the human body.

Intelligent or self-learning fuzzy control systems as a form of direct-adaptive control employ a measure of control performance relative to a desired trajectory ('performance index') to guide modifications to on-line generated fuzzy control rules [2]. It is important to distinguish this approach from self-tuning control schemes where the fuzzy rule base is fixed and controller gains or scaling factors are adjusted on-line. In our application the scaling factors are kept fixed. The fuzzy control system then learns on-line how to control each individual process presented to it starting with a completely blank rule base [3].

It appears as if the authors are pioneering medical application of self-learning fuzzy control. Initially this was applied to neuromuscular block during surgery. It was first presented as computer simulation studies only [4] but more recently demonstrated successfully in clinical trials [5, 6].

Methods

Self-learning fuzzy control requires another processing layer added to the conventional simple fuzzy controller (Figure 1).

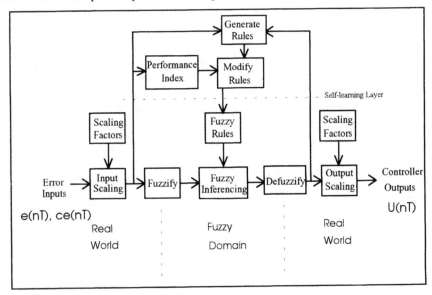

Figure 1 : Block diagram showing the self-learning layer added to a simple fuzzy controller to form a self-learning fuzzy controller.

The self-learning fuzzy control algorithm operates in the following way :-

At sample time nT,

1. Calculate current scaled error (e) and change in error (ce) values.

2. Add the modified generated rule to the fuzzy rule base at the cell pointed to by the scaled e and ce values at sample time (nT-DT-T), where DT is the process dead-time and T is the sample period (one minute in our application), with the output value given by :-

$$U_{nT-DT-T} + Perf(e_{nT}, ce_{nT}) \quad ....(1)$$

where U is the unscaled fuzzy output control term, *Perf* is the scaled performance index value according to the current scaled e and ce values. Note that the *Perf* scaling factor is inversely related to the average process gain.

In our application DT is one sample period (D=1), corresponding approximately to the transport of the drug in the patient's circulation to its action site. Upper and lower limits clearly apply to the output value of a modified generated rule before it is added to the rule base.

3. Calculate the current output value U(nT), defuzzification being by the centre of gravity algorithm, and apply the output scaling factor.

Our simplified approach to keep computational and memory requirements to a minimum in our research is to use a small 5 by 5 fuzzy rule base with fixed scaling factors. Each of the five input fuzzy terms for e and ce are evenly distributed over the universe of discourse with assigned symmetrical triangular membership functions having 25% overlap. The assignment of triangular membership functions to input error terms prior to fuzzification was found to reduce system sensitivity to process noise. Our fuzzy inference engine was found to perform well using simple max-product operations.

Clinical Application

In our preliminary investigation we have applied this technique to atracurium-induced neuromuscular block during surgery. Patient responses to atracurium are considerably variable with a 5:1 range in drug sensitivity, high nonlinearity and time-varying in nature due to changes in patient temperature and blood loss during the course of a surgical procedure. A pharmacokinetic-pharamcodynamic patient model for atracurium infusion was utilised for computer simulation studies [7]. This permitted establishment of suitable scaling factors for the fuzzy controller. It was also possible to test its performance with simulated difficult conditions such as high process noise and variable patient characteristics. The patient simulator also permitted off-line testing of the physical control system prior to its clinical validation [8].

A closed-loop computer system for atracurium-induced neuromuscular block was developed based on a general purpose PC (HP200LX palmtop, IBM compatible) connected to a Graseby Medical 3400 infusion pump and Relaxograph (Datex) EMG-based monitor via RS232 serial links. Following comprehensive off-line validation of the physical control system and approval from local ethics committee, we conducted clinical validation of the intelligent control system. A sample clinical trace is shown in Figure 2, demonstrating its effectiveness in maintaining stable surgical operating conditions. An added benefit of this control system is that reversal of neuromuscular blockade can be achieved as soon as the surgical procedure finishes.

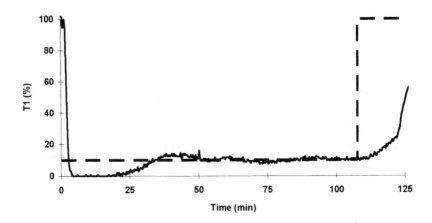

Figure 2 : Sample clinical trace obtained with our self-learning fuzzy controller showing stable neuromuscular block at T1=10% level over 75 minutes.

Discussion

We have therefore found our simplified approach to self-learning fuzzy control to perform well, showing good promise for application to other uncertain, non-linear and time-varying processes in medicine such as control of blood pressure, depth of anaesthesia and multivariable circulatory management of intensive care patients.

Acknowledgement

The authors wish to thank Graseby Medical Plc for supporting this research effort.

References

[1] Thomas D. et al, "Fuzzy Logic Control - A Taxonomy of Demonstrated Benefits", *Proc IEEE* 1995; 83(3): 407-421

[2] Procyk T. et al, "A Linguistic Self-organising Process Controller", *Automatica*, 1979; 15: 15-30

[3] Shenoi S. et al, Implementation of a Learning Fuzzy Controller, *IEEE Control Systems* 1995; 73-80

[4] Linkens D. et al, "Self-organising Learning Control and its Application to Muscle Relaxant Anaesthesia", *Computer Methods and Programs in Biomedicine* 1990; 33(3) : 119-134

[5] Mason D. et al, "Self-learning Fuzzy Control of Atracurium-induced Neuromuscular Block During Surgery", *Med Biol Eng Comput* <in review>

[6] Ross J., Mason D. et al, "Self-learning Fuzzy Control of Muscle Relaxation", *British Journal of Anaesthesia* 1997 <in press>

[7] Mason D et al, "Automated Delivery of Muscle Relaxants Using Fuzzy Logic Control", *IEEE Engineering in Medicine and Biology* 1994; 13: 678-686

[8] Mason D. et al, "Development of a Portable Closed-loop Atracurium Infusion System: Systems Methodology and Safety Issues", *Int J Clin Monit & Comput* <in press>

Temporal Reasoning and Planning

Planning and Scheduling Patient Tests in Hospital Laboratories

Constantine D. Spyropoulos, Stavros Kokkotos and Catherine Marinagi

Software and Knowledge Engineering Laboratory
Institute of Informatics and Telecommunications
National Centre for Scientific Research "Demokritos"
15310 Aghia Paraskevi, Greece
e-mails: [costass | stavros | katerina]@iit.nrcps.ariadne-t.gr

Abstract. Planning and scheduling patient tests is one of the most important functions within hospitals. The objective of this function must be to decrease patient discomfort, to minimize patient stay in hospital as well as to maximize equipment utilization. We propose an integrated planning and scheduling approach, which takes advantage of both hospital domain structure knowledge and generic planning techniques. Our approach is based on the dynamic distributed planning/scheduling paradigm that allows the creation of concise resource allocation plans to service test requests, while trying to distribute the load and reduce communications overhead, thus increasing the performance.

1 Introduction

One of the most important hospital functions is the performance of tests, to assist the diagnosis. Usually the laboratories are responsible for scheduling their own tests, with little or no cooperation between them. As a result patients are required to wait between tests, or even requested to visit the hospital again. The situation is reflected in the lack of research or commercial systems and methods for managing tests as a whole. Instead there is considerable activity in single laboratory management [14] as well as in areas like overall hospital management [10,15], bed allocation, emergency departments and operating theaters [7,16]. Overall test planning should receive more attention, because it influences heavily the length of stay for inpatients, therefore affecting the hospital cost, especially in countries where hospital fees are based solely on diagnosis [4,5,15]. Moreover, good test planning will reduce number and length of visits for outpatients and enable better utilization of hospital equipment.

There exist some approaches and systems to overall test scheduling [5,6,15]. One of their disadvantages is that they are based solely on scheduling techniques, ignoring the required planning. Planning is the creation of an ordered set of activities that allow the transition from an initial state to a given goal, while scheduling is the assignment of resource availability over time periods to satisfy constraints imposed by given actions. Smith [12] notes that scheduling approaches do not exploit state dependent constraints, while planning approaches do not use the problem or domain structure. Furthermore, he remarks that planning systems are more general, while scheduling leads to better performance. Recently, there is a gradually increasing motivation to integrate planning and scheduling approaches, even for traditionally scheduling domains, such as job-shop [12], to improve flexibility and performance.

Laboratory tests encompass both planning and scheduling features. Tests have temporal constraints, require resources over time periods and may be performed on several different devices, often resulting in different temporal constraints (scheduling), but there also exist incompatibility issues between tests, medical procedures that demand ordering of the tests in pre-specified queues and tests can be analyzed into steps (planning). A mixed methodology, based on the advantages of both planning and scheduling, would be the best solution. The ideal situation would allow cooperative overall planning and scheduling of tests, to obtain the best results.

In the present paper we present a novel approach to hospital laboratory test planning and scheduling, built upon a temporal planner and a dynamic distributed planning/scheduling methodology. The planner allows additional complexity to the domain modeling, like analyzing tests into steps and defining test incompatibilities, while the dynamic distributed planning/scheduling approach is expected to significantly reduce the overhead of scheduler communication and cooperation.

In section 2 we define the hospital laboratory test domain, and specify the basis for the rest of the discussion, by presenting related work on combined planning and scheduling approaches as well as on patient test scheduling. In section 3 our approach is described, while in section 4 we present our concluding remarks.

2 Background

2.1 Hospital Laboratory Test Modeling

The world of laboratory tests consists of *laboratories, equipment, laboratory personnel, patients, doctors, requests* and *tests*. Doctors examine patients and issue requests, prescribing tests to be performed. A request may contain more than one test for the same patient. Requests contain temporal constraints, in the form of start and due dates/times for the tests. Laboratory personnel perform the tests, either on the patients or on samples, using various devices from the existing laboratory equipment. Each laboratory is able to perform a pre-defined set of tests.

A test can be decomposed into an ordered set of *steps*, with predefined temporal relations between subsequent steps. Steps consist of *actions*. For every resource involved in the step (i.e. equipment, laboratory technicians as well as the patient) there exist a set of three actions: An action that prepares the involved resource, called *initialization* for equipment or *preparation* for patients and personnel, an action that uses the resource, called *busy*, and an action that allows the resource to return to its initial situation, called *reset* for equipment or *rest* for patients and personnel. Temporal constraints, define the order of the actions. Relations between steps as well as relations between actions may be uncertain. All actions are characterized by their *duration*. Laboratory devices have a maximum capacity, which defines the number of tests and actions that can allocate the device simultaneously.

For example consider a simple X-ray test consisting of 2 main steps: X-ray and film development. Film development can start 0:00-0:30 after the end of the X-ray step.

The X-ray step uses 3 resources: technician, patient, and X-ray device. The patient gets undressed (preparation 0:05), 0:00-0:05 later the X-ray is taken (busy 0:12) and immediately (0:00) afterwards the patient is dressed again (rest 0:05). The X-ray device has to be prepared by the technician (initialization/preparation 0:03), and 0:00-0:05 later the X-ray is taken (busy 0:12). Complex tests can be modeled, to be performed continuously or in distinct steps, involving several devices and personnel.

2.2 Approaches to Planning and Scheduling

Research prototype systems that support a mixture of planning and scheduling and can reason about resources have already been developed. Because there exists no standard terminology on the used resource types we accept the following definitions:

- *Unsharable reusable* is a resource that can be used by only one action at a time. The action returns it after it finishes.
- *Sharable reusable* resource is a set of equivalent aggregated resources with a maximum capacity. Actions borrow part of this resource and return it back.
- *Consumable* is a resource for which an initial quantity is available to be consumed so that its availability is decreased.
- *Producible* is a resource of which additional units are produced (usually by consuming quantities of other resources) so that its availability is increased.

SIPE [17] was the first planner to handle consumable/producible, besides unsharable reusable resources. FORBIN [1] uses pools of discrete objects that can be used, consumed or produced. It employs a heuristic scheduler, which tries to create a schedule from a given partial plan each time an expansion of a task has to be chosen. If the schedule is viable the system accepts the choice and continues with the next task. O-PLAN [2] treats consumable/producible and unsharable/sharable reusable resources uniformly. The search space is pruned by calculating optimistic and pessimistic resource profiles. This approach seems to be ineffective for reusable resources [3] and unsound with respect to managing resource conflicts [8].

IxTeT [8] proposes a sound and complete approach to manage sharable reusable as well as unsharable reusable and consumable/producible resources. It uses a clique-search algorithm on interval graphs that derive from the temporal constraint network, to detect resource constraint conflicts. The parcPLAN system [3] uses Boolean meta-variables whose values are the constraints of the problem in order to integrate temporal and resource reasoning at a global level. The parcPLAN system deals with sharable reusable resources, such as robot arms. Smith [12] suggests an integration framework for planning and scheduling where each scheduling decision defines a localized planning sub-problem. The solution of this sub-problem imposes more temporal constraints used for subsequent scheduling.

In the test scheduling domain there are only a few approaches to overall test management within a hospital. The approach described in [5,6] follows a distributed scheduling approach. Instead of having a single scheduler to decide for every aspect of the system, like in centralized scheduling, this approach assigns schedulers to laboratories, equipment types or even devices. These schedulers perform the resource allocation for a part of the hospital. Requests are decomposed into steps, and these steps are forwarded to the appropriate schedulers. Cases involving more than one scheduler, like when a patient must visit two or more laboratories, require extensive communication between schedulers, to eliminate conflicts.

3 A Patient-wise Test Planning and Scheduling Approach

3.1 Dynamic Distributed Planning/Scheduling

Overall test management in a hospital environment is a distributed problem. In [5,6] the distribution is based on laboratory or equipment, defining them as independent units. However our understanding is that a twofold distribution is involved: equipment-wise and patient-wise distribution. The patient-wise distribution derives from the observation that each request for tests involves only one patient, and that in the majority of cases the tests in a request are interdependent. Equipment-wise distribution usually leads to better resource utilization, but may require extensive communication overhead to establish a commonly acceptable schedule, while the results are not always the best for the patient. For this reason we introduce the idea *of dynamic distributed planning/scheduling*, based on patient-wise distribution.

The basic idea behind dynamic distributed planning/scheduling in test management is that every request is handled as an independent entity, instead of breaking it to partial requests as in distributed scheduling. In distributed scheduling there exists a constant number of schedulers assigned to specific sets of resources. In the dynamic distributed planning/scheduling, however, there can exist no constant number of planners/schedulers, because the number of unserviced requests cannot be defined a-priori. For this reason planners/schedulers are automatically generated (spawned) every time a new request is entered into the system. Each planner/scheduler is assigned to a request and "dies" when the request has been served. For this reason we call our approach dynamic.

3.2 Design Architecture of the Planning and Scheduling System

The proposed approach is based on a modular design architecture. This architecture allows distribution of the planning and scheduling load to several computer platforms and tries to minimize communication between the planners/schedulers. This design architecture is pictured in Figure 1.

Users (doctors, nurses, hospital front desk, laboratory technicians, etc.) enter their requests for test prescriptions, temporal constraints, equipment busy times (e.g. for maintenance), etc. These requests are stored into the *common database*, which contains and organizes information about the allocation of resources to requests, the full timetables of equipment, patients and personnel, as well as static information, like patient data, personnel data, lists of equipment for each laboratory, etc.

The *common knowledge base* records scheduling methods, like best fit, worst fit, etc. It also contains activity representation schemes, which describe activities (e.g. tests) and includes information about preconditions and effects, durations and analysis into lower level activities (e.g. steps of tests) along with temporal distances. It also includes lists of facts that contradict among themselves under restrictions, which are consulted during plan construction to detect conflicts. Finally the common knowledge base contains heuristic medical rules, imposed by hospital personnel when planning tests, based on their experience. These rules represent information such as correlation of steps of different tests or incompatibilities among tests.

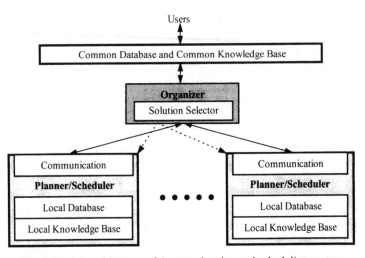

Fig. 1. Design architecture of the test planning and scheduling system

The central part of the system is the *organizer*, which acts as central control, dispatcher and communications channel. The organizer is responsible for generating the planners/schedulers according to the request load and returning their results to the common database. The data flow inside the organizer is as follows:

- The organizer recognizes the arrival of a new request to the common database.
- If more than one computer platforms are connected to the system, the organizer examines and specifies the one with the less load, onto which it generates a new planner/scheduler. Then it passes the relevant information about the request from the common database and knowledge base to the planner/scheduler (request details, timetables of concerned resources, details of concerned tests, medical practices for these tests, scheduling methods).
- The planner/scheduler generates a set of solutions to the problem. The number of the generated solutions is defined by the system administrator. The solutions may contain uncertainty. This means that certain actions may be scheduled for execution during time periods with uncertain bounds.
- The organizer receives the solutions and activates its *solution selector*. This module performs the following tasks:
  ◊ Rejects invalid solutions. Invalid solutions are generated because the planner/scheduler is isolated from the common database after its activation. As an example consider the following scenario: Planner/scheduler PS1

commences its execution at time T1 and PS2 starts at T2>T1. From T2 onwards PS2 is not updated on common database evolution. At time T3>T2 PS1 returns its solution, allocating a device D1. At time T4>T3 PS2 finishes. Some of the solutions generated by PS2 require D1 for the period which PS1 has already allocated it. These solutions are considered invalid and rejected. For this reason the planners/schedulers must generate more than one solution. In the generic case the solution selector checks the allocated capacity of the requested resources against the currently free capacity.

◊ Consolidates the uncertain times of the valid solutions. During this phase all uncertainty is eliminated from the resource allocation time periods.

◊ Selects the best solution, which is the solution with the most merit. After extensive discussions with hospital and laboratory managers, the merit of a solution has been defined as the objective function of Equation 1, which is an improvement over the one proposed in [5,6]. The weights W define how much we are interested in equipment utilization (W_E) or patient comfort (W_P). The weights W_{EB} and W_{PB} define our interest in equipment/personnel and patient busy time respectively, while W_{EF} and W_{PF} define our interest in their free time. The weights are complimentary: $W_E+W_P=1$ and $W_{EF}+W_{EB}=1$ and $W_{PF}+W_{PB}=1$. For example large W_{PF} means that we want to reduce the patient's stay in hospital, by reducing his/her idle time. The sums represent the total free or busy times for the set of devices or personnel used in the request (E_F or E_B) or for the patient (P_F or P_B), over periods of time extending for predefined time intervals before and after the request.

• The organizer sends the best solution to the common database. In case no valid solutions have been found the organizer directs the planner/scheduler to try again, else it discontinues the planner/scheduler execution.

$$OF = \min\left(W_E * \left(W_{EF} * \sum_E \sum E_F + W_{EB} * \sum_E \sum E_B\right) + W_P * \left(W_{PF} * \sum P_F + W_{PB} * \sum P_B\right)\right)$$

Equation 1. Objective function determining the merit of a solution

3.3 The Planner/Scheduler Module

The core of the *planner/scheduler module* is TRL-Planner [9], a domain-independent temporal planning system, that produces hierarchical, partially ordered plans and supports user interaction. It is built upon the TRLi [11] temporal reasoning system that supports both symbolic and quantitative temporal information. TRLi is an interpreter of the TRL temporal logic, which expresses temporal information as *temporal references* to predicates. Examples of temporal references are the temporal point T, the temporal interval <T1,T2> and the temporal instance [T1,T2]. TRLi's temporal inference rules are realized by constraint solving techniques. These are achieved by appropriate calls to the Symbolic Constraint Solver SCS, that accepts a set of temporal constraints and builds a consistent constraint graph, which is stored as a list of consistent and simplified constraints. SCS handles arithmetic constraints of the form X Cnstr Y, where X, Y are simple terms (i.e. variables and integers) or compound terms (i.e. terms of the form T+n or T-n, where T is a simple term and n is an integer). The operator Cnstr takes values from the set {=,<, >, ≤, ≥}. Detailed descriptions of TRLi and TRL-Planner are given in [9,11].

TRL-Planner has been applied to practical problems such as cargo handling operations for chemical carriers [9]. In the present case TRL-Planner is enhanced with scheduling capabilities in order to solve localized scheduling sub-problems and produce a set of alternative solutions.

TRL-Planner uses three sub-modules. These are the local database, the local knowledge base and the communications module. The local database and knowledge base contain information copied from the common database and knowledge base, which concerns the particular request. Therefore communication overhead is reduced. The communications module handles all communication between the TRL-Planner and the common database and knowledge base.

TRL-Planner generates the plan backwards, starting from goals, allowing both planning by achieving goals and planning by expanding activities [9]. It reads the current state of the world, including both static and temporal data contained in the local database, and starts producing a plan consulting the local knowledge base when needed. It generates a set of solutions, each represented as a temporal constraint graph, where activities may have uncertain temporal references and may be partially ordered. In case that a localized scheduling sub-problem is encountered during plan generation, a scheduling methodology is applied. For example, when a resource can be allocated between alternative free intervals, a best fit method can be applied. If the plan generation process backtracks then an alternative scheduling method is applied.

TRL-Planner enables the representation of different types of activities. These are described using a uniform representation schema, A=<N,D,T,Cd,E,Cst>, where activities, preconditions and effects are labeled by temporal references.

- N is the *parameterized name* of an activity.
- D is the *duration* of an activity that may be uncertain.
- T is the activity *type*. The schema can encode different types of activities: *Macro actions* are decomposed into a set of sub-actions. The execution order of sub-actions is determined through temporal constraints described in the sub-actions temporal constraints list. *Primitive actions* can not be further decomposed. *Scheduled events* have a known time of occurrence.
- Cd is the list of *preconditions*. These are distinguished into *assumptions* (A) and *subgoals* (S). Assumptions must be true for the particular activity to be selected. A subgoal, which is not already achieved, can be achieved by selecting an activity having a primary effect that matches with the subgoal.
- E is the list of *effects*, distinguished in *primary effects* (PE) that satisfy subgoals of other activities, and *general effects* (GE) that represent side effects.
- Cst is the *temporal constraints list*. It contains temporal constraints between time points appearing as variables in the schema.

3.4 An illustrative example

In the present section we describe a simple example. Details are eliminated because of lack of space. Assume that two tests, pancreas ultrasound and angiography, have been prescribed by Dr. Fox for Mr. Adams. The request consists of two goals:

[10:30,15:00] : angiography_test_completed(test31, mrAdams, drFox, TechnicianA, Device1, Device2)

[11:00,15:00] : pancreas_ultrasound_test_completed(test32, mrAdams, drFox, TechnicianB, Device3, Device4)

The temporal references of the goals are temporal instances which state that the angiography should be completed at some time between 10:30 and 15:00 and pancreas ultrasound should be completed at some time between 11:00 and 15:00. These goals are given in an arbitrary order.

Both the database and the knowledge base contain details of the domain such as the definition of unsharable reusable and sharable reusable resources, as well as the initial conditions, such as resource reservations. For example:

resource(x_ray_device, integris_3000_philips)
resource(doctor, drFox)

<9:00, 10:30>   : reserved(x_ray_device, integris_3000_philips)
<[9:50,10:00],10:30>   : reserved(doctor, drFox)
<Ta,9:00>   : reserved(patient, mrAdams)
<15:00,Tb>   : reserved(patient, mrAdams)

Tests are encoded as macro actions. The steps of each particular test are the sub-actions into which the test is decomposed. The temporal relations between steps are included in the Sub-actions Temporal Constraints list.

N   : <T1,T2> : angiography_test(Test_num, Patient, Nurse, Doctor, Technician, Device1, Device2)
D   : D1
T   : macroaction (Subactions:
         <T1,T3> : catheterism_&_pour_shading_liquid(Test_num, Patient, Nurse)
         <T4,T5> : x_ray_test(Test_num, Patient, Technician, Device1)
         <T6,T7> : film_development(Test_num, Patient, Device2)
         <T8,T2> : check_results(Test_num, Patient, Doctor)
         Subactions_TemporalConstraints : T3≤T4, T6≥T5, T6≤T5+30, T7≤T8)
Cd   : A :
         S : <Ts1,Ts1> : patient's_case_history_taken(Patient, Doctor)
E   : PE : <T2,T2> : angiography_test_completed(Test_num, Patient, Nurse, Doctor, Technician, Device1, Device2)
         GE :
Cst : Ts1≤T1

N   : <T1,T2>   : pancreas_ultrasound_test(Test_num, Patient, Nurse, Doctor, Technician, Device1, Device2)
D   : D2

```
T    : macroaction(Subactions:
       <T1,T3> :  pancreas_ultrasound(Test_num,Patient,Technician,Device1)
       <T4,T5> :  film_development(Test_num, Patient, Device2)
       <T6,T2> :  check_results(Test_num, Patient, Doctor)
       Subactions_TemporalConstraints : T4≥T3, T4≤T3+30, T5≤T6)
Cd   : A :
       S  : <Ts1,Ts1> :  patient's_case_history_taken(Patient, Doctor)
E    : PE : <T2,T2>   :  pancreas_ultrasound_test_completed(Test_num, Patient,
                         Nurse, Doctor, Technician, Device1, Device2)

       GE :
Cst  : Ts1≤T1
```

Steps of tests are also encoded as macro actions. Each step is analyzed into a predefined set of sub-actions, depending upon the resources, which are used. Resource availability is checked through assumptions and resource reservations are entered into the knowledge base through general effects.

```
N    : <T1,T2>  :  x_ray_test(Test_num, Patient, Technician, Device)
D    : D1
T    : macroaction (Subactions:
       <T1,T3>   :  x_ray_equipment_initialization(Test_num, Device)
       <T4,T5>   :  x_ray_equipment_busy(Test_num, Device)
       <T6,T7>   :  x_ray_equipment_reset(Test_num, Device)
       <T8,T9>   :  x_ray_patient_preparation(Test_num, Patient)
       <T4,T10>  :  x_ray_patient_busy(Test_num, Patient)
       <T11,T2>  :  x_ray_patient_rest(Test_num, Patient)
       <T1,T7>   :  x_ray_personnel_busy(Test_num, Technician)
       Subactions_TemporalConstraints : T4≥T3, T4≤T3+5, T5≤T6, T7≤T2, T9≤T4,
                   T10≤T11)
Cd   : A  : <T1,T7>  :  available(x_ray_device, Device)
            <T8,T2>  :  available(patient, Patient)
            <T1,T7>  :  available(personnel, Technician)
       S  :
E    : PE : <T2,T2>  :  x_ray_test_completed(Test_num,Patient,Technician,Device)
       GE : <T1,T7>  :  reserved(x_ray_device, Device)
            <T8,T2>  :  reserved(patient, Patient)
            <T1,T7>  :  reserved(personnel, Technician)
Cst  :
```

The sub-actions into which steps are decomposed are primitive actions. Their duration is usually an integer but it can also have an uncertain value. For example:

```
N    : <T1,T2>  :  x_ray_equipment_initialization(Test_num, integris_3000_philips)
D    : 3
T    : primitive
Cd   : A  :
       S  :
E    : PE : <T2,T2>  :  x_ray_equipment_initialization_completed(Test_num,
                                                   integris_3000_philips)

       GE :
Cst  :
```

Medical rules are also included in the knowledge base. For example:

<T1,T2> : pouring_of_shading_liquid_patient_busy(Test_num,Patient,Nurse):-
<T3,T4> : pancreas_ultrasound_patient_busy(Test_num, Patient),
$T3 \geq T2+30$.

The plan is generated hierarchically. The upper level contains the tests. This level is expanded to produce a partially ordered plan of test steps. The steps are expanded to allocate resources, apply medical rules and handle temporal constraints. In Figure 2 one of the produced solutions is pictured, after consolidating the uncertain time periods. Not all available information is pictured in this figure, for better clarity.

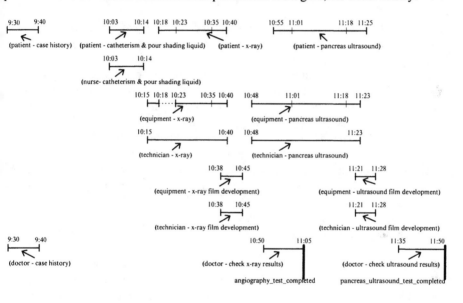

Fig. 2. Graphical representation of a Test Execution Plan

4 Conclusions

In the present paper we presented a novel approach for patient test management in hospital laboratories, based on a combination of planning and scheduling methods. The planning component allows modeling of complex tests, that can be decomposed into steps, which are performed separately as series of actions. Actions are served by sets of devices and specialized personnel. The scheduling component handles the temporal relations and constraints between tests, steps and actions.

Since the hospital environment is highly distributed, our approach is based on the idea of dynamic distributed planning/scheduling, that dynamically creates planner/schedulers over several platforms and assigns them to requests. Thus the load is distributed over several computers while the communication overhead is reduced, because each planner/scheduler handles a whole request spanning several laboratories. Communication between planners/schedulers, needed only in case of simultaneous demands for the same resources, is handled by an organizer module.

Based on the proposed approach the prototype HOSTESS system has been developed in cooperation with 01-Pliroforiki and the General Athens Hospital "G. Genimatas" [13]. HOSTESS is currently under B-Testing. Due to hardware availability limitations during the testing the same computer (SUN 330) serves as database server (INGRES) and planner/scheduler platform. Its response time, when configured to generate 2 alternative solutions, is in the order of 45 seconds to 1 minute, under the load of one of the largest hospitals in Athens. In the near future we expect to commence testing using 2 or 3 planner/scheduler platforms, which will be more modern computers. We expect that the performance of HOSTESS will increase by at least 50%.

From the testing, up to now, we have reached the conclusion that simultaneous requests, which require the same resources leading to conflict between planners/schedulers occur only in simple cases, like X-rays or blood tests. For these cases mainly we need multiple solutions. We chose to configure the system to generate multiple solutions, instead of starting again the planning process, because it is much cheaper, in terms of performance and computing resources, to generate alternatives to an existing plan rather than tune the whole process again, including reading the initial state. Multiple solutions increase the possibility of a valid one. In our test case 2 solutions proved adequate. In all other cases, with very few conflicts, the dynamic distributed approach almost eliminates the need for communication between planners/schedulers. The creation and destruction of processes (planners/schedulers) is not time consuming in modern computers and operating systems. Thus the only overhead worth mentioning is the reading of the world state from the database and knowledge base and the storing of the solution to the database.

For the future we intent to extend our approach to handle different types of resources and tests, such as batch analyzers and tests or tests that extend over a duration of several days. Furthermore we plan to extend the knowledge base so that more complicated medical rules can be integrated into the system. Currently we are only capable to represent medical rules that relate the performance of different activities, determining their temporal distance.

Acknowledgements

The HOSTESS system was developed during the R&D project PAVE 92BE45 "Development of an Integrated Environment for Management, Scheduling and Control of Hospital Operations", funded by the Greek General Secretariat for Research and Technology. In the project participated 01-Pliroforiki and the General Athens Hospital "G. Genimatas". Prof. G. Vassilacopoulos from Pireaus University, Greece, offered his support and his insightful comments while reviewing the system.

Reference

1. Dean T.L., Firby R.J., Miller D. "Hierarchical Planning Involving Deadlines, Travel Time and Resources", Computational Intelligence, Vol. 4, pp. 381-398, 1988.

2. Drabble B., Tate A. "The Use of Optimistic and Pessimistic Resource Profiles to Inform Search in an Activity based Planner", 2nd International Conference on AI Planning Systems AIPS-94, Chicago, IL, pp. 243-248, 1994.

3. El-Kholy A., Richards B. "Temporal and Resource Reasoning in Planning: the parcPLAN approach", European Conference on AI'96, pp. 614-618, 1996.

4. Fetter R. B. "Diagnosis Related Groups: Understanding Hospital Performance", Interfaces, Vol. 21, No. 1, pp. 6-26, 1991.

5. Kumar A. D., Kumar A. R., Kekre S., Prietula M. J., Ow P. S. "Multi-agent Systems and Organizational Structure: The Support of Hospital Patient Scheduling", 3rd Int. Conference on Expert Systems and the Leading Edge in Production and Operations Management, S. Carolina, pp. 551-566, May 1989.

6. Kumar A. D., Ow P. S., Prietula M. J. "Organizational Simulation and Information Systems Design: An Operations Level Example", Management Science, Vol. 39, No. 2, pp. 218-240, 1993.

7. Kuzdrall P. J., Kwak N. K., Schmitz H. H. "Simulating Space Requirements and Scheduling Policies in a Hospital Surgical Suite", Simulation, pp. 163-171, 1981.

8. Laborie P., Ghallab M. "Planning with Sharable Resource Constraints", 14th International Joint Conference on AI - IJCAI'95, pp.1643-1649, 1995.

9. Marinagi C.C., Panayiotopoulos T., Vouros G.A., Spyropoulos C.D. "Advisor: a Knowledge-based Planning System", International Journal of Expert Systems Research and Applications, Vol. 9, No. 3, pp. 319-353, 1996.

10. Moustakis V. S., Orphanoudakis S. "Requirements Definition for an Integrated Hospital Information System", EURINFO '88 Conference, Athens, Greece, North-Holland, pp. 852-858, May 1988.

11. Panayiotopoulos T., Gergatsoulis M. "A Prolog-like Temporal Reasoning System", 13th IASTED International Conference on Applied Informatics, Innsbruck, Austria, IASTED-ACTA PRESS, pp. 123-126, Feb. 1995.

12. Smith S.F. "Integrating Planning and Scheduling: Towards Effective Coordination in Complex, Resource-Constrained Domains", Italian Planning Workshop 1993, Keynote Address, Rome, Italy, Sept. 1993.

13. Spyropoulos C.D., Kokkotos S., Ioannidis E., Palaskas Z., Zerva E.Z., Kampourelis T. "Development of an Integrated Environment for Management, Scheduling and Control of Hospital Operations - Final Report 1.0", Technical Report, N.C.S.R. "Demokritos", February 1996.

14. Sullivan W. G., Blair E. L. "Predicting Workload Requirements for Scheduled Health Care Services with an Application to Radiology Departments", Socio-Economic Planning Science, Vol. 13, pp. 35-39, 1979.

15. The EDITH Initiative, "The EDITH Manifesto", GESI, Via Rodi 32, 00195 Rome, Italy, 1994.

16. Vassilacopoulos, G. "A Simulation Model for Bed Allocation to Hospital Inpatient Departments", Simulation, Vol. 45, No. 5, pp. 233-241, 1985.

17. Wilkins D.E. "Can AI Planners Solve Practical Problems", Computational Intelligence, Vol. 6, pp. 232-246, 1990.

Temporal Abstractions for Diabetic Patients Management

Cristiana Larizza[1], Riccardo Bellazzi[1], Alberto Riva[2]

[1] Dipartimento di Informatica e Sistemistica, Università di Pavia, Pavia, Italy
[2] IRCCS Policlinico S.Matteo, Pavia, Italy

Abstract. This paper outlines how Temporal Abstractions can be used to analyze and interpret longitudinal data coming from diabetic patients monitoring. We use temporal abstraction mechanisms to provide an abstract description of the patient's state useful to interpret the therapeutic response to the current protocol and to provide proper suggestions.

1 Introduction

Several medical domains require the capability to analyze and interpreting a large number of longitudinal data, coming from long-term monitoring of chronic patients. These data present some common features, that can be summarized as follows:

1. long-term monitoring generates a huge amount of data, coming from several, nearly-similar individuals.
2. the information is usually both of qualitative and quantitative nature.
3. the quantitative data are prone to measurement errors, due to the fact that they are collected by different people, often in different environments, and using different experimental settings.
4. the data are in general drawn on an irregular time grid, since the timing of the observations may depend on some individual factors, like the patient's compliance, or on some environmental constraints, like the physician's schedule of out-patients visits.

As a consequence, the physician must interpret such information on the basis of a comprehensive analysis, by extracting the relevant features from multi-variable time series and by combining historical with time-oriented data. In this context, several authors have recognized that a decision support system for long-term monitoring of chronic patients should allow to exploit all the available heterogeneous information, combining classical statistical techniques, like time series analysis, with methods coming from the AI field, like Temporal Abstractions (TAS) [11, 4, 7, 6, 3, 8].

Our goal is to demonstrate that more accurate data analysis and interpretation can be carried out by moving from raw data to an abstract description of the patient's behavior, which can be obtained through the TA methods. In particular, we want to stress the fact that TAs are not only useful for highlighting dangerous situations, or for explaining complex episodes, but may also be exploited to interpret the patient's history as a sequence of abstracted events.

We are applying the herein presented methodology to the long-term monitoring of insulin dependent diabetes mellitus (IDDM) patients. The basic goal of IDDM therapy and monitoring is to control the Blood Glucose Level (BGL), keeping the controlled variable within an interval of nearly-normal values. A tight control of BGL may avoid both IDDM short-term and long-term complications, as shown by the recent DCCT study [5].

As stated by several authors [11, 4], current information technologies may be exploited to improve the quality of chronic patients care by a) increasing the rate of information exchange between patients and physicians, b) providing patients and physicians with support tools for taking proper decisions. This work focuses on the latter point, although it is part of an overall project devoted to the Telematic Management of Insulin-Dependent Diabetes Mellitus (T-IDDM project) [2]. More details on the architecture and on the methodologies applied in the project can be found in [2, 9, 10].

2 Monitoring diabetic patients

IDDM patients control their glucose metabolism using several daily insulin injections. The patient performs self-monitoring of BGL at home, usually before meals, and reports the monitoring results on a diary. The accuracy of the patient's self-care is very important, since the onset and development of diabetic complications is strictly related to the degree of metabolic control that can be thus achieved [5]. Unfortunately, tight metabolic control involves 3 to 4 insulin injections per day, accurate home BGL monitoring, and an increase in the probability of hypoglycemic events. Out-patients follow a therapeutic protocol that is assessed by physicians on the basis of periodical visits, and are usually allowed to slightly modify the treatment in dependence of their health status and of occasional life-style modifications.

Data set information content
Usually, a patient diary contains the data record described below:

Day	Day Time	BGL	Glycosuria	Regular Insulin	NPH-Lente Insulin	Meal	Events

The *Day Time* field describes the measurement time, and may be quantitative, (e.g. "7.30 a.m.") or qualitative (e.g. "breakfast"). In the latter case, the patient usually refers to seven daily landmark periods, that we indicate with the term *time slice*, shown in the following table. The correspondence between the time slices and the quantitative day-time may be calculated on the basis of the patient's life-style.

Breakfast	Mid-Morning	Lunch	Afternoon	Dinner	Bed-Time	Night-Time

The BGL field contains the quantitative information on the measured BGL. This information is usually drawn from a reflectometer. The *glycosuria* field reports the level of glucose in the urine, as measured with the available measurement kit; glycosuria detects if, in the last few hours, the BGL has exceeded the glucose renal threshold (180 mg/dl). The glycosuria measurement is usually qualitative, and dependent on the measurement kit used. In general, it is possible to derive three qualitative levels from such measurements: *absent, traces, present*. The *Regular Insulin and NPH-Lente Insulin* field contains the Insulin units taken by the patients. The *meal* field should contain the carbohydrates contents of each meal in grams. In general, this information is missing, and it is necessary to resort to the patient's diet predefined by physicians, without knowing the real carbohydrate intake of that meal. Finally, the *event* field may contain information on the occurrence of symptomatic hypoglycemia episodes, physical activity, fever or other significant events. Unfortunately, often also this field is missing.

It is hence clear that the analysis of home monitoring data should rely on these seven time-stamped data fields, that possess all the characteristics and problems outlined in the introduction. Even the time-stamped nature of the data has to be considered in a fuzzy interpretation, being the time slice, and not hours and minutes, the time scale used.

In clinical practice, the physician usually tries to combine the seven patterns in order to detect relevant episodes. For example, the *Somogy effect*, defined as a response to hypoglycemia while asleep with counter-regulatory hormones causing morning hyperglycemia, is detected by looking for "hyperglycemia at breakfast with absence of glycosuria", while the *Dawn effect*, a morning hyperglycemia unrelated to nocturnal hypoglycemia, is detected by searching for "hyperglycemia at breakfast with presence of glycosuria"

The potential usefulness of TAs in this data analysis context is therefore clear. A meaningful analysis can be carried out by combining the temporal patterns coming from all the available fields, trying to help physicians in aggregating and interpreting the data. As a matter of fact, several techniques for interpreting BGL time series have been described in the literature, from time series analysis [4] to TAS [11]. In the following sections, we will present the details of our approach.

3   The TA methods

Background

In order to monitor a disease progression or the effectiveness of a therapeutic protocol the physician may need to periodically observe and interpret a large set of clinical parameters. However, the difficult task of considering the overall mass of variables leads the clinician to carry out a mental data processing in order to create an abstract representation of the patient's history.

TAs are methods defined to solve the task of creating an abstract description of the course of longitudinal data by extracting their most relevant features.

In clinical monitoring, these methods can be used to transform the fragmentary representation of the patient's history into a more compact one by moving from a time-point to an interval based description. TA methods can be exploited to analyze one or more time series representing the course of clinical parameters and to generate a collection of episodes which represent sequences of patho-physiologically meaningful states. We adopted these methods to interpret the data sets collected in the daily diary by IDDM patients.

To conceptualize the TA problem solving method we defined an ontology which distinguishes two main categories of abstractions: a) BASIC abstractions for detecting predefined courses in a time series; b) COMPLEX abstractions for investigating specific temporal relationships between intervals. Both methods generate a sequence of intervals as output.

Method a) receives a sequence of time stamped data (*events*) as input and aggregates into intervals (*episodes*) the adjacent observations which follow meaningful trends (increase, decrease or stationarity) (TREND abstraction) or stay inside a specific range of qualitative values (STATE abstraction). When detecting STATE patterns in time series of numerical variables a preliminary qualitative abstraction has to be carried out [6]. The TREND abstraction allows a flexible definition of "fast" or "slow" trends, by specifying the minimum rate of change of the pattern to be detected. For example, if we analyze the time series of the BGL measurements in the BREAKFAST time-slice, we can resort to the STATE abstraction method to identify episodes like "hypoglycemia", "hyperglycemia" and "normal BGL", whose temporal extent is greater than or equal to one day. In an analogous way, we resort to the TREND abstraction method to detect patterns like "BGL decrease", "BGL stationarity" and "BGL increase".

Method b) receives as input two sequences of intervals which can be generated by methods of type a) or b) and searches for specific temporal relations between them. The relation between intervals can be any of the temporal relations defined by Allen [1]. The intervals resulting from a complex abstraction can be the union or the intersection of the episodes considered in the abstraction, in dependence of the specific temporal operator used. For example, given a generic complex abstraction defined as "a OVERLAPS b", the method generates all the intervals obtained by intersection of the episodes a and b.

The COMPLEX abstraction method can be used in two different ways: 1) to represent the persistence of complex clinical situations characterized by the behavior of several clinical parameters; 2) to detect compound data patterns of a single variable that cannot be immediately detected with the method a). An example of the first way of using this method is given by the detection of episodes of "Somogy effect". To perform this task we have defined an abstraction which, starting from the sequences of episodes of "hyperglycemia" and "glycosuria absent" at breakfast, extracts their *overlapping* intervals. An example of the second way of using the mechanism is given by the search for "metabolic instability" through the detection of peaks in the BGL time series. The peak is a pattern that cannot be directly extracted with the BASIC abstraction method, but its detection is possible with a two-step procedure. First, it is necessary to detect all the occurrences of "BGL increase" and of "BGL decrease"; then, it is necessary to extract the "BGL increase" intervals that *meet* a "BGL decrease" interval. The resulting abstractions are obtained through the union of the intervals detected.

It is important to notice that the combined use of BASIC and COMPLEX

Table 1. BASIC Temporal Abstractions.

TA type	finding	Temporal Abstractions
STATE	BGL	Hypoglycemia Normal BGL Hyperglycemia
	NPH Insulin	Low NPH Insulin Medium NPH Insulin High NPH Insulin
	Glycosuria	Glycosuria Absent/Traces Glycosuria Present
	Physical Exercise	Extra Physical Exercise No Extra Physical Exercise
TREND	BGL	BGL Increase BGL Stationarity BGL Decrease
	NPH Insulin	NPH Insulin Increase NPH Insulin Stationarity NPH Insulin Decrease

abstractions may allow the detection of a variety of patho-physiological states.

TAs in the diabetes domain

In order to allow a proper interpretation of the data, we subdivided the 24-hour daily period into a set of consecutive non-overlapping time slices. This process is a first type of abstraction, that generates a qualitative time scale on the basis of the information about the patient's life-style, in particular the meal times. The relationships between actions (insulin intakes) and effects (BGL measurements) are built using the concept of *competent time slice*: an action in a certain time slice will be competent for the BGL measurements in the time slices that it directly affects. For example, an intake of regular insulin will be competent for the time slices that cover the subsequent six hours. Therefore, when a problem is detected in a particular time slice t, the possible adjustments will be the ones affecting the actions in the time slices that are competent over t.

Once the time slices have been generated, following the ontology defined for the TAs problem solving method, we have defined a set of BASIC and COMPLEX abstractions for each time slice. For example, the TAs defined for the *Breakfast* time slice are shown in Tables 1 and 2.

Exploiting the BASIC and COMPLEX abstractions, we derive from the raw data a set of relevant episodes, that can be used to build an abstract description of the patient's evolution. To perform this task, we suggest the following procedure:

• **detection of interesting episodes**: the simplest analysis consists in the

Table 2. COMPLEX Temporal Abstractions.

Definition	TA
Hyperglycemia OVERLAPS Glycosuria Absent	Suspected Somogy Effect
Hyperglycemia OVERLAPS Glycosuria Present	Suspected Dawn Effect
Hypoglycemia OVERLAPS High Evening NPH Insulin	Induced Hypoglycemia
BGL Increase MEETS BGL Decrease	Metabolic Instability

analogous of descriptive statistics on the raw data: the most relevant episodes are found following the definition of TAs, shown to the physician and summarized through simple statistics (counts, durations, periodicity);

• **modal day extraction**: the BGL *modal day* (BG-MD) is a characteristic daily BGL pattern that summarizes the typical patient's response to the therapy in a specific monitoring period; it can be used to evaluate the protocol performance over the selected time interval, even when the information is poor (e.g. data on meals missing). Several approaches for deriving the BG-MD have been presented in the literature, from time series analysis to belief maintenance systems [4, 9]. In our approach it is possible to derive the BG-MD, by calculating the probability distribution of the STATE abstractions defined for the BGL finding, as shown in [9]. This operation is simply performed by counting the number of occurrences of the state episodes, weighted by their time span. By using the same procedure it is possible to extract the typical insulin regimen that is followed by the patient, called *control actions modal day* (CA-MD); in this case the analysis is performed on the NPH and regular insulin STATE abstractions.

Furthermore, modal days can be derived on every episode that can be detected on a single measurement. So, we can define the Somogy effect modal day, the Dawn effect modal day, and so on. In such a way, it is possible to characterize the patient's behavior with a collection of modal days, that describe it from different perspectives.

Typical patient behaviors can be found also by counting the occurrence of complex episodes, having a minimum time span greater than one day. For example, the counts of metabolic instability episodes, defined on a minimum time span of three days, can be summarized by calculating the percentage of time spent in the episode with respect to the total monitoring time.

Other interesting results can be obtained through the time span distribution of the episodes; for example it could be of interest to know the number of increasing BGL episodes lasting for more than three days.

It is clear that a great number of patient behaviors can be defined, and that the relevant ones have to be selected according to the physician's preferences and the data availability.

• **time series analysis of abstracted episodes**: a more ambitious task is to derive meaningful time series from the episodes sequence, as well as causal models of the abstract behaviors. To achieve this goal, we have identified a method based on three steps:

1. We restrict our analysis to the episodes of a time slice with a minimum time span of one day. We identify a number of *state variables*, representing episodes that are mutually exclusive, whose value must be detected on each day. For example, on each day of the analysis in which a BGL measurement is available we can identify the state variable BGL that can assume the levels "hypoglycemia", "normal", "hyperglycemia", and the state variable BGL-TREND that can assume the levels "increasing", "decreasing", "stationary". In an analogous way, we identify the state variables NPH-LEVEL, NPH-TREND and GLYCOSURIA-LEVEL.

We define the *abstract state* AS as the description of the patient's behavior in one day, given by the union of the state variables levels in that day. We construct the time series of the ASs along the daily time axis.

An example of AS is the following:

Day	Time Slice	BGL	BGL-TREND	NPH-LEVEL	NPH-TREND	GLYCOSURIA-LEVEL
01-01-1992	Breakfast	Normal	Increase	Low	Decrease	Present

We transform the ASs time series by moving from the *day time scale* to a *transition time scale*. This is obtained by detecting the times corresponding to a state transition and by compressing the original AS time scale into one characterized by different consecutive states.

As an example, we can start from the following sequence of ASs at breakfast:

Day	BGL	BGL-TREND	NPH-LEVEL	NPH-TREND	GLYCOSURIA-LEVEL
02-01-1992	Hypoglycemia	Increase	Low	Decrease	Present
03-01-1992	Hypoglycemia	Increase	Low	Decrease	Present
04-01-1992	Hypoglycemia	Increase	Low	Decrease	Present
05-01-1992	Normal	Stationary	Medium	Increase	Absent
06-01-1992	Normal	Stationary	Medium	Increase	Absent
07-01-1992	Normal	Decrease	Medium	Stationary	Absent
08-01-1992	Hyperglycemia	Normal	Low	Decrease	Present

to obtain the following one:

Transition	BGL	BGL-TREND	NPH-LEVEL	NPH-TREND	GLYCOSURIA-LEVEL
1	Hypoglycemia	Increase	Low	Decrease	Present
2	Normal	Stationary	Medium	Increase	Absent
3	Normal	Decrease	Medium	Stationary	Absent
4	Hyperglycemia	Normal	Low	Decrease	Present

2. We perform a further analysis on the ASs time series in order to reduce, if possible, the AS dimension. If, for example, the therapy protocol has not been modified, the two state variables NPH-LEVEL and NPH-TREND are not informative and can, therefore, be discarded. The next step consists in investigating the existence of causal relationships among this reduced set of state variables. In particular, it is interesting to verify if it is possible to derive a model of the BGL episodes in dependence of the actual AS. This step can be conveniently performed, in a probabilistic setting [9], by extracting from the AS transitions the table of the conditional probabilities of the next BGL given the present AS.

It is important to notice that ASs time series analysis can be performed when the time elapsed between the different transitions is nearly constant. Otherwise, the transition time scale will be built on an irregular time grid; this, in general, may lead to a mis-interpretation of the data.

4   A case study

Let us consider the case of a 21 years old male patient, affected by IDDM from puberty. This patient underwent a treatment with two injections of NPH insulin at dinner and breakfast and three injections of regular insulin at breakfast, lunch and dinner. We concentrate our attention on the data measured at the breakfast time slice over a period of 131 days.

The BGL measurements and the *competent* NPH insulin dosages are shown in Fig. 1. By looking at these time series, it is clear that BGL has a highly oscillating behaviour, and that the therapeutic protocol was frequently modified during the monitoring period. We can perform a deeper inspection of this data by resorting to TA methods. The TA analysis performed is described below:

• **detection of interesting episodes**: in the considered period, we found the episodes reported in Table 3.

Table 3. The TAS episodes detected in the monitoring period (131 days).

TAS	# Occurrences	Total Duration (days)
BASIC		
Hypoglycemia	9	9
Hyperglycemia	27	83
High NPH Insulin	4	14
Low NPH Insulin	8	24
Glycosuria Absent/Traces	28	80
Glycosuria Present	29	51
BGL Increase	42	59
BGL Decrease	46	60
NPH Insulin Increase	20	20
NPH Insulin Decrease	15	17
NPH Insulin Stationarity	21	93
COMPLEX		
Suspected Dawn Effect	29	51
Suspected Somogy Effect	25	32
Metabolic Instability	36	96

From this table it is possible to notice that, during the monitoring period, the patient is in the hyperglycemia state for 63% of the time, and that about

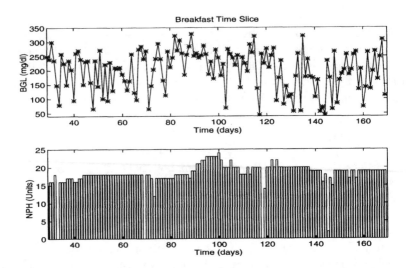

Fig. 1. Breakfast BGL measurements and their *competent* NPH insulin (dinner) dosages.

2 hypoglycemic episodes happen each month. Moreover, BGL measurements are highly unstable, showing a large number of increasing and decreasing episodes. The patient frequently modified the protocol, as shown by the increasing and decreasing episodes of NPH insulin: in about 28% of the time the patient has changed the NPH dose. The number of Suspected Somogy and Dawn effect episodes is relevant, and in particular, Suspected Dawn effect lasts for 39% of the monitoring time. The duration of the metabolic instability episodes indicate that, for 73% of the time, the course of BGL shows high oscillations; this fact is probably due to the very frequent insulin protocol modifications.

• **modal day extraction**: among the various *modal days* that can be extracted from these data, it is of interest to consider the BG-MD and the CA-MD, as well as to calculate the time span distribution of the morning hyperglycemia episodes (see Fig. 2).

MODAL DAYS					
BG-MD			CA-MD		
	mean	sd		mean	sd
Hypoglycemia	0.07	4.87e-04	Low	0.18	1.1e-03
Hyperglycemia	0.63	1.8e-03	Medium	0.72	1.6e-03
Normal	0.3	1.6e-03	High	0.10	7.23e-04

The BG-MD confirms the high percentage of hyperglycemia episodes, while the CA-MD shows a prevalence of medium dosages (between 18 and 20 Units).

Moreover, the histogram of hyperglycemia time spans shows a high number of episodes with duration greater than 3 days; in particular an episode lasts for 19 days.

The lower histogram in Fig. 2 indicates that the patient tried to improve the BGL control by continuously modifying the protocol; probably this was the main

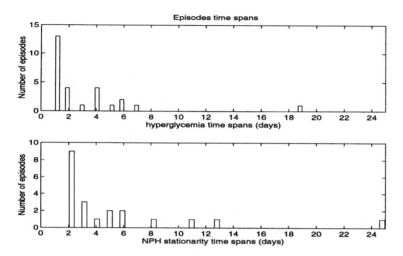

Fig. 2. The histogram of hyperglycemia and NPH stationarity time span distribution.

reason for his metabolic instability.

• **time series analysis of abstracted episodes**: following the steps described in the previous section, we have defined an AS composed by the set of state variables reported above. Then, starting from a day time scale on which we had 131 states (the monitoring period spans 131 days), we obtained a series of 114 states on the transition time scale. The percentage of compression of the AS series is low (13%) mainly because of the recurrent oscillations in the BGL time series. This generates a regular transition time-scale, and therefore allows us to apply AS time series analysis. In this case it is not possible to further reduce the AS dimension, since the patient frequently modified the NPH protocol.

We obtained some interesting results, both in finding the causal relationships among the variables, and in deriving a time-dependent model.

In the following table the counts of BGL states in dependence of the NPH-LEVEL state are shown. The corresponding probabilities appear in parentheses.

BGL	NPH		
	Low	Medium	High
Hypoglycemia	2 (0.0952)	3 (0.0566)	4 (0.1081)
Normal	6 (0.2857)	17 (0.3208)	7 (0.1892)
Hyperglycemia	13 (0.6190)	33 (0.6226)	26 (0.7027)

As the NPH level moves to the High value, the probability of dangerous events increases (hyper and hypoglycemia), showing that high NPH dosages are likely to have negative consequences, increasing metabolic instability.

If we derive the probability of the next BGL level given the previous one, we obtain the following table:

BGL_{s+1}	BGL_s		
	Hypoglycemia	Normal	Hyperglycemia
Hypoglycemia	0	5 (0.1613)	4 (0.0548)
Normal	1 (0.1111)	8 (0.2581)	22 (0.3014)
Hyperglycemia	8 (0.8889)	18 (0.5806)	47 (0.6438)

This table confirms the previously described analysis, showing that the probability of "changing" the current BGL state is quite high; for example if the current BGL level is hypoglycemia, the probability of having hypoglycemia on the next day is 0.

Other interesting information can be derived by counting the occurrences of BGL state episodes in dependence of the more frequent ASs found in the AS sequence. As shown below, when the NPH-LEVEL is *medium* and *stationary*, the BGL-TREND state variable influences the probability of the next BGL state.

BGL_{s+1}	AS_s			
	BGL	BGL-TREND	NPH-LEVEL	NPH-TREND
	Hyperglycemia	Decrease	Medium	Stationary
Hypoglycemia	0 (0.00)			
Normal	9 (0.64)			
Hyperglycemia	5 (0.36)			
	Hyperglycemia	Increase	Medium	Stationary
Hypoglycemia	0 (0.00)			
Normal	2 (0.20)			
Hyperglycemia	8 (0.80)			

Finally, it is interesting to know which conditions trigger hypoglycemic events. By analyzing the ASs that happen before a hypoglycemic event, it is possible to notice that: in 55% of the episodes the BGL was normal; in 45% of the episodes the NPH-LEVEL was high; in 78% of the episodes the NPH-LEVEL was high or normal; in 67% of the episodes the BGL-TREND was decreasing; in 34% of the episodes the NPH-LEVEL was high and the BGL-TREND was decreasing.

These data show once more that the BGL-TREND state variable is a significative feature for predicting BGL, and that above a certain threshold the NPH-LEVEL increases the risk of hypoglycemic events.

5 Conclusions and future work

Traditionally, TAs have been used to summarize the patient's behavior over a predefined time interval; in this paper we have exploited TA methods to interpret long-term monitoring data to explain the dynamics of the patient's evolution. In particular, we suggest several procedures for performing a TA *analysis*: i) *detection of interesting episodes*, ii) *modal day extraction* and iii) *time series analysis of abstracted episodes*.

The diabetes domain is a natural field of application for the above presented techniques, providing a huge amount of data, coming from patients' home monitoring. We have shown with a case-study that TA analysis is a valuable instrument for exploring such longitudinal data, and for searching for relationships among significative events.

We plan to include the here presented analysis techniques in a distributed system for IDDM patients management. In this context, we are interested in automatically deriving a number of therapeutic rules to be given to the patients, for improving their metabolic control. In the future we will exploit the possibility to resort to machine learning techniques in order to derive causal models and sets of rules for the patient to follow during home monitoring.

Acknowledgements. This work is part of the EC project HC-1024, T-IDDM, Telematic Management of Insulin-Dependent Diabetes Mellitus.

References

1. Allen J. F.: Towards a general theory of action and time. Artificial Intelligence **23** (1984) 123–154
2. Bellazzi, R., Cobelli, C., Gomez, E., Stefanelli, M.: The T-IDDM project: Telematic management of Insulin Dependent Diabetes Mellitus. Proc. of Health Telematics '95, M. Bracale, F. Denoth eds., Ischia (1995) 271–276.
3. Bellazzi, R., Larizza, C., Riva, A.: Cooperative Intelligent Data Analysis: an application to diabetic patients management. Proc. of IDAMAP '96, a workshop of ECAI 96, Budapest (1996) 1–6
4. Deutsch, T., Lehmann, E.D., Carson, E.R., Roudsari, A.V., Hopkins, K.D., Sönksen, P.: Time series analysis and control of blood glucose levels in diabetic patients. Comp. Meth. and Programs in Biomed. 41 (1994) 167–182.
5. The Diabetes Control and Complication Trial Research Group. The effect of intensive treatment of diabetes on the development and progression of long-term complications in insulin-dependent diabetes mellitus, The New England Journal of Medicine **14-329** (1993) 977–986
6. Larizza, C., Bernuzzi, G., Stefanelli, M.: A General Framework for Building Patient Monitoring Systems. Lecture Notes in Artificial Intelligence, P. Barahona, M. Stefanelli and J. Wyatt eds., Springer Verlag, Berlin (1995) 91–102
7. Keravnou, E.: Temporal asbtraction of medical data: Deriving periodicity. Proceedings of IDAMAP '96, a workshop of ECAI 96, Budapest (1996) 43–60
8. Miksch, S., Horn, W., Popow, C., Paky, F.: Therapy Planning Using Qualitative Trend Descriptions. Lecture Notes in Artificial Intelligence, P. Barahona, M. Stefanelli and J. Wyatt eds., Springer Verlag, Berlin (1995) 197–208
9. Riva, A., Bellazzi, R.: High level control strategies for diabetes therapy. Lecture Notes in Artificial Intelligence, P. Barahona, M. Stefanelli and J. Wyatt eds., Springer Verlag, Berlin (1995) 185–196
10. Riva, A., Bellazzi, R.: Learning Temporal Probabilistic Causal Models from Longitudinal Data, Artificial Intelligence in Medicine 8 (1996) 217–234
11. Shahar, Y., Musen, M.A.: Knowledge-Based Temporal Abstraction in Clinical Domains. Artificial Intelligence in Medicine 8 (1996) 267–298

Temporal Scenario Recognition for Intelligent Patient Monitoring

Nicolas Ramaux, Dominique Fontaine[a] & Michel Dojat[b].

[a]*Université de Technologie de Compiègne, HEUDIASYC, URA CNRS 817, Compiègne, France.*

[b]*Institut National de la Santé et de la Recherche Médicale, INSERM Unité 296, Créteil, France.*

email:{ramaux, fontaine}@hds.utc.fr, dojat@im3.inserm.fr

Abstract *: The recognition of high level clinical scenes as they are developing is fundamental in patient monitoring. In this paper, we propose a technique to recognize on the fly a session, i.e. the clinical process's evolution, by comparison to a predetermined set of scenarios, i.e. the possible behaviours for this process. We use temporal constraint networks to represent both scenario and session. Specific operations on networks are then applied to perform the recognition task. An index of proximity is introduced to quantify the degree of matching between two temporal networks and used to select the best scenario fitting a session. We explore the application of our technique to the recognition of typical scenarios for mechanical ventilation management.*

Key Words: Temporal Reasoning, Constraint Network, Monitoring, Mechanical Ventilation.

1. INTRODUCTION.

Interpreting data over time is an essential task to diagnose and control processes. The time course of a process, determined from the evolution of a set of representative parameters, is central to predict its future behaviour and to choose actions over time to influence this process. The work presented in this study deals with the same recurrent question [2, 4]: how to recognize dynamically from discrete medical data, high level clinical scenes as they are developing? To answer this question, we propose scenario recognition as a technique to reason about time in dynamic systems when no mathematical model of the process is known to determine completely its behaviour. We apply it to intelligent patient monitoring.

We propose to recognize on the fly the time course of a clinical process by comparison to a predetermined set of possible behaviours for this process. These predetermined behaviours are named scenarios. The recognition of the scenario S (or a part of S) states that the observed time course of the process (called a session S) corresponds to S. This recognition allows us to anticipate forthcoming events from the partial instanciation of the recognized scenario, and to intervene on the process for instance to keep it out of specific expected situations.

For example, a simple scenario S0 excerpt from the management of mechanical ventilation may be the following sequence (see Figure 1):

Part 1: a progressive increase in the respiratory rate appears after a long period of stable ventilation. The last suctioning of the endotracheal tube is reported two hours before. Since no specific events are reported.

Part 2: Few minutes later, an alarm (high respiratory rate) is raised on the ventilator. The patient is then disconnected from the ventilator for suctioning and reconnected to the ventilator. His/her ventilation is erratic during few minutes.

Part 1 suggests that bad ventilation is due to the partial obstruction of the endotracheal tube and Part 2 that bad ventilation is due to the stress generated by the disconnection/reconnection process.

A computerised system capable of recognising gradually the scenario S0, may increase automatically the mechanical assistance before suctioning, to support the increase in the patient's work of breathing due to the partial obstruction of the endotracheal tube. It may adapt the assistance to prevent short stress after reconnection and finally replace an adequate value of assistance when the episode S0 comes to a end.

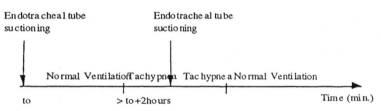

Fig. 1. A typical scenario (s0) excerpt from mechanical ventilation management. It indicates a progressive obstruction of the endotracheal tube followed by ventilation instabilities after suctioning.

The goal of this paper is to propose a technique to recognize automatically from a session a scenario such as S0. S0 will be used as a running example for the rest of the paper. We report the mechanisms used to represent and match a scenario S and a session Σ. Firstly, we present basic definitions for scenario and session. In Section 3, we review the approaches proposed in literature for scenario recognition. Sections 4 and 5 detail respectively how we represent scenarios and sessions and the mechanisms we propose for scenario recognition. Section 6 describes an example of the application of our approach to medical scenario recognition. Then, we discuss several aspects of our work for intelligent patient monitoring and we conclude on the work under development.

2.   SCENARIO AND SESSION: DEFINITIONS.

Our approach is based on two entities: the session and the scenario which are represented by temporal constraints between events occurrences. We take the notions of event, state, time-point and time-interval as primitives. We define a model of change in which events happen at time-points and initiate and/or terminate states which represent a property whose value holds during a time-interval. Similarly to the Event Calculus [12], events occurrences initiate a change in our description of the world.

Session and Scenario have the following definitions:

Session (Σ): This temporal structure represents the real evolution of the observed process in a working situation. The session is perceived via sensors generally with delays and imprecision. The perceived raw data are filtered, processed and finally classified into discrete values, which determine the states of the process. The states succession defines the dynamic of the process's behaviour. Temporal abstractions may be used to construct a concise view of the time course of the process.

Scenario (S): A scenario models an expected evolution of the process. Scenarios are defined by a domain expert who knows, by experience, the probable behaviours of the process in typical working situations and may label them as abnormal or normal. The scenarios are represented with a high level language based on domain concepts familiar to the expert.

According to the type of applications envisaged, two different interpretations for scenario may be considered:

- a scenario models *a class of behaviours*. This definition may be related to the general notion of *Script* [19], which describes a stereotyped sequence of events in a particular context; or to the notion of *Chronicle*, a primitive in the classical temporal logic of McDermott [15], which represents a complete possible history of the process. A chronicle is a way events might go. Scenario recognition is then equivalent to a classification problem: how to match a class (a scenario) with a given pattern (a session)?

- a scenario models *a real previously encountered situation*. A scenario is then considered as an unique case stored in memory (a case base). As proposed with case-based reasoning (CBR) technique, recognition of a scenario consists here in retrieving the previous case from memory and adapting it to fit the session [22]. In CBR, the temporal dimension of scenarios and sessions is generally missing. Recent extensions to introduce time in CBR have been proposed [18]. However, temporal reasoning capabilities remain limited and time does not appear as its main issue.

Clearly, the scenario recognition allows one to act preventively on the process to avoid failures. We do not assume that all the possible situations for a process are modelled and stored in the scenario base. To be efficient in control process, the scenario recognition must be performed on the fly while the session is developing. To be compared, sessions and scenarios must be expressed in the same language.

3. SCENARIO AND SESSION: CONSIDERED AS TEMPORAL NETWORKS.

We consider scenarios as temporal entities modelling a class of behaviours. Temporal representation is then central in our approach. Based on classical work in Artificial Intelligence on temporal logic, two primitives may be used to represent time: *intervals* or *points* [1, 24]. Constraint propagation in the interval algebra is NP-hard. In contrast, point algebra, which is equivalent to a restricted interval algebra, allows one to use propagation algorithms sound, complete and polynomial in time and space [24]. Moreover, point algebra facilitates the management of numeric constraints which is essential in patient monitoring.

We have identified three main point-based approaches to represent scenarios and sessions associated with corresponding temporal reasoning methods. Lévy [13] proposes to represent scenarios and sessions with linear sequences of time-stamped events. Scenario recognition consists in finding a pattern (the complete scenario) in a chain of characters (an ordered collection of events representing the session). With this model it is not possible to introduce uncertainty attached to the temporal occurrence of events. For instance we can not express the fact that two events, e_1 and e_2, should appear in any order but before a third one, e_3.

Scenarios may be represented using temporal constraint networks whose vertices represent time-stamped events and whose edges represent temporal constraints. The more the temporal constraints are relaxed, the more the scenario is general. These constraints may be numeric [3] or symbolic [23] leading to constraint propagation algorithms in $O(n^3)$ or $O(n^2)$ respectively. These two approaches deal with conjunctive temporal constraints and the management of disjunctive constraints is NP-hard [3]. Based on temporal constraint propagation, Dousson et al. [7] model a scenario as a network which contains a set of events e_i and windows of relevance $w(e_i)$, indicating all the possible occurrence dates of possibly forthcoming events e_i. Sessions are represented as a linear sequence of events.

Following [8], we consider both scenario and session as *temporal constraint networks* (see Figure 2). These networks are represented by $G_s = (V_s, E_s)$ and $G_\Sigma = (V_\Sigma, E_\Sigma)$ where V and E are respectively the sets of vertices and edges of each network. The mechanism of recognition consists in matching two temporal networks: one network for the session and one network for the scenario. Then, we dispose of a battery of standard algorithms developed in network theory, to perform operations on sessions and scenarios such as the matching task. For instance we use the well-known path consistency algorithm proposed by [14] to verify the coherence of the networks and to solve the recognition task.

Our model allows us to manage uncertainty attached to the ordering and occurrence of the events that compose the session.

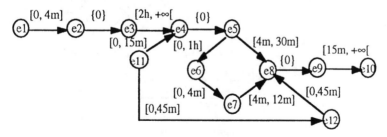

Fig. 2. A temporal network

The figure 2 shows the temporal network that represents the scenario S_0 described above and shown on Figure 1. e_i stands for occurring events and the edges are labelled with numerical temporal constraints. e_1 and e_2 bound disconnection of the patient during suctioning. e_3 and e_4 bound a normal ventilation state. e_5 and e_8 initiates and terminates respectively a tachypnea state. e_6 and e_7 bound patient's disconnection. e_9 initiates and e_{10} terminates a normal ventilation state. e_{11} and e_{12} bound the progressive increasing of respiratory rate. m and h stand for minutes and hours respectively.

4. SCENARIO AND SESSION FOR SUPERVISION TASK.

As indicated on Figure 3, the dedicated module to scenario recognition is a component of our supervisor for patient monitoring.

4.1. THE SUPERVISOR.

The supervisor takes raw data from the controlled process by means of several sensors. Numerical data are classified to obtain symbolic values describing the process and useful to diagnose its current state. Temporal abstractions (such as qualitative trends calculation [16] or aggregation [6]) are performed on numeric and symbolic values, to assess high level concepts describing the time course of the process. The scenario recognition module is fed with information obtained from external sources (laboratory, nurses, ...) and with events generated by the temporal abstraction module. The output of this module is a set of partially or totally recognized scenarios, ordered according to a calculated temporal proximity index [17]. The partial recognition of a scenario generates a set of expected events which are taken into account by the action planning module to intervene on the process. Depending on the situation, the action planning module 1) adapts data processing, 2) proposes to the user a set of actions to perform on the process or 3) acts directly on the process in case of a closed-loop system. For the medical application described in this paper, the controlled process represents a mechanically ventilated patient and actions are performed to adapt the ventilator's settings according to the patient's needs.

This paper describes the scenario recognition module. This module contains a scenario base and specific mechanisms to find the scenarios fitting a session.

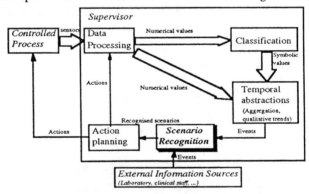

Fig. 3. The global architecture of our supervisor for patient monitoring. Each rectangle represents a specific function of the supervisor.

4.2. SESSION AND SCENARIO REPRESENTATION.

To represent scenario and session, we introduce two basic domain-independent entities: state and event. State and Event refine the general concept of TemporalObject [6] which links a property and a temporal existence. They are similar to the notion of *time-objects* introduced in [11] with a set of temporal, causal and structural relations. A state state(Value, Ival) represents a property whose value (Value) holds during the validity interval Ival associated to it. For instance, an assertion such as RespiratoryRateTrend(increasing, [t1, t2]) means that the respiratory rate increases during the period included between the instants t1 and t2. Event and state are basic temporal objects and are subclassed to introduce more specific objects (VentilationDiagnosis or RespiratoryState for instance).

4.2.1. SCENARIO REPRESENTATION.

Scenario is represented by using a temporal constraint network. Temporal constraints C_{ij} between two time-stamped events e_i and e_j are expressed with equalities or inequalities between their respective event occurrence dates t_i and t_j:

$$C_{ij} = t_j - t_i \in V_{i=1}^{n} [b_i, b_{i+1}] \quad b_i, b_{i+1} \in \Re \cup \{+\infty, -\infty\}.$$

Each scenario contains a conclusion part triggered when the scenario is recognized or rejected. The triggering has for effect the introduction of a new set of events or states used to pursue the reasoning. A scenario is formed of four parts: name, type (abnormal, ...), body (state, events and temporal constraints), and conclusion.

Conclusion part is triggered if temporal constraints between events and states, which appear in the scenario's body, are verified in the session. In the following example, the conclusion states that the tube has been obstructed and his/her secretions are abundant. States or Events are used to represent s_0, for instance states are used to represent patient's respiratory states and respiratory rate trends. Events are used to indicate the patient's disconnection from the ventilator.

```
Name :
ProgressiveEndotrachealTubeObstructionFollowedByUnstabilitiesAfterSuctioning
Type: Abnormal
Body:
                    States
        RespiratoryState(normal, [t3, t4])
        RespiratoryState(tachypnea, [t5, t8])
        RespiratoryState(normal, [t9, t10])
        RespiratoryRateTrend(increasing, [t11, t12])
                    Events
        Disconnection(t1)
        Reconnection(t2)
        Disconnection(t6)
        Reconnection(t7)
                    Temporal constraints
        t2-t1 ∈ [0, 4]
        t3-t2 ∈ [0, 0]
        t4-t3 ∈ [120, +∞[
        t5-t4 ∈ [0, 0]
        t11-t4 ∈ [0, 15]
        t6-t5 ∈ ]0, 60]
        t8-t5 ∈ [4, 30]
        t7-t6 ∈ [0, 4]
        t8-t7 ∈ [4, 12]
        t12-t8 ∈ [0, 45]
        t9-t8 ∈ [0, 0]
        t10-t9 ∈ [15, +∞[
        t12-t11 ∈ [0, 45]
Conclusion:
        EndotrachealTubeState(Obstructed, [t5, t6])
        SecretionTendency.Value = high
```

Fig. 4. Representation of the scenario s_0.

The figure 4 represents the complete scenario s_0. Before its incorporation into the scenario base, each scenario is transformed into a point algebra network and then the minimal labelling network[1] is computed (see Figure 5). For each state introduced into the scenario's definition, two events are incorporated automatically corresponding to its initiation and termination. For instance, RespiratoryState(normal, [t₃, t₄]) implies the introduction of two DiagnosticVentilation events: DiagnosticVentilation (t₃, initiates, RespiraytoryState = Normal), DiagnosticVentilation (t₄, terminates, RespiratoryState = Normal).

4.2.2. SESSION REPRESENTATION.

The session is incrementally built from the coming events. Each time a proposition change is detected by the temporal abstractions module, two events are generated. For instance, when at time t_5 RespiratoryState changes from Normal to Tachypnea, two diagnosis are introduced into the session: d_1 = DiagnosticVentilation (t₅, terminates, RespiraytoryState = Normal) and d_2 = DiagnosticVentilation (t₅, initiates, RespiraytoryState = Tachypnea). The date t_5 may be imprecise due to the response time of the complete chain including sensors, data processing, classification and temporal abstraction. t_5 is included into a temporal interval ($t_5 \in [bs, be]$).

5. SCENARIO AND SESSION: TEMPORAL MATCHING.

In the process of scenario recognition we compare a set of scenarios to the current session.

We consider that s is a solution of G, s ∈ sol(G), where G=(V, E), s ={(vᵢ, tᵢ)}, i ∈ {1,...n}, n=card(V), v_i ∈ V and t_i ∈ $\Re$ (date of occurrence of ei associated to vi) iff ∀c_{ij} ∈ E, $t_j - t_i$ ∈ C_{ij}.

Two solutions $a = \left\{\left(v_1^a, t_1^a\right), \left(v_2^a, t_2^a\right), \dots, \left(v_n^a, t_n^a\right)\right\}$ and $b = \left\{\left(v_1^b, t_1^b\right), \left(v_2^b, t_2^b\right), \dots, \left(v_k^b, t_k^b\right)\right\}$, are compatible comp(a,b), iff

comp(a,b) ⟺ ∀i ∈ {0,.., max(n,k)} if $v_i^a = v_i^b$ then $t_1^a = t_1^b$.

Let $G_s=(V_s, E_s)$ and $G_\Sigma=(V_\Sigma, E_\Sigma)$ be the respective networks associated to the scenario S and the session Σ, we define three possible relations:

- *satisfaction*: Σ satisfies S if *one can be sure* that the events of Σ satisfy the temporal constraints of S:
  sat(Σ, S) ⟺ ∀a ∈ sol(G_Σ), ∃b ∈ sol(G_s) / . comp(a,b)

- *compatibility*: Σ is compatible with S if *it is possible* that the events of Σ satisfy the temporal constraints of S:
  comp(Σ, S) ⟺ ∃a ∈ sol(G_Σ), ∃b ∈ sol(G_s) / . comp(a,b)

- *incompatibility*: Σ is incompatible with S if one can be sure that the events of Σ do not satisfy the temporal constraints of S:
  incomp(Σ, S) ⟺ ∀a ∈ sol(G_Σ), ¬∃b ∈ sol(G_s) / . comp(a,b)

---

[1] This operation consists in finding the minimal constraint network minG which has the same solutions as the network G.

To determine the relation corresponding to a couple session/scenario we use standard operations on temporal networks. Compatibility (resp. Incompatibility) is established if the minimal network F, obtained from the *fusion*[2] of G_s and G_r leads to a *coherent*[3] (resp. *incoherent*) network. Moreover, if F is included into G_r satisfiability is demonstrated [8]. Clearly, the relation between a session and a scenario is evolutive, function of a the progressive construction of the session. Fontaine [8] proposes an algorithm based on the concept of *updated scenario* to recognize incrementally the session on the fly: each time an event predicted by a scenario occurs, its occurrence date is taken into account and the temporal constraints are updated. The Figure 5 outlines the different steps of the scenario recognition.

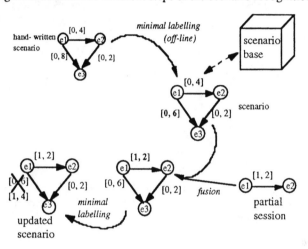

Fig. 5. The different steps to build and recognize a scenario.

The first minimal labelling changes the constraint c_{13} initially set to [0,8] to [0, 6]. The operation of fusion between the partial session and the scenario places c_{12} initially set to [0,4] to [1,2]. Then the minimal labelling modifies c_{13} to [1,4].

The hand-written scenario is transformed into a minimal point algebra network and stored into our scenario base. This scenario is then retrieved to be matched on the fly to the partial session. The operations of fusion (between session and scenario) and minimal labelling are performed to construct the updated scenario. The recognition of a scenario is stopped when the action planner decides that this scenario is no longer relevant (change of context or incompatibility) or when the scenario is totally recognized.

---

[2] The fusion operation of G1 and G2 consists in computing the intersection of two overnetworks of G1 and G2.

[3] A minimal network is coherent if and only if it has at least one solution.

6. AN EXAMPLE OF MEDICAL SCENARIO RECOGNITION.

We illustrate the use of our technique with the gradual recognition of a part of the scenario s_0 previously described (Figures 1, 2 and 4).

Time origin is the occurrence date of the first disconnection, e_1. An agenda stores the expected events. At time $t=0$, the events in our agenda are e_2 and e_3, both expected between 0 and 4 min.

Event	Interval
e_2	[0, 4m]
e_3	[0, 4m]

This agenda is updated only when an expected event occurs or when the system clock reaches a time equal to the smallest upper bound of the set of expected time intervals.

Hence, at time $t=0$, the supervisor concludes that if no events occur this agenda should not be updated before 4 min. At $t=2$ min., the supervisor is informed that e_2 occurred between 1 and 3 min. after e_1. The session and the updated scenario networks are:

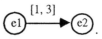

The representation of updated scenario networks is restricted to the session's nodes. The updated agenda is:

Event	Interval
e_3	[0, 2m]

At $t=3$ min, the supervisor is informed that e_3 occurred simultaneously with e_2. The session's network is

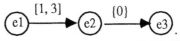

After detecting e_3, the events e_4, e_5 and e_{11} appear in the agenda. The expected time interval for e_{11} has been previously calculated during the minimal labelling and is equal to: $[45m, +\infty[$.

Event	Interval
e_4	$[2h, +\infty[$
e_5	$[2h, +\infty[$
e_{11}	$[45m, +\infty[$

50 min. after the occurrence of e_3, the supervisor is informed that e_{11} occurred between 44 and 46 min. after e_3.

The session (left) and updated scenario networks (right) become:

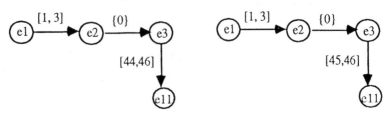

After the occurrence of e11, the agenda is :

Event	Interval
e_4	[70m, +∞[
e_5	[70m, +∞[
e_{12}	[0, 45m]

Each time a new event appears in the session, the agenda is updated with the same technique as detailed above. For each scenario partially recognized, the outputs of the scenario recognition module is the agenda which contains the expected events.

In our previous example, we have recognized the normal ventilation (e_3) following the reconnection of the patient (e_2) and the beginning of the increase in the respiratory rate (e_{11}). The scenario recognition module predicts that the increase in the respiratory rate will last no longer than 47 minutes (e_{12}). The ventilation will remain normal for 70 minutes (e_4) and will be followed by a tachypnea (e_5).

7. DISCUSSION

In medical domains several approaches have been proposed to allow computerised interpretation of physiological parameters over time. With the Résumé system [20], Shahar et al. propose a knowledge-based framework to build automatically, from raw data, high level temporal abstractions. Similarly, in NéoGanesh, a closed-loop system for artificial ventilation control [6], uses two specific abstractions mechanisms, *aggregation* and *forgetting*, to dynamically interpret ventilation parameters and define the actions to perform in real-time on the ventilator. In Vie-Vent [16], Miksch et al. introduce sophisticated methods for qualitative trends descriptions of monitoring data. TrenDx, [10], detects data consistent with a set of domain-specific predetermined patterns called trend templates. All these approaches are built with specific goals: match efficiently data against patterns for TrenDx, interpret data and define therapeutic actions in real-time for Vie-Vent and NéoGanesh, and generate temporal abstractions for Résumé.

In this paper we propose clinical scenario recognition as a technique for temporal reasoning in intelligent patient monitoring. Clinical scenario recognition is complementary to the techniques described above: the session we want to recognize might be constructed using similar techniques. The notion of clinical scenarios (or clinical scenes) to reflect physiological processes was introduced previously in [2]. Our main innovation is to consider both scenario and session as temporal networks. The consequence of this choice is to provide us with:

• a high level of *temporal expressiveness* for session and scenario representation. Temporal constraint networks offer a natural way to express uncertainty linked to the date of occurrence of events. Relative temporal ordering of events can be introduced both in session and scenario. Generally, in process supervision all the pertinent events are time-stamped. This corresponds to the approach proposed in [7]. However, in the medical domain some events are not automatically recorded and their occurrence date is only known with uncertainty and relatively to other events. For instance, the supervisor may be informed by the clinical staff that the pulse rate dropped between half an hour to one hour before the starting of the severe tachypnea.

• an *uniform representation* for sessions and scenarios. This allows us to order the recognized scenarios according to the temporal proximity index defined by [17]. Moreover, similarly to case-based reasoning, scenarios could be automatically learnt from recorded sessions.

The use of temporal networks for scenario representation has been proposed [9] to tackle another problem relative to process monitoring: planning a useful/optimal sequence of measurements to discriminate among competing scenarios. This approach is mainly concerned with qualitative scenarios and then use an interval-based algebra.

The drawback of our approach is its computational cost. However, we are interested in applications such as ventilation management where real time constraints are not too hard (response time between 1 sec. to 1 min.). Thus, we believe that a scenario recognition module can be integrated successfully into a ventilation supervisor.

8. CONCLUSION AND FUTURE WORK

Scenario recognition seems well-suited for patient monitoring tasks. We are currently implementing such a module and evaluating its real-time performances. In order to facilitate the recognition process, we must organise the scenario base according to specific relations between scenarios such as causality, inheritance or similarity. Scenario recognition generates information about the predicted behaviour of the controlled process. More knowledge has to be incorporated into the action planner module to deal with these predictions in order to act preventively on the process to avoid undesirable situations.

The construction of the scenario base is a crucial point. We elaborate, in collaboration with clinicians, typical clinical scenarios from data obtained with a computerised system used in ICU for the automatic control of mechanical ventilation [5].

Systems providing automated support for guideline-based clinical care need to recognize user's intentions and plans to achieve them [21]. Our future work includes applying temporal scenario recognition to this task.

9. REFERENCES

[1] J. F. Allen, *Maintaining knowledge about temporal intervals*, Communications of the ACM, 26 (1983) 832-843.

[2] A. I. Cohn, S. Rosenbaum, M. Factor and P. L. Miller, *DYNASCENE: An approach to computer-based intelligent cardiovascular monitoring using sequential clinical "scenes"*, Meth. Inform. Med., 29 (1990) 122-131.

[3] R. Dechter, I. Meiri and P. Judea, *Temporal constraints networks*, Artif. Intell., 4 (1991) 61-95.

[4] D. DeCoste, *Dynamic across-time measurement interpretation*, Artif. Intell., 51 (1991) 273-341.

[5] M. Dojat, A. Harf, D. Touchard, M. Laforest, F. Lemaire and L. Brochard, *Evaluation of a knowledge-based system providing ventilatory management and decision for extubation*, Am. J. Respir. Crit. Care Med., 153 (1996) 997-1004.

[6] M. Dojat and C. Sayettat, *A realistic model for temporal reasoning in real-time patient monitoring*, A.A.I., 10 (1996) 121-143.

[7] C. Dousson, P. Gaborit and M. Ghallab, *Situation recognition: representation and algorithms*, 13th International Joint Conference on Aritificial Intelligence (1993), Chambéry (Fr), 166-172.

[8] D. Fontaine, N. Ramaux *An approach by graphs for the recognition of temporal scenarios*, IEEE Transactions on Systems, Man and Cybernetics (1997) (to appear).

[9] J. Gamper and W. Nejdl, *Proposing measurements in dynamic systems*, 14th International Joint Conference on Aritificial Intelligence (1995), Montréal (Ca), 784-790.

[10] I. J. Haimowitz and I. S. Kohane, *Automated trend detection with alternate temporal hypothesis*, International Joint Conference on Artificial Intelligence (1993), Chambéry (Fr), 146-151.

[11] E. T. Keravnou, *Temporal diagnosis reasoning based on time-objects*, Artif. Intell. in Med., 8 (1996) 235-265.

[12] R. A. Kowalski and M. J. Sergot, *A logic-based calculus of events*, New Generation Computing, 4 (1986) 67-95.

[13] F. Lévy, *Recognizing scenarios: a study*, Workshop on diagnosis from first principles (DX-94) (1994), New Paltz.

[14] A. K. Mackworth, *Consistency in networks of relations*, Artif. Intell., 8 (1977) 99-118.

[15] D. McDermott, *A temporal logic for reasoning about processes and plans*, Cognitive science, 6 (1982) 101-155.

[16] S. Miksch, W. Horn, C. Popow and F. Paky, *Therapy planning using qualitative trend descriptions*, 5th conference on Artificial Intelligence in Medicine Europe, AIME'95 (1995), Pavia (IT), 197-208.

[17] N. Ramaux and D. Fontaine, *Recognizing a temporal scenarios by calculating a proximity index between constraint graphs*, International Conference on Tools in Artificial Intelligence (ICTAI'96) (1996), Toulouse (Fr), 464-467.

[18] S. Rougegrez, *Similarity evaluation between observed behaviours for the prediction of processes*, First European workshop on case-based reasoning (1994), 59-64.

[19] R. C. Schank and R. P. Abelson, *Scripts, plans, goals and understanding*. (Erlbaum, Hillsdale, N J, 1977).

[20] Y. Shahar, *A knowledge-based temporal abstraction in clinical domains*, Artif. Intell. in Med., 8 (1996) 267-298.

[21] Y. Shahar and M. A. Musen, *Plan recognition and revision in support of guideline-based care*, Technical Report KSL-94-70, Stanford University, 1994.

[22] S. Slade, *Case-based reasoning: a research paradigm*, Artif. Intell. Mag., 12 (1991) 42-55.

[23] P. Van Beek, Reasoning about qualitative temporal information, Artif. Intell., 58 (1992) 297-326.

[24] M. Vilain and H. Kautz, *Constraint propagation algorithms for temporal reasoning*, AAAI (1986), Philadelphia, 377-382.

Medical Planning Environment

Danielle Ziébelin
INRIA-Rhône-Alpes
655 avenue de l'Europe
F38330 Montbonnot Saint Martin
e-mail : Danielle.Ziebelin@imag.fr,

Annick Vila
Laboratoire EMG-EFSN
CHU B.P 217X
F38043 La Tronche
e-mail : Annick.Vila@imag.fr

1. Medical planning decision

Electromyography (EMG)is a set of electrophysiological techniques allowing to define neuromuscular disease diagnosis. The electromyographic diagnosis is carried out from a systematic acquisition of numeric and symbolic data. It is decomposed into a set of well defined steps : formulation of hypotheses and specialised examination procedure suited to the patient under study, evaluation of test and procedure results, validation or questioning of the current hypothesis, elaboration of a conclusion. The domain of EMG is broad, covering more than a hundred existing diagnoses, exploiting knowledge belonging to various kinds of data, including about four thousand tests of nervous or muscular structures. The complexity of EMG examination of course raises problems, specially for novice practitioners. Most often, they exceed or fall short of what is required. In the first case, they propose heavy, costly and painful examination for the patient by fear of forgetting tests. In opposition, in the second case, they tend to propose an insufficient examination procedure, without considering for example case of associated pathologies. To cope with this complexity of the EMG diagnosis, we are developing a knowledge based system, MYOSYS, which takes into account the expert experience from the symptoms evocation until the tests procedure elaboration. Our objective is to provide an optimal test procedure for a given diagnosis.

2. Knowledge representation

To modelise and implement medical planning reasoning, we required the representation of three types of knowledge : reasoning knowledge represented by tasks, operational knowledge represented by methods and medical concepts represented by entities.
- *Tasks* : a task describes the different actions to be executed by the EMGer, and associates the adequate hierarchical reasoning strategy. The automatic medical reasoning is based on recursive decomposition of complex tasks in more elementary subtasks.
- *Methods* : methods constitute the leaves of these recursive task decomposition strategies. They refer to internal basic inference or to external software programs and describe their instructions of use.
- *Entities* : entities are introduced to represent knowledge manipulated by the tasks (and methods) and describe the input and output information needed for task and method execution [Marino &al 90].
The complete knowledge is represented under object form. The knowledge concerning entities is an object-centred knowledge base management system, Shirka, [Rechenmann & 91], based on a notion similar to frames. To represent the knowledge concerning tasks and methods, a specific object centred model has been defined. This model relies on the same elementary object centred concepts. Therefore the uniform object centred knowledge representation allows to apply the same reasoning mechanisms to tasks, methods and entities. The classification mechanism is used in general to reason about object class hierarchies[Marino&al 90]. It is also used by the

task engine to reason about tasks. In the following, we first expose with Shirka elementary object centred concepts. This immediately shows how entities are represented via object classes. Afterwards, the object centred representation of tasks and methods is explained.

3. Entities representation

Shirka is an object-centred knowledge base management system that relies on the class-instance shift. A class, in the same way as its instances, is defined in a scheme via its set of slots. A slot is in turn defined by a list of facets, and a facet by a list of values. Such a value is either a scheme or a reference to a scheme. Every slot is typed via the facet $a (or $list-of, for slots that support multiple values). This facet associates an elementary type (such as integer, real, ...) or a complex type (an object class) to the slot. An object is called complex if the type of at least one of his slots refers to an object class (figure 1). The description of a slot might be completed by other facets that constrain the domain of the slot value or that define ways to infer this value. The classes are organised in acyclic graphs, in class hierarchies. Classes describing different medical concepts are organised in different hierarchies. Via inheritance a class in the hierarchy transmits the knowledge and constraints defined for its slots to all its subclasses (figure 1). This knowledge might be precise and completed in the subclasses, but not contradicted. We identified three types of concepts : initial concepts representing input entities at the beginning of the planning process (symptoms, signs, favoring factors ...), some concepts representing deduced information (disease, hypotheses, tests procedures, tests results), and secondary concepts allowing to precise the former one, for example anatomy concepts and topography which precise the localisation of a symptom, of a pain, or the localisation of a test [Johnsen & al 94].

```
{ symptom
      kind-of           =        clinical-sign
      apparition-site list-of anatomy
      group             is-astring
                        domain   paresthesiæ, cramp, pain, palsy
      ... }
```

Figure 1 : A simplified class scheme and the associated class hierarchy, describing the class *symptom*. The figure shows that *symptom* is a complex object: the slot *apparition-site* refers with *anatomy* to another object class. This figure presents only a subset of the symptom' slots and facets.

4. Representation of tasks and methods

Medical planning reasoning might be defined at different abstraction levels by different, more or less specific task descriptions. At a low abstraction level, the task is sufficiently precise, so that a problem solving strategy can be associated to the task description. The set of input and output entities and the problem solving strategy constitute the most essential parts of a task definition. The problem solving strategy describes how a complex task can be decomposed into more elementary subtasks. Each subtask may be in turn a complex task, or refer to a method ; in this case it is directly solved through the execution of an associated software program. The *control flow* describes how the subtasks are to be chained to solve the complex task itself. Different operators are available to combine subtasks: *sequence, parallel, iteration, choice* and *user-task*. A subtask is a user-task if the user indicates the result of the task.

```
{evoke-and-localise
            kind-of         =        task;
      &input  patient-sign  list-of  clinical-sign;
```

345

```
&output patient hypotheses    list-of    hypotheses;
        patient-factors       list-of    favoring-factors;
strategy:choice(evoke-from-neuroanatomy,evoke-from-topography);
...}
```

Figure 2 - Simplified definition of the *evoke-and-localise*. This complex task describes an evocation and a localisation of disease hypotheses. The input data are the **clinical** signs of patient. The outputs of this task represent the **hypotheses** and the **favoring factors of each hypothesis**. The solving **strategy** consist in solving a choice of two subtasks.

Figure 2 gives an example for a task description. As tasks are modelled by object classes, they are organised in hierarchies. Each global problem is modelled inside a separate class hierarchy. This organisation provides a way to structure for each task the available problem solving strategies using operators : choice, sequence, iteration, parallel. Each class inside this hierarchy models the task at a different abstraction level, and associating the adapted problem solving strategy. Depending on the characteristics of the entities that form a precise problem context, the choice of the adequate problem solving strategy can therefore be supported by a classification process over the hierarchy of tasks. An example for task classification is given in figure 3.

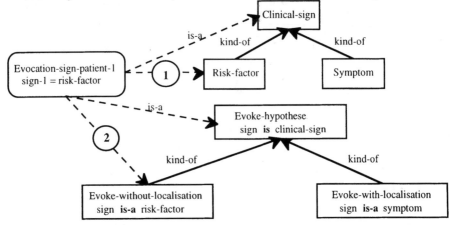

Figure 3 : Example for the classification of tasks. This example shows in the lower part the simplified class hierarchy concerning the task *evoke-hypothesis*. The *sign* to analyse are represented by a *clinical-sign*. But the more specialised evocation types (Evoke-without-localisation, Evoke-with-localisation) are only adapted to more specific types of clinical-signs. When an evocation has to be done (*evocation-sign-patient-1*) the initial sign (*sign-1*) is provided (upper left). The classification of sign-*1* inside its proper class hierarchy, shown in simplified form in the upper right, allows to determine what specific evocation type can be executed.

As indicated above, the recursive task decomposition strategies finally refer to methods. Also methods are defined via object classes. These classes describe the input / output entities of the methods and associate direct means to solve them.

5. The task engine

The task engine exploits the knowledge base for automatically solving problems. Different phases are distinguished in the problem solving process and in the task engine's functioning:
- The *instantiation phase*: the class corresponding to the initial task to execute is instantiated ; its input entities are determined.

- The *classification phase*: according to the characteristics of these input entities, the solving strategy is chosen ; this is done applying the classification mechanism that determines which subclasses are appropriate in the specific problem context. Missing input information can be inferred or asked to the user during classification. The constraints concerning this information are then verified. The task-instance is finally attached to the chosen subclass.
- The *input completion and validation phase*: missing input entities or parameters are obtained and the preconditions defined for the task verified.
- The *execution or decomposition phase*: the solving strategy associated to the problem description is executed. Each sub-task refers in turn either to a complex task, which is executed applying recursively the same algorithm, or to a method and with the method a software program, that is directly executed. The execution of a subtask is integrated in the global problem solving process as defined in the execution-context that links it to the complex task.
- The *output completion and validation phase*: the global output entities are synthesized. The constraints concerning them are verified.
- Finally a *general view* of all the output entities is shown to the user.
  A task may fail during any of these phases, either because the selected specialisation was a bad one, or because some constraints concerning input or output were not satisfied, or because one of its subtasks failed, or furthermore because of a user's intervention. Then the task engine backtracks: it turns back to the last decision point in order to explore another branch of reasoning.

6. Conclusion

To help the novice practitioners and cope with the complexity of the EMG test procedure elaboration, we developped MYOSYS, an hierarchical planning environment. Building an EMG knowledge base consists in formalizing and structuring medical concepts and actions. The knowledge modeling to be done concerns tasks i.e. possible problems, methods corresponding to elementary part of resolution and medical entities. All are represented under object form structured in separate class hierarchies and are accessible for the user. At each step of the resolution process an adequate placement of the instance in the corresponding class hierarchy has to by found, depending on the input/output entities of the task and on its strategy. The identification of this placement can be supported by classification and plan recognition techniques.

7. Bibliography

[Johnsen & al 94]   Johnsen B., Vingtoft S., Fuglsang-Frederiksen A., Barahona P., Fawcett P., Jakobsen L., Liguori R., Nix W., Otte G., Schofield I., Sieben G., Talbot A., Veloso M., Vila A., *A common structure for the representation of data and diagnostic processes within clinical neurophysiology*, Proc. Conf. MIE 94 12th international congress, Lisbon, Portugal, may 94.
[Marino & al 90]   Marino O., Rechenmann F., Uvietta P., *Multiple perspectives and classification mechanism in objet-oriented representation*. Proc. of ECAI' 90, Stockholm, Sweden.
[Rechenmann 91]   Rechenmann F., *Modelling tasks and methods in knowledge-based PDE solver"*, Proc. IMACS'91, Dublin, Irlande, 22-26 juin 1991.

Strengthening Argumentation in Medical Explanations by Text Plan Revision*

Fiorella de Rosis[1], Floriana Grasso[2] and Dianne C. Berry[3]

[1] Dipartimento di Informatica, Università di Bari, Italy
e-mail: derosis@gauss.uniba.it
[2] Department of Computing & Electrical Engineering, Heriot-Watt University,
Edinburgh, UK, e-mail: floriana@cee.hw.ac.uk
[3] Department of Psychology, University of Reading, UK
e-mail: d.c.berry@reading.ac.uk

Abstract. Explanations are an important by-product of medical decision-support activities, as they have proved to favour compliance and correct treatment performance. To achieve this purpose, these texts should have a strong argumentation content and should adapt to emotional, as well as to rational attitudes of the Addressee. This paper describes how *Rhetorical Sentence Planning* can contribute to this aim: the rule-based plan discourse revision is introduced between Text Planning and Linguistic Realization, and exploits knowledge about the user personality and emotions and about the potential impact of domain items on user compliance and memory recall. The proposed approach originates from analytical and empirical evaluation studies of computer generated explanation texts in the domain of drug prescription.

1 Introduction

Explanations are an important by-product of any medical decision support activity, as they substantiate the system suggestions by favouring, at the same time, compliance and correct treatment performance. To achieve their goals, these messages have to be formulated in a clear and convincing way, and their arguments have to be adapted to the addressee. Whenever possible, they have to be generated by exploiting information from already established sources, rather than requiring ad hoc data collection.

In the last few years, several text generation systems have been designed in order to produce effective explanations. In these systems, the generation process is made up of a phase of *Text Planning*, in which information content and order and rhetorical structure are established, followed by a phase of *Linguistic Realisation*, in which the plan is translated into an understandable, coherent message [7]. More recently, the limitations of this approach have become apparent, and several authors are now investigating how to bridge the gap between the

---

* This work was partially supported by a British-Italian Collaboration in Research and Higher Education Project, which involved the Universities of Reading and of Bari, in 1996.

two phases. Methods proposed introduce, between Text Planning and Linguistic Realisation, a phase which is usually denoted as *Sentence Planning* [8, 10]. In this intermediate phase, *local* refinement techniques are applied to increase the quality of the generated text. For example: aggregating clauses or elements internal to a clause, defining how to realise rhetorical relations, or the salience nucleus/satellite and so on [11, 2, 13].

It is our opinion that, although there is a real need for style refinement in complex text generation (especially when existing information sources are employed), this new phase of *Plan Revision* should also be aimed at strengthening argumentation in the text: this requires developing methods which consider the emotional state of the addressees, as well as their knowledge. This claim is indirectly supported by Dalianis and Hovy: "text length (i.e. redundancy of words) is not the best measure of readability of aggregated texts. Instead, a better measure is internal (structural) coherence" [2]. Sentence optimisation then originates not only from linguistic needs, but also (in some cases, mainly) from rhetorical ones.

On the other side, the importance of argumentation in medical explanations has been proved by several experimental psychologists, who have argued that "enlistment of the patient by the physician is promoted by the use of inclusive language, that is, language that explicitly recognises patients' competence and thus treats them with respect. We believe that such language increases the physician's (and possibly also the prospective system's) chances of having the patient hear the diagnosis and treatment recommendations" [5].

In her paper about the generation of *empathetic responses* in a dialogue about medical treatment, Haimovitz [6] argues that, to produce texts suited to the direct and the indirect users' needs, sentences with a given information content should be generated so as to "stress favourable information while downplaying or offsetting unfavourable information". This effect can be obtained by exploiting knowledge about the indirect user's *concerns* and *worries*, in addition to domain knowledge about the possible *impact* of information items. A *very sensitive test* or a *non invasive treatment* are examples of favourable information, whereas *a very long hospital stay* or *a painful procedure* are examples of an unfavourable one. The *cost* of an utterance is calculated as a function of the addressee's characteristics (for example: anxiety about pain); the *accent* of a sentence is then modified by joining sentences with appropriate conjunctions, or by introducing *detensifier* or *intensifier* adverbs.

The work reported in this paper is the continuation of a European Research Project OPADE which was aimed at designing and prototyping a decision support system in the domain of drug prescription. A text generator was designed as part of that Project, from a corpus of explanations provided by doctors. Texts generated were submitted to informal and formal evaluations, which confirmed their interest but also revealed a number of limitations in the method developed. In this paper, after briefly describing the structure of our generator (Sect. 2), we will examine these limitations (Sect. 3). We will then prove that they cannot be solved by a purely stylistic revision of the text, but require a more complex *Plan Revision and Refinement*, which exploits knowledge about the domain, as well as about the addressee (Sect. 4). We will then outline (in Sect. 5) a method which solves part of these problems. Some consideration about the limitations of this approach will conclude the paper (Sect. 6).

2 The Context

The explanation component of OPADE generates a text which illustrates the prescription by retrieving information from a set of heterogeneous databases: a medical record, a drug database and a prescription record. The generation process combines hierarchical Text Planning with a Linguistic Realisation based on Augmented Transition Networks [3]. The message produced is adapted to the Speaker (the doctor who made the prescription) and to the addressee (the patient, a nurse or a doctor's colleague): two user models represent the main attitudes of the two users. Adaptation of the message is made in the planning phase (by introducing in plan operators conditions about the context), as well as in the Linguistic Realisation (by attaching similar conditions to ATN's arcs). The discourse plan is represented in OPADE as a tree, whose leaves correspond to primitive communicative actions; a communicative goal and a rhetorical relation are associated with its intermediate and root nodes. An example of the top part of a plan tree is shown in Fig. 1. This plan includes the following main

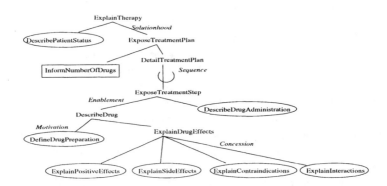

Fig. 1. An example of the top part of a discourse plan

components (which are encircled with an oval):
- A *Persuade about the need of treatment*, realised by means of a description of the health problems that the prescription intends to solve.
- A *Request to perform the treatment*, with information about the number of drugs in the prescription.
- A detailed description of the treatment plan. Drugs are considered in sequence, by introducing, for each of them: (i) a *Request to administer the drug*, with a description of its characteristics; (ii) a *Persuade that the drug is useful and not harmful*, with an illustration of its positive effects (efficacy) and of the negative

ones (side effects, contraindications, interactions with other drugs), and (iii) an *Enable to administer the drug correctly*, with a detailed description of administration modalities. An example of text generated from this plan in shown in Fig. 2. This text is subdivided (for explicative purposes) into *discourse segments* which are the expansion of the encircled goals in Fig. 1. A sample of texts generated was evaluated by

Comments to the drug prescription for Mr Fictif

DS1 You have been diagnosed as suffering from a mild form of what we call 'angina', that is a spasm of chest resulting form over-exertion when hearth is diseased. In addition, you have elevated cholesterol.

DS2 To solve these problems, there are two drugs I would like you to take.

DS3 The first one is Aspirin, which is a analgesic, that is it relieves the pain.

DS4 This drug has been shown to reduce the risk of hearth attack and prevents abnormal blood clotting within five minutes.

DS5 The only problem is that this drug can be associated with some side effects. The first one is bleedings, that is a slight hemorrhage; it can be a serious side effect but occurs infrequently. In the unlikely event that this occurs, I suggest you to stop treatment. The second one is allergic reaction; it can be a serious side effect but doesn't happen commonly; it occurs especially when the patient is suffering from what we call 'atopic disease', that is a hypersensitivity to substances having a basis of hereditary predisposition. In case you notice that this problem occurs, you should stop treatment.

DS6 I must also prevent you that this drug may interfere with many others. One interaction is with Vitamin K inhibitors; this could cause increased bleeding risk. Therefore, please follow carefully your prescription, do not take other drugs without telling your physician and do not stop treatment without your physician's advice.

DS7 You have to take this drug by mouth; take it with water, at regular intervals. If you miss a dose, do not modify rhythm or quantity of the following ones. Regarding administration of this drug, the treatment steps are the following. The first one is a attack treatment. The dosage is 1 gr in 2 intakes for 1 day. You have to take one tablet of 500 mg at 8 am and one tablet of 500 mg at 8 pm. The second one is a maintenance treatment. The dosage is 500 mg in 1 intake for 7 days. You have to take one tablet of 500 mg at 20.

DS8 The second drug I will give you is Glyceril Trinitrate...

......

DSf These are the main treatment suggestions I wanted to give you. If you need any more information, please do not hesitate to ask me directly.

Fig. 2. An example of text generated from OPADE

representatives of OPADE's final users: in this informal evaluation, explanation texts were considered as very interesting for both patients and health professionals, especially considering that, in general, this type of information is only provided verbally (if at all). Subsequently, we performed two more formal evaluation studies. In a first *analytical evaluation*, we compared the artificial texts with the corpus of explanations that were employed to define the generation method. In a second, *empirical study*, we evaluated the efficacy, on the addressee, of texts built by varying information content and order. The two studies highlighted several limitations in the generated texts, and provided a number of cues on how better texts might be obtained.

3 Limitations of Texts Generated

3.1 Comparison with the Corpus of Explanations

Our corpus of explanations included 36 texts, produced by 6 doctors on 4 clinical cases (two cases of angina in a male and a female aged patient, a case of tuberculosis and a case of subacute thyroditis). Although the computer generated explanations reproduce the overall characteristics of these texts, several elements contribute to increase the *argumentative strength* of natural messages, and are not reproduced in the artificial ones.

Enlistening Techniques in the 'Persuade about the need of treatment'.
This goal is obtained by linking the two discourse segments *Describe Patient Status* and *Expose Treatment Plan* by a rhetorical relation (RR) of Solutionhood.
This RR may become a Concession when the patient is not seriously ill, conveying the idea that, although the disease mildness might let one presume that treatment is not needed, this is not the case:
Ex1: This condition is mild, *but* we have to treat it. . . .
On the other side, the Description of the patient's health status contains a RR of Elaboration Object-Attribute, whose nucleus is the name of the diagnosis and whose satellites are its severity and certainty. The value of these satellites influences the nucleus description. For example:
Ex2: *Unfortunately* you have an infection. . ., (when the severity is *high*).

Persuasion Elements in the 'Request to perform the treatment'.
The goal *Request to perform the treatment* is achieved, in our generator, by a simple sentence which indicates the number of drugs in the prescription. In the corpus of texts examined, elements of persuasion are introduced, in this segment, by means of several techniques:
(1.) To predispose favourably the addressee towards the Request: by anticipating the positive aspects of treatment, when it has a high expected effectiveness or when it is, at least, expected to have a positive effect on symptoms:
Ex3: *So, the good news* is that we do have tablets that are very effective against TB. . .
Ex4: With the treatment we'll give you, *we can bring all these things back to normal.* . .
Ex5: We can give you something *to make you feel more comfortable.* . .
(2.) To prevent a non collaborative attitude: by anticipating aspects on which a high compliance is needed, especially when treatment is long and complex:
Ex6: We have to undertake *quite a long course of treatment.* . .
(3.) To promote remembering of significant items: by synthesising information items which are common to several drugs, *before* detailing the treatment:
Ex7: . . . two drugs which are very similar: *they both aim to open the blood vessels up.*
Ex8: I'm going to ask you to take *two tablets.* . .
Ex9: . . . *some tablets to take twice a day.* . .
Ex10: . . . and you will have to take them *for some months.*
or by means of a *final synthesis* of this detailed description:
Ex11: So, in summary, we'll give you *tablets to help the spasm of the blood vessels.* . .
(4.) Persuasion elements in the 'Request to administer the drug'. This purpose is achieved by associating treatment to procedures or drugs with which patients are familiar and that they know to be *harmless*:
Ex12: The drug that I'm going to ask you to take is Aspirin, *just ordinary Aspirin.* . .
or by emphasising positive aspects of treatment:
Ex13: . . . one *small* dose of. . .
(5.) Strengthening or attenuation techniques in the 'Persuade that the drug is not harmful'. In this case, positive aspects are overemphasised by means of particular linguistic markers and negative aspects are offset by using *aggregation* techniques to avoid repetitions :
Ex14: *The only possible side effect* this may have is to. . .
Ex15: *Again,* it's very unlikely to happen; *Again,* I would like you to reassure that. . .
Ex16: *Occasionally,* they can disturb you in your sleep.

3.2 Cues from Evaluation Studies

At the University of Reading, several studies were made to investigate whether and how the order of presentation of information and the level of detail influence the effectiveness of explanation, measured in terms of how good the explanation is, perceived likelihood of taking the medication and memory of information. To this aim, several texts were prepared, by combining differently the following components of an OPADE explanation: description of the patient health status, prescription, description of drug, side effects and contraindications. Experiments were repeated by varying number and seriousness of side effects. The results of these studies are described elsewhere [1]: here, we refer only those of them which are relevant to this paper.

The first finding is that the optimal order of presentation of information cannot be established in a rigid way, but depends on the overall explanation content. In particular, participants in the study overall recalled more information about drug administration when it was presented before information about side effects. However, when the explanation described only a few side effects, participants remembered more information about side effects if the information was presented before, rather than after, the information about drug administration. There was no effect of order when the explanation described a large number of side effects. Therefore the optimal order of information within the explanation can only be determined once the number of side effects has been established.

The second finding concerns the perceived likelihood of taking the medication and the evaluation of how good the explanation is, as a function of side effects' seriousness: if the text includes *negative information*, the need for additional explanatory information increases. Thus the decision about the level of detail of the explanation is a function of the overall information content: details have to increase according to the *negativity* of information elements in the text, such as the severity of the disease or of the side effects of drugs.

4 Some Hints on How to Solve the Mentioned Problems

We identify two limitations in current text generation methods, that reduce argumentation strength in the texts produced: (i) Text Planning is a one shot process which does not take into account the impact that the text 'as a whole' will have on the addressee; (ii) the subsequent phases disregard the rhetorical nature of the text. Let us justify more deeply our claim.

4.1 Text Planning Shortcomings

In hierarchical Text Planning, information content and presentation order are established as a function of the main communicative goal, of hypotheses about the mental states of the Speaker and the addressee and of domain knowledge.

In their decision on whether to apply a specific plan operator, top-down plan expansion methods consider only the values of information items which relate to the discourse segment which is being planned. The overall content of the text is not known until planning has been completed. For example: when the subtree concerning one of the side effects of a specific drug is being expanded, the planner doesn't yet *know* how many side effects the drug will have and whether these side effects will be serious, frequent and so on. The discourse structure and its content will be established entirely only when the plan will have been completed: problems mentioned in Sect. 3 will only then become manifest.

4.2 Sentence Planning Shortcomings

As we mentioned in the Introduction, the need for an intermediate phase between Text Planning and Linguistic Realisation is acknowledged by most researchers in the domain, and the tasks this phase is supposed to undertake have been specified by several authors. Among them, a fine grained local discourse structuring, which includes decision about inclusion/exclusion of discourse markers, a sentence content delimitation, an internal sentence organisation, with aggregation, reference and lexical choice [8]. Concepts involved in this phase are essentially linguistic-stylistic ones: focus, pronominalisation, preposition phrases, etc.

We think that, in most of these tasks, rhetorical concepts should be considered as well, and that other rhetoric-driven tree-restructuring tasks need to be performed. For example:

1. adding empathy to sentences: by stressing positive concepts (Ex12,13,14), offsetting negative ones (Ex16), marking a non-aggregation choice (*again* in Ex15) or showing an empathetic or enlistening attitude (Ex2).

2. treatment of repetitions: *aggregation* is defined as the process of removing redundant information in a text without loosing any information [2]. The aim of this process is to obtain more fluent and easy to read texts. So from the three sentences: *Tom loves Mary, Dick loves Mary, Harry loves Mary*, aggregation will produce the sentence: *Tom, Dick and Harry love Mary*, which is much more fluent, and undoubtedly natural. But, let us suppose that this was an argumentative text, aimed at convincing the addressee of the kindness of Mary. The text will be much more effective if repetition is employed (and possibly emphasised with an emphatic punctuation): *Tom loves Mary! Dick loves Mary! Harry loves Mary!* which means: *Everybody loves Mary, who couldn't?*

The decision on whether to aggregate repetitions or to emphasise them should therefore be made by considering the global aim of the sentence, not only its readability. Ex15 reveals that doctors are guided by this concept in their decisions. In addition, rhetorical aspects can help to decide, when aggregating, the order in which items should be presented to maximise the argumentative effect.

3. introducing opening or closing summaries: Examples from 3 to 11 showed how these summaries can be employed to predispose favourably the addressee or to promote memory of relevant facts.

4. changing information ordering: the result of studies by psychologists at

Reading showed that the information ordering established by the planner has sometimes to be revised, according to the overall discourse content; the same applies to the next item:

5. revising information detail: (see findings about side effects).

6. changing rhetorical relations: Ex1 is a typical case in which a rhetorical relation of Solutionhood can be less effective than a Concession when addressees have to be persuaded to undertake an action aimed at solving a problem that they perceive as minor.

Some of these tasks require a *Plan-Tree Refinement*, in which the main decisions of the plan (information order and content, RRs, communicative goals) are respected: we name this class of tasks *Rhetorical Sentence Planning*, to contrast them with current Sentence Planning techniques.

Another class of tasks introduces deeper changes in the plan structure and could be called *Plan-Tree Revision*.

5   Some Implementation Attempts

Rhetorical Sentence Planning and plan revision tasks require **upgrading knowledge** that is commonly employed for text generation. The Addressee mode, which usually includes general characteristics (eg. age, family status) and a large variety of *rational* attitudes (knowledge, beliefs, goals) is extended with domain-related, emotional aspects of personality, such as *hostile towards treatment* or *anxious*. This broadening of the user modelling sphere of interest corresponds to a trend in the domain of human-computer interaction, which claims that extrarational aspects of human beings should be considered in designing *believable* computer systems [4, 12]. Domain knowledge has to be upgraded as well, by attaching to the data items (object-attribute-value triples) one or more labels defining the semantic properties which may be relevant in the domain (eg. *favourable for compliance, relevant for correct treatment* and so on).

Both Rhetorical Sentence Planning and Plan Revision make a wide use of these knowledge sources, and can be represented as sets of tree-rewriting rules which apply to discourse subplans. For each rule:

The left-hand side is a logical combination of conditions on the communication goal and the RR associated with the root, the semantic properties of information associated to the leaves and the addressee's attitudes.

Examples of semantic properties of information are the following:
- *unfavourable* item: Severity (?disease, serious)
- *favourable* item: Efficacy (?drug, high)
- *relevant-for-compliance* item: Duration (?treatment, short)
- *relevant-for-correct-treatment* item: AdministrationForm (?drug, tablets).

Examples of addressee's attitudes:
- Compliance (?drug-treatment, low)
- Anxiety (?pain, high).

The right-hand side is a tree-restructuring algorithm which varies according to the task to be performed.

5.1 Some Examples of Rhetorical Sentence Planning Rules

Adding Empathy to Sentences.

R1 IF the subtree 'Persuade that the drug is not harmful' includes sub-subtrees whose leaves are 'favourable' items with equal values AND the patient is pain-anxious THEN emphasise these leaves.

The emphatization algorithm depends, in this case, on the Rhetorical Relation associated to the root node: it may consist of adding intensifier or detensifier adverbs or adjectives or in generating compound sentences in which the components are joined by a contrasting conjunction (as in [6]). Operations of this type may solve problems like those in Ex2 and Ex13, Sect. 3. In the first of them, a RR of Elaboration Object-Attribute is associated with the root. In this case, the two *Inform* are merged into a unique sentence, which is introduced by an appropriate expression: an intensifier (*the good news is that*) in case of favourable information, a detensifier (*unfortunately*) in case of unfavourable information. A similar transformation is applied to the second tree, by introducing the detensifier adjective *small*. These transformations are adapted to the addressee and exploit a semantic knowledge of the domain.

Rhetorical Aggregation.

R2 IF the subtree 'Persuade that the drug is not harmful' includes sub-subtrees whose leaves are unfavourable items with equal values AND the patient is pain-anxious THEN aggregate repetitions of unfavourable items in these subtrees.

This algorithm is applied to subtrees whose root-node is associated with an Ordinal Sequence or a Logical RR: repetitions in the text usually originate from these subtrees. To illustrate it, let us consider a segment of an OPADE's text:

However, I must inform you that this drug may cause some side effects. The first one is nausea; it is serious, it occurs infrequently, in a strong form, in sensitive patients. The second one is headache; it is serious, it occurs infrequently, in a strong form, in sensitive patients. The third one is insomnia; it is not serious, it occurs frequently, in a strong form, in sensitive patients....

The algorithm is made up of four main steps:

step 1: finding subtrees such that the RR associated to the root is an Ordinal Sequence or a Logical. In our example, this step extracts, from the plan tree in Fig. 1, the SubTree shown in Fig. 3. This subtree is made up of several *similar* (in their structure) sub-subtrees;

step 2: classifying leaves. The classification is made in two stages:

• identification of the *main nucleus* of each sub-subtree (according to the focusing structure) and labelling of these leaves as *objects*; labelling of remaining leaves as *characteristics*.

In our example, there are three nuclei (one in each element of the Sequence), corresponding to nausea, headache and insomnia; and four characteristics for each of them: severity, frequency, intensity and risk-category.

• classification of objects according to the values of their characteristics, and identification of characteristics whose values are the same in all objects (uniform

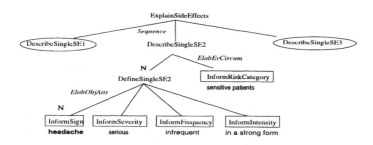

Fig. 3. A portion of the plan tree to explain side effects of a drug

characteristics) or only within a class (class-uniform characteristics).
In our case, frequency and severity are class-uniform characteristics; risk-category
and action are uniform characteristics.

step 3: deciding which characteristics to aggregate.

In our example, *strong* intensity is an unfavourable item, *infrequent* frequency is
a favourable one; the first one is therefore aggregated, the second one is dupli-
cated.

step 4: restructuring the subtree:

4.1: prune uniform characteristics and add a new root and a new child leaf of
this root for each of them;

4.2: rearrange the nuclei in the original Ordinal Sequence according to classes
of *similar* objects; for each class which contains more than one object, create a
new intermediate node and define an Ordinal Sequence among objects within it;

4.3: apply recursively 4.1 and 4.2 within each class.

Figure 4 shows how the subtree in Fig. 3 is transformed by this algorithm. If
some empathy is added to sentences, the following text will be generated:
*However, I must inform you that this drug may cause some side effects. A first group
of them includes nausea, which occurs infrequently and only in particularly sensitive
patients, and headache which, again, occurs infrequently and only in particularly sensitive patients; these side effects are both serious. Then, you may have insomnia: it is
not serious but can be frequent; however, once again I would like to reassure you that
it occurs only in particularly sensitive patients. All these side effects can occur in a
strong form.*

5.2 Some Examples of Plan Revision Rules

Our attempt to solve the text revision problems outlined in Sect. 4 is far from
being a general purpose one: more study is needed to better understand how to
read a text plan in order to discover its argumentative deficiencies. For the time
being, we have defined some *ad hoc*, strictly domain-dependent rules whose right
sides include the following tree transformations: introduction of new subtrees or
new intermediate nodes, change of the relative order of subtrees or change of the
RR associated to a node. For example:

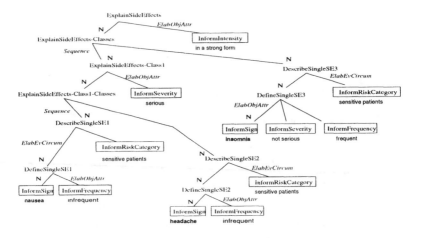

Fig. 4. The subplan tree of Fig. 3 after the treatment of repetitions

R3 IF the leaves of the subtree 'Persuade about the need of treatment' include several favourable items AND the patient has a 'hostile' attitude towards drug therapy THEN substitute the RR of Solutionhood with a Concession, in the main root of the tree (Ex1)

R4 IF at least one leaf in the subtree 'Request to administer the drug' is a favourable item AND the patient has a 'hostile' attitude towards drug therapy THEN substitute the 'Request to perform treatment' with a new subtree, to emphasise these items. (Ex3,4,5)

R5 IF at least one leaf in the subtree 'Enable to administer the drug correctly' is an item relevant for correct treatment AND the patient is aged THEN introduce a new subtree before the Enable, to emphasise these items. (Ex8,9,10,11)

6   Conclusions

We share Hovy and Wanner's opinion that "the generation process is even more complex than originally viewed, and that this complexity centrally affects the planning procedures" [8]. The tree-rewriting rules that we propose in this paper are domain-dependent heuristics, derived from analysis of empirical data. A domain-independent improvement in the discourse generation process could only be obtained by reconsidering Text Planning as a conjunctive and non serially decomposable problem, in which strong interactions between subgoals exist [9]. This would require representing *communicative actions* in a more fine-grained way than at present, by specifying their negative as well as their positive effects. In argumentative texts, in particular, graduality in the persuasion process could be obtained by introducing degrees of goal adoption and degrees of belief holding in the mental model of the addressee. Let us take, for example, the case of an 'Inform about side effects', as a leaf of the subtree of 'Persuade that the drug is useful and not harmful'. If the side effect is serious, this act will reduce

the addressee's intention to perform the treatment, that was increased by the previous subgoals of 'Persuade about the need of treatment' and 'Persuade that the drug is not harmful'. The combination of several, serious side effects will then produce a 'negative precondition' for the 'Enable to administer the drug correctly', which depends on their number.
With the Text Planning techniques that are applied at present, we claim that several plan revision tasks are needed to counteract negative effects of not considering subgoal interactions: sentence planning is only one of them. We acknowledge the importance of style refinement, but we contend that other, more argumentative tasks are important as well, and that knowledge about the domain and about the addressee plays a crucial role in all of them. In the medical field, this knowledge concerns not only what addressees presumably know, want or prefer, but also emotional factors such as, for instance, fear about disease prognosis or anxiety about pain.

References

1. D. Berry, I. Michas and F. de Rosis: Evaluating explanations about drug prescriptions. Submitted to Psychology and Health.
2. H. Dalianis and E. Hovy: On lexical aggregation and ordering. Proc. of 8th International Natural Language Generation Workshop (INLG-96), Poster session (1996) 29-32.
3. B. De Carolis, F. de Rosis, F. Grasso and A. Rossiello: Generating recipient-centered explanations about drug prescription. Artificial Intelligence in Medicine 8(2) (1996) 123-145.
4. F. de Rosis, F. Grasso, C. Castelfranchi, I. Poggi: Modelling conflict resolution dialogues between believable agents. Working notes of the ECAI-96 Workshop on: Modelling conflicts in AI (1996).
5. D. Forsythe: Using ethnography in the design of an explanation system. Expert Systems and Applications 8(4) (1995) 403-417.
6. I. Haimowitz: Modeling all dialogue system participants to generate empathetic responses. Computer Methods and Programs in Biomedicine 35 (1991) 321-330.
7. E. Hovy: Automated discourse generation using discourse structure relations. Artificial Intelligence 63 (1993) 341-385.
8. E. Hovy and L. Wanner: Managing sentence planning requirements. Working notes of the ECAI-96 Workshop on: Gaps and Bridges, New directions in planning and language generation (1996) 53-58.
9. R. Korf: Planning as search: a quantitative approach. Artificial Intelligence 33(1) (1987) 65-88.
10. M. Meteer: Bridging the generation gap between text planning and linguistic realization. Computational Intelligence 7(4) (1991) 296-304.
11. O. Rambow and T. Korelsky: Applied text generation. Proc. of 3rd Conference on Applied Natural Language Processing, Trento (1992) 40-47.
12. S. Reilly and J. Bates: Natural negotiation for believable agents. School of Computer Science, Carnegie Mellon University, CMU-CS-95-164, June 1995.
13. L. Wanner and E. Hovy: The HealthDoc Sentence Planner, Proc. of 8th International Natural Language Generation Workshop (INLG-96) (1996) 1-10.

An Ontological Analysis of Surgical Deeds

A. Rossi Mori [a], A. Gangemi [a], G. Steve [a], F. Consorti [b], E. Galeazzi [c]

[a] Reparto Informatica Medica, Istituto Tecnologie Biomediche, CNR , Roma, Italy [1]
[b] IV Clin. Chirurgica and [c] Dottorato Informatica Medica, Univ. La Sapienza, Roma, Italy

We collected a set of words, suffixes, and idioms regarding actions in surgical procedures, ie. "deeds" as defined in a CEN European Prestandard; we then searched for their definitions in different authoritative sources and we performed an ontological analysis of this material according to the ONIONS methodology. The result was a formal model on surgical actions, as an extension of our previous model ON8.5, using Ontolingua with "frame ontology".
We worked out criteria to assist domain experts in organizing hierarchies on surgical actions, according to structural, technical and functional points of view.

1. Introduction

In this paper we present an analysis of surgical deeds, which is the outcome of an original approach to ontology, involving:
1) systematically capturing taxonomic knowledge from authoritative sources,
2) treating such knowledge by a methodology using linguistic and conceptual tools,
3) representing it formally by i) a set of ontologically committed primitives and ii) a set of axioms on those primitives.

1.1. "Surgical Deed" and "Surgical Procedure" in CEN ENV 1828

The starting point for our analysis has been the European Prestandard CEN ENV1828 [CEN95]; it defines *surgical deed* as "deed which can be done by the operator to the patient's body during the surgical procedure", with the note that the surgical deed "shall be described without reference to any specific human anatomy or interventional equipment".

It provides about 60 examples of deeds, arranged in 14 clusters (examples of clusters are: to open, to pass through, to install; examples of deeds included in the cluster "to install" are: to implant, to inject, to insert, to transfuse, to transplant). In existing classifications and nomenclatures, concepts of deeds exceeds 500 (cf. [Bernauer96]). The Prestandard also introduces a description for *surgical procedure* (table 1).

The CEN distinction between *procedure* and *deed* mainly depends on the empirical criterion of *instantiatability*: if a surgical "action" is specific to a certain structure (human anatomy or interventional equipment) it is a procedure, otherwise it is a deed. On the other hand, most actions are naturally performed only on certain *kinds* of structures; thus, which is the sufficient instantiation for an action to be a procedure? (or the sufficient generality to be a deed?). The criterion of *sufficiency* is obviously left to intuition. Moreover, as our Ontolingua translation shows, CEN's constraints depend on standalone categories, which are not parts of any formal theory.

Starting from these difficulties, we defined an ontology of surgical actions, providing a theory to explicitly motivate categorial choices as well as criteria for instantiation. We also show that a comprehensive and consistent theory greatly enhances the definition of constraints for classifying the kinds of actions carried out by surgeons.

---

[1] send mail to ARM, viale Marx 15, I-00137 Roma; angelo@color.irmkant.rm.cnr.it

Table 1. Definition of surgical procedure in CEN ENV 1828, here translated in Ontolingua [Gruber93] as a standalone item, ie. not as a part of any general formal theory

```
(define-class cen-surgical-procedure (?c-sp)
"a surgical procedure is determined in CEN by some instance of human anatomy,
pathology, or interventional equipment, which may act as direct or indirect object, as
well as means. It includes at least one direct object, as well as at least one
instance of human anatomy, and has deeds made during it"
  :def  (and (exists (?d ?x ?y)
                  (and (deed ?d)
                       (during ?d ?c-sp)
                       (has-direct-object ?c-sp ?x)
                       (or (human-anatomy ?x)
                           (pathology ?x)
                           (interventional-equipment ?x))
                       (human-anatomy ?y)))
             (=> (has-indirect-object ?c-sp ?z)
                 (or (human-anatomy ?z)
                     (pathology ?z)
                     (interventional-equipment ?z)))
             (=> (has-means ?c-sp ?z)
                 (or (human-anatomy ?z)
                     (pathology ?z)
                     (interventional-equipment ?z)))))
```

1.2. Relevance of Ontology in Formal Models

The project GALEN-IN-USE [GALEN92-96] is populating a formal model on surgical procedures by a cooperative effort; experts from 4 centers in Europe (including one in Rome) are building a comprehensive model from rubrics of various coding system, in collaboration with Victoria University in Manchester [Rossi Mori95, 96b]. In our center, we initially instructed domain experts to use a limited list of well-defined deeds and to force each new word they were encountering into one existing concept; but they felt that rule too limiting on their expressiveness. We decided then to let experts be free to introduce any new deed, but we also asked to place them in the context of existing ones, ie, to put each new deeds as subordinate to one or more existing ones possibly working out the differences towards them.

At the same time, we started to build a robust ontology on deeds, to formally describe similarities and differences among available concepts and towards the new ones.

Parallel work on this issue was made by another partner in the GALEN-IN-USE Project [Bernauer96], merging the current "Generic Process Model" with deeds that could be identified in the German version of ICPM [Kolodzig94], yielding a structure organizing deeds under about 20 major aspects. However, many deeds can be organized under different legitimate aspects; eg. *smoothing* is a kind of *removing* and *reshaping*; *wiring* is a kind of *connecting, immobilising* and *device-application*.

A major issue is therefore to adopt a well-structured and stable representation of deeds, which can be only obtained by a thorough understanding of original intended meaning of deeds within a framework of general theoretical *paradigms*.

We maintain that a correct approach for this issue is *ontological analysis and integration*, which are supported, for example, by our ONIONS methodology [for ontology in general: Guarino95; for ONIONS: Steve96a, Gangemi96a; for ontology and KB: [van Heijst97]; for ontology libraries in medicine: [Falasconi94]).

Moreover, an ontological methodology may help clarifying the choice of primitives of representation (what concepts are to be modelled as predicates?, what is a role vs. a sort or a property?, cf. [Guarino94, Steve96b]); finally, tangleness of collected hierarchies is another point of attack for ontological integration, which can define flexible criteria of identity according to different aspects, viewpoints, contexts.

1.3. Relevance of a Methodology for Ontological Analysis

In current ontology literature, few Authors address the problem of defining a methodology for ontological analysis, being mostly concerned with representational issues (for a critique: [Gangemi96]; for some work on methodology: [Uschold96, Steve96b]). Indeed, there are well defined and used methodologies for knowledge acquisition [eg, Schreiber92, Shadbolt93], but these are meant mainly for acquiring task-specific, operational problem-solving knowledge rather than multi-functional domain knowledge, ie. the purpose of ontological *analysis*. Moreover, they do not treat at all ontological *integration* of knowledge sources. In the following we show why we need analysis and integration of sources.

It is relatively easy to envisage criteria to group a large number of deeds and to relate them, at least in a first approximation; eg, using as characteristics: (1) "movement with respect to organism", and (2) "physical state of the moved substance", we have:

	taking away from organism	insert into organism
fluid	drainage, aspiration, ...	instilling, puncturing, inject, transfuse, ...
solid	remove, extirpate, -ectomy, ...	install, implant, transplant, ...

But this method is not appropriate to produce a really stable and complete structure, even if it provides an useful understanding and a preliminary organization of the field.

A more precise and analytic process has to be followed, extracting principles and primitives that are ontologically grounded to domain-independent paradigms, in order to be coherent with a comprehensive and stable framework. Criteria such as *taking away, inserting, solid structure*, have to be put in the context of general theories at several degrees, for example *taking away* calls for a theory describing *movement*, and —more generally— *actions, intentional events, processes*. The taxonomy of theories which allow integration constitutes a hierarchy of semantic fields structured by some semantic operators (logically, a hierarchy of sorts and relations, and a set of axioms; conceptually, a set of concepts and a set of relations for defining concepts).

This procedure of understanding and integrating criteria in an ontological framework is part of a comprehensive methodology of ontological analysis, briefly presented in § 2.

2. Materials and Methods

Building the ontological model on surgical deeds corresponds, for our group, to two parallel activities:

- to extend the branch on surgical procedures of our integrated model for medical taxonomic sources, ON8.5 [Steve96b];
- to adapt our methodology for ontological analysis, ONIONS [Gangemi95], to the particular features of this study, integrating it with the CEN-MOSE approach [CEN96, Rossi Mori96a].

Deeds are expressed by single words (with the exception of a few suffixes or idioms), because all explicit information about particular structures, devices and functions was removed from the phrases in the original corpora, according to the definition of "surgical deed" in CEN ENV 1828 (see § 1.1).

We had consequently the problem to preserve a *systematic, reproducible approach* to compositional analysis, compatibly and in parallel to our methodology for ontological analysis.

Therefore we describe in this paragraph how we used two kinds of original materials:
- the top level of ON8.5, generated trough the ONIONS methodology;
- various terminological corpora —sources of phrases and authoritative sources of definitions— from which we arranged three kinds of intermediate resources:
  - a list of deeds;
  - a collection of definitions for a subset of these deeds;
  - a hierarchy of deeds, made according to definitions and extended by using knowedge from experts.

2.1. Terminological and Definitional Sources

a) sources for deeds: ENV 1828 [CEN95] and major coding systems: ICD-9-CM [HCFA88], ICD-10-PCS [Averill95], SNOMED Int'l [Rothwell93].
Suffixes were isolated when reasonably independent, eg, *-ectomy, -tomy, -plasty*.
We kept all kinds of actions, even very specific, eg, *fundoplication, cannulating*.
We made no distinction on grammatical forms of a word, ie, verbal forms (eg, infinitive, past participle), suffixes, noun phrases (eg, verbal substantive, deverbal noun) were considered as the same deed.
We collected about 200 deeds, from which we selected only the ones regarding actual actions performed by surgeons; ie, we did not consider:
1 meta-expressions on enactment of procedures, eg, *terminate, cancel, suspend, repeat*
2 too general actions, eg, *change, operation*;
3 healthcare activities, eg, *therapy, prevent, diagnosis, control* (see § 3.2).

b) sources for definitions or explicit interpretation hints:
- a systematic source on surgery, ie, an early report on ICD-10-PCS [Averill95];
- dictionaries of medicine [Dorland's94, Wiley86, Stedman's95]
- a computer-based dictionary of English, hierarchically structured [Wordnet96]
- the English dictionary adopted for CEN standards [Oxford95]
Only definitions relevant to surgery were considered, for a total of 142 definitions.

c) additional informal knowledge: we extracted further knowledge, embedded in implicit or explicit organization of textbooks and coding systems, specially SNOMED, also by discussions with domain experts in Rome.

2.2. Methods
Our methodology is not automatic nor objective, but it defines how to analyze the ontology of the sources and how to build an integrated formal ontologic model.

Preliminary Phase
We extracted words, suffixes and idioms of deeds from various coding systems (§2.1a); they are preferential sources for terminological phrases, because in principle they are authoritative, intersubjective, maintained, complete of relevant items and tested by users. For most deeds we found adequate definitions into dictionaries (§2.1b); we added to our list of deeds also the superordinate ones used in these definitions. In some source we were able to extract partial hierarchies. When we encountered more than one sense for the same word, we introduced new entries; analogously, when our experts were not able to see any difference between the meanings of two words, we collapsed them provisionally into a single entry, so that each entry in our list represents a precise, distinguishable concept within each source respectively.
Results of this phase are: a list of deeds, a collection of local definitions, and some local and temporary hierarchies among deeds.

Extension and Refinement Phase

Extension and iterative refinement of the model are the output of three activities performed in parallel and deeply depending on each other.

Activity A: maintenance of hierarchy. We used the differentiating characteristics from available definitions —and informal discussions with the experts— to arrange the related subset of deeds in a hierarchy and to revise it when appropriate according to feedback from the other two activities. For remaining deeds, we asked the experts to place them in the above hierarchy and to make explicit, if possible, differentiating characteristics between parents and children. Difficult and intriguing issues from the three activities were discussed also with external experts. Results were twofold: the hierarchy and the set of *descriptors* (differentiating characteristics) used to organize it.

Activity B: systematization according to the ontological model ON8.5. The model ON8.5 has been developed through our ONIONS methodology from a set of medical taxonomic sources (eg, SNOMED, ICD-10, UMLS). Descriptors from Activity A have been, when possible, directly integrated in the common framework of general theories used in previous top-level model building; otherwise, they had been referred to additional theories, implying a model rearrangement. Such theories are not considered in every part, but only to the extent they provide the minimal structure for creating a framework which allows for integration of criteria. Extension of ON8.5 implies the ontological opportunity of introducing some new connective concepts, eg. a local top-level for surgical deeds, which makes such distinctions as mereologically-oriented vs. topologically-oriented deeds, or function-changing vs. morphology-changing deeds.

Activity C: maintenance and refinement of formal model. According to previous work, we organized the branch on surgical procedures in sorts, relations (inheritable or not), properties, roles, contexts, description frames, viewpoints, general and contextual rules. The model is currently represented in order-sorted logic and Ontolingua. We used representation primitive categories of ON8.5, which commits to structural concepts, structuring concepts, roles (for details: [Steve96b]). Tests are being carried out to implement this ontology in a snepslog-based [Shapiro92] language.

3 . Results

The core result of our process of analysis consist in the extension of ON8.5; the current Ontolingua model covers about one hundred deeds. *Surgical procedure* in CEN ENV1828 corresponds to "surgical-procedure" in ON8.5, and *surgical deed* roughly corresponds to "surgical-telic-event" (§ 3.1) or "surgical-act" (§ 3.3).

Here we also introduce the organizing criteria to explain and order such deeds, as derived from our ontological model (§ 3.2).

3.1 Definition of Surgical Telic Event in the model ON8.5

The application of ON8.5 top-level has provided the formal definition of telic events involved in surgical procedures (table 2).

This definition includes all partial definitions inherited from being a sub-class of:

```
: TelicEvent: Action: Activity: Process: Object.
```

The ontology of telic events requires ordering situations temporally as well as contextualizing them by the second-order predicate IST (*is-true-in*, [McCarthy94]).

This has been implemented through a metalinguistic approach, which allows quantifiers to range over a logical expression taken to be true within a context.

Table 2. Formal definition, expressed in Ontolingua, of surgical-telic-event *in ON8.5.*
Predicates preceded by a ° are properties (unary predicates representing structuring
concepts), while those preceded by a * are roles:

```
(define-class surgical-telic-event (?ste)
"surgical telic events are dynamic objects in the biologic world, have biologic or
material structures as substrates within a time interval, are carried out by surgeons,
have signs or conditions as goals, are constitutive phases of healtcare activities, have
inherent surgical acts, may use instruments or means, and typically carry out a change
along two or more consecutive situations"
   :def (and (telic-event ?ste)
             (exists (?msign ?cond ?surg ?str ?mdev ?mc1 ?mc2 ?s1 ?s2 ?cha ?pha ?ha ?*sa)
                (and (medical-sign ?msign) (*physical-agent ?pha)
                     (condition ?cond) (*surgeon ?surg) (*surgical-act? *sa)
                     (or (material-structure ?str)
                         (biologic-structure ?str))
                     (medical-device ?mdev) (healthcare-activity ?ha)
                     (situation ?s1) (situation ?s2) (*chemical-agent ?cha)
                     (meta-concept ?mc1) (meta-concept ?mc2)
                     (°intervallistic ?ste) (°dynamic ?ste)
                     (°depends-on-biologic-layer ?ste)
                     (is-constitutive-phase-of ?ste ?ha)
                     (has-constitutive-phase ?ste ?*sa)
                     (performs ?surg ?ste)
                     (embodies ?str ?ste)
                     (or (is-instrumental-for ?mdev ?ste)
                         (is-instrumental-for ?cha ?ste)
                         (is-instrumental-for ?pha ?ste)
                     (or (is-goal-of ?msign ?ste)
                         (is-goal-of ?cond ?ste))
                     (precedes ?s1 ?s2)
                     (=> (ist ?s1 "(constrains ?mc1 ?ste)")
                         (ist ?s2 "(constrains ?mc2 ?ste)")))))))
```

Nesting and Sequencing of Phases

A surgical procedure is a part of a *healthcare activity* (eg, *control* or *prevent* a disease,
perform a precise diagnosis). Surgeons manipulate *structures* (body parts, substances,
devices) to fix damaged *functions* (including aesthetical function) or induce *functional*
reactions from organism. Finally, surgeons exploit means instrumental to the above
changes (ie. devices and chemical or physical agents) to perform *technical* actions.

Most deeds therefore consist in *changes* to a structure (eg, adding, removing or
transforming it) to achieve a functional effect in the same or another structure (eg,
elimination of a pathological function, to avoid further consequences in the organism).

ON8.5 provides *mereological* (phase) and *actantial* (cause or goal) relations to express
the dependencies among various kinds of action: a *technical action* is a constitutive
phase (as well as a cause) of a structural action. A *structural action* in turn is a phase
of a *functional action*, that is a constitutive phase of (as well as it has as goal) a
healthcare activity .
These points of view correspond to classes of criteria to organize deeds (§ 3.2).

Moreover, surgical telic events can be considered as sequences of constitutive phases.
For example, *remove* and *insert* are constitutive phases of *replacement*, while *remove*
from a *donor* is an additional constitutive phase of *transplant*. Analogoulsy, *sampling*
could be intended as *disconnecting* a portion and *remove* it.
We modelled this dependency by introducing the "surgical act", as explained in § 3.3.

3.2. Mereological and Actantial Dependencies Among Deeds
Intuitive considerations on points of view correspond to constraints in table 2, and they lead to a set of criteria to describe and organize deeds.

Point of View Regarding Structures and their Context
The "structural" point of view considers situations in the time span of a surgical action, and focuses on actual changes in properties of the *structure* which embodies the action ('direct object' in CEN), or on its regional *context*; it corresponds to the *ist* metalinguistic constraint on properties of structures, ranging over a context (a *situation*) and a *meta-concept* containing a logical expression about the situation.

Table 3 presents some informal interpretation hints (the preferred interface to experts) to organize surgical telic events in relation to the *structuring* concepts that change from a situation to another. Such structuring concepts are organized in ON8.5 as: *mereological* concepts (part-whole relations); *topological* concepts (connexity relations); *morphological* concepts (qualitative and quantitative relations on matter).

Our model then distinguishes surgical telic events focalizing primarily to:
- *mereological* properties (ie to regional context) of the structure involved;
- *morphological* properties of the structure involved;
- *topological* properties of the structure involved, eg. regarding its connections to other structures, or its topological *genus* (various kinds of holes).

Further criteria (not in table 3) depend on specialization of those structuring concepts:
- kind of structure involved (body part, device or substance);
- physical state of the structure (eg. fluid, solid).
- for quantitative properties, "increase" vs "decrease" in number or size;
- for extended topological properties, weak or strong connexity.

A surgical telic event may encompass various constitutive actions which change different properties; eg, *sampling* amounts to *disconnect* portions or non-essential elements of a biologic structure and to *remove* them from the organism (see § 3.3).

table 3. Properties of structures changed by a structural point of view
(with examples and notes on the right)

shape	reconstruct, reduce a fracture
size	dilate, lengthen
physical state	vaporize, melt
hygienical state	sterilize
having holes	(temporary) patency/closure, clamp (vessel), stomy
connexity of parts	split, fragment, sampling (portions), fix (fracture)
connection to other structures	anastomosis
being a part of patient	remove, drain, insert (temporarily), harvest
being a part of region	transfer
having anchors	fixation, -pexy, release
position of anchors	advance (a tendon)

Point of View Related to Functional Outcome of the Procedure
The "functional" point of view considers the situation after the surgical procedure, and focuses on functional changes *to be achieved* by the "structural action" above; it corresponds to possible *ist* metalinguistic constraints on biologic functions (in case of complex, encapsulated goals). In table 4 we present the criteria to organize actions in relation to the functional outcome of the procedure.

Additional criteria to further organize deeds from a functional point of view (not in table 4) consider the degree of restoration or loss of performance, referred to:

- a structure (either a body part, a body system, or the whole organism), and
- the kind of reference situation (ie, a pathological or normal situation).

table 4. Potential functional changes of a structure
(with examples and notes on the right)

loose functional role	isolate functionally
adapt to other function	by transfer or morphological changes (make a reservoir)
restore original function	(totally, partially); functional repair
assist existing function	by installing prosthesis
no relevant change in function	for acquisition of information or sampling

Point of View Related to the Technical Aspect of the Procedure

A third point of view (table 5) regards the "technical" way to perform an operation (ie, how the surgical telic event is actually performed); it corresponds to the *is-instrumental-for* constraint in table 2, ranging over the telic event and either a *chemical agent, a physical agent* or a *device*. Note that sometimes the use of a device determines particular structural surgical actions: eg, "to clamp a vessel" implies not only the use of the instrument, but also *compression* and *closure* of lumen (see §4.2).

table 5. Means exploited in the instrumental point of view;
the effect is not explicit in the deed (examples of deeds are on the right)

chemical agents	alcoholization
physical agents	warming, compression
devices	cut, drill, clamp, inject

3.3. Surgical Acts and Sequences of Constitutive Acts

Further studies on surgical actions have required an understanding of the telic events which have the role of *constitutive acts* within a surgical telic event, called *surgical acts* in our model. Some of such acts as *move, separate, destroy*, etc. have been defined: *move* definition is shown in table 6. The ontological definition of *surgical act* is made in order to impose less constraints as possible: for instance, what embodies a *move* is a generic *structure*, since either *body parts*, or *substances*, or *artifacts*, or

Table 6. Formal definition of the surgical act "move"
as stipulated within the ontology on surgical procedures

```
(define-class move (?m)
"a move as a surgical act is a telic event embodied in a structure which is in one
region of an organism. Such an event has the goal of having that structure in a
different region of that (or another) organism. A moving entails a moving from a
position and a moving to another position, temporally ordered: this is intended here
as old and new situations."
  :def (and (*surgical-act ?m)
            (=> (*surgical-act ?m)
                (exists (?p ?r1 ?r2 ?s1 ?s2 ?org1 ?org2)
                    (and (structure ?p) (region ?r1) (region ?r2)
                         (situation ?s1) (situation ?s2)
                         (organism ?org1) (organism ?org2)
                         (is-part-of ?r1 ?org1)
                         (or (is-part-of ?r2 ?org1)
                             (is-part-of ?r2 ?org2))
                         (precedes ?s1 ?s2)
                         (=> (ist ?s1 "(and (has-position ?p ?r1)
                                          (embodies ?p ?m))")
                             (ist ?s2 "(has-position ?p ?r2)")))))))
```

abnormal structures can be moved surgically. Moreover, a *structure* has a generic *position* to a *region*, since a region is meant to be the *contextual around* which is focalized constructively: the region can be the *whole* of the structure, or can *contain* it, or can be even *adjacent to* it, etc.

On the other hand, when a surgical telic event is defined through some of its surgical acts, more specific items are to be represented (ie., specific type restrictions are made). The final goal of having surgical acts analyzed is to define an algebra of surgical procedures, that could be integrated in a more general algebra of procedures.

4. Discussion

Discussion is organized in 2 parts. First we explain the rationale of our methodology. Second, we see how points of view influence analysis and systematization, and how the basic properties of a surgical procedure could be better understood.

4.1. On Ontological Analysis and Modeling Methodologies

Support of cooperative modelling requires a methodology for early discovery of potential sources of conflicts among modellers, early reconciliation, minimization of interactions by focusing on anticipated issues, etc.

It is hard to integrate cooperative efforts —not only in GALEN-IN-USE, but also among CEN standards on various subject fields and among CEN standards and other initiatives— without a unique, ontologically based framework.

Timely discovering of uniform (stable) principles is crucial to establish guidelines and to perform integration among independently developed fragments of models.

Issues on integration. Ontological analysis is a craft; but this does not prevent to state reasonable principles and guidelines for a rigorous and intersubjectively controllable work. ONIONS guides the knowledge engineer to answer the following main issues:

1　*corpus formation*, ie, strategies for finding valuable sources, checking for their terminological organization and their definitions (if any), possibly sampling or chunking them to the needed extent, etc.;

2　*rearrangement of concepts extracted from terminologies* (dictionaries, taxonomies, nomenclatures, semantic networks, formal languages) within possible hierarchies and through informal discussions. The outcome should include *explicit criteria* used for the various hierarchical rearrangements;

3　*integration of criteria*, according to general and domain theories triggered from literature. Such general theories are accepted to the extent they provide the minimal structure to create a framework for integration of criteria. Minimal structure should include a minimal *top level* as well;

4　*formal modelling*, ie., assignment of concepts resulting from 1, 2, and 3, to some representational primitives (sorts, roles, relations, properties, etc.), syntactically organized in a formal language (predicate logic, Ontolingua, KIF, conceptual graphs, etc.) and with explicit logical semantics. This should account for axiomatic treatment of the ontology;

5　*implementation of the formal ontology*, and its testing with experts.

Ambiguity of NL and precision of the model. Words are our initial experimental material, but we analyze definitions and additional information in order to discover principles as much language independent as possible: we *conceptualize* words.

We considered any word with different senses (eg "reduce" fracture vs "reduce" volume) as two independent concepts to be modelled. But there are subtler cases of context-dependent shifts on sense; routine mapping from actual words-in-context (eg from medical records) to our model has to be carefully made for each terminological phrase, on the basis of ontologic constraints and not by similarity of wording.

4.2. On the Organization of Surgical Deeds

Our results on surgical deeds provide:

* principles and general issues; they could also be an input for the planned revision of the CEN standard, or for the enhancement of the top-level ontology in GALEN;
* the representation of individual deeds; it could also be validated and integrated in the model of surgical procedures being developed by the GALEN-IN-USE project;
* informal descriptions of plausible points of view for practical use by domain experts (presented in three tables, according to the domain ontology).

As shown in § 3.2, a deed explicitly refers to one or more points of view; but in most cases, specially if embedded in a particular context, a given phrase evokes by default in the mind of surgical specialists a complete healthcare process, and a set of potential transformations between viewpoints. In other words, knowledge on the process from one view puts strong constraints on other views.

Relations between a surgical telic event and the involved structures and processes apparently depend on linguistic *focalization*; eg, "repair femur with 2 pins" focuses on a body part (*femur*) embodying the event, on a surgical act (*repair*) and on a device (*pin*) having the role of instrument (*with*). A different focalization appears when the instrumental word (*with*) is paraphrased so that the implicit "insert 2 pins in femur" explicitly emerges. This last phrase focuses on the device (*pin*) and a different surgical act (*insert*), keeping the body part (*femur*) as a positional reference.

Actually, the two phrases are both partial views of the same complex domain conceptualization which accomplishes a surgical telic event (say: *bone repair*) embodied in a body part (*femur*) through the main phase consisting of a technical act (say: *exploit pins*), let alone other possible phases.

In other words, the *same* intervention can be represented from different points of view, producing different constructs and formally different representations (table 7). Note that for a specialist, different views are often transformable into each other.

table 7. Dual views of some surgical telic events [cf Rossi Mori96b]

structural action	technical action
repair femur with 2 pins	inserting 2 pins in femur
destroy a nerve by neurolytic fluid	injecting neurolytic fluid
release bowel	lysing peritoneal adhesions
dilatation of artery	perfoming a balloon catheterization
increase temperature of tumor mass	warming blood

Table 3 to 5 were consequences of these considerations (the fourth point of view on healthcare activities is not discussed in this paper). Depending on task, a procedure can be described by a set of criteria according to any of those viewpoints.

This modelling activity could be a spin-off point to actual knowledge acquisition (ie. connections between multi-functional domain ontologies and problem-solving methods [cf. Musen92]).

An independent axis of description is obtained by the introduction of surgical acts (§ 3.3), that allow to express a deed by a sequence of more elementary acts, on the same or different structures.

5. Conclusions

Cooperative modelling adds severe problems of coherence to the difficult task of formal modelling. Integration of independent efforts is practically impossible without sharing a unique goal: a stable ontological foundation.

CEN initiatives on medical terminologies produce a first approximation of criteria to organize concepts within particular subject fields in healthcare; but a fixed schema cannot satisfy the raising needs of integration of multiple purposes and views.

Nevertheless, we showed that their results on surgical procedures can be the starting point to perform a subsequent ontological analysis, to:
1. discover and make explicit deep ontological principles;
2. interpret the principles within a solid general framework (eg, our model ON8.5).

Our methodology uses coding systems as sources for well-organized knowledge, in order to assure coverage and an intersubjective approach. We also used authoritative definitions to anchor our compositional analysis to a recognized basis.

In this paper we outlined a set of criteria for surgical experts, suitable to let them express different points of view; the various perspectives lead to different subsets of primitives and multiple organizations among them.

Our results can be used by the European Standardization Body to revise the standard on surgical procedures, as well as by the GALEN-IN-USE project, that is populating a formal model on surgical procedures. Finally, by suitable application of our criteria, end-users can build specialized hierarchies for their particular tasks.

Our approach can be generalized to analyze and integrate semi-formal models ("*categorial structures*" in [CEN96]) developed by independent initiatives. Their results can fit into an incremental mosaic, and endorsement by CEN could assure adequate exploitation of the model as a whole, within terminological systems for advanced information systems in healthcare [Rossi Mori96a, Rossi Mori95].

Acknowledgements Work partially supported by the Committee on Information Sciences of CNR, under the Program on "Strumenti Ontologici e Linguistici per la Modellizzazione Concettuale" (Ontological and Linguistic Tools for Conceptual Modelling), 1994-1996.
Work also partially supported by European Union, under the IV Framework Program (Project GALEN-IN-USE); actual cooperative modelling of rubrics from coding systems on surgical procedures, including discussions with other European Centers, was a stimulating environment for develement of ideas presented in this paper.

References

Averill RA, Mullin RL, Steinbeck BA, Goldfield NI, Grant T. The development of the ICD-10 Procedure Coding System (ICD-10-PCS), 1995. available from: 3M Health Information Systems, 100 Barnes Road, Wallingford CT 06492.

Bernauer J. Merged list of deeds from GRAIL and German version of ICPM. GALEN-IN-USE, Internal Document, 1996

CEN ENV 1828:1995. Health care informatics — Structure for classification and coding of surgical procedures. Brussels: CEN, 1995

CEN ENV 12264:1996. Medical Informatics — Categorial structure of systems of concepts — Model for representation of semantics. Brussels: CEN, 1996

Dorland's Illustrated Medical Dictionary 28th ed, WB Saunders Co., Philadelphia 1994

Falasconi S Stefanelli M. A Library of Medical Ontologies. in N Mars (ed), *Workshop on Comparison of Implemented Ontologies, ECAI 94*, 1994

372

GALEN and GALEN-IN-USE documentation 1992-96, available from the main contractor A Rector, Medical Informatics Group, Dept. Comp Sc, Univ. Manchester, Manchester M13 9 PL, UK (e-mail galen@cs.ac.man.uk; home page http://www.cs.man.ac.uk/mig/galen)

Gangemi A, Steve G, Rossi Mori A. Cognitive Design for Sharing Medical Knowledge Models. in Kaihara (ed.), *Proceedings of MEDINFO-95*, 1995

Gangemi A, Steve G, Giacomelli F. ONIONS: An Ontological Methodology for Taxonomic Knowledge Integration. In van der Vet (ed.) *Proc Workshop on Ontological Engineering, ECAI96*, 1996

Gruber T. A Translation Approach to Portable Ontology Specifications. *Knowledge Acquisition* 1993; 5:188-220

Guarino N, Carrara M, and Giaretta P. An Ontology of Meta-Level Categories. In J Doyle, E Sandewall and P Torasso (eds.), *Principles of Knowledge Representation and Reasoning: Proc. of the Fourth International Conference (KR94)*. Kaufmann, San Mateo, 1994.

Guarino N Ontologies and Knowledge Bases: Towards a Terminological Clarification- in *Proc 2nd Int'l Conf on Building and Sharing Very Large-Scale Knowledge Bases* , 1995

HCFA: Health Care Financing Administration, U.S. Department of Health and Human Services. *International Classification of Diseases, 9th rev. Clinical Modifications (ICD-9-CM), vol. 3 - Procedures*, DHHS-HCFA, 1988

Kolozig Ch, Thurmayr R, Diekmann F, Raskop AM (eds). Internationale Klassifikation der Prozeduren in der Medizin, Blackwell, Berlin 1994

McCarthy J, Buvac S. Formalizing Context. Stanford Tech Note STAN-CS-TN-94-13, 1994

Musen M. Dimensions of Knowledge Sharing and Reuse*Comp Biom Res* 1992;25:435-67

Oxford. The Concise Oxford Dictionary of Current English, Clarendon Press Oxford, 1995

Rossi Mori A, Galeazzi E, Agnello P, Steve G, *Terminological modelling in CEN/TC251/ WG2 and GALEN: the example of surgical procedures*. in Proc. AMICE 95 "Strategic alliances between patient documentation and medical informatics", Amsterdam, 1995a

Rossi Mori A. Coding systems and controlled vocabularies for hospital information systems. *Int J Biom Comp* 1995;39:93-8

Rossi Mori A. Towards a new generation of terminologies and coding systems. in J Brender et al. (eds), Medical Informatics Europe '96, IOS Press, Amsterdam 1996, 208-12

Rossi Mori A, Galeazzi E, Consorti F, An Ontological Perspective on Surgical Procedures. JAMIA 1996; symp suppl: 115-9 (1996b)

Rothwell DJ, Coté RA, Brochu L (eds), *SNOMED International*, Northfield, IL: College of American Pathologists, 1993, 3rd ed.

Schreiber AT, Wielinga B, Breuker JA (eds.). KADS: A Principled Approach to Knowledge-Based Systems Development. Academic press, London 1992

Shadbolt N, Motta E, Rouge A. Constructing Knowledge Based Systems. IEEE Software, 10, 6, 1993

Shapiro SC, Rapaport WJ. The SNePS Family. In F Lehmann (ed.): Semantic Networks in Artificial Intelligence, Pergamon, Oxford, 1992: 243-275.

Stedman's Medical Dictionary, 26th edition, Williams & Wilkins, Baltimore 1995

Steve G, Gangemi A. Modelling a Sharable Medical Concept System: Ontological Foundation in GALEN. in Artificial Intelligence in Medicine Europe, AIME95

Steve G, Gangemi A, Rossi Mori A. Knowledge Integration of Medical terminological Sources: An Ontologic mediation. In S.Ali(ed.): *Proc FLAIRS 96 Track on Information Interchange*, 1996a

Steve G, Gangemi A. Ontological Commitment in the ONIONS Methodology. in B Gaines, G van Heijst (eds), *Proc. of KAW (Knowledge Acquisition Workshop) 96*, 1996b

Uschold M, King M. Towards a Methodology for Building Ontologies. IJCAI95 Workshop on Basic Ontological Issues in Knowledge Sharing, 1995

van Heijst G, Schreiber ATh, Wielinga BG. Using Explicit Ontologies in KBS Development. *International Journal of Human-Computer Studies*, to appear, 1997

Wiley: International Dictionary of Medicine and Biology, 3 voll., Churchill Livingstone, New York, 1986

Wordnet, available from http://www.cogsci.princeton.edu/~wn/

Building Medical Dictionaries
for Patient Encoding Systems: A Methodology

C. Lovis [1], R. Baud [2], AM. Rassinoux [3], PA. Michel [2], JR. Scherrer [2]
University State Hospital of Geneva, Switzerland
[1] Department of Internal Medicine
[2] Division of Medical Informatics
Vanderbilt University, Nashville, USA
[3] Division of Biomedical Informatics,

Abstract

One of the most critical problems of automatic natural language processing (NLP) is the size of the medical dictionaries. The set of compound medical words and the often used possibility to create new terms render the exhaustivity of medical dictionaries beyond question. The structure of such dictionaries is usually composed of two parts : the first one generally contains morphological and sometimes syntactical information necessary to identify, on a grapheme level, a given word in a sentence whereas the second part is often devoted to conceptual knowledge associated with the recognised word. It is only when these two prerequisites are fulfilled that an attempt to understand the meaning of a whole expression is possible. The approach developed in this paper shows the pragmatic method used to implement a powerful analyser dedicated to help physicians or coding clerks to encode medico-economic information about patients using international classifications like ICD. It describes how to build medical dictionaries that can help the application of morphological and conceptual analysers (encoders). The methods used have proved to be efficient for various classifications as well as for multiple languages as the system presently supports French, German, English and Dutch for the full ICD-10 classification.

1 Introduction

The necessity of encoding medical diagnoses is essential for community-based research, clinical epidemiology and medical economics. There is a real lack of tools ensuring good quality and exhaustivity of diagnosis encoding. *Chute et al.* reported that only up to approximately 60% of encoding fully matches the original diagnosis [1]. *Jollis et al.* showed that correlation ratio's between claims and clinical databases ranged from 0.09 to 0.86 [2]. We analysed and manually re-encoded more than 3'000 consecutive diagnoses issued directly from the department of Medicine's discharge letters and found similar results [3]. To overcome these problems and contribute to the establishment of a database with a good representation of patients case mix, we decided to closely associate the coding activity carried out by the physicians in charge of the patients with the redaction of the discharge summary. As this leads to increased work for the physicians, we have built a system that is user-friendly, fast and easy to use, and that can be used for medical management of patients and for research purposes, as well as for reimbursement purposes. The system is part of the *Diogene 2* open and distributed architecture with PC's terminals and distributed UNIX relational databases. It is based on a natural language analyser interface to help physicians find the correct ICD codes. The need to morphologically recognise any word of a sentence before being able to analyse the meaning of the whole expression and the need to have at least one concept attached with any morphological unit is the first step to achieve before any NLP system can have a practical use. This step is concomitant with the computational handling of inflectional morphology, as treated by *Koskenniemi* [4].

It has been shown that the human « *natural language processor* » in the brain can cope with non-programmable computation [5]. This fascinating discovery supports the idea of dealing with word segmentation methodology for NLP systems. Wittgenstein considers, at first, that language is a mirror of the world, and separates the *reference* from the *meaning*. Later, he considers language related to established knowledge, where the meaning of a word is defined by its *usage* [6]. The linguistic sign *(« le signe »)*, as defined by *Saussure*, is a form *(« le signifié »)* associated with a signification *(« la valeur du signifiant »)*. This relation is arbitrary, but « a sign can be characterised by its relation » [7]. Therefore, some words can be considered as referring to a single signification, like *nose* whereas others are an association of signs, like *restless*. The well-suited medical language is a good subject to apply such principles, because this sublanguage is very stable among languages and makes extensive usage of latino-greek root words. The word segmentation technique is especially powerful with such words. Such an approach has already been studied, by *Norton and Pacak* at the NIH about the *-itis* termination in medical words [8], later with forms denoting surgical procedures (*-ectomy, -stomy, -tomy, -rrhaphy, -plasty* and *-pexy*) [9]; by *Suzanne Wolff* from the Linguistic String Project in New York [10] developed a very attractive way to cope with compound words for NLP, but it is mainly for latino-greek linguistic elements . *Dujols et al.* have done an interesting research on the suffix *-osis*. This suffix can have different meanings, according to the various affixes that precede it in a word. They described a methodology and an implementation able to retrieve the correct meaning of *-osis* [11]. These groups have demonstrated the power, necessity and feasibility of handling word decomposition.

2 Thesauri and Terms Sources

We limited the domain of accuracy of our analyser to the ability to recognise natural language used by physicians in the fields of diagnosis and procedures, especially in the fields covered by international classifications. The system currently supports SNOMED 2, ICD-9, ICD-9CM, ICD-10 and ICPC, but all examples and discussion will be based on ICD-10.

To build the basic terms dictionaries, we used different sources of information. First of all, the classification itself. The ICD-10 classification can be obtained in machine readable form in *WordPerfect* format. Approximately 3 man/months were needed to transform this format into a relational database format and validate all links intrinsically found in ICD, like exclusions. We used multilingual mapping to help us validating the results. From these files, all words have been extracted and individualised. This results in dictionaries of terms, approximately >40'000 for French, or >35'000 for German. To these basic dictionaries, we add various sources of known medical expressions mapped to their ICD equivalent, like *Chevalier's Thesam* for French, or the alphabetical ICD hierarchy. Other sources, including SNOMED or UMLS can also be used. The result of the aforementioned is called *terms source*.

3 Building Dictionaries

3.1 Step 1 : Normalisation

The normalisation is performed for each language, by looking at the corresponding terms source and all words are normalised. Normalisation of terms consists of correcting all grammatical and typographical errors and grouping all lexical variants in one unique representation. This representation is language dependent, and consists typically of *lexical type, gender, inflexions* for French or *type, inflexions* for English. The *inflexions* group and *type* of terms vary between languages, like plurals for English, French and German or genitive forms for German.

Example :

Terms source	abrasif, abrasifs, abrasives, abrasion, abraser, abbrasion
Grammatical correction	abrasif, abrasifs, abrasives, abrasion, abraser
Normalisation	adj: abrasi.f,fs,ve,ves
	nfe: abrasion,s

After the normalisation of dictionaries, the French terms source has been decreased to approximately 25'000 entries, whilst the German one has been decreased to approximately 17'000 entries. This step is essential, as it renders the dictionary, in each language, independent of the morphological variations that can be used for a given term. A typographic normalisation is also carried out, especially for German [12].

Example :

Initial element	Typographic normalisation	*Terms examples*
f	ph	Fantasm = phantasm
β	ss	blaβ = blass
k	c	karzinom = carcinom
ä	ae	Nähe = Naehe

3.2 Step 2 : Segmentation

Our dictionary is not exclusively composed of full words, but mostly of segmentation units. By this, we mean any linguistic element that cannot be fragmented into smaller units without losing its original meaning. There are many different elements that may compose a word, including prefixes (like *hyper-, pseudo-*), suffixes (like *-therapy, -ectomy*) or inflections (like *-s* or *-ies* for plura*l*) amongst others. In these morphosemantems, we also include unique words, like *kidney*, eponyms like *Addison* or trademarks like *Ciproxin™*, etc. A given unit may have kept its original meaning (like *andro* – male) or may have undergone a semantic sludge. To illustrate this situation, we can take *-méno* that means nowadays, *menstruation*, as used in *menopause* or *dysmenorrhea*, instead of *mên = moon* in Greek. The prior meaning was related to the cyclic analogies between moon and menstruation. Building the dictionaries was achieved in two steps : we first included all latino-greek elements with their meanings. Then, any given new word that could not be correctly segmented whilst keeping its meaning, was added to the dictionary as a new morphosemantem. In this form, the new root acquires all the characteristics as any other morphosemantem and can therefore be used as a new segmentation unit. So, we consider any new word as a potential new morphosemantem. The process of segmentation was carried out manually to ensure a good quality dictionary and to avoid the noise generated by an automatic segmentation process.

This allows us to correctly analyse, for example : « crise addisonienne » where the concept is, in fact, Addison disease and permits us to build dictionaries with exponential recognising capabilities whilst keeping particularisation possibility to any peculiar word for linking it to a meaning determined by the medical usage. This property is very important for dealing with words like anatomy, which is not the combination of ana- (already) and -tomy (to cut). Contrary to the approach of S. Wolff [10], we do not use rules to ensure that, for example, all words ending in -tomy are confined in a surgical procedure conceptual category. This allows us to deal more easily with words like postmastectomy, referring to the period after the surgical procedure, and not to the surgical procedure itself.

Examples :

Terms source	antalgie	
Normalisation	antalgie,s	
Segmentation	ant_algie,s	ant_ is a negation
Terms source	antiarythmisant	
Normalisation	antiarythmisant,s,e,es	
Segmentation	anti_a_rythmisant,s,e,es	double negation
Terms source	antihyperlipidémiant	
Normalisation	antihyperlipidémiant,s,e,es	
Segmentation	anti_hyper lipid émiant,s,e,es	negation and semantic elements

Beyond the power of representation of this step and the implicit ontology model that has been built, the way to do allows all the various meanings that can be in a unique term, or morphologically subsumed to a term, to be picked up, and therefore renders the dictionary quite independent from the different ways physicians use to express themselves.

Example :

a search with antihypertenseur would be something like :
anti*   link to aggregate « anti, against, etc ... »
hyper*   link to aggregate « hyper, increase, etc ... »
tenseur*   link to aggregate « tenseur, tension, etc ... »

After this step, the French dictionary decreased to approximately 17'000 terms. All the work was also done manually, due to the noise generated by the various automated approaches we tested. Normalisation and segmentation are evaluated at around 2 man/months per language treated.

3.3 Step 3 : Aggregation

This step enables the building of a first level implicit ontology representation of segmented elements. The segmented elements, that represent a kind of atomic concept, are grouped following semantic similarities. These similarities include lexical variants (*lateral - latero*); nouns or adjectives (*cortex - cortical*); synonyms or analogous semantic contents (*heart - myocarde*); abbreviations (*mb - member - membrane*); logos (*AMI - acute + myocardial + infarction*) and so on.

Examples :

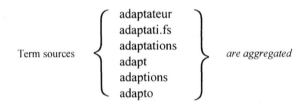

The aggregation step only includes elements found in the terms sources. No external terms, synonyms or links are added up to this step.

3.4 Step 4 : Adjunction

New words or elements are then added to the dictionaries obtained in order to increase the power of morphological analysis. The choice of added terms is mostly, but not exclusively, domain dependent. Examples of such terms include synonyms, or analogous terms, like *alligator* for *crocodile*, short cuts not found in the classification but often used like *op* for *operation*; eponyms like *Rendu-Weber-Osler-Sutton disease* for *Hereditary hemorragic telangiectasies* or drug specialities like *amoxicillin* for *penicillin*. Feedback from users essentially contributes to increasing the adjunction's dictionaries.

3.5 Step 5 : Expression Linking

The source classification is analysed using the aggregated dictionary and a links dictionary is built between the elements found in each aggregation group and the terms found in the expressions of the classification. Whereas the previous steps were done manually by a physician and a computer scientist, the linking is done automatically.

Examples :

Term source	adaptation	
	F43	Réaction à un facteur de stress sévère, et troubles de l'adaptation
	F43.0	Réaction aiguë à un facteur de stress
	F43.1	État de stress post-traumatique
	F43.2	Troubles de l'adaptation
adaptation	F43.8	Autres réactions à un facteur de stress sévère
is linked to	F43.9	Réaction à un facteur de stress sévère, sans précision
	Z55.4	Mauvaise adaptation éducative et difficultés avec les enseignants et les autres élèves
	Z56.5	Mauvaise adaptation au travail
	Z60.0	Difficultés d'ajustement aux transitions entre les différentes périodes de vie

4 Words Representation

This internal representation of a words dictionary has been developed to permit a fast morphological recognition of parts of words, therefore making the real-time segmentation analysis possible as well as a pretty good resistance to typographical errors. This representation is based on a character oriented tree model, using only uppercases and typographic normalisation. If only uppercase is used, there is a maximum of 36 alternative characters at each level ('A'..'Z' and '0'..'9'). Therefore, the worst results search for a 10 character long term is $log_2 36 * number\ of\ chars$, which means ap-

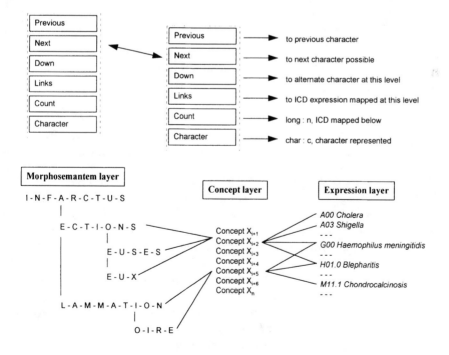

Fig. 1. Character-tree representation

proximately 60 iterations. This number is stable independently of the size of the dictionary and can be greatly improved if a good match algorithm is used. This method is also interesting because partial matches can indicate information on all links below the last match, therefore allowing the morphological treatment to be immediately used for segmentation analysis. The construction of this representation needs 500 to 600 milliseconds on a Pentium 100 MHz for with a set of 20'000 medical words (round 150'000 characters). In that case, 70'000 nodes have been generated, what means that approximately half of all words have partial common morphological representation.

5 Word Mapping Analysis

The major step of the natural language analysis is the morphological terms recognition. This recognition needs huge dictionaries to avoid having unknown terms in the sentence analysed, but needs also to be able to recognise new compound words frequently used in medicine. The dictionaries and their structures, as explained above, allow us to process fast and efficient mapping between terms in the written sentence with elements of the dictionaries. This analysis is based on a highly recursive morphological treatment to identify all known elements of a word or a sentence, then computing *performance indexes* choose the best element associations that represent the word.

Examples : analysis of neurolipoatrophie

Solutions found	54	
Performance index	Recognition	
-6	NEURO LIPO ATROPHIE	*3 semantic, no char lost*
	00011 0002 00000003	
-7	NEUROL I P O ATROPHIE	*2 semantic, 3 char lost*
	000111 / / / 00000002	
-7	NEURO LIPO A TROPHIE	*3 semantic, 1 char lost*
	00011 0002 - 0000003	*maybe negation*
etc ...	etc ...	*etc ...*

In this case, it must be noted that the word *neurolipoatrophie* does not exist in the ICD-10 classification, nor has been introduced into the dictionaries. Despite this, the word has been correctly segmented and semantic elements have been clearly identified. The implemented heuristics consist in minimising the lost characters whilst maximising the length of the semantic terms found. The links in ICD-10 found with this recognition are the following :

G12.2	*Maladies du neurone moteur*
G60.0	*Neuropathie héréditaire motrice et sensorielle*
G64	*Autres affections du système nerveux périphérique*
G71.1	*Affections myotoniques*
M89.0	*Algoneurodystrophie*

This analysis and methodology is actually operating for the ICD-9-CM and ICD-10, in German, French and English.

6 Conclusions

The use of powerful segmentation processing linked with semantic representation have prove to be highly efficient for the implementation of a natural language encoder. Such a representation with a tree-based model of runtime dictionaries allows a very fast morphological analysis with semantic recognition to be carried out on a PC based computer. This programme, called *Lucid*, is presently used in several Hospitals and supports the WHO's International Classification of Diseases version 9 and 10 in French, English and German. A Dutch version of ICD-10 has also been implemented. The present development phase consists of implementing and exploiting an explicit ontology for our concept layer. This phase should greatly improve the quality of retrieval.

Acknowledgments
We wish to thank Dr *Maurice Chevalier* for his work on the French *Thesam*, Dr *Werner Ceuster* for providing the processed Dutch version of ICD-10 and Dr *Vincent Griesser* for helpful criticism on managing ICD links.

References

1. Chute CG, Atkin GE, Ihrke DM. An empirical evaluation of concept capture by clinical classifications. In : Proceedings MEDINFO 92 (Ed. Lun KC, Degoulet P, Piemme TE, Rienhoff O), North-Holland, Amsterdam, 1992, pp.1469-1474
2. Jollis JG, Ancukiewicz M, DeLong ER, Pryor DB, Muhlbaier LH, Mark DB. Discordance of databases designed for claims payment versus clinical information systems. Ann Intern Med, 119:844-850, 1993
3. Lovis C, Michel PA, Borst F, Baud R, Griesser V, Scherrer JR Medico-Economic Patient Encoding in the University Hospital of Geneva. *Proceedings*
4. K. Koskenniemi. Two-level model for morphological analysis. PhD Thesis. University of Helsinki, 1983
5. K. Matsuno. Semantic commitments as a mode of non-programmable computation in the brain. Biosystems (Netherlands), 27/4: 235-239, 1992
6. LJJ. Wittgenstein. Philosophical Investigations.Oxford: Basil Blackwell, 1953
7. F. de Saussure (1915). Cours de linguistique générale. Bally & Sechehaye, Ed. Payot, 1966
8. MG. Pacak, LM. Norton, GS. Dunham. Morphosemantic Analysis of -ITIS Forms in Medical Language. Meth Inform Med, 19: 99-105, 1980
9. LM. Norton, MG. Pacak. Morphosemantic Analysis of Compoud Word Forms Denoting Surgical Procedures. Meth Inform Med, 22: 29-36, 1983
10. S. Wolff. The Use of Morphosemantic Regularities in the Medical Vocabulary for Automatic Lexical Coding. Meth Inform Med, 23: 195-203, 1984
11. P. Dujols, P. Aubas, C. Baylon, F. Grémy. Morphosemantic Analysis and Translation of Medical Compound Terms. Meth Inform Med, 30: 30-35, 1991
12. Brigl B., Mieth M., Haux R., Glück W. The LBI-method for automated indexing of diagnoses by using SNOMED. Part 1. Int J Bio Med Computing, 37: 237-247, 1994

A Semantics-Based Communication System for Dysphasic Subjects⋆

Pascal Vaillant

Thomson-CSF/LCR, Computer Science Group,
Domaine de Corbeville, 91404 ORSAY CEDEX, FRANCE
Phone: (+33) 1 69 33 93 25, Fax: (+33) 1 69 33 08 65
E-mail: vaillant@lcr.thomson.fr

Abstract. Dysphasic subjects do not have complete linguistic abilities
and only produce a weakly structured, topicalized language. They are
offered artificial symbolic languages to help them communicate in a way
more adapted to their linguistic abilities. After a structural analysis of
a corpus of utterances from children with cerebral palsy, we define a
semantic lexicon for such a symbolic language. We use it as the basis
of a semantic analysis process able to retrieve an interpretation of the
utterances. This semantic analyser is currently used in an application
designed to convert iconic languages into natural language; it might find
other uses in the field of language rehabilitation.

1 Introduction

The field of Assisted Communication for speech impaired people now offers a
wide range of material or logical devices that produce audible sentences for the
user. Few systems, though, provide a good communication for subjects whose
language abilities, and not only speech ones, are impaired.

We have tried to tackle the problem of understanding asyntactic utterances
produced by speech and language impaired people through a technique of semantic analysis. This principle has been implemented in a computer application, PVI (*Prothèse Vocale Intelligente*), allowing users to communicate through
sequences of icons translated into French sentences. The same principle had already inspired the COMPANSION system [3], which converts, with different AI
techniques, sequences of uninflected words into English sentences.

In this paper, we will expose in a first part what are the language disabilities
we have to cope with, situate them in the frame of language disorders, and see
what type of discourse disorganization they produce by examining a corpus.

In a second part, we propose a specific technique of semantic analysis able
to analyse this type of discourse. We make some hypotheses on the structure of
the language, draw a model able to represent it, and then expose the operations
one can perform on this model.

⋆ This work has taken place in the frame of the PVI (*Prothèse Vocale Intelligente*)
project, funded by AGEFIPH and Thomson-CSF. It has involved constant cooperation of the Rehabilitation Centre of Kerpape (Lorient, Brittany, France).

We briefly describe the application in which the technique has been implemented. The application itself is described in more detail in [9].

We finally give some elements of evaluation of the system, as they emerge both from quantitative (benchmarking) and qualitative (on-site) evaluation.

2 Consequences of Dysphasia on the Language

2.1 Context of our Study

Speech and language disorders among children can be so miscellaneous in their nature as a simple language acquisition delay or a severe and permanent language deficit.

1. Language acquisition delay may be correlated with some types of mental retardation, or in some cases with social or psychological troubles. Children in this case present some symptoms like lack of phonological or syntactical control, appearing mainly though as mistakes of the same nature as typical childhood language mistakes — not as a systematic deviant linguistic behaviour.
2. A permanent language deficit may be a consequence of:
   (a) a general developmental trouble like *autism*;
   (b) a cerebral lesion acquired during childhood — in this case the language disorder is referred to as *acquired aphasia*;
   (c) a specific language development disorder: *dysphasia*.

The subjects we are working with, children with cerebral palsy, suffer from a global language deficit due to stable cerebral lesions, consequence of a pre- or perinatal accident (e.g. prolonged anoxia).

It has been shown [4] that these children present language disorders which are very close to those of developmental dysphasia. In a clinical perspective, the diagnostic methods are the same, and the rehabilitation guidelines are the same in respect to the proper linguistic troubles. That is why we will further use the term of dysphasia as a set of clinical symptoms, which can be used to characterize the subjects in our study.

The techniques described in this paper have been implemented in communication help software for these children. We will present the types of speech and language troubles observed among the subjects, as these troubles may externally appear.

2.2 Nature of the Language Troubles

The subjects present various symptoms of speech disability, that may be classified roughly into two main categories:

1. speech troubles: phonatory, or articulatory, they hinder the utterance of speech strictly speaking;

2. language troubles: they show themselves in the use of language as manipulation of linguistic signs.

Speech troubles occur at different levels as a consequence of the neuromotor troubles characteristic of cerebral palsy. They can be of phonatory nature (impossibility to form proper sounds in the oral cavity: *dyslalia*), and of articulatory nature (lack of control of the muscles which govern articulation: *dysarthria*).

Language troubles of the subjects possibly affect many linguistic competences. They are symptomatically similar to those observed for dysphasic subjects. We may distinguish:

1. **Semantic troubles**
   They often affect the emergence of abstract concepts and categories. Some subjects are unable to group into a single concept several instances of a category. Some may form improper categories, for example confuse concepts belonging to the same semantic domain.
   More scarcely, one may observe, like in adult aphasia, troubles of lexical access: missing word or jargon.
2. **Syntactic troubles**
   Most widespread, they appear in the subjects' communication as a more or less flagrant destructuration of the utterances. The children reach a stage in the development of syntactic competence and cannot progress beyond that stage. This implies weak grammaticality, and frequently goes along with subjects' preference to short utterances. Furthermore, two noticeable trends have emerged from corpus analysis:
   First, no, or very few, morphosyntactic information is inserted in the message: absent or improper flexion, no "grammatical words". For example, coordination is seldom explicitly conveyed by a particle, neither are semantic relations like attribution, property ... The subjects tend to use only "meaningful" words, producing telegraphic-style utterances.
   Second, the order of the words or symbols in the utterances is not systematically determined by regular rules of grammatical nature. It is chiefly guided by the focus of the message, leading to topicalized utterances. Concepts do not go through a linear encoding of a deep syntactic structure.
   These observations led us to consider semantic analysis as the appropriate way to get the meaning of these utterances.

There are different symptom clusters in situations of dysphasia; but the two main and most widespread symptoms are phonological (speech) and syntactical (language) disorders. This study has been led with a purpose of pragmatic communication aid, more than in a speech therapy perspective. Hence we will focus on the syntactical disorders and the methods proposed to make up for them.

2.3 Adaptative and Augmentative Communication

To make up for those difficulties in using language, rehabilitation centers use a set of vicarious symbolic systems generically referred to as AAC (*Adaptative and Augmentative Communication*) [7].

Several artificial languages have been developed for educational, rehabilitation or communication purposes. These languages are grounded on the preserved linguistic capabilities, which mainly consist in loose categorization and semantic association. They do not rely on any rigid structure, as syntax is beyond the reach of the language impaired patients. These languages are symbolic or iconic and include Bliss, Communimage and Grach.

1. The Bliss pictographic alphabet [1] is composed of ideograms which can be assembled with atomic ideographic elements. It is the most elaborate of the three, and may represent some abstract notions.
2. The Communimage icon set is composed of highly representative figurative drawings.
3. The GRACH symbol set is also of an iconic nature, although more stylized than the Communimage.

Those languages offer:

1. an easier access to meaning, as many of these systems use figurative icons. Even the Bliss alphabet is based on a non-arbitrary relation between a symbol and its signified concept;
2. correlated to the previous point, a more limited set of symbols, excluding in particular subtleties for abstract notions, and excluding "empty", i.e. grammatical words;
3. absence of a specified syntax, the iconic or pictographic language offering simply a set of isolated symbolic conventions with very few dialectal pressure (i.e. collectively set habits of using them).

The discourse that these symbolic systems allow the subjects to produce is thus essentially based on semantics.

The utterances have an underlying semantic structure representing their meaning, where the semantic units are linked to the others through casual relations. This meaning is expressed by the mere sequence of symbols corresponding to the semantic units, as there is no way to express the type of casual relations. There is a directionality in the semantic structure which is expressed by the order of the symbols in the sequence.

While these iconic languages can be interpreted by medical staff, the process of automating their interpretation through computer appears to have several benefits, including giving a correct feedback on patients (which can serve rehabilitation purposes) and enabling them to communicate with a broader environment, not restricted to their family and medical staff. Because these language have a finite set of semantic contents, automatic processing also appears feasible.

3 Semantic Analysis

Therapists or parents of language impaired children generally understand the children's messages because they reconstruct the global meaning by attributing a correct semantic role to every word or symbol. We tried to formalize this process so as to be able to implement it in a communication help software.

The first step is to ground our work material on the phenomena observed in the corpus. We collected a corpus reflecting the spontaneous use of symbolic languages (mainly Bliss and Communimage) by language-impaired children. This corpus is a set of icon sequences (average length of four) which constitute single "utterances", each one being usually interpreted by a Bliss-skilled nurse. Examples of utterances in the corpus are: I/PUT/FLOWER/TABLE, I/WANT/SLEEP, I/WANT/EAT/FISH/CAKE, ANIMAL/PLAY/BALL ...

Study of the corpus led to consider two main semiotical facts:

1. paradigmatic structures: some sets of icons obviously form semantic categories, as they may appear in the same contexts (e.g. the category of "*meals*", which all come with the pictogram for "*eating*");

2. syntagmatic structures: some icons very systematically appear along with some complemental icons, within the same sequence, which belong to regularly the same categories (typically the pictogram "*to eat*" with an icon representing an animal or human being, and with another icon representing a meal). *Syntagmatic* structures don't mean *syntactic* structures, as no compulsory order is always respected, but they form "frames" which represent the basic context associated to a particular icon.

These facts were to support a representation of the iconic language which is exposed below:

3.1 Cognitive and Linguistic Postulates

The language we are trying to analyse has the following two main characteristics:

1. It is generated from a lexicon of invariant, meaningful words or symbols.
   Following linguistic evidence [8], we organized the lexicon into *ad hoc* categories arising from corpus studies, *taxemes*. These taxemes are groups of symbols which have a common semantic base and may be used in the same contexts, e.g. the taxeme of beverages. Every taxeme is part of a *semantic domain*. The domains give a frame for general semantic consistency of the utterances.
   The semantic content of a terminal in the lexicon is thus composed of:
   (a) a semantic domain;
   (b) a semantic category: the taxeme;
   (c) some specific semantic content distinguishing it from the other members of the same taxeme.

2. The utterances of the language are short sequences with no formal structure where the main semantic units are disposed in a topicalized order.
   They have an underlying semantic structure representing their meaning, where the semantic units are linked to the others through casual relations. This meaning is expressed by the mere sequence of symbols corresponding to

386

the semantic units, as there is no way to express the type of casual relations. There is a directionality in the semantic structure which is expressed by the order of the symbols in the sequence.

It could be argued whether these postulates on the nature of the language of dysphasic subjects are not oversimplifications of complex disorders of the manipulation of syntactic structures. However we have adopted them as a good approximation for short sequences of symbols.

Having thus pointed out the properties of the subjects' language, postulated out of corpus evidence, we may define a model fit for implementation.

3.2 Formalization

In order to manipulate the semantic content of the symbols, we use a structural description based on semantic features. Every symbol has generic features inherited from the domain and the taxeme it belongs to, and specific features identifying it inside the taxeme.

A feature is defined as a simple attribute-value couple, where the value is always an atom. In most cases in our lexicon, the elementary features we use have a binary value: +1 or −1.

The number of features used to define the content of one symbol is not set a priori, but depends on the needs to distinguish it from other symbols. This approach, which is the approach of *differential semantics* [8], is based on the corpus only, and ensures compatibility with assessed semiotic phenomena. It has the drawback of setting combinatory problems when the size of the lexicon grows, but we have been dealing up to now with a small corpus and have not met the problem yet.

The meaning content of an utterance is represented by a network in which the vortices are semantic units and typed arcs are casual relations, like in Fig. 1. Topicality is represented by an order defined on the vortices of the network.

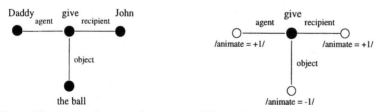

Fig. 1. The semantic network   Fig. 2. A potential casual structure

The basic operation chosen to represent dynamic manipulation of semantic data is *unification* [6]. A semantic relation in a network is the actualization of a potential structure where some variables are left uninstantiated. These potential structures are typical casual structures, observable in the corpus, which are "fossilized" in the lexicon (like in Fig. 2). The semantic information borne by these structures is represented as selectional features, which condition the unification of a symbol as the casual filler of another.

3.3 Heuristics for Automatic Understanding

Natural Language Understanding systems are classically based on a first step being the parsing of formal structures. [2] defines a dependency parser for free word order languages such as latin, but it still relies on syntactic (to be exact, morphological) information.

Our aim in this study is to provide a good analysis of a language which has a limited expressive power, but provides no syntactic information to guide understanding. As we have postulated (3.1.2.) that this language is flatly generated from a semantic network where the organization is provided by semantic relations, we shall logically extract information from the sequences by trying to identify these semantic relations, in order to find back a semantic network.

This is done by trying to match the best case fillers to every potential casual structure attached to a symbol in the sequence.

The input to analyse is a sequence of symbols $s_1, s_2, ...s_n$, where every symbol in the sequence has a set of intrinsic features defining its semantic content: $\mathcal{IF}(s_i) = F$ (F is a set of semantic features).

Some symbols in the sequence are "predicative" symbols, i.e. a potential casual structure may be attached to them. The casual structure is a set of casual relations, each of which has a set of selectional features attached to it:

$$\mathcal{CS}(s_i) = \{< c_1, F_1 >, < c_2, F_2 >, ... < c_k, F_k >\}$$

(where c_j is the type of a casual relation, and F_j is a set of semantic features).

We note the set of selectional features attached to the (predicative) symbol s_i for the case c_j: $\mathcal{SF}(s_i, c_j) = F$ (which is equivalent to $< c_j, F > \in \mathcal{CS}(s_i)$).

We define the "value" of a case-filling unification, i.e. the value of the symbol s_k as a filler for the case c_j of the predicative symbol s_i, as the *semantic compatibility* of the intrinsic features of s_k to the selectional features of s_i for the case c_j:

$$\mathcal{V}(s_i, c_j, s_k) = \mathcal{C}(\mathcal{SF}(s_i, c_j), \mathcal{IF}(s_k)) \tag{1}$$

The relation of semantic compatibility of a set of semantic features to another is itself defined as:

$$\mathcal{C}(F_1, F_2) = \frac{\sum_{f_i \in F_1 \cap F_2} \mathcal{X}(f_i, F_1, F_2)}{\text{number of elements in } F_2} \tag{2}$$

where $\quad \mathcal{X}(f_i, F_1, F_2) = +1$ if f_i has the same value in F_1 as in F_2, $\quad\quad\quad\quad\quad = -1$ otherwise.

This relation is asymmetric: it measures the degree of fitness *of* the set F_2 *to* the set F_1.

An *affectation* A of a set of candidate symbols $S = \{s_{i1}, s_{i2}, ...s_{ij}\}$ as case-fillers to the predicative symbol s_i is an application of the set of cases of s_i ($\mathcal{CS}(s_i) = \{< c_1, F_1 >, < c_2, F_2 >, ... < c_k, F_k >\}$) into the set of candidate symbols:

$$A = \{< c_x, s_{iy} >\}, \text{ where } x \in [1, k] \text{ and } y \in [1, j].$$ (3)

We define the global value of an affectation A of the symbols $s_{i1}, s_{i2}, \ldots s_{ik}$ as case-fillers of the predicative symbol s_i as the sum of the values of every single unification:

$$\mathcal{V}(s_i, \{< c_1, s_{i1} >, < c_2, s_{i2} >, \ldots < c_k, s_{ik} >\}) = \sum_{j \in [1,k]} \mathcal{V}(s_i, c_j, s_{ij})$$ (4)

Hence, the search of a best interpretation of the sequence is the search, for every predicative symbol of the sequence, of the best affectation of other symbols as its case-fillers, i.e. the search of a maximum for the value defined above:

$$\max_{A} \mathcal{V}(s_i, A)$$ (5)

3.4 Implementation

Sample PROLOG code is provided to illustrate the implementation.

Intrinsic features of the symbols are defined in the internal database:

```
feature(Sym,(Att,Val)).
```

So are the predicative symbols' selectional features, attached to their casual relations:

```
case(Sym,Cas,(Att,Val)).
```

The semantic compatibility of a set of semantic features to another is calculated based on the number of selectional features satisfied by the presence of the corresponding intrinsic features (with the same value):

```
compatible_ratio(L,[],(0,Den)) :-
  length(L,Den).

compatible_ratio(L1,[(Att,Val)|L2],(Sum,Den)) :-
  member((Att,Val),L1),!,
  compatible_ratio(L1,L2,(Psum,Den)),
  Sum is Psum+1.

compatible_ratio(L1,[(Att,Val2)|L2],(Sum,Den)) :-
  member((Att,Val1),L1),!,
  Val1 =\= Val2,
  compatible_ratio(L1,L2,(Psum,Den)),
  Sum is Psum-1.

compatible_ratio(L1,[(_,_)|L2],(Sum,Den)) :-
  compatible_ratio(L1,L2,(Sum,Den)).
```

```
compatible_float(L1,L2,Real) :-
  compatible_ratio(L1,L2,(Sum,Den)),
  Real is Sum/Den.
```

The semantic value of an affectation is the sum of the semantic values of every single unification of a symbol to a case:

```
affectation(Pred,[],_,0).
```

```
affectation(Pred,[Cas|Lc],[Sym|Ls],Score) :-
  bagof((SelAtt,SelVal),
        case(Pred,Cas,(SelAtt,SelVal)),
        LselFeat),
  bagof((IntAtt,IntVal),
        feature(Sym,(IntAtt,IntVal)),
        LintFeat),
  compatible_float(LselFeat,LintFeat,UnifScore),
  affectation(Pred,Lc,Ls,Pscore),
  Score is Pscore+UnifScore.
```

The search of the best affectations is then the result of a *quick sort* algorithm.

3.5 Other Elements of the Analysis Process

With the analysis technique described in 3.3, there potentially could be a correct interpretation of any sequence of symbols, provided that the total number of casual relations in the casual structures reaches the number of symbols in the sequence minus one. As a matter of fact the search for a maximum always yields a result, even if the maximum is negative.

Pragmatically, this is unrealistic and might lead to utter nonsense. The data given in the corpus show that a minimal isosemy is present in any utterance, guaranteeing its consistency.

We have thus introduced a first constant, the *acceptability threshold*. Individual semantic unifications whose values do not exceed this threshold are rejected.

Similarly, the topicality of the utterances makes it unlikely that long distance semantic attachments exist between two symbols which are not in a close vicinity in the sequence. This locality constraint becomes relevant as soon as sequences are 4 or 5 symbols long. To take it into account, we have defined a second constant, the *locality* constant, which represents the fading of semantic relations with the linear distance in the uttered sequences.

Practically, this constant will intervene in the calculus of the value of a semantic unification at the power of n, n being the distance between the two semantic units within the sequence.

This constant is a rough way of modeling the effect of distance in semantic relations inside a text (in a broad sense). We use it successfully on our small examples.

Both the acceptation threshold and the locality constant have been defined by iterative tries based on the corpus.

4 The Application

The technique of semantic analysis described above has been implemented in an adaptative and augmentative communication application: PVI (*Prothèse Vocale Intelligente*, i.e. Intelligent Voice Prosthesis), available as a software program for portable computers. This application has a broader scope which also includes assisting the subjects for pictogram input, taking into account their motor disabilities, as well as generating correct sentences in natural language (French) from the semantic networks obtained after the analysis.

As the differential semantic description appears to be common both to symbolic languages and natural language, it provides the basis for conversion of one language into another. To convert a semantic representation into natural language assumes that the process of semantic analysis can be somehow reversed, a processing phase called lexical choice. It consists in determining which words can be formed from the network of semantic features yielded by the semantic analysis. This is mainly a matter of reorganizing the semantic content into relevance islands. These islands are determined by the proper description of an object or an action. For instance, every feature describing the same object will be grouped into a single word - if such a word exists - no matter which icon they come from. This is performed through a natural language dictionary described with the same semantic features as the icon vocabulary, and a set of heuristics.

Of course, in natural language, even simple utterances have to follow syntactic well-formdness principles. This is why conversion between symbolic and natural language cannot rely purely on semantic knowledge but has to include syntactic information in the late stage of translation. Syntactic information is incorporated into syntactic trees in the formalism of Tree-Adjoining Grammar [5]. This accounts for a predicate-centered syntactic representation accepting various modifiers which fit the basic phenomena encountered. More complex syntactic phenomena such as long-distance dependencies fall out of our scope.

As a whole, the PVI application should be a completely transparent application with a customizable, graphical front-end for the user, and a natural language front-end for the interlocutors, ideally acting as a filter between agrammatical pictographic designation and natural language.

Sample utterances treated by the application:

```
?- transfer([i,eat,meat],Sentence).
Sentence = "Je mange la viande"                    "I eat the meat"
?- transfer([meat,i,eat],Sentence).
Sentence = "Je mange la viande"                    "I eat the meat"
?- transfer([fork,i,eat],Sentence).
Sentence = "Je mange avec la fourchette"           "I eat with the fork"
?- transfer([fork,i,eat,meat],Sentence).
Sentence = "Je mange la viande
avec la fourchette"                                "I eat the meat with the fork"
?- transfer([i,give,cat,meat],Sentence).
Sentence = "Je donne la viande au chat"            "I give the meat to the cat"
```

```
?- transfer([i,give,cat,daddy],Sentence).
Sentence = "Je donne le chat à Papa"        "I give the cat to Daddy"
```

5   Evaluation

The system has been submitted to a benchmarking test: a set of 200 icon sequences, reproducing in their structure a number of spontaneously uttered patterns, has been given as input for content analysis and language generation.

The results were indexed into the four following categories, depending on their correct analysis but also on the "naturalness" of the French sentence produced: (I) Correct analysis, correct generation; (II) Correct analysis, clumsy generation; (III) Incomplete or clumsy analysis; (IV) Incorrect analysis.

The results were the following: category I: 147 sequences; category II: 15 sequences; category III: 15 sequences; category IV: 18 sequences.

When we decide to consider "acceptable" the sequences which were either correctly analysed and generated, or correctly analysed but imperfectly generated (and still comprehensible), that is when we merge categories I and II, we thus get an acceptability rate of 80.5 % on this benchmark.

This of course must not be taken for a global acceptability level of the PVI system by the user in an ecological situation. During on-site evaluation, which was conducted during five months with six individuals subject to cerebral palsy in the rehabilitation center of Kerpape (Brittany, France), a certain number of problems linked to real-life situations were unveiled:

1. unexpected answers from the system, even if they are a minority, very soon get the user frustrated and nervous, since the actual input of the sequence of icons by a person suffering from motor disabilities is rather long (it may be counted in minutes). A bad result is thus immediately resented as a frustrating waste of time;

2. lack of vocabulary can not easily be overriden by hand gestures or segments of words, as it is the case during direct communication — or else the missing element in the sequence will lead to nonsense. We have been asked with emphasis to increase the initial vocabulary of the system (grossly 300 icons) whose limits are reached very soon;

3. problems of interface ergonomy are sometimes crucially important for users who have only a few interface points with the system.

However, these critiques might be interpreted as an encouragement to develop a promising prototype, whose principles have been validated, and to adapt it to the realities of difficult ecological situations.

6   Conclusion

We have proposed and implemented a semantic analyser which performs manipulation of symbolic knowledge. It has proved to be successful in the interpretation of weakly structured utterances of symbols.

Further reflexion will aim at taking into account other semantic phenomena. Very interesting ones are contextual meaning effects, which should be described by *dynamic* manipulation of semantic features.

Another arising topic of interest is the more detailed theoretical study of how visual (icon or pictogram) semantics and language semantics intersect and interact wih each other.

The technique exposed in this paper was designed to cope with a specific problem of language alteration for dysphasic subjects, but its availability might open new perspectives. Language prostheses have a great potential for the rehabilitation of language impaired patients. In particular, its adaptation to adult traumatic aphasia, with the experience in the field of rehabilitation for these cases, might bring promising results.

References

1. C. K. Bliss. *Semantography*. 1965.
2. M. Covington. Parsing discontinuous constituents in dependency grammar. *Computational Linguistics*, 16(4): 234–236, 1990.
3. P. W. Demasco et K. F. McCoy. Generating text from compressed input: an intelligent interface for people with severe motor impairments. *Communications of the ACM*, 35(5): 68–78, 1992.
4. C.-L. Gérard, M. Dugas, et P. Lacert. Dysphasia and early focal brain injury. Hypothesis for postlesional cerebral reorganization. In *First international symposium on specific speech and language disorders in children*, University of Reading, U.K., 1987.
5. A. K. Joshi, L.S. Levy, et M. Takahashi. Tree adjunct grammars. *Journal of Computer and System Sciences*, 1975.
6. M. Kay. Unification. In M. Rosner et R. Johnson (eds), *Computational Linguistics and Formal Semantics*. Cambridge University Press, Cambridge, 1992.
7. L. L. Lloyd, R. W. Quist, et J. Windsor. A proposed Augmentative and Alternative Communication model. *AAC Augmentative and Alternative Communication*: 172–183, 1990.
8. F. Rastier. *Sémantique Interprétative*. Formes Sémiotiques. PUF, Paris, 1987.
9. Pascal Vaillant et Michaël Checler. Intelligent voice prosthesis: converting icons into natural language sentences. In *Montpellier'95. 4th International Conference "Interface to Real & Virtual Worlds" Proceedings*, Montpellier, 1995. EC2 & Cie, 9 rue Denis-Poisson, 75017 Paris — France.

Multilingual Decision-Support for the Diagnosis of Acute Abdominal Pain: An European Concerted Action (COPERNICUS 555)

C. Ohmann, H.P. Eich, E. Keim and the COPERNICUS Abdominal Pain Study Group

Theoretical Surgery Unit, Department of General and Trauma Surgery, Heinrich-Heine-University, Düsseldorf, Germany

1. Introduction

Acute abdominal pain (AAP) is a frequent clinical problem with the necessity for urgent management decisions (1). Treatment varies considerably between countries and centers with major differences in outcome. It has been shown that clinical care can be improved by standardized computer-supported documentation and computer-aided diagnosis (2). It is the aim of the Concerted Action (CA) to develop software in national languages providing support for documentation and diagnosis in acute abdominal pain, to distribute the program to Eastern European countries and to introduce it into clinical routine. The program will be used to study the diagnostic accuracy, the distribution and presentation of diseases, the spectrum of diagnostic and management procedures and the outcome. The quality of care in Eastern Europe in AAP will be assessed and if necessary, strategies for improvement will be developed. In the project a new informatic approach is introduced dealing with the multilingual problem of software design in medicine.

2. Methods

The CA covers a 3 years period starting from the 1st of January 1995. Till now 28 participating centers from 18 countries are involved mainly from Eastern Europe. The CA is coordinated by the Theoretical Surgery Unit of the Heinrich-Heine-University in Düsseldorf. The project plan covers 8 phases: preparatory phase, software engineering, development of national data dictionaries, evaluation of national data dictionaries, preparatory phase for introduction of software, introduction of software in clinical routine, clinical application of software and final evaluation. The software for diagnostic support of AAP has been developed by object oriented analysis, design and programming (3,4). The program consists of three components: a data dictionary, a clinical data base and the knowledge-based system (figure 1).

The data dictionary is aimed at providing consistent data over time and among multiple users, making all medical terms known to all parts of the system and leading to standardized recording of patient data (5). In the clinical data base, all patient data are stored. The clinical data can be entered via a documentation program with form-based data entry (6). The knowledge-based system covers different knowledge modules, such as scoring systems and rule-based systems developed with automatic rule generation from prospective data bases. The procedure of knowledge acquisition is not the topic of this paper and is discussed elsewhere (7,8). This work deals mainly with the provision of multilingual decision-support by adequate software design.

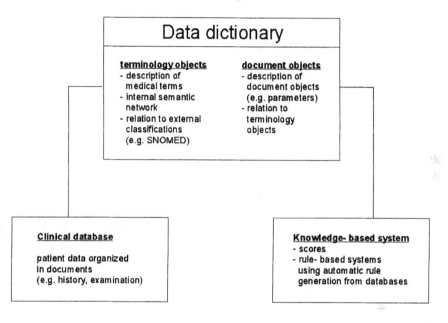

Figure 1: **Informatical conception**

The data dictionary conception is based on a two layer model (figure1, (6)). The first layer covers the terminology objects characterized by the description of the medical terms, an internal semantic network connecting medical terms and relations to external classifications (e.g. SNOMED). The second layer covers all document objects. It contains a description of the document objects (e.g. parameters to be documented) and relations to terminology objects. Blood pressure for example is placed in the semantic network as a medical term (terminology object) and is part of the clinical examination. It is defined as a parameter in the section of document objects by the method of investigation (RIVA ROCCI), the parameter type (continuous) and the valid range. The actual value of the patient (e.g. 120 mmHg) is stored in the clinical data base together with the identification number of the parameter.

The data dictionary program consists of two modules, a data dictionary editor and a data dictionary translator. With the data dictionary editor terminology and document objects can be entered, edited or deleted. In addition, internal and external relations between terminology objects can be defined and displayed. The data dictionary translator is used to perform the translation of terminology and document objects into different languages. In figure 2 an example of a translation of the parameter „location of abdominal pain, at onset" into the German language is demonstrated. The data dictionary translator has been used to translate the original versions of the data dictionaries (English, German) into the different Eastern European languages.

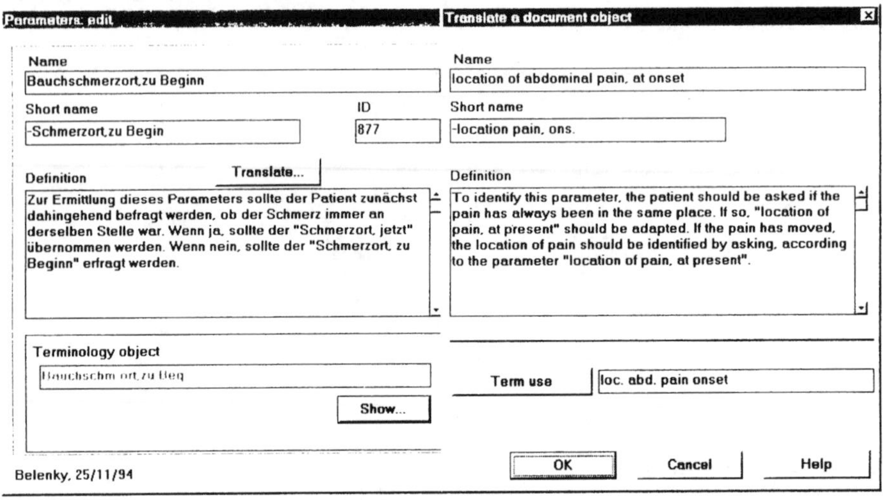

Figure 2: **Data dictionary translator**
Screen mask of a translation of a german document object into an english document object (location of abdominal pain, at onset)

In the program conception a clear cut distinction is made between the documentation program and the knowledge-based system on one hand and the national data dictionary on the other hand. The documentation and the knowledge module are uniform and identical for all the program versions. In order to get functioning programs in the different languages a national data dictionary is linked to the uniform program module. In order to get another version in a different language one has simply to exchange the national data dictionary. All software modules have been developed for IBM-compatible PC's with Windows 95 and Borland C++.

3. Results
Using the data dictionary editor a German and English data dictionary for AAP has been developed with 580 terminology objects, 501 document objects and 2136 links between terminology objects. These original data dictionaries have been translated by national representatives in Düsseldorf into the following Eastern European languages: Hungarian, Estonian, Lithuanian, Latvian, Polish, Slovak, Romanian and Belarussian. The national data dictionaries have been evaluated by national representatives and experts. The different data dictionaries have been linked to the documentation program and to the knowledge-based system. Figure 3 shows a screen mask of the history in the

Belarussian version. The different national programs have been presented to the project participants in a project meeting (June 96) and have been discussed and evaluated. The software has been approved and will now be introduced into clinical routine. Data collection will start at the 1st of January 1997.

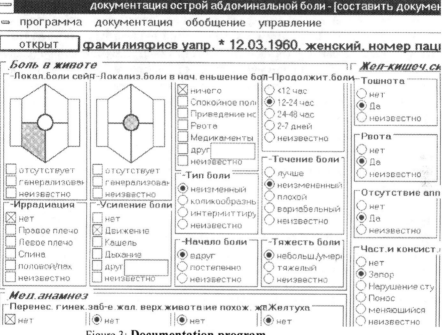

Figure 3: **Documentation program**
Part of a screen mask of the history (Belarussian version)

4. Discussion

The data dictionary approach in clinical information systems and knowledge-based systems can now be considered as a standard (5,6,9). It is an optimal approach to control consistency of data entry and to assure adherence to international standards. In addition, structured report generation, screen mask generation and interactive data entry may be supported by a data dictionary (e.g. (10)). Another major feature is the support of multilingual documentation. In our design only terminology objects and document objects have to be translated once together with the definitions. There is no need to translate internal and external relations. If a term has been translated, such as acute appendicitis, it can be used in many clinical documents (e.g.ultrasound, diagnosis) or in the knowledge-based system (e.g. diagnostic score, computer-aided diagnosis). The software design is very efficient and a new national version can easily be generated. Once the terminology has been translated it is possible to expand the program to other modes of computer-aided decision support (e.g. guidelines, algorithms) and to produce new national versions. In the design of the data dictionary it is differentiated between medical terms and document objects (6). Medical terms are considered rather stable and independent of concrete clinical documentations. For example the medical term „severity of pain" can be characterized as an attribute of pain and described as the perceived intensity of pain. No more information is necessary from the view point of terminology, except that the severity of pain „is part of" pain (internal relation) and to which SNOMED and UMLS term this medical term is related. Much more difficult is the use of a medical term under clinical circumstances. Severity of pain may be documented by the categories „mild", „moderate" and „severe", where severe pain is defined by pain which causes the patient obvious stress. Another mode of documentation would be to assess severity of pain on a visual analogue rating scale with values from zero (best) to 10 (worth). In our design terminology and document objects are distinguished in order to separate basic knowledge and terminology issues from a concrete documentation of parameters. This clear cut structure is an advantage to existing data dictionaries which do not distinguish between medical terms and documents objects.

5. Acknowledgement

The work was supported by grant of the European Union Copernicus program (project 555).

6. References

1. Hoffmann J, Rasmussen OQ: Aids in the diagnosis of acute appendicitis. Br. J. Surg. 76: 774-779 (1989)
2. Adams ID, Chan M, Clifford PC, Cooke WM, Dallos V, Dombal FT de, Edwards MH, Hancock DM, Hewett DJ, McIntyre N, Sommerville PG, Spiegelhalter DJ, Wellword J, and Wilson DH. Computer-aided diagnosis of acute abdominal pain: a multicentre study. Br. Med. J. 2193: 800-804 (1986)
3. Coad P and Yourdon E. Object Oriented Analysis. Prentice Hall, Inc., New Jersey (1991)
4. Coad P and Yourdon E. Object Oriented Design. Prentice Hall. Inc. New Jersey (1991)
5. Linnarson R and Wigertz O. The data dictionary: a controlled vocabulary for integrating clinical data-bases and medical knowledgebases. Meth. Inform. Med. 28: 78-85 (1989)
6. Ohmann C, Belenky G, Platen C. Integration of a data dictionary and a clinical database in an expert system for acute abdominal pain. In: R.A. Greenes, H.E. Petterson, D.J. Protti (editors): Proceedings of the Eigth World Congress on Medical Informatics (MEDINFO 95). North Holland, Amsterdam, 943-946 (1995)
7. Ohmann C, Moustakis V, Yang Q, Lang K. Acute Abdominal Pain Study Group: Evaluation of automatic knowledge acquisition techniques in the diagnosis of acute abdominal pain. Artif. Intell. Med. 8: 23-36 (1996)
8. Ohmann C, Yang Q, Franke C, and the Abdominal Pain Study Group. Diagnostic scores for acute appendicitis. Eur. J. Surg. 161: 273-281 (1995)
9. Prokosch HU, Dudek J, Junghans G, Marquardt K, Sebald P and Michael A. WING-Entering a new phase of electronic data processing at the Gießen University Hospital. Meth. Inform. Med. 30: 289-296 (1991)
10. Bernauer J. Designing a terminology controlled interface for report generation. In: T. Timmers, B.I. Blum (editors): Software Engineering in Medical Informatics. North Holland, Amsterdam, 441-462 (1992)

Medical Concept Systems, Lexicons and Natural Language Generation

Judith C. Wagner, Christian Lovis, Robert H. Baud, Jean-Raoul Scherrer

Medical Informatics Department
University Hospital of Geneva, Switzerland

Natural Language Generation (NLG) and Medical Concept Representation can function to mutual benefit. NLG tools need a concept representation system for their semantics, whilst compositional and language independent Medical Concept Representation systems need NLG of readable expressions for composed concepts. To meet these needs, the roles of both sides and their links must be clearly defined. In particular, a clear distinction between concepts, terms and lexical items is necessary. The benefits of linking multilingual lexicons with a concept system are described, together with an architecture designed to integrate NLG within a set of terminological services.
Keywords: Natural Language Understanding; integration of KBS and patient medical record.

Introduction

The importance of using controlled medical vocabularies or standardised terminologies as an underlying base for a whole range of applications in the medical informatics domain has been widely recognised. Whilst the necessity for co-ordinating and integrating these terminologies is uncontested, the approaches differ. Most of the approaches tend to be primarily term-oriented, but increasingly this is supplemented by a conceptually oriented approach[1-3]. The next step is towards deep representations, which are compositional on a conceptual level, such as in the GALEN project[4].

Today, concepts are, in most cases, represented by terms, but the distinction between term and concept is often unclear. This creates various problems when dealing with the terminological variety already in the English language[5], and it becomes crucial in a multilingual context. Differentiation on this level is mandatory, especially for Natural Language Processing purposes[6,7].

Natural Language Generation for Medical Concept Representation

One of the key features of a conceptual model is to be language independent. In a purely conceptual model, a given concept could be represented by any arbitrary identifier. For use within an application, however, concepts must be represented in a language by an expression. For an atomic concept, this mapping can be realised by assigning string(s) to the concept. Such a string may consist of a simple or a multi-word term. A simple concept-to-term mapping is not, however, sufficient for generating or recognising all terminological variants of a concept. Moreover, it does not allow different terms to be used as required by a specific domain or application, as the semantic model does not take into account the context dependency for the usage of given terms. Most significantly of all, the more a model becomes compositional, the less it is possible to maintain such a mapping. Such an approach defeats the generative nature of the model: a deep representation model of medical concepts needs a tool for generating natural language, allowing a natural language expression to be composed from the sub-parts of its compositional concepts. This necessity will become more evident the more medical concept representation systems become semantic-oriented and generative.

Knowledge Structures for Natural Language Generation

In contrast to the analysis of natural language, NLG is essentially a process of choices. This includes for example the selection of words for concepts and the selection of syntactic structures as the 'frame' for putting these words together. Hence, the links between concepts and words, and between semantics and syntax are prevailing aspects in this process. We will concentrate below on mechanisms for linking concepts to words.

Lexicons and their content

As mentioned earlier, lexical choice is a central element in the generation process[8]. Therefore, the lexicons are a central knowledge structure for any natural language processing tool. 'No longer is the lexicon simply the repository for thematic rules and certain grammatical exceptions. It is rather being seen as a rich theoretical construct with its own complexity and formal properties. There is little agreement on how to proceed with constructing a lexical framework...'[9:1]. Lexicons are defined as that part of the grammar of a language containing the lexical entries for all the words and/or morphemes in the language. They may also contain other information such as morphological, syntactic information etc., also in form of 'lexical rules'.

Terms: linking concepts to words

When using a language-independent basic representation, it is important to link the words in different languages to the semantics in order to use them for expressing the concepts. In our work[10], the link 'word-to-concepts' is inverted: we do not have an inventory of the words of a language which are then linked to grammatical and semantic information. Instead, we have an 'inventory' of concepts - the CORE model - linked to language 'units', expressing these concepts in several languages. This allows synonymous terms of the same language, as well as the terms of different languages, to be linked via the model. These language 'units' may consist of single words or morphemes (such as prefixes), in which case they are similar to classic lexical items. However, they may also be constituted of specific word forms (e.g. words in plural, such as 'platelets' for the laboratory value within 'elevated platelets'). They may also embody multi-word terms, which are an important and frequently met element in medical language (e.g. 'body structure' - 'structure du corps'- 'Körperstruktur'). The difficulty of deciding whether to split compound terms within the conceptual representation into their constituent parts or not has been recognised[2]. In fact, a medical concept representation can not be lead to a granularity where every concept corresponds to a word. This is especially true when dealing with different languages, as words exist at different levels of granularity.

Multi-word terms introduce specific problems: it is not possible to assign grammatical information such as the lexical category, subcategorisation facts and morphological or syntactic irregularities to these items in the same way as they can be assigned to discrete words in a traditional lexical entry. 'Pathological body structure' is not a noun, but a noun phrase consisting of 'structure' as head, a noun premodifier ('body') and an adjectival premodifier ('pathological').

Any natural processing system needs information about the underlying phrase structure for the correct morphological or syntactic handling of these items. This has two consequences: 1. the grammatical information for terms is different from the information in traditional lexicons. 2. the terms annotated to concepts have to be put down to words in order to assign the respective information to them.

Annotations: linking a domain model to the lexicons

For linking concepts, terms and words, we propose the following structure, comprising three different layers (Fig. 1):

- A conceptual **model** of the domain, including the basic and composite concepts, composite concepts being defined by basic concepts and semantic links.
- **Annotations** of concepts, linking concepts to the several synonymous terms for a concept. If such an annotation consists of a multi-word term, it has to be decomposed in a deep syntactic representation, referring to lexical entries. In the case of annotation by a single word or morphemes, the annotation can directly point to a lexical entry.
- **Lexicons**, assigning different grammatical properties to a lexical item.

Concept annotations link concepts to phrases, that is to instantiations of phrasal categories by words. Independently of this, the properties of words are described in the lexicons.

Acquisition of the knowledge

The distinction of three layers as proposed is also sensible with respect to the acquisition of the contents: The annotation of concepts by terms should be done by the modellers, at least in their own language, as they are best placed to know to which terms a new concept is associated. On the contrary, the modeller is unlikely to be the provider of the linguistic information about words and terms. The decomposition of multi-word terms to a deep representation can be achieved by a parser. Finally, for the assignment of linguistic properties to lexical entries we can refer to available dictionaries, at least partially.

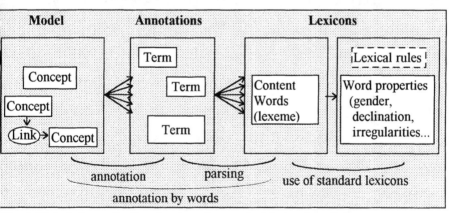

Fig. 1. Links between the three layers and ways of achieving these links.

A Multilingual Natural Language Generation Component

As part of the GALEN project, we have implemented a multilingual NLG tool which is based on the structures described above[11]. This tool is working for the English, French, German, Dutch and Italian languages. Experiments have also been done for other languages. Within this tool, we apply Conceptual Graph operations[12] using the definitions of concepts, in order to adapt the level of granularity to the availability of terms in each language, and to the desired language style[13] (Fig. 2). Furthermore, graph operations, allow semantic or syntactic graphs for multi-word terms to be integrated within the graph serving for generation, and therefore allow these terms to be handled correctly.

[cl_SurgicalDeed,[rel_isCharacterisedBy([cl_performance,[rel_isEnactmentOf([cl_Extrac ting,[rel_playsClinicalRole([cl_SurgicalRole,[rel_actsSpecificallyOn([cl_Calculus,[rel_ha sLocation(cl_Ureter)]]),rel_hasSpecificSubprocess([cl_SurgicalApproaching,[rel_hasSurg icalOpenClosedness([cl_Route,[rel_passesThrough(cl_SkinAsOrgan)]])]])]])])])])]]
english: 'percutaneous extracting of a ureteric calculus'
french: 'extraction d''une lithiase urétérale par voie percutanée'
german: 'perkutane Extraktion einer Lithiasis des Ureters'
dutch: 'percutane extractie van een urethersteen'

Fig. 2. Example of multilingual generation from the GALEN model.

Conclusion

With the ongoing evolution of medical concept representation systems, and the necessity of multilingual aspects of informational supports as well as user-interface, the use of Natural Language Generation tools will become pervasive in future. The results obtained within the GALEN project are very encouraging as they show the feasibility of a) designing a language independent model of medical knowledge and b) generating phrases in several languages from this model. Provided that concepts, terms and lexical items are strictly separated, the possibilities for generating natural language expressions in one or several languages are manifold. Adapting natural language expressions to contexts, users or domains, without losing the link to controlled vocabularies, becomes possible.

References

1. Masarie FE, Miller RA, Bouhaddou O, Giuse NB, Warner HR. An Interlingua for Electronic Interchange of Medical Information: Using Frames to Map between Clinical Vocabularies, *Comp Biomed* 1991; 24: 379-400.
2. McCray AT, Nelson SJ. The Representation of Meaning in the UMLS. *Methods Inf Med* 1995; 34(1/2):193-201.
3. Friedman C, Huff SM, Hersh WR, Pattison-Gordon E, Cimino JJ, The Canon Group's Effort: Working Toward a Merged Model. *J Am Med Informatics Assoc* 1995; 2(1):4-18.
4. Rector AL, Solomon WD, Nowlan WA et al.. A Terminology Server for Medical Language and Medical Information Systems. *Methods Inf Med* 1995; 34(1/2): 147-57.
5. McCray AT, Srinivasan S, Brown AC. Lexical Methods for Managing Variation in Biomedical Terminologies. *Proc Annu Symp Comput Appl Med Care* 1994; 235-239.
6. Friedman C, Cimino JJ, Johnson SB. A Schema for Representing Medical Language applied to Clinical Radiology. *J Am Med Informatics Assoc* 1994; 1(3): 233-248.
7. Baud RH, Rassinoux A-M, Wagner JC et al. Representing Clinical Narratives Using Conceptual Graphs. *Methods Inf Med* 1995; 34(1/2): 176-186.
8. Nogier J-F, Zock M. Lexical choice as pattern matching. *Knowledge-Based Systems* 1992; 5(2):200-212.
9. Pustejovsky J (ed). *Semantics and the Lexicon*. Dordrecht: Kluwer Academic Publishers, 1993.
10. Baud R, Lovis C, Rassinoux A-M, et al. Towards a Medical Linguistic Knowledge Base. In: Greenes RA et al. (eds). *MEDINFO 95*. Proceedings. Amsterdam: North-Holland,1995; 8-12.
11. Wagner JC, Solomon WD, Michel P-A et al. Multilingual Natural Language Generation as Part of a Medical Terminology Server. In: Greenes RA et al. (eds). *MEDINFO 95*. Proceedings. Amsterdam: North-Holland,1995; 100-104.
12. Sowa JF. *Conceptual Structures: Information Processing in Mind and Machine*. Reading, MA: Addison-Wesley Publishing Company, 1984.
13. Wagner JC, Baud RH, Scherrer J-R. Using the Conceptual Graphs Operations for Natural Language Generation in Medicine. In: Ellis G et al. (eds). *Conceptual Structures: Applications, Implementation and Theory*. Berlin: Springer-Verlag, 1995; 115-128.

Image and Signal Processing

Distributed Plan Construction and Execution for Medical Image Interpretation

N.Bianchi*, P.Bottoni**, C.Garbay***, P.Mussio**, C.Spinu***

* ElectroTechnical Laboratory, 1-1-4 Umezono, Tsukuba, Ibaraki, 305 Japan
email bianchi@etl.go.jp
** DSI - University of Rome, via Salaria 113, 00198 Rome, Italy
email {bottoni,mussio}@dsi.uniroma1.it
*** Lab. TIMC, Institut Bonniot, 38706 La Tronche, France
email: Catherine.Garbay@imag.fr

Abstract

Research in the field of medical image interpretation inspired a multi-agent planning model in which a population of agents reaches global goals pursuing local plans and producing partial results. Cooperation is achieved by collecting results, reanalysing the reached state and starting new plans; local plans are generated and executed in a distributed way. The state is composed of a directed graph, describing the currently obtained results and of an attributed string, concatenating the trace of the performed operations with the current plan. A model of agent and agent generation is presented and an example of application given in the field of liver biopsy interpretation.

1 Introduction

Physicians derive high level synthetic descriptions from images and express them in a specialised subset of natural language. To automatically derive such a description, image processing and analysis tools are used following a plan not foreseeable in advance and depending on properties of the image at hand: the goal of a process is not clearly stated in terms of a precise state to reach, but rather it is incrementally refined during analysis [BMP94]. This situation requires new control techniques in contrast with the classical position on planning problems: establishing a sequence of actions from the current state to a well defined state, the goal [LTW93].

Typical to most medical images is the variability of local properties such as light intensity and noise characteristics: an image can be partitioned into subimages, each one being homogeneous with respect to some of these properties or to a given operation. Each zone can then be treated by a different version of a tool performing the operation, tuned to its specific properties [SGC95]. Given the results obtained so far, the control problem is twofold: to determine which operation to perform next and how to perform it. Several goals may be pursued together and the obtained results may be not sufficient to complete a task, but can subsequently be exploited in the achievement of unrelated tasks.

Such considerations suggest a multi-agent model of planning where agents pursue local plans, i.e. have to complete a task limited to a certain part of a global process state, having a limited knowledge of this state and producing partial results. The global goal of the image interpretation emerges from cooperation between agents. Cooperation is achieved by collecting results, re-analysing the reached state and starting new plans. This mechanism is decentralised: more and more specialised local plans are generated and executed in a distributed way. This contrasts with those methods of planning where focus is on how to distribute to multiple agents the realisation of centrally established plans [KR93] or, to the contrary, on how to make multiple agents participate in coordinating and deciding upon their actions [Dur88].

2 A Scenario for Biopsy Interpretation

The image descriptions used by physicians are situated in specific contexts (hepatology, osteology) and obtained according to conventional rules, established by the community of physicians. This community collectively determine the types of patterns significant for their tasks when appearing in a class of images. In [BCL96], such types of patterns are called the *characteristic structure types* and their instances *characteristic structures*.

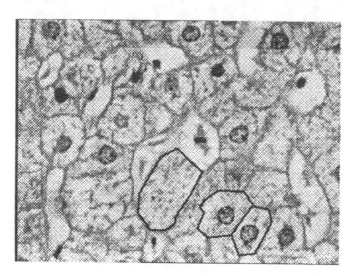

Fig. 1. The green component of a biopsy

Figure 1 shows the results of a biopsy interpretation by a hepatologist: three hepatocytes have been manually outlined, bounded by their membranes. Two of them contain a nucleus, which has been manually circled with a dotted line. Such a description is not universal, on the contrary it is situated in the context of liver studies, and reflects hepatologists' specific knowledge. Here, characteristic structure types are cell types (hepatocyte) and biological structures (sinusoid) as well as their components (hepatocyte nucleus, non hepatocyte nucleus, membranes). A hepatocyte is a nearly hexagonal structure with mean colour red, and whose texture is finely grained. Usually, a hepatocyte contains a round, heavily coloured nucleus. A sinusoid is an irregular, usually elongated, structure with uniform texture and mean colour white. A sinusoid may contain some cells of different types, e.g. Ito cells. For this reason, some structures may appear inside the sinusoid and some of these structures may appear as small nuclei. Being a biopsy the result of a slicing action, nuclei can be absent or present in part, while sinusoids and other cells may be present or not.

In general, medical image interpretation is multi-goal (e.g. the pathologist looks for hepatocytes, sinusoids and other cells). A medical image interpretation may fail with respect to one or more goals (no structure of a given type are found), or be partially successful (there is uncertainty on the interpretation of one or more structures), or be fully successful.

In interpreting an image, physicians use both images and descriptions. They operate on images to improve their readability and to extract characteristic structures and on descriptions to classify characteristic structures. Both activities require local as well as contextual information. The result of such an activity is therefore a set of descriptions and a set of images which materialise part of the descriptions to highlight some structures. For example, Fig.2 is the materialisation of hepatocytes and sinusoids found in Fig.1 using the control model described in the next section.

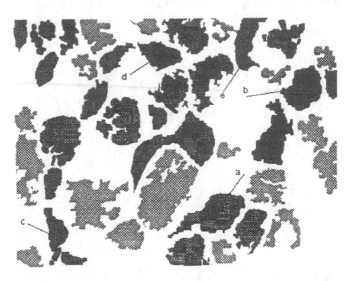

Fig. 2. The final classification of the system: Hepatocytes (light grey and light texture) and Sinusoids (dark grey, heavy texture and black). Labels indicate reclassified zones.

3. Distributed Evolution of State

3.1 State and Evolution of the Interpretation Process

The result of an interpretation activity is represented by the *result graph*, a directed graph in which nodes are images or descriptions, and an edge denotes an action performed on the source node and resulting in the target node. A result graph is obtained via planning-execution cycles.

Planning consists of deciding on a course of action before acting [CF82] and developing explicit goal/plan/subgoal structures as part of the control process [CL93]. Planning requires knowledge not only of the data but also of the already performed actions and of the foreseen ones. To this end, we give a name to each action and describe its success or failure by attributes denoting nodes in the result graph the action was tried on and nodes on which it succeeded.

Each action is described by an attributed symbol (its name and its attributes): a *plan* is a string of attributed symbols describing actions to be performed and a *trace* is a string of attributed symbol describing actions already performed. The pair (result graph / trace-plan string) defines the *state* of interpretation process.

The interpretation process itself is described as a sequence of states. Given a state, we define the action to reach the next one by rewriting rules. The application of a rewriting rule results into either evolution of the result graph or evolution of the plan. Plan evolution is a form of meta-reasoning and the rules governing it are called metarules. A metarule generates a new plan on the fly, according to the current process state, as stated by conditions and functions on the current result graph and trace.

Each set of rules or metarules is denoted by the same name which identifies the actions it describes. Let R be the set of rule names, MR the set of metarules names and S=R∪MR. Plan and trace can be interpreted as strings of names of set of rules and metarules, i.e. strings on S. A new property is necessary to associate names and sets of (meta)rules: with each name from S, a value table is associated specifying the (meta)rules with that name.

Rules and metarules have a syntactic part <<A,X>;C> and a semantic part <γ,φ>, where A is the antecedent, X the context and C the consequent. γ (condition) is a predicate on the attributes of A and X; φ (semantic action) is a set of functions to evaluate the attributes of C.

In a *rule* r, A, X, and C are labelled graphs. A rule is applied to a result graph rg only if its antecedent matches rg, i.e. an instance IA of A is found in rg, an instance IX of X in rg, and the condition holds. Applying a rule produces a new result graph where old antecedent nodes are present, nodes are added with the correct associated values, or values of existing nodes are updated, and dependency among results is tracked.

In a *metarule* mr, the antecedent A is the symbol ◊, marking the beginning of the plan string, and the context X is a pair <G, M>, with G a graph and M a set of symbols in S. The consequent C is a string ◊∘p with p a string on S. Functions in φ are used to compute the value of table for names in the plan. Formally, mr:<<◊,<G, M>>;◊∘p>. A meta-rule is applied to a state (rg,τ◊π) only if its antecedent matches the state, i.e. an instance IG of G is found in rg, an instance IM of M in τ, and the condition holds. Applying a meta-rule produces a new plan where p is inserted before π.

Rules and meta-rules are applied by the following rewriting mechanism: given a state, (meta)rules are scheduled which allow the determination of the next state. A plan is composed of fragments [May92], delimited by #∊S. Actions with names in a fragment are tried concurrently, while an action in the next fragment can be executed only if all actions in the current fragment have been completed. Using fragments, trace and plan are strings on S∪{#}. The symbol ∘ is used as a separator between names in the same fragment.

3.2. Distributed Rewriting of Plans and Results.

We model the planning-execution cycle as the coupling of two rewriting processes, taking place on a result graph and on the plan string. The two processes are executed concurrently in a completely local fashion: for each (meta)rule to be executed an agent is created. Thus, an agent is created with the task of completing a subplan. Such an agent acts only having available a partial view of the result graph and of the process trace at the time of its creation.

Let rg' be a result graph and rg a subgraph of rg', τ the current trace and ac a (meta)rule from the current plan. An agent's initial state is defined by (rg, τ, ac) and its behaviour is informally specified as follows: if ac is a metarule and its antecedent matches rg and τ, the agent will create a new subplan as specified by ac and will instantiate new agents to execute it; if ac is a rule and its antecedent matches rg, it will produce a new result graph. In both cases, upon completion of the subplan competing to it, the agent will report the obtained results to its originator, which will update its own copy of rg' and τ.

3.3 Local Adaptation of Plans

Given a result graph rg, a *zone* is a collection of nodes from rg, together with a set of restrictions on the values of the attributes of the nodes. Typically, if a node in a result graph denotes an image, a zone will contain a subimage; if a node denotes a tuple, a zone will be some component of the tuple.

The unfolding of a planning process is realised by the use of metarule sets to identify relevant zones in the result graph and to generate subplans adapted to different zones. We distinguish two types of metarule sets, indicated by mrStr and mrSeg. A set of type mrStr, with a number ns of mutually exclusive metarules, allows the plan to be adapted according to the identification of a certain situation from a set of possible ones. A singleton of type mrSeg allows adaptation of rules to different zones, trying to identify all the relevant zones in the current state.

For mrStr, a set of metarules is defined such that only one of them will succeed and the plan will proceed in a univocal way. For mrSeg, a single metarule is used to compute zones and start several simultaneous rules on different parts. The two mechanisms are combined to generate complex plans. Metarules of type mrStr and mrSeg can be further refined, so as to generate several fragments. A typical case is when they place in the plan not only rules to be performed on zones, but also metarules allowing the computation of the continuation, based on the newly obtained results. A *continuation metarule* is often used to recombine a set of zones into a single value of the domain.

4. The Variable Agent Organisation

As discussed in section 3, for each (meta)rule an agent is created. Each agent is provided with a state variable which initially specifies a global process substate at the time of agent creation. An interpretation process starts with an agent associated with the initial meta-rule interpreting the initial state, and generating the initial plan together with the initial population of agents.

4.1. Agent Types

Three types of agents are defined: Managers, Schedulers, Executors. A *Manager* agent (Fig.3a) has a generic control cycle specified by Interpreter described in section 4.2. A Manager's task is to evaluate a metarule, generate a subplan and execute it by creating the agents necessary to manage this subplan, collect results from these agents and report to its originator. A *Scheduler* (Fig.3b) is in charge of managing the concurrent activation of agents executing a same type of rules. Such an agent is needed when a symbol in R∪MR denotes a non-singleton set of (meta)rules.

An *Executor* (Fig.3c) executes an operation on a node or a zone, as specified by a rule. These agents are created with initial states for their execution (shown with thicker boxes in figure 3): a portion of the result graph, and a specification of the plan and the actions (rules or meta-rules) to execute. As regards Scheduler agents, they are provided with a list of the agents to create. All agents are equipped with communication tools to report to their originator and to receive reports from the agents they have originated.

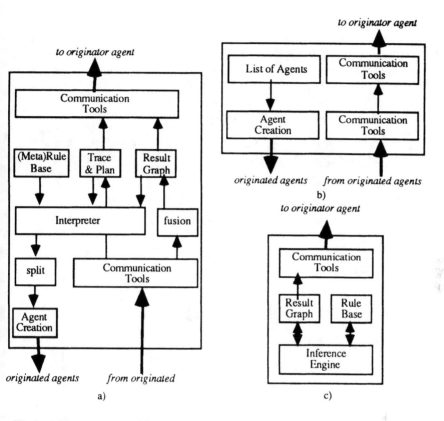

Fig.3. a) Manager Agent Model; b) Scheduler Agent Model; c) Executor Agent Model

4.2. Management of planning and execution activities

The process is started by a Manager agent executing Interpreter (Tab.1) on an initial node i_0, with a starting mr0. The Manager: a) establishes the process initial state b) deliberates the plan to be executed, interpreting mr0 by a call to DeliberatePlan which updates plan by inserting the names of sets of (meta)rules to be performed.

Table 1. The procedure describing the Interpreter of Manager agents

```
Procedure Interpreter(results, trace, metarule)
/* Initialisation */
    state← <results, trace°metarule>
/* initial deliberation determines a new plan (state) */
    state← DeliberatePlan(state)        /generates detailed initial plan*/
/*execution cycle */
/* Application of plan determines updating of plan, trace and result graph*/
    while (halt-condition(state) is false)
        state ← ApplyPlan(state)
    endwhile
    Return(newResults(state),newTrace(state))
```

Next, Manager checks the halt condition: if the condition is not satisfied ApplyPlan is called. For example in [BMP94] *halt-condition* checks that either 1) the next action in the plan has already been applied twice with equal results; or 2) no action has to be applied (plan is empty). ApplyPlan extracts the first fragment from the plan. It generates an agent for each name -denoting a set of either rules or metarules- in the fragment. If a generated agent is a Manager or a Scheduler, it will generate other agents. Managers and Schedulers also record their children activities. On their side, children agents must record their parents' address to communicate back their results to them via completion messages. A parent agent collects its children completion messages and uses them to produce a description of the results of its global activity. In its turn it will send such a description as a completion message to its parent.

5. Application to Biopsy Interpretation.

In this section a semiautomatic biopsy interpretation process -refined from [MPB91]- is discussed, taking as example Fig.1.

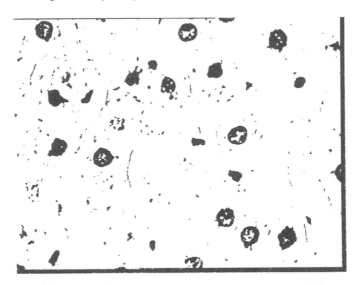

Fig.4. The set of Candidate Nuclei i_{CN} in the biopsy shown in Fig.1

A Manager MA1 is first created with a state given by s_0=<BIOPSY10, $\lambda°$ ◊ CellStr>: BIOPSY10 is a 512 × 384 image in the output format of three colour RGB images from a Sony camera DCX_M2PH; CellStr is the name of one metarule defining the strategy proposed by histologists for biopsy interpretation. MA1 created MA2, which is now in a state where four data structures have been obtained from the original image and it is about to evaluate EvStr2 to assess how to combine information in the different descriptions. These data structures describe candidate Nuclei (DescCN -see Fig.4), candidate Hepatocytes and Sinusoids (DescCHS -see Fig.5), White Zones (DescCW -see Fig.6) and Membranes (DescCM) each being the description of some property of BIOPSY10. Such a state is represented as:

$$s=<\{BIOPSY10, DescCN, DescCHS, DescCW, DescCM\}, NucleiStr \#$$
$$HepSinStr°WhiteZoneStr°MemStr°◊ EvStr2>$$

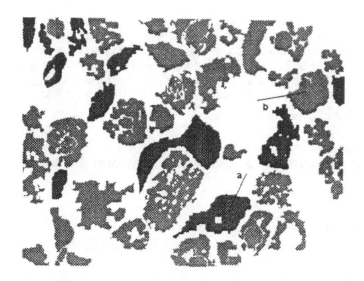

Fig.5. Classification of Candidate Hepatocytes (light grey) and Sinusoids (dark grey) after completion of the first fragment generated by EvStr1. Zones a and b will be reclassified.

Fig.7 summarises the subsequent evolution of the process. Bold rectangles denote generated subplans, light rectangles metarules and an oval denotes a rule to be applied to the result graph. Arrows denote generation, and labels indicate specific mechanisms exploited by metarules. Set of arrows labelled with Or indicate that several alternatives are considered of which only one produces the represented plan. Set of arrows labelled with And indicate that several versions of a same rule are produced and applied concurrently. A metarule failure is understood to produce the nil alternative.

Fig.6. White Zones in Fig.1 with area$\geq$190. Zone b will be used to classify Sinusoids

MA2 generates a manager for EvStr2 evaluation which deliberates by checking the condition for re-evaluation of the obtained results.

In this case the condition is the presence of candidates of at least two different types and re-evaluation takes into account their geometrical and topological relations. If the check is positive, EvStr2 adds to the plan the names of sets of metarules specialised to contextual re-examination of candidates. EvStr2 is a set of meta-rules of type mrStr. In particular its metarules define 8 alternatives (only the first two are here shown, the other 6 exhaust the other possibilities):

EvStr2:
Syntactic part:
<<◊,<{DescCN,DescCW,DescCM},∅>>;◊NucPresStr°WhitePresStr°MemCutStr# FusStr>

<<◊,<{DescCN,DescCW,DescCM},∅>>;◊ NucPresStr°WhitePresStr°# FusStr>
Semantic part:
γ1: (NotEmpty(DescCN) ∧ NotEmpty(DescCW) ∧ NotEmpty(DescCM)
γ2: (NotEmpty(DescCN) ∧ NotEmpty(DescCW) ∧ Empty(DescCM)
F1: ...

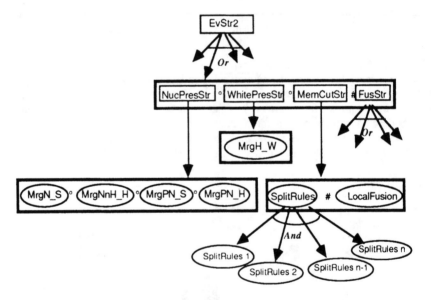

Fig. 7. Partial unfolding of the interpretation process on BIOPSY10.

In this case, nuclei, white zones and membranes were found and the new state is:

s=<{BIOPSY10,DescCN, DescCHS, DescCW, DescCM }, NucleiStr # HepSinStr
°WhiteZoneStr°MemStr° ◊ NucPresStr°WhitePresStr°MemCutStr# FusStr>

During application, NucPresStr and WhitePresStr exploit context provided by previously identified Nuclei and White zones to refine the classification of candidate Hepatocytes and Sinusoids stored in DescCHS. Thus, NucPresStr activates rules for merging information provided by classification of structures in DescCN as Nuclei of Hepatocytes and of structures in DescCHS as Sinusoids. The latter are reclassified as Hepatocytes if they contain a Nucleus (rules MrgN_S); Nuclei of non Hepatocytes cause re-classification of Hepatocytes as Sinusoids (rules MrgNnH_H); Possible Nuclei within Sinusoids are turned to Nuclei of non Hepatocytes (rules MrgPN_S) and Possible Nuclei within Hepatocytes are turned to Nuclei of Hepatocytes. Similarly, rule MrgWH combines information on White Zones and Hepatocytes to reclassify some of these as Sinusoids. This refinement implies both reclassification and merging of structures. For example, Fig.2 shows that the structure "a" of Fig.5 is reclassified as a Hepatocyte because of the presence of a Nucleus of Hepatocyte inside it.

This result can be refined by the use of MemCutStr which exploits long edges in DescCM to separate fused structures in DescCHS. In particular, Fig.8 shows the edges found according to MemStr in the zone around the neck of the structure "a" of Fig.5.

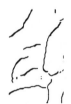

Fig. 8. Edges in a window around the neck of structure a in Fig.5 (Larger size than original)

On the contrary, structure "b" is reclassified as a Sinusoid because it contains a Non-Hepatocyte Nucleus and is a white zone, as shown in Fig.6. Metarule MemCutStr is of type mrSeg, restricting the use of edges to zones of uncertainty, expressed as:

MemCutStr:
Syntactic part
<<◊,<DescCHS, ∅>>; ◊ SplitRules# LocalFusion>
Semantic part
γ: ExistBigAreas(DescCHS,threshold)
F: {   zones=BigAreaZones(DescCHS,threshold);   table(splitRules)=∅;
  foreach zone ∈ zones
    table(splitRules)=AddTbl(table(splitHepRules), Specialise(templSplitRules, zone));
  endfor   }
The set of splitting rules resulting from specialisation of the templates is:
SplitHepRules:
Syntactic part (for i=1, ..., |zones|)
<<DescCHS°DescCM,λ,>; DescCHS$_i$ref>
Semantic part (for i=1, ..., |zones|)
γ$_i$:   ExistLongEdge(DescCM, zone$_i$)
F$_i$:   DescCHS= Split(DescCHS, DescCM, zone$_i$)

Subsequently, LocalFusion merges the refined classifications into a single data structure to be exploited by FusStr. FusStr is the continuation metarule for EvStr2; it merges the refined descriptions by the rule Fusion, producing a global description (DescFus). The final trace and plan string is now:

$$\tau°\pi = \text{NucleiStr \# HepSinStr ° WhiteZoneStr ° MemStr° NucPresStr \#}$$
$$\text{WhitePresStr°MemCutStr\# FusStr ◊}$$

while the global result graph is shown in Fig.9. In this case FusStr does not prescribe

415

any continuation. Now, since all the managers generated from CellStr have completed their actions, the halt condition is true (plan is empty). The manager for CellStr terminates, archiving the set of obtained images and descriptions.

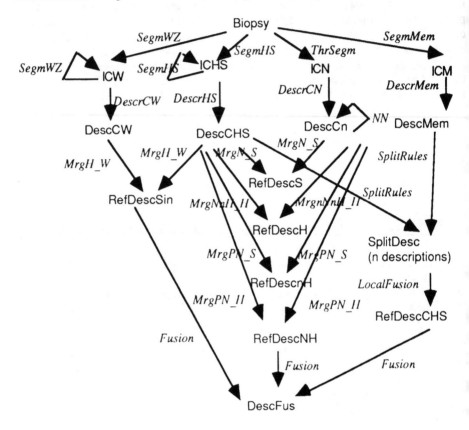

Fig. 9. The global result graph of the interpretation process.

6. Discussion and Conclusions

The paper has presented an original approach to develop flexible management of distributed plans, providing a unified frame to integrate deliberative and opportunistic control. Deliberative control accounts for adaptation to situations, by dynamically determining which operation to perform next, based on the state of the process. Opportunistic control accounts for local variability of data to operate on, by tuning operations to zones, each one being homogeneous with respect to a given operation.

20 biopsies have been analysed with plans derived from CellStr. These biopsies contained 784 identifiable objects (642 hepatocytes and 142 sinusoids) according to the histologist who collaborated with us. On the 20 images the system singled out 706 objects, of which it agreed with the histologist on 467 hepatocytes (89.1%) and 163 sinusoids (89.5%). As to sinusoids, they are often split by the system due to the presence of other structures. So we found an excess of 21 sinusoids (14.7%).

The advantage of adaptation and dynamicity in plan definition is highlighted by considering that, on the average, about 10% of the correctly classified Hepatocytes and 25% of the correctly classified Sinusoids are classified during the execution of the subplan generated by EvStr2. These results are interesting because they show that the weak points are in segmentation, even if our approach allows some recovery. The present procedure can be exploited in a semi-interactive tool in which the histologist can complete the segmentation interactively.

From the theoretical point of view, the main contribution of the work lies in an adaptive definition of the planning process. The way the plan is developed is not goal directed: there is no global goal defined, nor any decomposition of goals into subgoals. Rather, plan elaboration obeys a constructivist approach according to which decisions are incrementally taken, based on evolution of the result graph. As a consequence, plan and problem structures are strongly coupled, and a goal emerges as the successive achievements of locally distributed goals. No form of negotiation or communication among agents [RG85] is required, nor is a conflict referee [Geo83] required. Rather, results of individual plans are all considered acceptable, and possibly subsequently re-evaluated.

7. Acknowledgements

Work supported by the Galileo/Galilée Project for France-Italy cooperation. Thanks to Centro Studi Medicina Teoretica for providing images and to Dr. E.Arosio of CSMT for expertise on biopsy interpretation.

8. References

[BCL96] P.Bottoni, M.F.Costabile, S.Levialdi, P.Mussio, "Visual Conditional Attributed Rewriting Systems in Visual Language Specification", *Proc. IEEE Symp. on Visual Languages*, pp.156-163, 1996

[BPG94] O.Baujard, S.Pesty, C.Garbay, "MAPS: a language for multi-agent system design", *Expert Systems*, 11(2):89-98, 1994

[BMP94] P.Bottoni, P.Mussio, M.Protti "Metareasoning in the determination of image interpretation strategies", *Pattern Recognition Letters*, 15:177-190, 1994

[CF82] P. Cohen and E. Feigenbaum, eds., *The Handbook of Artificial Intelligence*, Vol.3. Kaufman, 1982.

[CL93] N. Carver and V. Lesser, A planner for the control of problem-solving systems, *IEEE Trans. on Sys, Man and Cyb.*, 23(6):1519-1536, 1993.

[Dur88] E.H.Durfee, *Coordination of Distributed Problem Solvers*, Kluwer, 1988

[Geo83] M.Georgeff, "Communication and action in multi-agent planning", *Proc. Natl. Conf. on AI*, 125-129, 1983.

[KR93] J.Katz, J.S.Rosenschein, "Plans for multiple agents", *Computers and Artificial Intelligence*, 12(1):5-35, 1993

[LTW93] H.Lee, J.Tannock, J.S.Williams, "Logic-based reasoning about actions and plans in artificial intelligence", *Knowl.Eng.Rev.*, 8(2):91-121, 1993

[May92] B.Mayoh, "Templates, fragments and skins", in G.Rozenberg, A.Salomaa, eds., *Lindenmayer Systems*, Springer, 497-514, 1992

[MPB91] P.Mussio, M.Pietrogrande, P.Bottoni, M.Dell'Oca, E.Arosio, E.Sartirana, M.R.Finanzon, N.Dioguardi, "Automatic cell count in digital images of liver tissue sections", *Proc. 4th IEEE Symp. on CBMS*, pp.153-160, 1991

[RG85] J.S.Rosenschein, M.R.Genesereth, "Deals among rational agents", *Proc.9th IJCAI*, 91-99 1985

[SGC95] C.Spinu, C.Garbay, J.M.Chassery, "A cooperative and adaptive approach to medical image segmentation", in P.Barahona, M.Stefanelli, J.Wyatt eds., *Artificial Intelligence in Medicine*, Springer, pp.379-390, 1995

Improved Identification of the Human Shoulder Kinematics with Muscle Biological Filters

Jean-Philippe Draye[1,*], Guy Cheron[2,**], Davor Pavisic[1], Gaëtan Libert[1]

[1] Polytechnical Faculty of Mons, *"Parallel Information Processing"* Laboratory
Rue de Houdain, 9 - B7000 Mons (Belgium)
[2] Free University of Brussels, Laboratory of Biomechanics
Avenue Heger, 28 - B1050 Brussels (Belgium)

Abstract. In this paper, we introduce new refinements to the approach based on dynamic recurrent neural networks (DRNN) to identify, in humans, the relationship between the muscle electromyographic (EMG) activity and the arm kinematics during the drawing of the figure eight using an extended arm. This method of identification allows to clearly interpret the role of each muscle in any particular movement.
We show here that the quality and the speed of the complex identification process can be improved by applying some treatments to the input signals (i.e. raw EMG signals). These treatments, applied on raw EMG signals, help to get signals that are better reflections of muscle forces which are the real actuators of the movements.

1 Introduction

Human movements are a fascinating field of research. One can only be filled with wonder in front of the accuracy, the speed and the grace of human movements. Briefly, we can describe the cause-and-effect sequence of events that takes place for a human movement to occur as [11] : *(i)* registration and activation of the movement command in the central nervous system; *(ii)* transmission of the movement signals to the peripheral nervous system; *(iii)* contraction of the muscles that develop tension with concomitant generation of electromyographic (EMG) signals; *(iv)* generation of forces at synovial joints; *(v)* regulation of these forces by the anthropometry of the skeleton; *(vi)* movement of the rigid skeletal segments in a manner that it is recognized as the functional movement desired by the central nervous system.

In this paper, we will be interested in the relationship between the electromyographic (EMG) signals (which are a reflection of the command signals sent by the central nervous system to the muscles) and the movements of the skeletal systems. If we refer to the model presented below, we are interested in understanding the relationship between steps *(iii)* and *(vi)*.

---

* J.P. Draye is also a Senior Research Assistant of the Belgian National Fund for Scientific Research (F.N.R.S.)
** G. Cheron is also with the Department of Neurosciences at the Université de Mons-Hainaut (B7000 Mons - Belgium)

We will then apply different treatments on raw EMG signals in order to get signals that are better reflections of the muscle forces (which are the real actuators of the movement). These improvements will lead to a better and faster identification of the relationship we are concerned about.

2 The considered application

We will restrict the application of the neural networks to the identification of the kinematics of the human arm during complex movements in free space. A conventional identification system to handle this task is very difficult to design. Indeed, this one would have to take all the concepts of biological motor control into account but even like that, the quality of the identification would be poor because we still ignore many of these concepts (such as the real pathway of informational signals between the muscles and the central nervous system or some movement invariances). Several techniques have been proposed to solve this complex problem using techniques such as the theory of optimization, the identification using mathematical high-order functions or statistical correlation between EMG and limb movements. Unfortunately, all these techniques require important approximations on the EMG signals and/or provide poor simulation results.

2.1 Related works

The identification of the EMG-kinematics relationship has been considered by several researchers essentially to solve the problem of *distribution* i.e. *how are the large number of muscle forces distributed among relatively few joints ?* (this problem is sometimes referred as redundancy, it is linked to the ill-posed problem).

There have been essentially three strategies that researchers have followed

- **Studying the relationship between EMG and muscle force.** Inman *et al* in 1952 [7] first observed changes in myoelectric signal amplitudes according to variations in the applied muscle load.
- **Estimating individual muscle forces by means of mathematical optimization theory.** One can obtain an acceptable mechanical description of individual muscle forces in human movements only by solving an indeterminate system of equations; this latter fact, along with kinematic invariances of movements, has led to the use of mathematical optimization theory [3]. As explained before, one major problem is that the cost function to be minimized (or maximized) cannot be known exactly *a priori.*
- **To correlate EMG and joint positions or moments.** Pedotti in 1977 [10] made a qualitative investigation of EMG and joint moment correlations for the lower limbs during level walking. Although his study, which included seven muscles, was inconclusive, it did illustrate the complexity of the problem.

Sepulveda *et al* estimate that despite the lack of progress the third strategy has the greatest potential; they were the first to use an artificial neural networks algorithm for correlating EMG and joint kinematics and dynamics in human gait [11]. They proposed a feedforward neural network to solve the distribution problem : it was able to converge and slight perturbation to all EMG inputs led to similar output predictions. They also noticed several limitations : their model does not include physical arrangement of muscles, force-velocity relation or sensory feedback information. The most severe drawback was that feedforward neural models did not include temporal relationships (i.e. parameters at time $t+1$ are a function of what happened at time t) although the learning algorithm did present the training patterns in sequential order.

Facing the interesting results of artificial neural methods in solving biomechanical tasks but, also, the drawbacks of feedforward networks, we concentrate our research on the application of recurrent dynamic networks to EMG-human arm kinematics relationship identification.

2.2 Methods

Four male right-handed subjects between 21 and 25 years (mean weight : 73 kg and mean height : 179 cm) were asked to draw as fast as possible four series of figures eight with the right extended arm in free-space (the initial directions of the movements were up-right, up-left, down-left, down-right respectively). They were asked to perform the movement repetitively (5-10 cycles) at a self-determined frequency (generally from 0.7 to 1.2 kHz).

The movements of the arm were recorded and analyzed using the optoelectronic *ELITE* system (including 2 TV cameras working at a sampling rate of 100 Hz.

Surface EMG patterns of seven muscles were measured using telemetry. Muscle activity was recorded using pairs of silver-silver chloride surface electrodes on the following muscles : posterior deltoid external and internal (PDE and PDI), anterior deltoid (AD), median deltoid (MD), pectoralis major superior and inferior (PMS and PMI) and latissimus dorsi (LD). Surface electrodes were positioned at the approximated geometrical center of the muscle belly with an interelectrode distance of 2.5 cm. From previous experiences with the analysis of fast unidirectional movements of the arm which revealed quite large differences in shoulder muscle activation patterns (with respect to amplitude and to relative timing), it can be concluded that cross-talk between these muscles is small. Raw EMG signals (differential detection) were amplified (1,000 times) and bandpass filtered (10-2000 Hz). After this, the EMGs were digitized at 2 kHz, full-wave rectified and smoothed by means of a third order averaging filter with a time constant of 20 ms.

Four infra-red reflecting markers were attached to the arm (on the shoulder, the elbow, the wrist and the index finger), the three-dimensional spatial position of these markers were computed by the *ELITE* system. As the movements were performed with the extended limb, the information from the four markers is partly redundant. The reconstruction of the movement of the arm by the *ELITE* system using the trajectories of the four markers confirmed the visual inspection that the upper arm, forearm, hand and index finger acted as a rigid link. Thus, we used the data with the best definition related to the representation of the figure eight : the position of the index marker.

The artificial neural network is a fully connected 20 neuron network which is governed by the following equations [5] :

$$T_i \frac{dy_i}{dt} = -y_i + F(x_i) \quad \text{with} \quad x_i = \sum_j w_{ji}\, y_j \tag{1}$$

where y_i is the state or activation level of unit i, $F(\alpha)$ is the squashing function (sigmoid-like function) and x_i the total input of the neuron. Immediately, we can notice that our model presents two types of adaptive parameters : the classical weights between the units and the time constants T_i. These ones will act like a relaxation process. The correction of the time constants will be included in the learning process in order to increase the dynamics of the model. It has been proved that these adaptive time constants have a very good influence on the network frequential behaviour, on its dynamical features and on its long-term memory capacities (for more details and the complete learning algorithm, see [4]). The network was trained to reproduce the arm trajectory performed by the subject in response to the EMG signals. Each training was associated to only one subject and for only one type of electrode location.

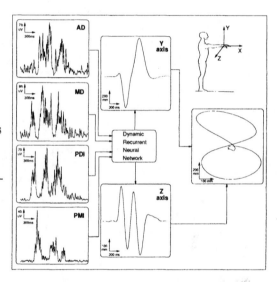

Fig. 1. *Input-output organization of the DRNN.*

2.3 Results

Among the twenty fully connected neurons of the DRNN, eighteen receive the inputs (all the different EMG signals) and two of them give the output (the coordinates Y and Z, see Figure 1). We only train the network with these two latter coordinates because they define the action plane. The amplitude of the movement according to the rostro-caudal axis (X axis) is very weak and is mainly due to the skeletal constraint. In this case, this passive movement could not have been identified by the DRNN on the basis of the EMG signals (mainly related to the voluntary movement).

We have already proved that DRNNs are successful in identifying the complex mapping between full-wave rectified EMG signals and upper-limb trajectory (see [2]. We have shown that the quality of the identification of the mapping allows to clearly interpret the role of each muscle in any particular movement. We have developed a method to prove the plausibility of the identification using artificial lesions and error vectors. Moreover, our neural model is able to reproduce unlearned trajectories when it is previously trained with the figure eight; that means that the information content in the combination of the seven EMG signals is, in the case of the figure eight, sufficiently relevant to reach the generalization ability.

This also means that the figure eight is an ideal movement for the learning process of the DRNN. The particular curve implicates throughout the movement a permanent change of its direction combining clockwise and counterclockwise rotation. This highly learned trajectory enables the DRNN to identify neural constraints [8] such as the covariation between geometrical (the curvature) and kinematics (the tangential velocity of the arm) parameters of the movement [12] (more details can be found in [2]).

3 Improvement of the simulation model

The application presented in the previous section consists in the identification of the relationship between the *raw* EMG signals sent to the arm muscles and the related arm kinematics. This section is devoted to the presentation of different treatments that we can apply on raw EMG signal in order to get a signal that is a better reflection of the muscle force. Indeed, forces generated by the muscles are the real actuators of the movements. As we will see, these improvements in the quality of the input signals lead to a better and faster identification of the relationship we are concerned about.

The improvements will be divided in three different categories : filtered EMG input signals, sign-adjusted EMG input signals, muscle forces using biological filters.

3.1 Filtered EMG input signals

Neural delays and muscle lag are essential characteristics of muscles. Although the axon velocity is quite high (50 m/s), the minimal reflex response time from a foot sensor (afferent + efferent pathways $\approx$ 2 m) is about 40 ms. Similarly, a centrally initiated command will also take about 40 ms to reach a distal muscle. This means that triggering of the first motor unit takes 40 ms with a further electromechanical delay in the start of the muscle twitch, followed by the lag due to the low-pass characteristics of the muscle twitch itself [9]. Thus, the peak tension from the very first motor unit might not be reached for a further 50 to 110 ms, followed by delays in the recruitment of further motor units. The EMG signal (recorded by the electrode which is generally located over the middle of the muscle) is always slightly delayed behind the neural pulse trains. There is thus an electromechanical delay between the time that the EMG signal is recorded and the time it takes for the electrical wave to propagate along the muscle fibers to each tendon at a velocity of about 4 m/s. Electromechanical delays can add another 20 ms to neural delays. The propagating force arrives at the tendon in the form of a twitch which has been analyzed as a critically damped, second-order, low-pass system with cut-off frequency around 5 Hz [9]. Such a transfer function of the muscle will cause a further lag in the buildup of tension.

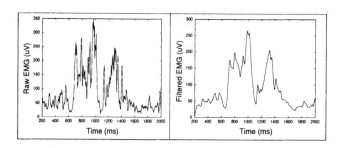

Fig. 2. *Raw EMG signal of the anterior deltoid (left) and its filtered version (right) at 5 Hz.*

The first obvious preprocessing that one could apply to the EMG signals is of course to model this transfer function. This treatment is illustrated on Figure 2 where the raw EMG signal of the anterior deltoid (left) and its filtered version (right) at 5 Hz are plotted versus time.

3.2 Sign adjusted EMG input signals

One important problem arises when using raw or filtered EMG signals. Indeed, the interpretation of a particular burst of a muscle EMG activation can be very difficult for an identification process. Let us take the example of the part of figure eight trajectory depicted on Figure 3. The experimenter begins to draw the trajectory at time $t = 0$ and lets his (her) arm going down

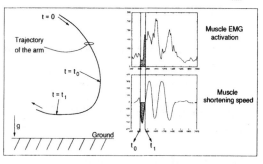

Fig. 3. *Illustration of the concept of passive burst.*

toward the ground thanks to the action of the extensor muscles (which preferential field is directed toward the bottom). Due to gravity, the speed of the limb increases and at time $t = t_0$ the central nervous system sends a command to slow down the movement. This slowing down is induced by the activation of muscles which have a flexor preferential field (their action is directed toward the top). When such a muscle is activated, its effect is not to move the limb upward but to slow down the movement downward. The action of such a muscle is depicted on right-up corner of the figure. The speed of shortening of this particular muscle is also depicted just below. We note that the burst occurs when the speed of shortening of the muscle is negative : that means that the muscle was lengthening when the activation happened. We can also note that, at time $t = t_1$, the muscle speed of shortening becomes positive : the muscle acts again in its preferential field and the limb begins to move upward. One solution to help the identification system to identify *active bursts* (the limb move in the direction of the preferential field of the muscle) or *passive bursts* (the limb is slowed down in the opposite direction of the preferential field of the muscle) is to look at the speed of muscles. When the speed is negative, we can consider that the burst as a brake action and *invert it*.

The corrected EMG signal is constructed using the following procedure. When the speed becomes negative, we revert the EMG activation. Nevertheless, in order to keep a continuous signal, we do not flip the signal with respect to the X axis but with respect to the line that joins EMG activation of the instants of null speed. The resulting EMG signal (dashed line) has been named the *sign-adjusted EMG signal*.

3.3 Muscle forces using biological filters

The different preprocessing methods described in the previous section attempt to get closer reflections of the force generated by muscles. We will present here a much more efficient way to obtain these force signals by using biological filters. These filters will be applied to raw EMG signals to give muscle forces and will be derived using two well-known muscle models : Lumped parameter models and cross-bridge models.

Lumped Parameter models - Hill models The filters are based on descriptions which resulted in muscle models that were composed of viscoelastic elements. The most widely applicable of these models is that of A. V. Hill.

They can be described as follows [6] : muscle is composed operationally of three elements (see Figure 4) : *(i)* a contractive element (CE) that acts as an active force generator; *(ii)* an elastic element (SE) that represents the combined stiffness of tendon and cross-bridges in series with the force generator; *(iii)* a second elastic element on parallel with the previous two elements (PE) that represents the passive tissue contribution to

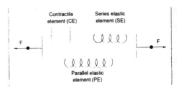

Fig. 4. *Schematic representation of Hill model structure.*

muscle force. Hill has proved that this model explained the force-velocity relation of a muscle. This relation consists of separate equations for lengthening and shortening muscle.

424

Cross-bridge models Together with the tension-velocity, there exists a tension-length relation of a muscle; this latter one will be derived using cross-bridge models. Muscle force exhibits a pronounced length dependence which can be explained by the sliding filament theory. As muscle length changes, the relative overlap of the actin and myosin filaments in each sarcomere changes because of telescoping of the sarcomere structure; this overlap determines the maximum number of available cross-bridges at any given muscle length. Figure 9.12a shows the idealized length-tension curve measured during steady-state isometric contraction when the muscle is fully active.

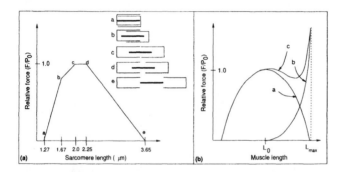

Fig. 5. *Force-length relation. (a) isometric force length relation of a sarcomere and the corresponding sarcomere geometry responsible for this effect. (b) the generalization to the force-length relation of a muscle.*

In contrast to lumped-parameter models which try to reproduce macroscopic behaviour with discrete mechanical elements, cross-bridges models strive to incorporate the known micro-structure of the sarcomere together with metabolic kinetics of muscle to predict macroscopic variables such as whole muscle force, stiffness, shortening velocity, energy consumption, heat liberation, etc.

Concerning the force-length relation of a muscle, it is the perfect image of the same relation of a sarcomere (see Figure 5a, curve *a*) except that we must take into account the passive tissue contribution to muscle force. Indeed, when a muscle is fully extended, the sarcomere can not develop a force anymore but the passive elasticity of the tissue gives rise to an increasing force which tend to infinity (see Figure 5b, curve *b*). The complete force-length relation is obtained by the cumulative effect of curve *a* and *b* (i.e. their addition) : curve *c*.

Computation of the muscle biological filters This section is devoted to the description of our muscle filter model (the reflection of our EMG to force processing approach).

The main attribute of this muscle filter model considered here is based on two different complex filters which are used in series : a *static filter* (active and passive) and a *dynamic filter*. The first one represents the idealized tension-length relationship (see Figure 5), the second one the idealized force-velocity curve. The current activation level of each muscle during the complex movement is defined by a normalization of the absolute EMG value in percentage of the maximal voluntary contraction (MVC) of the muscle tested in the primary position of the studied movement (extended arm at horizontal).

Classically, the total tendon force F^T is defined by the following *product* relationship [1] : $F^T = a F_0^M F_l F_v \cos\alpha$ where F_0^M is the peak isometric force at rest length, F_l the force-length component, F_v the force-velocity component, α the pennation angle and a the normalized activation level which is bounded by the inequality : $0 \leq \alpha \leq 1$. The pennation angle α gives the angle between the position of the muscle (defined by its two tendons) and its effective action direction. For simplicity, we do not take α into account because this coefficient remains constant throughout the figure eight movement.

In order to determine the filters, we have to compute the actual length of the different muscles; this one is calculated on the basis of current kinematics data that provide the shoulder angles in 3D space. These experimental data are combined with a set of musculotendon actuator parameters [13].

Static filter : The static filter is divided into two components : the *active tension static filter* (ATSF) and the *passive tension static filter* (PTSF).

The *active tension static filter* (ATSF) is defined by the relation : ATSF= $k_0 L^2(t) + k_1 L(t) + k_2$ where $L(t)$ corresponds to the current length of the musculotendon actuator and k_0, k_1, k_2 are the parameters of the idealized parabolic function (which corresponds to the curve a of Figure 5).

The *passive tension static filter* (PTSF) is defined as : PTSF= $p_0 L^2(t) + p_1 L(t) + p_2$ where $L(t)$ corresponds to the current length of the musculotendon actuator and p_0, p_1, p_2 are the parameters of the idealized parabolic function (which corresponds to the curve b of Figure 5). The component PTSF is only taken into account if $L(t) > L_0$ (see Figure 5).

Dynamic filter : The dynamic filter includes only one component due to the force-velocity relationship. This relation is denoted DTF : *dynamic tension filter.*

Force computation : The expression of the force has been given below. Nevertheless, we will prefer a more simple expression to calculate the different forces using the three filters : ATSF, PTSF and DTF using the expression : $F = [(\text{EMG} \times \text{ATSF}) + \text{PTSF}] \times \text{DTF}$. The interpretation of this relation is quite simple : the raw EMG signal must, in a first phase, be modulated by the active force-length relation (thus modulated by the ATSF filter); this latter term must be increased by the passive PTSF if the length of the muscle is greater than L_0. This latter value is then modulated by the force-velocity relation (DTF filter) to give *an approximation* of the muscle force.

We wish to emphasize that this procedure gives an approximation of the real force and not its absolute value. Each approximated force is equivalent to the real force times an unknown constant (this constant is the same for all the muscles). Nevertheless, if the computed values are relative, the different ratios between the muscles are absolute and it is these different ratios that are important for the DRNN identification.

Type of inputs	Root mean square error
Raw EMG	$14.5\ 10^{-3}$
Filtered EMG	$11.4\ 10^{-3}$
Sign adjusted EMG	$7.4\ 10^{-3}$
Force	$5.9\ 10^{-3}$

Table 1. Root mean square error according to different types of inputs.

3.4 Results

The results of the computation of the real muscle forces and their use as inputs of the DRNN identification are depicted in the following figures (Figures 6). After having trained the network for 5,000 epochs (with each type of inputs), we computed the mean trajectory for each type of training to get the curves of Figure 6 (left curves) For each mean trajectory, we took the error vectors between the experimentally recorded trajectory and the simulated one (see Figure 6, curve b of the top figure). We then shifted these error vectors in order that their origins coincide with (0,0) (Figure 6, right). The improvements in the quality of the simulated curve can be visually observed.

The root mean square amplitude of these vectors can be computed. Table 1 shows that identification process benefits from the EMG input signals prepro-cessing.

4 Conclusion

The present results show that dynamic recurrent neural networks are successful in identifying the complex mapping between full-wave rectified EMG signals and upper-limb trajectory. Moreover, it has been proved that the quality of the identification of the mapping will allow to clearly interpret the role of each muscle in any particular movement. Our method succeeds whereas several others estimating individual muscle forces by means of mathematical optimization theory, study of the mechanical action of each muscle, ...) have failed or gave poor results to solve the complex problem of muscular redundancy.

We have shown in this paper that the quality and the speed of the complex identification process can be improved by applying some treatments to the input

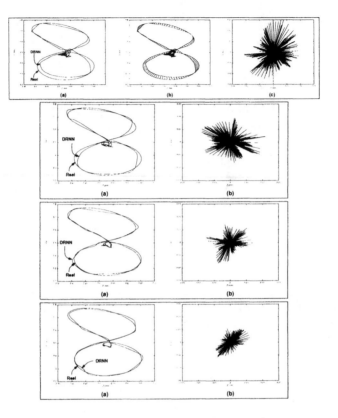

Fig. 6. *From top to bottom : training with the raw EMG as inputs, with filtered EMG as inputs, with sign adjusted EMG as inputs and with the forces as inputs.*

signals (i.e. the raw EMG signal). These treatments, applied on raw EMG signals, help to get signals that are better reflections of muscle forces which are the real actuators of the movements.

There are number of research avenues that have potential in future applications of the dynamic recurrent neural network approach. This type of simulation studies can be of great importance in the fields of basic motion research, preventive health care, pre-surgery simulation, physical rehabilitation and sport performance. For example, the network could be trained on pathological EMG and movement data on one patient prior to orthopedic surgery. Then, it could be possible to simulate, by changing some of the EMG inputs of the previous learned network, the effects expected by surgery. In the same way, the DRNN would be particularly helpful in physical rehabilitation where it could be used to realize a rehabilitation training program including an appropriate selection of muscle activations as well as the adequate temporal and spatial combination of antagonist muscles.

The performance of this neural identification also reinforces the idea that the study of the relationship between EMG signals and kinematics will lead to insight into the formation of the central motor pattern and in particular will help to understand the *internal models* acquired by the brain through motor learning.

References

1. A.S. Bahler. The series elastic element of mammalian skeletal muscle. *American Journal of Physiology*, 213:1560–1564, 1967.
2. G. Cheron, J.P. Draye, M. Bourgeois, and G. Libert. Dynamical neural network identification of electromyography and arm trajectory relationship during complex movements. *IEEE Transactions on Biomedical Engineering*, 43(5):558–552, 1996.
3. R.D. Crowninshield and R.A. Brand. A physiologically based criterion of muscle force prediction in locomotion. *Journal of Biomechanics*, 14:793–801, 1981.
4. J.P. Draye, D. Pavisic, G. Cheron, and G. Libert. Adaptive time constants improve the prediction capability of recurrent neural networks. *Neural Processing Letters*, 2(3):12–16, 1995.
5. J.P. Draye, D. Pavisic, G. Cheron, and G. Libert. Dynamic recurrent neural networks : a dynamical analysis. *IEEE Transactions on Systems, Man, and Cybernetics- Part B: Cybernetics*, 26(5):692–706, 1996.
6. A.V. Hill. The heat in shortening and the dynamics constants of muscle. In *Proceedings of the Royal Society of Biomechanics*, volume 126, pages 136–195, 1938.
7. V.T. Inman, H.J. Ralston, J.B. Saunders, B. Feinstein, and W.B. Wright Jr. Relation of human electromyogram to muscular tension. *Electroencephalography Clinical Neurophysiology*, 4:187–194, 1952.
8. J.T. Massey, J.T. Lurito, G. Pellitzer, and A.P. Georgopoulos. Three-dimensional drawing in isometric conditions : relations between geometry and kinematics. *Experimental Brain Research*, 88:685–690, 1988.
9. H.S. Milner-Brown, R.B. Stein, and R. Yemm. The contractile properties properties of human motor units during voluntary isometric contractions. *Journal of Physiology*, 230:359–370, 1973.
10. A. Pedotti. A study of motor coordination and neuromuscular in human locomotion. *Biological Cybernetics*, 26:53–62, 1977.
11. F. Sepulveda, D.M. Wells, and C.L. Vaughan. A neural network representation of electromyography and joint dynamics in human gait. *Journal of Biomechanics*, 26(2):101–109, 1993.
12. J.F. Soechting and C.A. Terzuolo. Organization of arm movements in three-dimensional space. Wrist motion is piecewise planar. *Neuroscience*, 23(1):53–61, 1987.
13. J.E. Wood, S.G. Meek, and S.C. Jacobsen. Quantization of human shoulder anatomy for prosthetic arm control. I. Surface modeling. *Journal of Biomechanics*, 22(3):273–292, 1989.

A Society of Goal-Oriented Agents for the Analysis of Living Cells

Alain Boucher[1], Anne Doisy[2,3], Xavier Ronot[2,3] and Catherine Garbay[1]

[1] Laboratoire TIMC/IMAG, Grenoble, France
[2] DyOGen (UPRES n° EA 2021), INSERM U309, Grenoble, France
[3] Laboratoire de Neurobiologie du Développement, E.P.H.E., Montpellier, France
Authors can be joined at:
Institut Albert Bonniot, Domaine de la Merci, 38706 La Tronche Cedex, France
E-mail: Alain.Boucher@imag.fr

Abstract. This paper presents a new model for the segmentation and analysis of living cells. A multi-agent model has been developped for this application. It is based on a generic agent model, which is composed of different behaviors: perception, interaction and reproduction. The agent is further specialized to accomplish a specific goal. Different goals are defined from the different components of the cell images. The specialization specifies the parameters of the behaviors for the achievement of the agent's goal. From these goal-oriented agents, a society is defined, and it evolves dynamically as the agents are created and deleted. An internal manager is integrated in the agent to control the behavior's execution. It makes use of an event-driven scheme to manage the behavior priorities. The present design is mainly oriented toward image segmentation, but includes some features on tracking and motion analysis.

1 Introduction

Cell migration is a major event in tissue formation and remodeling during physiological processes and diseases (embryogenesis, wound healing, ...) as well as in pathological situations (invasion and metastasis of tumor cells). Quantitative analysis of the cellular deformation and motion can improve knowledge on the cell's migratory properties and then, help to differentiate and control physiological and pathological situations affecting the migration. In this paper, a goal-oriented approach to study living cells is presented. It is based on a multi-agent system combining multiple behaviors within a generic agent model. The model is similar to the one developped by Guessoum and Dojat [13]. Each agent is specialized to accomplish its own tasks, which are modeled as several behaviors, combining segmentation activities and social organization.

Three main aspects are known to be associated with the motion problem: image segmentation, object tracking and motion analysis. Most research on visual motion aims at either one or another of these aspects [20], [22]. For a long time, segmentation has been seen as the problem of applying edge or region detectors to an image [21], especially in cytology [12]. The segmentation of cell images has been considered by many researchers and has been a difficult problem [7], [18], [24], due to the contrast quality and to the deformable structure of the cell. To attempt to solve these difficulties, several methods have been tried, like active contours methods [17], [14], [16]. Two successive progress lines are now emerging. First, the use of a priori knowledge [18] and models allow to cope with the difficulty of moving image segmentation. Secondly, most of the research work concluded to the necessity of a cooperation between methods, and their adaptation to the local situations in the image [8].

These conclusions lead to the consideration of a multi-agent system [11]. Behavior-based systems have received much attention for the past years, and have given rise to different models [6], [19], [23], which integrate the abilities of the separate behaviors. A cooperative and data-driven system has been designed by Bellet [2], where edge and region growing methods co-operate in a multi-process system for low level image segmentation. Some knowledge-based systems have also been developed, where agents use problem-related knowledge [1], [3], to adapt to application needs. Our approach combines behavior-based approaches with the introduction of a priori knowledge to specialize the agents.

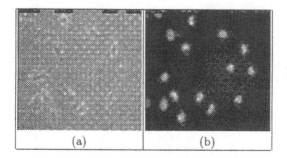

Fig. 1. Images of murine fibroblasts L929. (a) Image of cells observed in phase contrast. (b) Image of nuclei observed by fluorescence. Both images are acquired simultaneously. An image sequence is a set of pairs of images.

Cultured cells of murine fibroblasts were used for experimentation. An imaging workstation has been used to acquire the cell image sequences. It comprises an inverted microscope (Axiovert 135M, Carl Zeiss) equipped with a temperature and CO_2 controlled chamber and a SIT camera (C2400-08, Hamamatsu). This apparatus is connected to an image analyser (SAMBA^{TM} 2640, Unilog). Cell images have been acquired at regular intervals (15-30 minutes) for several hours. Both phase contrast (cells) and fluorescent Hoechst 33342 labeled (nuclei) images were registered (figure 1). More details on the acquisition methods can be found in [10].

2 System Design

2.1 The Multi-Agent Model

The system is comprised of a population of agents, which are dynamically created and deleted under the control of a scheduler. Each agent is meant to perform the segmentation of a given part of the image. This task is modelled as combining several subtasks: perception, interaction with other agents and reproduction. Each subtask is modelled as a specific behavior of the agent. The behaviors are controlled by an internal manager. The system is divided into several levels (figure 2). The **scheduler** manages the execution of the agents, which are implemented into a single Unix process. The **internal manager** makes use of priorities to control the agent's behaviors. It also manages these priorities, depending on incoming events. The agent **behaviors** perform the segmentation and control the exploration of the images. The user is above the system, and can interact through the scheduler. He can create or delete agents, modify their priorities on execution time or configure the agents before their execution through a configuration file. The environment, at the bottom level, includes the input images, their characteristics, and the results.

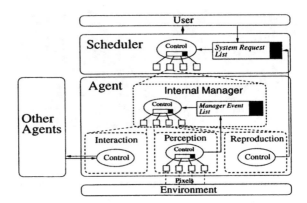

Fig. 2. Multi-agent system model.

2.2 The Scheduler

The scheduler's goal is to manage all the agents in the system. It is built like an internal operating system. All the agents in the system are asynchronous and interruptible. They are scheduled for execution, one after the other, for a given time slice (figure 3). At each loop, the agent list is updated according to incoming requests, coming either from the user or from the agents. Two kinds of requests exist: create/delete an agent and modify its priority. The execution time depends

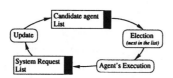

Fig. 3. Scheduler's control loop.

on two parameters, given by the scheduler to the agent: a time quantum and a priority. The execution time (time quantum x priority) can be used by the agent as it needs, but at the end of the allowed time, the agent is responsible for giving back the control to the scheduler. The time quantum parameter is fixed for all agents and is used by the scheduler to adjust the execution time of the agents according to the number of agents present at one time. This time is decreased as the number of agents increases. The priority mechanism provides the possibility to emphasize the execution on a particular type of agent. For example, one could want some agents, with more robust behaviors, to have twice the execution time as the other agents, less robust at a given time.

2.3   The Agent

The agent is composed of two levels (figure 2). The bottom level includes the different behaviors involved in the segmentation process. They work asynchronously and concurrently in the agent and are supervised by the internal manager, which is the higher level of the agent. This internal manager is the interface between the agent and the scheduler and between the behaviors in the agent. A complete discussion of this management scheme will be provided in section 3.4. Three different kinds of behavior exist: *perception* (normal / focalized region growing), *interaction* (merging / negotiation) and *reproduction* (into the same frame / toward the next frame). The normal growing is the basic behavior. It is responsible for analyzing the local environment, evaluating it, and labelling pixels using a region growing scheme. The merging behavior permits the fusion of two regions describing the same entity. Two agents communicate and decide to merge or not the two regions. The reproduction behavior is reponsible for the creation, at any time, of new agents surrounding the existing agent in the current frame or duplicating itself in the next frame. The focalized region growing and the negotiation behavior are explained in [5] and will not be elaborated further here.

3   Specialization to Living Cells

The cell images are segmented in four different zones, resulting in four types of agent specialization. Each agent is specialized, by a configuration file, for one type of segmentation. This specialization influence the way the different behaviors will perform their task. These four specialization types are:

1. The **nucleus** is the cell's heart. As its segmentation is rather easy, the corresponding agent plays a central role in the reproduction behavior by driving the image exploration strategy. Reproduction is thus considered as a prominent behavior for this agent and will be described into more details.
2. The **background** surrounds the cell and shows a noisy distribution of gray level intensities. The role of the corresponding agent is to help the cell delineation. Multiple agents of this type are created all around the cells and they merge to result in one single agent defining all the background. The merging behavior will thus be described in more details for this agent.
3. The **pseudopods** are cytoplasmic extensions of the cell. The cytoplasm is segmented along with the pseudopods. They represent the hardest part of the segmentation problem. They are poorly contrasted from the background, but their motion is important.
4. The **white halos** circle the cell and define a blurred frontier between the background and the cell. They are included in our definition of the cell.

The role of the corresponding agents, for the pseudopods and the white halo, is to achieve an accurate delineation of these components. Therefore, the perception behavior will be emphasized for these agents.

3.1 The Nucleus Agent

The image exploration strategy is based on the agents segmenting and tracking the cell nuclei. The nucleus agent is responsible for the creation of all other agents segmenting the cell. Two reasons explain this choice: the nuclei are easy to find with the fluorescence image and there is only one nucleus per cell (except during the mytosis process). The major criteria for their segmentation is an evolutive and adaptative thresolding. It is computed from the gray level of the current nucleus region and updated at each newly aggregated pixel (threshold = mean gray level x fixed factor). The mean gray level changes along with the segmentation process, as the threshold does. Therefore, it is computed dynamically as the situation evolved. The thresholding factor is user-defined.

In the current version of the system, the reproduction strategy is completely managed by the nucleus agents (figure 4). This strategy implies the creation of agents in one frame (spatial exploration) and in the next frame (temporal exploration). This strategy is dynamically elaborated, based on local rules, which express the application constraints. Indeed, the sequence exploration strategy is not predefined. It emerges from the agent activation and findings. Nucleus agents are launched first (figure 5a), based on seeds computed automatically from two user-defined parameters: a maximum number of seeds and a minimum distance between seeds. Indeed, the nucleus agents are launched at the brightest pixels, according to the nucleus image in fluorescence. Moreover, a minimum distance must be respected between seeds to avoid having all the agents started on the same nucleus. At the outset, nucleus agents launch background agent seeds surrounding them (figure 5b) because background takes longer to segment and because information from its segmentation is useful to later segment pseudopods

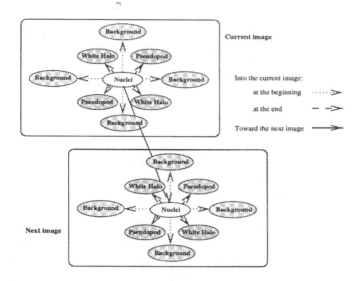

Fig. 4. System exploration stategy. A local plan is defined at the nucleus agent level.

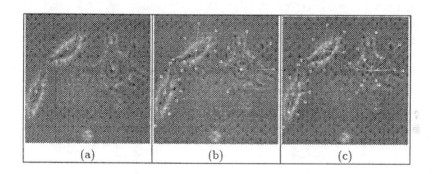

Fig. 5. System exploration strategy. (a) The nucleus agents are first created. (b) The background agents are created by the nucleus agents. (c) The pseudopod and white halo agents are finally created when the nucleus segmentation is finished.

and white halos. Nucleus agents in the subsequent frames are started when the current frame segmentation is judged sufficiently mature (bigger than a fixed size). In this way, the segmentation of all the frames is done through a pipeline. A specific link is created between the newly created agent and its initiator. Any agent knows which one launched it and can thus retrace its motion from his knowledge. The motion segmentation is based on links kept between agents on different frames. When the nucleus segmentations are finished, pseudopod and white halo agents are finally started around the existing nuclei (figure 5c). Their development is constrained by the nuclei and the background. The seeds' position are computed by the nucleus agent according to its local environment. In each direction, the gray level profile is analysed to estimate the best position for a new seed, according to its type. This preliminary exploration allows the launching of many agents on different shapes of cells.

3.2 The Background Agent

The goal of the background segmentation is to help the definition of the cell boundaries. The major criteria used for segmentation is the variance similarity. The background agent seeds are created all around the cell at the beginning of the nucleus agent life (figure 5b). They circle the cell and outline the search area for the other agents. Many background agents are launched. They segment and label pixels independently until they meet. Then, they go into a merging process. The merging behavior permits the fusion of two regions describing the same entity. It is launched when some pixels of a region are neighboring another region of the same type and with similar characteristics. An agent will then communicate with the other agent and request the merging of the two regions (figure 6). The merging process is activated only if there are enough neighboring pixels in a region. It will also favour the agent with an active perception behavior, to ensure that the region will continue to grow after the merging (figure 7). One of the two agents will then terminate, and the other one will continue the segmentation of the whole region. At the end, there will be only one agent for the complete background region.

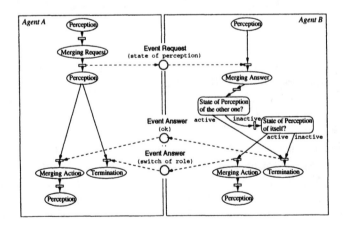

Fig. 6. Communications in a merging behavior modeled as a Petri's network [11].

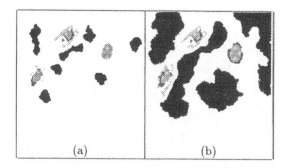

Fig. 7. Background agents merging. (a) The background agents are segmenting separately the area around the cell. (b) They merge and only one agent per region will continue the segmentation process.

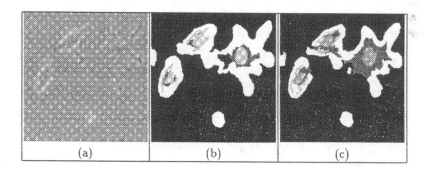

Fig. 8. Segmentation of a cell frame. (a) Cell frame. (b) Segmentation using only static criteria. (c) Segmentation using static and motion-based criteria.

3.3 The Pseudopod and White Halo Agents

The white halos and the pseudopods are hard to define exactly. There shapes are different for different cells. For their segmentation, a region growing method, based from the work of Bellet [2], is used. The perception behavior evaluates pixels with two different series of criteria, relying on static or motion-based information. Five static criteria are used for these two components: variance similarity, compactness, gray level similarity, gradient direction similarity and cell image thresholding. Four criteria based on motion information have been developped. Two motion information sources are used: the difference image, computed between two following frames, and the segmentation of the previous frame. Figure 8 shows the segmentation results for an image frame (figures 8d) segmented with static criteria only (figures 8e) and with both static and motion-based criteria (figure 8f). The background and the nuclei are generally well segmented. The pseudopods and the white halos show variable results.

3.4   The Internal Manager

The internal manager ensures the relation between the agent and the scheduler. It manages the agent behaviors and it is implemented as a control loop (figure 9). It selects the most appropriate behavior, with the highest priority, executes it and then adjusts the priorities of all other behaviors. This control loop is similar to the one presented for the scheduler (figure 3), except for the election of a new candidate. The scheduler will choose the agent to executed one by one, while the internal manager will always choose the behavior with the highest priority. All the behaviors in the agent are interruptible and they work asynchronously in the agent. Each behavior has a priority of execution. At each loop, the behavior with the highest priority is executed. During its execution, the behavior returns some events to the internal manager: by those events, the behavior tells the internal manager a fact that happened during its execution (figure 10). The events are further used by the internal manager to modify the priority of the other behaviors. Doing this, it can selects at each loop the most appropriate behavior for the current situation.

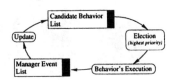

Fig. 9. Internal manager's control loop.

The agent basic behavior is perception and is always present. Its termination means the end of the agent's life, since its primary goal is segmentation. Other behaviors are activated depending on the events produced by this first behavior, and will produce other events themselves. They can also react to events from other agents. Figure 11 shows an example of this management scheme for the reproduction behavior. At the beginning of the agent's life, the perception behavior is the only one to be executed. When it starts, it sends an event to indicate its beginning. From this event, the reproduction behavior will be activated, to create other agent seeds. Later on, the perception behavior will send *size* events as the region grows. These events are used to increase the priority of a reproduction behavior toward the next image. This behavior will be executed when its priority will be high enough. At the end of the perception behavior's life, a new event is sent to indicate the internal manager to start a new reproduction behavior. This organization allows the management of heterogeneous behaviors within a single structure and with no direct communication between the different behaviors. Only the internal manager knows the complete situation and which behavior is the best suited for the current working status.

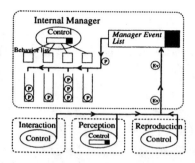

Fig. 10. Events sent by the different behaviors are used by the internal manager to compute and adjust the behaviors' priorities.

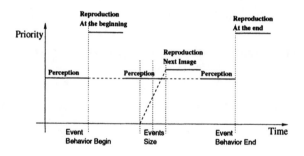

Fig. 11. Priorities' evolution in time for the reproduction behavior function of the incoming events in the agent internal manager.

4 Perspectives

The system is designed to study and analyse the cell motion. Figure 12 shows a typical application with the wound closure process. An artificial injury was done on a cultured cell monolayer of murine fibroblasts. Then, an image sequence was acquired to observe the wound closure. The a posteriori analysis of the sequence was performed by the system, to observe the cell migration. Currently, the cells have been tracked using their nuclei. At the end of a nucleus agent's life, a trace of its center of gravity is plotted in the tracking window. Lines are plotted to link one component in two successive frames, to show the displacement of the component between these frames. Further analysis allows to identify some parameters of this motion. More details can be found in [4]. The perspective of this work is to study the influence of various substances such as growth factors on the wound closure process. It would also be of interest to study cell migration using chemo-attractant substances or oriented gels leading to a contact guidance of cells [9]. It would thus be possible to analyse whether factors promoting autonomous migration of cells into a denuded area of a cell monolayer differ from those responsible for their chemotactic or biased migration [15]. These different models could provide a better knowledge of in vivo cell migration mechanisms involved in processes such as wound healing and tumor cell invasion.

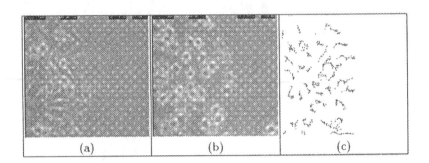

Fig. 12. The wound process. (a) Cell positions after an in vitro injury. (b) Cell positions after 13h. (c) Cell tracking over this period.

References

1. O. Baujard and C. Garbay. KISS: a multiagent segmentation system. *Optical Engineering*, 32(6):1235–1249, 1993.

2. F. Bellet, J.M. Salotti, and C. Garbay. Une approche opportuniste et coopérative pour la vision de bas niveau. *Traitement du Signal*, 12(5):479–494, 1995.

3. O. Boissier, Y. Demazeau, G. Masini, and H. Skaf. Une architecture multi-agents pour l'implémentation du bas niveau d'un système de compréhension de scènes. In *2ièmes journées francophones IAD et SMA*, 1994. Voiron (France).

4. A. Boucher, A. Doisy, X. Ronot, and C. Garbay. Cell migration analysis after in vitro wounding injury with a multi-agent approach. *Artificial Intelligence Review Journal.* under revision.

5. A. Boucher and C. Garbay. A multi-agent system to segment living cells. In *Proceedings of the 13th ICPR 96*, volume 3, pages 558–562, 1996. Vienna (Austria).

6. R. A. Brooks. Intelligence without representation. *Artificial Intelligence*, 47:139–159, 1991.

7. F. Cloppet-Oliva and G. Stamon. Segmentation coopérative région/contour pour une analyse automatique d'images de cellules en culture. In *Proceedings of 10e congrès RFIA*, volume 2, pages 1063–1072, 1996.

8. J.-P. Cocquerez and S. Philipp. *Analyse d'images : filtrage et segmentation.* Masson, 1995.

9. R.B. Dickinson, S. Guido, and R.T. Tranquillo. Biased cell migration of fibroblasts exhibiting contact guidance in oriented collagen gels. *Ann. Biomed. Eng.*, 22:342–356, 1994.

10. A. Doisy, S. Paillasson, P. Tracqui, F. Germain, F. Leitner, M. Robert-Nicoud, and X. Ronot. In vitro dynamics of chromatin organization and migration. *Cell Biol. Toxicol.*, 12:363–366, 1996.

11. J. Ferber. *Les systèmes multi-agents : vers une intelligence collective.* InterEditions, 1995.

12. K.S. Fu and J.K. Mui. A survey on image segmentation. *Pattern Recognition*, 13(1):3–16, 1981.

13. Z. Guessoum and M. Dojat. A real-time agent model in a asynchronous-object environment. In *Proceedings of MAAMAW*, pages 190–203, January 1996.

14. S.H. Gwydir, H.M. Buettner, and S.M. Dunn. Non-rigid motion analysis of the growth cone using continuity splines. *ITBM*, 15(3):309–321, 1994.

15. H. Kondo, R. Matsuda, and Y. Yonezawa. Autonomous migration of human fetal skin fibroblasts into a denuded area in a cell monolayer is mediated by basic fibroblast growth factor and collagen. *In Vitro Cell Dev. Biol.*, 29A:929–935, 1993.

16. F. Leitner, S. Paillasson, X. Ronot, and J. Demongeot. Dynamic functional and structural analysis of living cells : new tools for vital staining of nuclear DNA and for characterization of cell motion. *Acta Biotheoritica*, (43):299–317, 1995.

17. F. Leymarie and M.D. Levine. Tracking deformable objects in the plane using an active contour model. *IEEE Trans. on PAMI*, 15(6):617–634, 1993.

18. C.E. Liedtke, T. Gahm, F. Kappei, and B. Aeikens. Segmentation of microscopic cell scenes. *AQCH*, 9:197–211, 1987.

19. P. Maes. How to do the right thing. *Connection Science Journal*, 1(3), 1989.

20. S. Naudet, L. Nicolas, C. Faye, and M. Viala. Suivi temporel 3D d'objets en présence d'occultations dans une séquence d'images monoculaires. In *Proceedings of 10e congrès RFIA*, volume 2, pages 849–858, 1996.

21. N.R. Pal and S.K. Pal. A review on image segmentation. *Pattern Recognition*, 26(9):1277–1294, 1993.

22. F. Siegert, C.J. Weijer, A. Nomura, and H. Miike. A gradient method for the quantitative analysis of cell movement and tissue flow and its application to the analysis of multicellular Dictyostelium development. *J. Cell Sci.*, (107):97–104, 1994.

23. L. Steels. Cooperation between distributed agents through self-organization. In *DAI*, volume 1, pages 175–196. Elsevier Science, 1990.

24. K. Wu, D. Gauthier, and M.D. Levine. Live cell image segmentation. *IEEE Trans. on Bio. Eng.*, 42(1):1–12, 1995.

Methodology for the Design of Digital Brain Atlases

B. Gibaud[1], S. Garlatti[2], C. Barillot[1], E. Faure[2]

[1] Laboratoire SIM, Faculté de Médecine, Rennes , France
[2] Laboratoire IASC, ENS Télécommunications de Bretagne, Brest, France

Abstract. This paper deals with the development of computerized brain atlases addressing both research and clinical needs. The authors analyze in detail the potentialities of these systems and discuss the capabilities and limitations of the digital atlases currently being developed around the world. The authors propose to reconsider the concept of a brain atlas, regarding both its *content*, and the way it has to be *used and managed* in order to set up a more effective cooperation between the user and the system. Particular emphasis is put on the *evolutivity* and *reuse* issues, which are critical in this rapidly evolving field. These orientations result from both the authors' experience and the analysis of current trends in the field of neuroimaging. The general methodology is illustrated with examples related to computer aided surgical planning.

1. Introduction

The role of medical imaging in the neurological and neurosurgical practice, as well as in neuroscience in general, is becoming increasingly important. Indeed, the interpretation of the images plays a prominent role in diagnostic and therapeutic decisions, and quantitative image analysis is a major research issue in neuroimaging. Brain atlases [e.g. 1, 2, 3, 4] aim at assisting the interpretation of brain images by providing a priori knowledge about brain anatomy by means of anatomical plates obtained from *post-mortem* brains or *in vivo* images. These plates provide the anatomical substrate, from which more details about brain features (e.g. morphology, relationships with surrounding anatomical structures, function, variability) are accessible in textual or graphical form.

From an historical point of view, atlases were developed to overcome the limitations of the *in vivo* imaging techniques. However, in spite of the availability of modern and powerful imaging techniques such as Magnetic Resonance Imaging (MRI), atlases are still necessary for three major reasons: (1) The spatial resolution and the contrast of the images are limited: for example the different nuclei composing the thalamus cannot be distinguished on MRI images; (2) Through the anatomical substrate, it is often the *function* of the different brain areas that is relevant to the surgeon in order to select the best surgical approach. In most cases this information is not available (functional imaging modalities are not so widespread) and this information has to be retrieved from an atlas. (3) Brain atlases are still commonly used in the neuroimaging community, especially by people working on the mapping of human brain functions [5, 6]. A first explanation is related to the low spatial resolution of functional imaging techniques like Positron Emission Tomography (PET): indeed, the registration with patient anatomy (through MRI) cannot be very precise, so it may be more simple to relate functional information to anatomy by means of a reference atlas (e.g. Talairach) rather than the patient MRI data itself. A second explanation arises from the fact that PET experiments cannot be repeated many times on the same individual due to the use of radiopharmaceuticals. Therefore PET studies must be conducted onto several individuals in order to provide statistically significant results: registration to a common atlas is a simple way to merge results from different patients in a standardized way.

The digital nature of in vivo imaging techniques brings new capabilities to represent anatomical information in an atlas and to access to related knowledge. We have experienced some of them during the last decade. Our interest in the mid-80s was primarily focused on 3D representation of brain anatomy [7, 8], then on the registration of images between different patients [9, 10]. More recently we have studied how knowledge about the major anatomical features could be represented in a more explicit way (e.g. atlas plates, symbolic objects represented by frames, illustrations) [11, 12], and how access to this information could be managed in a way taking into account contextual information domain of interest and task of the user) [13]. Finally some aspects of the evolutivity of such systems have been studied, especially regarding schema evolution capabilities in Object Oriented databases [14].

These works, as well as the analysis of general trends concerning the management of information in the neuroimaging community have led us to reconsider the concept of a brain atlas, regarding both its *content*, and the way it has to be *used* and *managed*. This is the major subject of this paper. Section 2 analyzes in more details new capabilities induced by the digital nature of the images, and discusses the major trends arising from the recent literature on brain atlases. Section 3 presents our approach to this problem, with particular emphasis on the *evolutivity* and *reuse* issues. These two constraints strongly influence both the content of the atlas and the way it is used and managed. Finally, section 4 summerizes this general approach, and underlines some difficulties in putting this methodology into practice.

2. Current Status of Digital Atlases

Before analyzing the potentialities and added value of digital brain atlases, and reviewing current works in this field, it is useful to briefly recall the basic function of an atlas. The utilization of an atlas involves 3 steps (Fig. 1): (1) *spatial registration* between the image data to interpret and the anatomy of one or several individuals displayed on atlas plates; (2) *identification* of anatomical structures of the subject from the outlines and labels of the same structures within the atlas plates; (3) *access* to the knowledge associated to the anatomical structures.

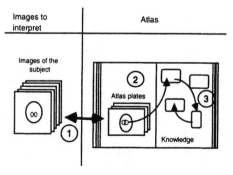

Fig. 1: Process of utilization of an atlas

Atlases are usually printed and thereby have severe limitations. Digital atlases offer a wide range of capabilities, which overcome these limitations.

• The first concerns *image display*. Brain anatomy is 3D, so the understanding of 3D data sets makes it necessary to use both surface representation and volume representation (cut planes in the three major directions of space). Printed atlases obviously cannot offer this flexibility (limited to 2D display, no possibility to redefine viewing angles).

• The second concerns *inter-individual variability*. The matching between two brains assumes that some warping model can be applied. Printed atlases impose warping models to be very simple (for example Talairach [1]). Computer-based atlases allow much more complex models to be used (e.g. non-linear rather than linear), leading to simpler use and better accuracy.

• The third is related to *extensibility*. As opposed to printed atlases, a digital atlas can be extensible: i) the number of atlas plates can be increased (which helps to overcome the inter-individual variability problem); ii) new warping models can be added; iii) the corpus of accessible knowledge can be extended.

• The fourth concerns the *flexibility of navigation* within the associated knowledge corpus; this allows for taking into account the goals and tasks of the user in order to guide the navigation towards the more pertinent information.

• The last concerns the *possible utilization of this knowledge by artificial cognitive agents* for decision-making. This is obviously not feasible with classical atlases and permits to free the user from computing tasks that computers do more efficiently than humans.

The development of computer-based atlases is motivated by this potential added value; three major categories of systems have been or are being developed.

(1) The first category is basically a transposition of paper-atlases, and may be called *computerised maps*. Some of these systems put emphasis on gathering encyclopaedic knowledge from neuroscience sub-areas. For example Toga has developed a 3D anatomical and functional atlas of the rat brain [15]. Other systems propose the integration of data from various atlases, such as the system developed by Nowinski: this system provides atlas plates from the Talairach et Tournoux, Schaltenbrand/Wahren and Ono atlases [16]. Finally, some systems are organized around 3D display tools: for example the system called "Digital Anatomist", proposed by Brinkley, provides 3D display of the anatomical features by means of both still and moving images, and offers designation facilities allowing their naming [17]. The "Voxel-Man" system developed by Höhne is based on the same concept with more enhanced facilities for editing the 3D model and retrieving related symbolic information [18]. These systems are more and more edited and distributed on CD-ROM; demonstrations are sometimes possible through Internet.

(2) The second category focuses on modeling the morphological inter-subject variability and on the design of warping models. The general principle consists of labelling precisely 3D data sets of one (or several) brains, and to estimate a displacement field between this reference brain and the particular brain to be matched, in order to assign the reference brain labels to the voxels of the unknown brain. The major issue is to make sure that this transformation guarantees the conservation of topological relationships between the labelled regions. Many methods have been developed, for example: [19, 20, 21, 22, 23, 24, 25].

(3) Finally, many atlas systems have been developed to support the automatic interpretation of anatomical images. They generally include symbolic knowledge about anatomy or imaging techniques in order to assist the delineation and labelling of these

features within morphological or functional images, for example: [26, 27, 28, 29, 30, 31, 32].

It is also important to mention collaborative efforts carried out in the context of the american Human Brain Project. Mazziota proposed the constitution of a multi-centric database, in order to build a probabilistic brain atlas [33, 34]. The "BrainMap" system developed by Fox at the University of Texas is accessible through the Internet and gathers many experimental results concerning cognitive studies from many laboratories (activation protocols, localization in the Talairach space, references of publications).

All these works have brought out significant contributions to the various aspects of brain atlas conception and use (more accurate models of the brain variability, 3D display and editing tools, computer-aided image interpretation techniques). Besides, projects like the Human Brain Project highlighted the interest of collaboration across disciplinary and geographic boundaries for brain research. Nevertheless, although claimed as important [34], evolutivity and reuse issues have not really been addressed yet. Finally, potentialities concerning the utilization of knowledge available from an atlas for automatic or assisted problem resolution (for example surgery planning) have not been really investigated yet. Projects like SAMMIE have tried to go into this direction, in particular for assisting the interpretation of Electroencephalography (EEG) or Magnetoencephalography (MEG), but achievements are still in their infancy [31].

This situation requires a more thorough analysis of the way knowledge is used by humans for the resolution of medical problems concerning the brain. Experiments carried out by Boshuizen and Schmidt [35] have shown that physicians make use of several kinds of knowledge, including both general knowledge (called biomedical knowledge) and situated knowledge derived from previous experiences. They also demonstrated that novices use more biomedical knowledge than experts do. However, in difficult cases where usual reasoning schemes may fail, experts use general knowledge as well. These works are very interesting with respect to our atlas problem. First, they reinforce the need of associating in an atlas several kinds of knowledge, namely general knowledge, and situated knowledge. Second, they suggest that the system should be designed in such a way that: (1) it provides the user with the most relevant knowledge, depending on the user's task and expertise level, and (2) it supports the emergence of new biomedical knowledge from the experience of past cases. This is the general orientation described hereafter.

Design and Use of Atlases

The general approach described here emphasizes the *evolutivity* and *reuse* issues. This concern tends to be more and more critical in the design of Information Systems in general, and are particularly relevant in the context of the management and use of brain related knowledge. Indeed, neuroscience is a very active research field [34], and many disciplines try to elucidate brain structure and functioning from different perspectives (e.g. anatomy, physiology, psychology, behaviour), which leads to an extreme fragmentation of knowledge. However it is generally admitted that multi-disciplinary research is very effective and fruitful, which assumes that knowledge and results must be shared in an appropriate way. Brain research is also very productive which means that this knowledge must be able to be *easily updated*, which obliges to consider evolutivity as a major concern in the design of brain knowledge management systems. The same arguments apply regarding clinical applications, since clinical processes and medical decisions oblige to integrate many components (patient specific anatomy, physiology, age, medical history, social condition) each of which referring to specific knowledge, and involving references to previous cases.

This approach articulates around three axes: (1) the first deals with the content of atlases (knowledge sources), (2) the second with the general organization of information processing (Decision-making and knowledge acquisition processes) and (3) the third with the way multi-disciplinary knowledge can be managed.

3.1 Knowledge Sources

Before describing in detail the different kinds of information a digital atlas should manage, it is necessary to introduce the terminology we are going to use in the following. The term *data* refers to any signifying entity used by an information processing agent. The term *information* refers to the meaning attached to a particular datum, which thereby depends on the cognitive background of the agent which interprets this datum [36]. The term *knowledge* is (as usual) more difficult to define: we will consider as knowledge any information allowing data to be interpreted and to which one wishes to attach a particular worth; this worth may arise from several origins: (1) abstraction level and capacity to synthesize a set of information; (2) level of consensus a piece of information is gathering; (3) applicability of a piece of information in a given context (solving power) and potential of reuse in other contexts.

These notions are very important with respect to evolutivity and reuse: the level of abstraction, applicability and degree of confidence play a major role in reuse. Moreover broadly accepted knowledge is likely to be more stable in time than uncertain one.

An atlas involves two fundamentally different kinds of information:

(1) biomedical knowledge concerning brain, characterizing the properties which are shared by most individuals, or within meaningful categories of individuals (such as right-handed people).

(2) Situated knowledge (cases): this information characterizes particular individuals, about which data have been recorded (e.g. images, physiological signals) and interpreted, in order to make their specific characters explicit.

One may feel appropriate to speak about these two kinds of information in terms of knowledge base and database. We prefer avoiding to do so in order to emphasize the conceptual difference between the two, rather than focusing on implementation issues.

3.1.1 Biomedical Knowledge

This general biomedical knowledge includes four major kinds of knowledge:

- *Conceptual knowledge* about one or more brain disciplines: it is usually organized in ontologies describing abstract brain entities (e.g. anatomical structures, functional systems, neurochemicals) or relationships between these entities (e.g. spatial relationships, neural connections, part-whole relationships). These entities are generally represented by means of object oriented models or frames.

- *Illustrations* (such as drawings or schemata) aim at making more explicit the meaning to be associated to the previous brain abstract entities. By definition they are indented to humans rather than artificial agents.

- *Numerical data, functions of space or time*: for example 3D probability maps represent the probability that a point belongs to a particular anatomical structure.

- *Decision models* include inference mechanisms or algorithms capable of deriving new information from existing one: for example a warping model which allows a brain to be mapped onto another, or an image segmentation algorithm, consisting of successive image processing operations, aiming at delineating and labelling a particular structure.

3.1.2 Situated Knowledge

This information depicts various aspects of the brain of particular subjects: anatomy, physiology, behaviour of the subject, characteristics of the individual himself (for example sex, manual dominance, age, pathology, if any). It may have been obtained in vivo, by means of imaging techniques (e.g. CT scanner, MRI, functional MRI, PET) or neurophysiological techniques (e.g. EEG, Depth electrodes recordings, MEG), or from cadavers (photographs of brain cryosections, histological or histochemical data).

This information about individual brains can take several forms:

- *numerical data, functions of space or time*: e.g. images or physiological signals.

- *instances of brain abstract entities,* whose attributes describe the specific characters of each brain (e.g. length and depth of a cortical sulcus, volume of grey matter within a gyrus), or relationships between these entities for example spatial relationships between anatomical structures. These objects describe in an explicit way some properties which are shown by images or signals, as a result of a manual or automatic interpretation process.

- *instances of application of a decision model*, for example describing the successive steps of an image processing procedure resulting in the labelling of a particular anatomical structure (interpretation process).

This information can be considered as knowledge, because according to previous definitions, one assigns a worth to it, and therefore wishes to keep it, in order to refer to it and reuse it. This value arises from several factors:

- a particular brain feature may be typical or atypical;

- some information may be difficult to obtain for technical or medical reasons: for example depth electrodes recordings can be obtained in very few patients (e.g. patients suffering some form of epilepsy requiring surgery). This kind of information is very precious although a very small part of it can be understood yet: indeed it provides a view of what is really happening inside the brain.

- complexity level of the description: the delineation, identification and labelling of brain features on images or signals bring a significant added value to the data because it establishes explicit relationships between this data and abstract brain entities. This added value is manifold and brings potentialities of reuse: (1) the result of this delineation may help another user or expert to achieve a similar task; (2) the description itself provides many ways for accessing the images (indexation of the data); the more complex the description is, the more various and specific these ways are; (3) it allows multivariate analysis to be done in the future in order to put in light interesting correlations.

- level of consensus they gather: an interpretation may always be wrong or uncertain. Validation by several experts increases the confidence one may have, and thereby augments the chances of reuse.

A major issue is to be able to clearly distinguish, each time it is feasible, the raw data (which are relatively objective) and the interpretations one may wish to record (which are necessarily subjective). Digital atlases allow to do that, whereas it is much more difficult with classical printed ones (for example on paper, the delineation of a region on an image generally hides the initial information, e.g. pixels values in an MRI image). This issue is also very important with respect to the system evolutivity: in effect, one may be able to interpret or re-interpret data, using some new knowledge appeared in the meantime: in a such case it is important to be able to use the original data, rather than processed ones.

3.1.3 Relationships Between Situated and Biomedical Knowledge

Biomedical knowledge and situated knowledge are complementary. As previously mentioned, the descriptions of particular subjects' brains refer to abstract brain entities, which have to be defined in a non-ambiguous way (notably to allow correct interpretation and reuse in other contexts). Conversely, situated knowledge explain general concepts by providing real world examples.

3.2 Decision and Knowledge Acquisition Processes

We are now presenting our general framework for managing information and knowledge in computerized brain atlases. It details the *decision-making processes* in which data are interpreted, leading to the production of new information, and the *knowledge acquisition processes* by which information (situated knowledge) is transformed into new biomedical knowledge. The analysis of decision-making processes will particularly focus on human-computer cooperation and on the management of multi-disciplinary knowledge.

3.2.1 Modeling of the General Approach

The general process of using and evolving an atlas is presented on Fig 2. It involves two major kinds of processes: decision processes which make use of current knowledge and produce new information, and knowledge acquisition processes which allow new knowledge to be created.

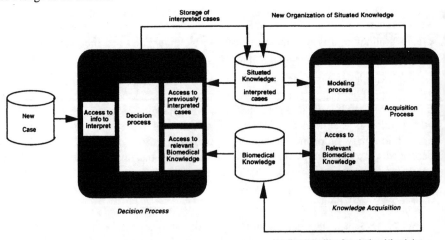

Fig. 2 : General framework - Decision processes and knowledge acquisition processes

1) *Decision processes* (Fig 2 - Left) usually consist of analyzing brain-related data acquired for clinical or research purposes, and interpreting them. These interpretations (for example in which anatomical structure a particular depth electrode is located) may be part of the resolution of a more global and more complex problem (in this case, locating an epileptogenic focus, in order to remove it by surgery). Such processes make use of:

- brain-related information concerning a particular individual (such as a 3D MRI dataset, neurophysiological data),

- general biomedical knowledge (brain abstract entities, decision models),

- information concerning previous cases (situated knowledge), which present similarities with the current problem.

These decision processes are active processes making connections between situated knowledge and the global framework and produces new information (interpretation) which becomes part of the information patrimony of the atlas.

2) *Knowledge Acquisition Processes* (Fig 2 - Right) aim at formalising new biomedical knowledge from available information (more abstract or more synthetic models):

- classification into categories (for example cortical sulci having similar structural and morphological characteristics),

- numerical models as probability maps (probability that a point belongs to a particular anatomical structure),

- deformable models resuming the morphological properties of a particular anatomical structure.

Of course, the validity of this new information has to be assessed. In particular it should not be contradictory with previous knowledge. Eventual conflicts must be detected and solved in one way or another. This new knowledge may authorize or require to update previous knowledge (and concern both general biomedical knowledge and situated knowledge). For this reason, schema evolution capabilities must be provided in order to achieve these modifications.

2.2 Decision-making Processes and Human/Computer Cooperation

The decision-making processes requiring use of a medical atlas cannot be formalised, they are what Simon calls "unstructured decisions". This means that the processes leading to the decision may be unknown to the user himself: they are usually very heuristic and progressive, and may require backtracking stages. Decision support systems address this kind of needs by providing multiple decision models (knowledge-based systems, image tools) and human computer interaction tools, allowing the most appropriate solution to be chosen interactively, case by case.

Tasks distribution between natural and artificial cognitive agents

Current digital atlases are purely reactive systems, limited to the supplying of the information requested by the user. A more fruitful approach is to design an *active* environment capable of augmenting his skills. Then, the interaction between the user and the system is based on a mixed approach. Users should be able to question the system and the system can offer hints to the user as well. The tasks and the control are distributed among the user and the system in an adaptive manner.

This distribution must be flexible and evolutive. Let us take an example, in order to show how the system contribution can be smoothly augmented. In this example four stages of development of the system are considered, in order to assist the identification of a given anatomical structure in a 3D MRI data set:

1. the system allows for the retrieval of other individuals' 3D MRI data sets ;

2. the system allows for the retrieval of those 3D MRI data sets in which the anatomical structure of interest has been delineated and labelled;

3. the system actually performs the superposition of a probability map concerning the anatomical structure of interest on the new 3D MRI data set;

4. finally, the system controls a segmentation algorithm which makes use of the probability map in order to achieve the delineation.

This example suggests how the boundary between automatic and human-controlled tasks can be shifted. The system architecture must be designed in such a way that this boundary can be moved very easily in order to enhance progressively the performances of the system (evolutivity).

Organization of cooperation

This cooperation should be organized in a way which is both flexible and natural to the user, allowing him to assess his reasoning, and validate his assumptions. It should allow him to interrupt the system's resolution process, choose another decision model, or do the resolution himself. The system would primarily be used for executing calculations within well-known and well-formalized tasks. However, artificial agents may also be involved to provide the user with the information he needs or even play a part in determining the appropriate cooperation level, taking into account the distribution of skills in the context of a specific problem.

This imposes that the relevance of available information should be explicitly and continuously assessed, which can be achieved by means of a task model [37]. The precision and the sophistication of this model depend on the kind of support the system is supposed to offer. Supporting the retrieval of relevant general biomedical knowledge and relevant previous cases can be achieved in a relatively simple way, relating this information with the general concepts involved in the user's task. If the system must contribute more effectively in solving sub-problems or be involved in the control of the cooperation, then it is necessary to develop much more complex models of the tasks and the skills of the (natural and artificial) agents involved (e.g. a priori distribution schemes, decomposition of tasks into sub-tasks) [38].

3.3 Managing Multi-disciplinary Knowledge

The necessity to manage multi-disciplinary knowledge has been underlined previously. A major issue is that knowledge production and maintenance is generally organized *vertically* (according to more and more specialized research fields), whereas utilization is primarily organized *horizontally* (i.e. multi-disciplinary). These two organization schemes lead to contradictory constraints: taking into account *evolutivity* constraints would lead to organize knowledge in separate ontologies, whereas multi-disciplinarity may orient to a more ad-hoc (specific problem driven) knowledge management.

Our approach to this problem takes into account the concern of evolutivity and reuse, and recommends to organize the knowledge base by means of multiple knowledge sources [39, 40] which can be partitioned by type (for instance, knowledge about tasks, methods and domains) and by level of abstraction (in our framework: neuroanatomy, neurology, neurophysiology, etc).

4. Discussion and Conclusion

We have proposed a general methodology for building and managing knowledge in digital brain atlases, in a way which guarantees evolutivity and facilitates reuse in different contexts: it can be summerized by a number of basic principles.

1. Information concerning particular brain instances is a form of knowledge, which is complementary to general knowledge (called biomedical knowledge). One should clearly distinguish several levels of interpretation of the data acquired about each brain instance, in order to allow these interpretations to be refined in the future, in the light of some new knowledge.

2. General biomedical knowledge should be organized in a vertical way (scientific disciplines). In effect, it is difficult (almost impossible) to design a single ontology that includes every aspect required to model the world. Dividing the world into distinct knowledge sources makes it easier to understand, to reuse and to update.

3. Knowledge based decision-making processes involve multi-disciplinary knowledge; t is therefore necessary to establish cross-speciality relationships.

4. Applications should as far as possible reuse existing knowledge rather redevelop it from scratch. This could save time and energy, and facilitate the maintenance and the evolution of this knowledge. Moreover it would allow the knowledge corpus to be built in an incremental way.

5. Cooperation between the user and the system should be user-centered because the decision-making processes are complex and not fully understood by the users themselves. The boundary between automatic and human-controlled tasks must be very flexible to upgrade progressively the system performance (evolutivity), and to achieve an optimal way of cooperation adapted to each situation (optimal reuse of available knowledge).

These principles provide general orientations. However putting them into practice raises many unsolved issues that one should not ignore. Evolving and reusing knowledge leads to face difficulties at four different levels: (1) at a geographical level, (2) at an organizational level, (3) at a semantic level, and finally (4) at a strategic level. Whereas the two first ones can be easily overcome, the two latter are far more fundamental.

• In the field of brain atlases, more and more information can be obtained in digital form, thus facilitating their communication between research labs or within the Healthcare system, through local and global networks (Internet).

• The second level is organizational. Indeed, in order to communicate or to share information, communicating parties have to share common objectives, in order to define the intention of communication and how it should take place. Regarding this issue, we can notice that many initiatives have been launched in the field of brain research to set up common frameworks between research labs (e.g. European projects such as SAMMIE, Human Brain Mapping project in the USA).

• The third obstacle arises from the various scientific disciplines concerned by brain research. Modeling brain related concepts within a given discipline is already a difficult task (due to the brain intrinsic complexity). Establishing models which are understood and valid across several disciplines is probably not feasible. In practice, trying to describe explicitly those concepts by means of multiple forms of representation (symbolic objects, illustrations, cases) should facilitate the understanding and the reuse by both natural and artificial cognitive agents in various research or clinical environments, or at least facilitate the detection of contradictions and mismatches. Setting up explanation mechanisms may be a good way to satisfy both the needs for concision (e.g. referring to the concepts rather than detailing them when both parties share a common understanding) and semantical accuracy (e.g. control that the associated semantics are not contradictory).

• Finally, one must be able to assess and manage the value and relevance of knowledge with respect to the goals of each organization. It becomes more and more difficult, because global networks considerably increase the possibilities of accessing existing knowledge. The problem is to find efficient ways of appropriation of this knowledge, which is particularly challenging in a multi-disciplinary context like brain research.

5. Bibliography

1. J. Talairach and P. Tournoux, *Co-Planar Stereotactic Atlas Of The Human Brain*. Stuttgart: Georg Thieme Verlag, 1988.
2. G. Szikla, G. Bouvier, and T. Hori, *Angiography of the human cortex*. Berlin, Heidelberg, New York: Springer Verlag, 1977.
3. G. Schaltenbrand and W. Wahren, *Atlas for stereotaxy of the human brain*, Thieme, Stuttgart 1977.
4. M. Ono, S. Kubik, and C. D. Abernathey, *Atlas of the cerebral sulci*. Stuttgart: Georg Thieme Verlag, 1991.
5. R. J. Seitz, C. Bohm, T. Greitz, P. E. Roland, L. Eriksson, G. Blomqvist, G. Rosenqvist, and B. Nordell, "Accuracy and precision of the computerized brain atlas programme for localization and quantification in Positron Emission Tomography", *Journal of cerebral blood flow and metabolism*, pp. 443-457, 1990.
6. A. C. Evans, T. S. Marrett, J. Torrescorzo, S. Ku, and D. L. Collins, "Mri-Pet Correlative Analysis Using A Volume Of Interest (Voi) Atlas", *J. of Cerebral Blood Flow and Metabolism*, vol. 11, pp. A69-A78, 1991.
7. C. Barillot, B. Gibaud, J.M. Scarabin and J.L.Coatrieux, "Three dimensional reconstruction of cerebral blood vessels", *IEEE computer graphics and applications* , 5, 12, pp. 13-19, 1985.
8. C. Barillot, B. Gibaud, O. Lis, L.M. Luo, A. Bouliou, G. Le Certen, R. Collorec and J.L. Coatrieux, "Computer graphics in medicine: a survey", *CRC Critical Reviews in Biomedical Engineering*, 15, 4, pp. 269-307, 1988.
9. D. Lemoine, C. Barillot, B. Gibaud and E. Pasqualini, "An anatomical-based 3D registration system of multimodality and atlas data in neurosurgery", IPMI 1991, London, Information Processing in Medical Imaging, *Lecture notes in computer science*, Vol 511, A.C.F. Colchester and D.J. Hawkes (Eds), Springer Verlag, pp. 154-164, 1991.
10. C. Barillot, D. Lemoine, L. L. briquer, F. Lachmann, and B. Gibaud, "Data fusion in medical imaging: merging multimodal and multipatient image, identification of structures and 3D Display aspects", *European Journal of Radiology*, vol. 17, pp. 22-27, 1993.
11. E. Montabord, B. Gibaud, C. Barillot, S. Garlatti, I. Kanellos, B.S. Wu, A. Biraben and X. Morandi, "An Hypermedia System to Manage Anatomical Knowledge about Brain". in: Lemke HU, Inamura K., Jaffe CC, Felix R. Eds., Computer Assisted Radiology, Springer-Verlag, pp. 414-419, 1993.
12. C. Barillot, B. Gibaud, E. Montabord, S. Garlatti and I. Kanellos, "An Information System to Manage Anatomical Knowledge and Image Data about Brain", SPIE Vol 2359, Visualization in Biomedical Computing, pp. 424-434, 1994.
13. E. Montabord, B. Gibaud and C. Barillot, "HYPER-YAKA: Hypermedia et base de connaisances sensible au contexte". Congrès "Langages et Modèles à Objets", Nancy, pp. 153-171, 1995.
14. J.H. Yapi , A. Lasquellec and B. Gibaud, "Evolution de schéma et migration d'instances. Prise en compte des besoins d'une application médicale". Congrès Bases de Données Avancées (BDA 96), Cassis (France), 1996.
15. A. W. Toga, "A Three-Dimensional atlas of structure/function relationships", *Journal of chemical neuroanatomy*, pp. 313-318, 1991.
16. W. L. Nowinski, A. Fang, and B. T. Nguyen, "Schaltenbrand-Wharen/Talairach-Tournoux brain atlas registration", SPIE Vol 2431, pp. 126-136, 1995.

17. J. F. Brinkley, K. Eno, and J. W. Sundsten, "Knowledge-based client-server approach to structural information retrieval: the digital Anatomist Browser", *Computers Methods and Programs in Biomedecine*, pp. 131-145, 1993.

18. K. H. Höhne, M. Bomans, M. Riemer, R. Schubert, U. Tiede, and W. Lierse, "A volume based anatomical atlas", *IEEE Comp. Graphics & Appl.*, vol. 12, pp. 72-78, 1992.

19. R. Bajcsy and S. Kovacic, "Multiresolution Elastic Matching", *CVGIP*, vol. 46, pp. 1-21, 1989.

20. F. L. Bookstein, "Thin-Plate Splines And The Atlas Problem For Biomedical Images", in *Information Processing in Medical Imaging*, *Lecture Notes in Computer Sciences Vol.511*, A. C. F. Colchester and D. J. Hawkes, Eds. Berlin: Springer-Verlag, pp. 326-342, 1991.

21. A. C. Evans, D. L. Collins, and B. Milner, "An MRI-based stereotactic atlas from 250 young normal subjects", *Soc. Neurosci. Abstr*, pp. 408, 1992.

22. J. C. Gee, C. Barillot, L. Le Briquer, D. R. Haynor, and R. Bacjsy, "Matching Structural Images of the Human Brain using Statistical and Geometrical Image Features", presented at SPIE, Visualization in Biomedical Computing, SPIE Vol 2359, pp. 191-204, 1994.

23. D. L. Collins, A. C. Evans, Holmes and T.M. Peters, "Automatic 3D segmentation of neuro-anatomical structures from MRI", in *Computational Imaging and Vision: Information Processing in Medical Imaging*, vol. 2432, Y. Bizais, C. Barillot, and R. Di Paola, Eds.: Kluwer Academic Publishers, pp. 139- 152, 1995.

24. G.E. Christensen, R.D. Rabbitt, M.I. Miller, S.C. Joshi, U. Grenander, T.A. Coogan, and D.C. Van Essen , "Topological properties of smooth anatomic maps", in *Computational Imaging and Vision: Information Processing in Medical Imaging*, vol. 2432, Y. Bizais, C. Barillot, and R. Di Paola, Eds.: Kluwer Academic Publishers, pp. 101-112, 1995.

25. G. Subsol, J.P. Thirion, and N. Ayache, "Une méthode générale pour construire automatiquement des atlas anatomiques morphométriques à partir d'images médicales tridimensionnelles : application à un atlas du crâne", presented at RFIA, Rennes, pp. 159-168, 1996.

26. E. Sokolowska and J. A. Newell, "Multi-Layered Image Representation: Structure and Application in Recognition of Parts of Brain Anatomy", *Pattern Recognition Letters*, pp. 223-230, 1986.

27. H. H. Zachmann, "Interpretation of cranial MR images using a digital atlas of the human head", in: Lemke HU, Rhodes M.L., Jaffe CC, Felix R. Eds., Computer Assisted Radiology, Springer-Verlag Berlin Heidelberg, pp. 283-4287, 1991.

28. I.C. Carlsen, M. Imme, M.H. Kuhn, K. Ottenberg and K.H. Schmidt, "Knowledge based Interpretation of cranial MR images", in: Lemke HU, Inamura K., Jaffe CC, Felix R. Eds., Computer Assisted Radiology, Springer-Verlag Berlin Heidelberg, pp. 277-282, 1991.

29. K. Natarajan, M. G. Cawley, and J. A. Newell, "A knowledge based system paradigm for automatic interpretation of CT scan", *Medical informatics*, vol. 16, pp. 167-181, 1991.

30. E. D. Lehmann, D. J. Hawkes, D. L. G. Hill, C. F. Bird, G. P. Robinson, and A. C. F. Colchester, "Computer aided interpretation of SPECT images of the brain using an MRI derived 3D neuro-anatomical atlas", *Medical Informatics*, vol. 16, pp. 151-166, 1991.

31. M. Staemmler, E. Claridge, and J. Cornelis, "SAMMIE - Software applied to multimodal images and education", presented at IMAC 93, Berlin, pp. 91-98, 1993.

32. G. P. Robinson, A. C. F. Colchester, and L. D. Griffin, "Model-Based Recognition of Anatomical Objects from Medical Images", in *Lecture Notes in Comp. Science: Information Proc. in Med. Imag.*, vol. 687, H. Barrett and A. Gmitro, Eds.: Springer-Verlag, pp. 197-211, 1993.

33. J. C. Mazziotta, A. W. Toga, A. C. Evans, and P. Fox, "A Probabilistic Reference System for the Human Brain", Application to the Human Brain Project: Phase I June 1993.

34. J. C. Mazziotta, A. W. Toga, A. C. Evans, P. Fox, and J. L. Lancaster, "A Probabilistic Atlas of the Human Brain: Theory and Rationale for its development", *Neuroimage*, pp. 89-101, 1995.

35. H. G. Schmidt and H. P. A. Boshuizen, "On Acquiring Expertise in Medecine", *Education Psychological Review*, pp. 205-221, 1993.

36. V. Prince, *Vers une informatique cognitive dans les organisations, le rôle central du langage*, Editions Masson, 1996.

37. V. O. Mittal and C. L. Paris, "Context: indentifying its elements from the communication point of view", presented at Workshop on Using Knowledge in its context, IJCAI, Chambery, 1993.

38. J. Willamowski, "Modélisation de tâches pour la résolution de problèmes en coopération système-utilisateur", Université Joseph Fourier Grenoble 1, 1994.

39. R. Simmons and R. Davis, "The Role of Knowledge and Representation in Problem Solving", in *Second Generation Expert Systems*, J. M. David, J. P. Krivine, and R. Simmons, Eds.: Springer Verlag, pp. 27-45, 1993.

40. S. Garlatti, E. Montabord, B. Gibaud and C. Barillot, "A methodological approach for object knowledge bases", Expert Systems 95, Cambridge, Edited by M.A. Bramer, J.L. Nealon, R. Milne, Research and Developments in Expert Systems XII, pp. 201-214, 1995.

Rule-Based Labeling of CT Head Image

Dubravko Ćosić and Sven Lončarić

Department of Electronic Systems and Information Processing
Faculty of Electrical Engineering and Computing, University of Zagreb
Unska 3, 10000 Zagreb, Croatia
E-mail: dubravko@zems.fer.hr, sven@zems.fer.hr

Abstract

A rule-based approach to the labeling of computed tomography (CT) head images containing intracerebral brain hemorrhage (ICH) is presented in this paper. Fully automated segmentation of CT image is achieved by the method composed of two components: an unsupervised fuzzy clustering and a rule-based labeling. The unsupervised fuzzy clustering algorithm outlines the regions in the input CT head image. Extracted regions are spatially localized and have uniform brightness. Region features and region-neighborhood relations are used to create the knowledge base for the rule-based system. The rule-based system performs the labeling of the segmented regions into one of the following labels: background, skull, brain, ICH, and calcifications. The rules are determined from the a priori knowledge about the relations between the CT image regions and their characteristics. The method has been applied to a number of real CT head images and has shown satisfactory results.

1   Introduction

Systems for analysis of medical images assist radiologists in diagnosis process resulting in a more accurate and faster diagnosis [1, 2]. An accurate quantitative analysis of ICH requires a correct classification of CT head images [3]. This paper presents a rule-based method for automatic classification of CT head images. The outline of the proposed method is presented in the following section. Results and conclusion are presented in Sections 3 and 4, respectively.

2   Methods and Procedures

The proposed procedure consists of two stages. The first processing stage or region extraction is performed by an unsupervised fuzzy clustering algorithm [4] which partitions the original image into a number of spatially localized regions having uniform brightness. Extracted regions are divided into three groups of regions: bright, dark, and gray regions. These results are input to the second processing stage which performs understanding of the image through the region labeling process. The rule-based system assigns a label from the predefined label set to each of regions. The label set contains five labels: background, skull, brain, ICH, and calcifications. The knowledge base of the system for image labeling consists of facts and rules. The facts are used to represent the properties of the particular input image and are determined by several region features and region-neighborhood relations. The region brightness (dark, gray, bright), the area, and the intensity variance are used as features for region description. The area is described by the number of pixels contained in the region. The intensity variance describes a variability in pixel brightness within the particular connected region. There are three possible variances: low, medium, and high. For example, the following fact represents a dark region with the area equal to 50 pixels and a low intensity variance.

region (*id* 2) (*neighbor* 5 7 8) (*area* 50) (*brightness dark*) (*variance low*))

In this example, the region identity number is equal to 2 and is adjacent to the regions with the identity numbers 5, 7, and 8. The relationships among the facts are represented by rules. The rules are determined from the knowledge about the relations between the CT image regions and their characteristics. The rules are independent units that are not procedurally linked to other rules. Every rule consists of a premise and a conclusion. The action specified in the conclusion is taken when a rule is considered and the expression in the premise is found to be true. The rules can be classified by means of a label which they assign to the selected region. There are rules for the background, skull, brain, ICH and calcifications labeling. Some of these rules are presented in the following subsections in if/then form which is the most appropriate way to represent a reasoning process. The rule-based expert system for image labeling has been developed using the expert system shell "C Language Integrated Production System" (CLIPS).

.1 Background labeling rules

The following rules define the properties of the regions which belong to the background area.

1. **if** region has only one adjacent region **and** adjacent region is background
   then region is background
2. **if** region is adjacent to skull **and** adjacent to background **and** not bright
   then region is background
3. **if** region is adjacent to brain **and** adjacent to background **and** not bright
   then region is background
4. **if** region has only one adjacent region **and** adjacent region is skull **and** is dark
   then region is background
5. **if** region is adjacent to background **and** adjacent to non-labeled region **and** non-labeled region is bright **and** is gray
   then region is background and adjacent non-labeled region is background
6. **if** region is dark **and** has the largest area among dark regions
   then region is background

2.2 Brain labeling rules

These rules define the properties of the brain regions.

1. **if** region is adjacent to skull **and** area > 1000 **and** is gray
   then region is brain
2. **if** region has only one adjacent region **and** adjacent region is brain **and** is not bright
   then region is brain
3. **if** region is adjacent to brain **and** is adjacent to non-labeled region **and** non-labeled region is bright **and** non-labeled region area < 20 **and** is dark
   then region is brain

2.3 Skull labeling rules

The skull area is determined according to the following rules.

1. **if** region is bright **and** has the largest area among bright regions
   then region is skull
2. **if** region is adjacent to brain **and** is adjacent to background **and** is bright
   then region is skull

2.4 Hemorrhage labeling rule

The hemorrhage area is labeled according to the following rule.

1. **if** region has only one adjacent region **and** adjacent region is brain **and** region area>19 **and** region is bright
   then region is hemorrhage

2.5 Calcifications labeling rules

Calcifications are determined by the following three rules.

1. **if** region has only one adjacent region **and** adjacent region is brain **and** region area<20 **and** is bright
   then region is calcification
2. **if** region has two adjacent regions **and** adjacent regions are brain **and** region area<20 **and** is bright
   then region is calcification
3. **if** region has three adjacent regions **and** adjacent regions are all brain regions **and** region area < 20 **and** is bright
   then region is calcification

3 Results

The system proposed in this paper has been used to perform segmentation of a number of real CT head images of size 128 × 128. In this section some segmentation results are presented.

The input CT head image is partitioned into a smaller regions by the unsupervised fuzzy clustering algorithm. The rule-based system performs the labeling of these regions into five labels: skull, ICH, brain, background, and calcifications. The results of the rule-based labeling are presented in Figure 1.

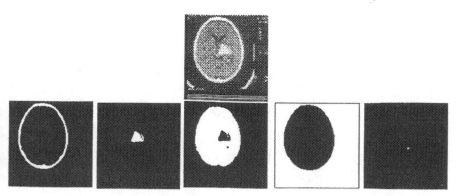

Figure 1: Original CT head image; skull, ICH, brain, background, and calcifications.

4 Conclusion

In this paper we have presented a rule-based approach to the labeling of CT head images containing ICH. The proposed approach to the labeling problem is computationally efficient. The rule-based approach to the labeling problem provides more flexibility for the solution of this problem. The rules are easy to construct and modify. They are relatively independent and can be changed without affecting other parts of the knowledge base. This provides a convenient framework for addition of new rules. The system has been applied to a number of real CT head images and has shown encouraging results.

References

[1] M. Garreau, J. L. Coatrieux, R. Collorec, and C. Chardenon. A knowledge-based approach for 3-D reconstruction and labeling of vascular networks from biplane angiographic projections. *IEEE Transactions on Medical Imaging*, 10:122–131, 1991.

[2] C. Li, D. B. Goldgof, and L. O. Hall. Knowledge-based classification and tissue labeling of MR images of human brain. *IEEE Transactions on Medical Imaging*, 12:740–750, 1993.

[3] S. Loncaric, D. Cosic, and A. Dhawan. Hierarchical segmentation of CT images. In *Proceedings of the 18th Annual Int'l Conference of the IEEE EMBS*. IEEE, 1996. Amsterdam.

[4] I. Gath and A. Geva. Unsupervised optimal fuzzy clustering. *IEEE Transactions on PAMI*, 11:773–781, 1989.

Characterisation of Tumorous Tissue in Rat Brain by in Vitro Magnetic Resonance Spectroscopy and Artificial Neural Networks

Torsten Derr[1], Thomas Els[2], Michael Gyngell[2] & Dieter Leibfritz[1]

[1]Universität Bremen, Institute of Organic Chemistry, Bremen, Germany

[2]Max-Planck-Institute for Neurological Research, Cologne, Germany

INTRODUCTION

Nuclear magnetic resonance (NMR) is a spectroscopy technique based on the fact that atomic nuclei oriented by strong magnetic fields absorb radiation at characteristic frequencies. NMR is used to gain qualitative and quantitative information from many metabolites in body fluids, like blood and urine, or biological tissue extracts simultaneously in one experiment. NMR spectra obtained from tissue extracts differentiate fifty and more metabolites in the tissue and reflect altered cellular metabolism before more gross morphological changes are manifest. This makes NMR potentially useful in the diagnosis and prognosis of brain tumors[1,2,3]. However, the spectra are generally complex and a lot of biological information is inaccessible to standard manual analysis due to problems with peak overlap and baseline noise. Therefore NMR data requires special techniques like Artificial Neural Networks (ANN) for correct classification.

In this study proton NMR spectra of tumorous and healthy brain tissue from rats were used to train a linear multilayer feed-forward network. The purpose of this study is the automation of tumor diagnosis and the differentiation of tumors using only NMR spectra as a source of information. Output sensitivities were calculated from the trained ANN to analyze the effect of each input factor on the classification result. This method allows the identification of signals (metabolites) in the spectrum that are most important for classification and class membership.

MATERIALS AND METHODS

Experimental brain tumors were induced into the nucleus caudatus of male Fisher rats (n=25, 250-350g body weight) by allotransplantation of tumor cells. 90 tissue samples were taken from funnel frozen brain of male Fischer rats (n=25, 200-350g body weight) with the induced tumors F98 glioma (16), RN6 schwannoma (20) and E376 neuroblastoma (26). For the extraction of low molecular weight compounds from the brain tissue, the biopsy samples were frozen in liquid nitrogen.

homogenized and extracted with perchloric acid. The chemical extracts were neutralized, centrifuged and lyophilized.

NMR spectroscopy was performed on a Bruker AMX360WB spectrometer. On the day of analysis the sample was redissolved in 0.5ml deuterated water. Proton NMR spectra with 32.000 data points were recorded at 298K using a standard water suppression pulse sequence.

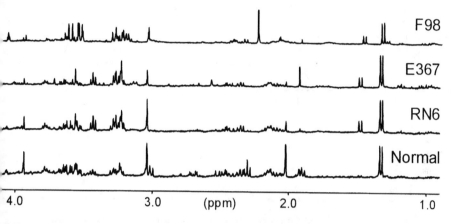

Figure 1: Typical proton NMR spectroscopic data from tissue extracts of F98 glioma, RN6 schwannoma and E367 neuroblastoma brain tumours compared to control tissue (normal).

ANALYSIS

The spectra were phased, baseline-corrected and normalized using standard algorithms. For ANN analysis the spectra were integrated at 0.04 ppm intervals in the range of 0.5-4.5 ppm giving 100 variables. The neural network was trained by Back-Error Propagation with Least Mean Squared cost function using 14 hidden nodes and four output nodes. A 'leave-one-out' method was used for sample classification after 1000 epoches of training.

For the identification of important signals in the spectra, sensitivity analysis of the neural network was used as a basis of inference of input-output relationships. A logarithmic sensitivity matrix[4,5] S was calculated from the trained network with ANN parameters described above:

$$S_{xy} = -\frac{\delta \ln(T_y - O_y)}{\delta \ln(I_x)}.$$

The first order output sensitivities S_{xy} between the xth node of the input I_x and the the yth node of the output layer O_y are evaluated, where T_y is the desired output (target).

RESULTS

The best ANN classification results were obtained, when the samples were put into four classes. Tissue from the edge of the tumor or necrotic tumorous tissue are regarded to be in the same class like pure tumor. Therefore, a four node orthogonal representation of classes has been chosen to be the target vector. Figure 1 shows typical proton NMR spectra of these four tissue types. Table 1 summarizes the results from ANN analysis. All spectra were assigned correctly, except one sample from the edge of the tumor, containing large amounts of healthy tissue, which was not classified.

Class	Correct	Wrong	Unclassified
F98	15/16	0	1/16
E367	20/20	0	0
RN6	26/26	0	0
Control	28/28	0	0
Total	98.9 %	0.0 %	1.1 %

Table 1: Results from Classification using the Leave-Out-One method.

Sensitivity analysis was carried out on a second training set consisting of F98 gliomas (16 samples) and healthy tissue (28 samples). The absolute sensitivity value of each input factor is correlated with the signal's importance for class membership. Figure 2 illustrates the sensitivity values for the F98 glioma class.

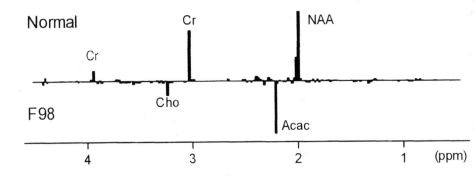

Figure 2: Sensivity parameters for F98 glioma tumors.

For these two classes major sensitivity values are assigned to N-acetyl aspartate (NAA), creatines (Cr), acetoacetate (Acac) and choline derivates (Cho). These peaks are supposed to have the biggest effect on the classification result. Other compounds like lactate at 1.33 ppm show little or no sensitivity and can be excluded from ANN input in further studies.

Sensitivity analysis of the other groups yielded the results listed in table 2. As expected, for the classification of different tumor types the NMR resonances related to substances NAA, creatine, myo-inositol, choline and alanine were found to be important.

No.	Chem. Shift [ppm]	Substance
1	2.019	N-Acetyl-Aspartate (NAA)
2	3.994	Creatine 1 (Cr)
3	3.538	myo-Inositol (m-Ins)
4	1.462	Alanine (Ala)
5	3.598	Glycine (Gly)
6	3.082	Creatine 2 (Cr)
7	3.285	Choline (Cho)

Table 2: Important signals of NMR detectable substances for the classification of different brain tumors.

CONCLUSION

The NMR data in this study was interpreted statistically without using molecular and spectroscopical prior knowledge. Only the class origin (tumour/healthy tissue) was used as additional information for the training pattern. The samples were consistently classified successfully. This indicates that sample classification can be automated. Sensitivity analysis of the input pattern can be used for interpretation of NMR spectra without adding any medical or biochemical knowledge. The substances NAA, creatine, myo-inositol, choline and alanine were found to be important, the concentration of lactate seems to be an unreliable parameter for this classification problem. These results are exactly in line with clinical findings and medical interpretation of tumor metabolism. This study demonstrated, that NMR spectroscopy in combination with ANN offers a promising potential for the diagnosis of brain tumors.

REFERENCES

. H. Bruhn, M.L. Gyngell et al., *NMR Biomed.*, **5**, 253, 1992
. R.J. Maxwell et al., *Proceedings of the Workshop on Neural Network Applications and Tools*, IEEE-Press, 18, 1993.
. S.L. Howells et al., *Magn.Reson.Med.*, **28**, 214, 1992
. R. Dorf, *Modern Control Systems*, Addision-Wesley Publishing Company, 1988
. J. Herts et al., *Introduction to the Theory of Neural Computation*, Addison-Wesley Publishing Company, 1991

An Application of Machine Learning in the Diagnosis of Ischaemic Heart Disease

Matjaž Kukar[1], Ciril Grošelj[2], Igor Kononenko[1], Jure Fettich[2]

[1] University of Ljubljana, Faculty of Computer and Information Science,
Tržaška 25, SI-1001 Ljubljana, Slovenia,
[2] University Medical Centre Ljubljana, Nuclear Medicine Department,
Zaloška 7, SI-1000 Ljubljana, Slovenia
e-mail: {matjaz.kukar, igor.kononenko}@fri.uni-lj.si,
{ciril.groselj, jure.fettich}@mf.uni-lj.si

Abstract. Ishaemic heart disease is one of the world's most important causes of mortality, so improvements and rationalization of diagnostic procedures would be very useful. The four diagnostic levels consist of evaluation of signs and symptoms of the disease and ECG (electrocardiogram) at rest, sequential ECG testing during the controlled exercise, myocardial scintigraphy and finally coronary angiography. The diagnostic process is stepwise and the results are interpreted hierarchically, i.e. the next step is necessary only if the results of the former are inconclusive. Because the suggestibility is possible, the results of each step are interpreted individually and only the results of the highest step are valid. On the other hand, Machine Learning methods may be able of objective interpretation of all available results for the same patient and in this way increase the diagnostic accuracy of each step. We conducted many experiments with four learning algorithms and different variations of our dataset (327 patients with completed diagnostic procedures). Our results show that improvements using Machine Learning techniques are reasonable and might find good use in practice.

1 Introduction

Ishaemic heart disease (IHD) is the most important cause of mortality in developed as well as in developing countries. Therefore improvements as well as the rationalization of diagnostic procedures and treatment of IHD are necessary.

The usual procedure in IHD diagnosis consists of four diagnostic levels containing evaluation of signs and symptoms of the disease and ECG at rest, sequential ECG testing during a controlled exercise, myocardial scintigraphy and coronary angiography as a final test. Because the suggestibility is possible, the results of each step are interpreted individually and only the results of the highest step are valid. The amount of data available for each patient in all diagnostic levels is too large to be efficiently and objectively evaluated by physicians.

The goal of a rational diagnostic algorithm is to establish the conclusive diagnosis of IHD and to plan the most appropriate management of the disease using only the necessary diagnostic steps. This can be achieved by taking into account and evaluating all the information collected by different diagnostic methods according to their importance and diagnostic value.

The performance of different diagnostic methods is usually described as classification accuracy, sensitivity and specificity:

accuracy   =   (true positive+true negative test results) / all patients
sensitivity   =   true positive test results / all patients with disease
specificity   =   true negative test results / all patients without disease

The reported average values of these measures, taken from 29 reports containing several thousands of patients are as follows [1]. Sensitivity for exercise ECG (5796 persons) is 72%, specificity 79%, and accuracy 74%. For exercise myocardial scintigraphy (2413 persons) they are 84%, 88%, and 85%, respectively. Coronary angiography is a reference method.

The goal of our study was to improve the diagnostic performance (sensitivity and specificity) of non-invasive diagnostic methods (especially myocardial scintigraphy) by evaluating all available diagnostic information using Machine Learning (ML) techniques. The results of coronary angiography were used as a definite proof of IHD presence.

2   The Problem and the Dataset

The function of the heart is pumping blood to all the organs of the body. For this task an uninterrupted supply of oxygen to the heart muscle is needed. This is achieved by sufficient blood flow trough the coronary arteries to the heart muscle – myocardium. In case of diminished blood flow through coronary arteries due to stenosis or occlusion, IHD develops. The consequence of IHD is impaired function of the heart and lastly necrosis of the myocardium – myocardial infarction.

During the exercise the blood flow through the body has to be increased. Therefore the delivery of oxygen to the heart muscle has to increase several times by increasing blood flow trough the coronary arteries.

In a (low grade) IHD the blood flow is sufficient at rest or during a moderate exercise, as perfusion of the myocardium is adequate, but insufficient during a severe exercise. Therefore, signs and symptoms of the disease develop only then.

There are four levels of diagnostics of IHD. First signs and symptoms of the disease are evaluated clinically and ECG is performed at rest. This is followed by the sequential ECG testing during controlled exercises. If this test is not conclusive, or if additional information regarding the perfusion of the myocardium is needed, myocardial scintigrapy is performed. Radioactive material which accumulates in the heart muscle proportionally to its perfusion is injected into the patient and the images (scintigrams) showing perfusion of the heart muscle during exercise and rest are taken. By comparing both sets of images, the presence, localization and distribution of the ishaemic tissue are determined. If an invasive herapy of the disease is contemplated, i.e. coronary artery bypass surgery, the diagnosis has to be concluded by imaging of the coronary vessels (injecting the contrast material into the coronary vessels and imaging their anatomy by x-ray coronary angiography).

In our study we used a dataset of 327 patients with performed clinical and aboratory examinations, exercise ECG, myocardial scintigraphy and coronary angiography. In 229 cases the disease was angiographically confirmed and in 98 cases it was excluded. The patients were selected from the population of approximately 4000 patients who were examined at the Nuclear Medicine Department in years 1991-1994. For the sake of our study we selected only the patients with complete diagnostic procedures (all four levels).

Our experiments were conducted on four problems, depending on the amount of clinical and laboratory data (attributes) available for learning (between 30 and 77 attributes).

3 Algorithms and Experiments

In our experiments we used the following algorithms: the naive Bayesian classifier [3], backpropagation learning of neural nets [4] with weight elimination [5] and algorithms for induction of decision tree Assistant-I and Assistant-R [2].

The learning task for ML algorithms was given as four problems, differing in amount of clinical and laboratory data available for each patient.
1. Signs and symptoms
2. Signs, symptoms and the exercise ECG
3. Signs, symptoms and the exercise ECG and scintigraphy
4. The exercise myocardial scintigraphy only

In the first two cases we compared our results with results obtained by the physicians from the exercise ECG only. The third and fourth step were compared with their results from the myocardial scintigraphy only. The experiments on each variation of our dataset was performed 10 times by randomly selecting 70% of instances for learning and 30% for testing and the results were averaged. Each system used the same subsets of instances for learning and for testing in order to provide the same experimental conditions. In Tables 1 and 2 the results of physicians and ML algorithms are presented and compared.

Table 1. Results obtained by physicians verified with coronary angiography

Physicians	Accuracy	Sensit.	Specif.
Exercise ECG only	65.1	89.3	57.1
Exercise myocardial scintigraphy only	83.8	83.7	85.7

Table 2. Results of Machine Learning algorithms. 1 = Signs and symptoms, 2 = Signs, symptoms, and the exercise ECG, 3 = Signs, symptoms, the exercise ECG, and scintigraphy, 4 = The exercise myocardial scintigraphy only.

	Naive Bayes			Neural net			Assistant-I			Assistant-R		
	Acc.	Sensit.	Specif.	Acc.	Sensit.	Specif.	Acc.	Sensit.	Specif.	Acc.	Sensit.	Specif.
1.	79.1	89.2	54.5	79.2	85.5	63.8	71.2	73.4	59.3	73.2	76.1	61.9
2.	79.7	89.3	57.1	81.6	88.5	65.0	70.5	73.2	59.3	73.1	76.8	61.0
3.	88.5	91.7	80.1	89.7	93.8	79.5	89.0	89.1	88.1	86.6	89.6	79.7
4.	87.3	90.2	80.1	88.4	92.6	79.1	87.2	88.9	83.2	84.0	87.4	73.5

464

4 Discussion

The results of our work are promising. The most significant result is the increase of specificity and sensitivity of the exercise myocardial scintigraphy by using other available information (signs, symptoms and exercise ECG). When compared with physicians' results of myocardial scintigraphy, Assistant-I showed the 2.5% increase in specificity and 5.5% in sensitivity. In practice two-fold rationalization could be expected. Due to higher specificity less persons without the disease would have to be examined with invasive and dangerous coronary angiography. Together with higher sensitivity this would also save money and shorten the waiting times of the sick patients The second interesting result is that by using ML techniques one can merely from the evaluation of signs and symptoms achieve the sensitivity of 89% and the specificity of 55% (Bayesian classifier) which is equivalent to the sensitivity and the specificity of the exercise ECG. This fact is well-known but it holds only for experienced physicians specialists. Less experienced physicians need the evaluation of the exercise ECG for reliable diagnostics. By using the ML techniques this could be avoided.

By using the evaluation of the exercise ECG together with the evaluation of the signs and symptoms the neural network increased the specificity for 8% while keeping the sensitivity on the same level (89%). This in turn implies that, if such system was implemented in practice, less persons without the disease would have to pass the myocardial scintigraphy or the coronary angiography.

However, it should be taken into account that the results of our study are obtained on a significantly restricted population and therefore may not be generally applicable to the normal population, i.e. the patients coming to the Nuclear Medicine Department. Further studies are needed to verify our findings. In particular, the on-line data gathering is necessary to obtain a representative dataset.

For future experiments the algorithms have to be adapted to control the sensitivity-specificity trade-off. We plan to incorporate the misclassification cost matrices into the learning algorithms of all four systems. This way a sensitivity-specificity point on the trade-off curve may be selected that fits the user requirements which would highly increase the usability of the systems for the medical diagnostic tasks.

References

1. C. M. Gerson. Test accuracy, test selection, and test result interpretation in chronic coronary artery disease. In C. M. Gerson, editor, *Cardiac Nuclear Medicine*, pages 309–347. Mc Graw Hill, New York, 1987.
2. I. Kononenko, E. Šimec, and M. Robnik-Šikonja. Overcoming the myopia of inductive learning algorithms with ReliefF. *Applied Intelligence*, In press, 1996.
3. I. Kononenko. Inductive and Bayesian learning in medical diagnosis. *Applied Artificial Intelligence*, 7:317–337, 1993.
4. D.E. Rumelhart and J. L. McClelland. *Parallel Distributed Processing*, volume 1: Foundations. MIT Press, Cambridge, 1986.
5. S. Weigand, A. Huberman, and D. E. Rumelhart. Predicting the future: a connectionist approach. *International Journal of Neural Systems*, 1(3), 1990.

Meta-level Learning
in a Hybrid Knowledge-Based Architecture

E. Christodoulou and E.T. Keravnou

Department of Computer Science, University of Cyprus
P.O.Box 537, CY-1678 Nicosia, Cyprus
{cseleni,elpida}@turing.cs.ucy.ac.cy

Abstract. A hybrid knowledge-based architecture integrates different problem solvers for the same (sub)task through a control unit operating at a meta-level, the metareasoner, which coordinates the use of, and the communication between the different problem solvers. A problem solver is defined to be an association between a knowledge intensive (sub)task, an inference mechanism and a knowledge representation formalism operated by the inference mechanism in order to perform the (sub)task. An important issue in a hybrid system is the learning aspect. It reflects the ability of the system to evolve on the basis of its experiences in problem solving. Learning occurs at different levels, learning at the meta-level and learning at the level of the specific problem solvers. Meta-level learning reflects the ability of the metareasoner to improve the overall performance of the hybrid system by improving the efficiency of meta-level tasks. Meta-level tasks include the initial planning of problem solving strategies, and the dynamic adaptation of chosen strategies depending on new events occurring dynamically during problem solving. In this paper we concentrate on meta-level learning in the context of a hybrid architecture. The theoretical arguments presented in the paper are demonstrated in practice through a hybrid knowledge-based architecture for the domain of breast cancer histopathology.

1 Introduction

Knowledge-based architectures for complex, real, domains, need to employ multiple problem solvers in order to perform their task efficiently and effectively. A particular problem solver is associated with a knowledge intensive (sub)task and comprises an inference mechanism which operates on a specific view of the given knowledge domain; it can therefore be abstracted in terms of a (sub)task, an inference mechanism and a knowledge representation formalism. A hybrid knowledge-based architecture integrates multiple problem solvers through a meta-reasoner for controlling the use of, and the communication between the different problem solvers. Each problem solver can either run on a stand alone basis, or in collaboration with other solvers associated with the same (sub)task, for achieving the required results. Hence the different solvers, for the same task, exhibit a "competitive-collaborative" behaviour. The decision as to which of the competitor solvers to deploy for a particular problem case is taken dynamically depending on specific meta-level requirements (time considerations, detail of the solution, etc.). If during problem solving the selected solver is shown to be unable to deliver the required, intermediate or final, results then other solvers can be used, to support or replace the failing solver. This means that decisions should be taken dynamically at different points during the problem solving activity, and this entails whether implicated solvers are used competitively or collaboratively. Such dynamic decisions can be quite complex, and are taken by the metareasoner. The metareasoner operates at a meta-level, the level above the specific problem solvers, and is responsible for carrying out essential and critical (meta-level) tasks of the hybrid system. Such tasks include the planning of the most appropriate problem solving strategy for a specific case to start with, and the reactive adaptation of chosen strategies in order to take into consideration new events occurring dynamically during problem solving. A problem solving strategy specifies the different problem solvers to be used and their relative activation patterns. The reactive adaptation of chosen strategies reflects the reactive behaviour of the metareasoner.

Learning constitutes a critical aspect of a hybrid knowledge-based architecture. Learning should occur at different levels, at the meta-level and at the level of the specific problem solvers. The latter refers to the ability of the (object-level) solvers to improve their reasoning mechanisms and to enhance their knowledge in order to increase their time efficiency and the correctness of their solutions. Different solvers may use different learning mechanisms depending on the knowledge representation formalisms and the inference mechanisms that they implement. Each solver could evolve on the basis of its accumulated experience independently of the other solvers. Learning at the meta-level reflects the ability of the metareasoner to improve the overall problem solving performance of the hybrid system and hence the overall effectiveness of its meta-level tasks on the basis of strategic experiences. Even though learning at the level of the problem solvers is an important aspect of a hybrid architecture, learning at the meta-level is of higher importance, because of the critical role assigned to the metareasoner. Meta-level learning aims to improve the initial planning of a problem solving strategy and the subsequent reactive adaptation of this strategy. Additionally, the metareasoner is responsible for supporting the different problem solvers in improving their problem solving performance, ie it should also support the object-level learning. For this purpose the metareasoner should transmit new, learned, information between the different problem solvers, in order to enable them to enhance their knowledge and improve their reasoning mechanisms.

In this paper we concentrate on meta-level learning. In section 2 the main tasks of the metareasoner are overviewed. The examples used in the sequel for illustration purposes are taken from a hybrid knowledge-based system, for the domain of breast cancer histopathology, developed by the first author. A short description of the system is also given in section 2. Learning with respect to each of the identified meta-level tasks is discussed in sections 3-5. Related research work is discussed in section 6 and finally section 7 concludes the discussion.

2   Main tasks of the metareasoner and meta-level learning

The central tasks of the metareasoner are the planning of problem solving strategies and the reactive adaptation of such strategies on the basis of events occurring
dynamically during the execution of the strategies, ie either externally to the system or in the context of the activated problem solvers. A problem solving strategy
is a plan of problem solver activations. It is planned on the basis of parameters
describing the problem case (meta-parameters) and on problem solver characteristics. Problem solver characteristics constitute part of the knowledge base of
the metareasoner; these could include information about the maximum/average
length of time needed by the solver to achieve a solution, information about
the complexity of the domain knowledge used by the solver, as well as information about the dependencies of the specific problem solver with other solvers.
Problem case meta-parameters could include the desired level of detail for the
computed solutions and the length of time for solving the problem. Based on
the combination of such parameters, a problem solving strategy is planned. This
means that before a specific problem solver is activated, a global evaluation of
the overall problem solving situation is carried out and an appropriate, initial
problem solving strategy is chosen or synthesised. During execution, a problem solving strategy may be shown to be ineffective/inefficient for the particular
problem case. Thus the execution of a strategy should be dynamically monitored
and reviewed throughout so that necessary adaptations, or replacement of strategy, are done in a timely and constructive way to minimize wastage. This task
falls under the main responsibilities of the metareasoner and reflects its reactive
behaviour. Another significant task of the metareasoner is to support the different problem solvers in their learning efforts for improving their performance.
The performance of a problem solver is improved when its knowledge and/or
reasoning mechanism are enhanced. This can be supported by communicating
back to the solvers new information learned dynamically during problem solving.

Meta-level learning provides ways for improving the effectiveness of the critical meta-level tasks. More specifically meta-level learning addresses the following:

- How to improve the planning of the initial problem solving strategy for a
  particular problem case, so that the most appropriate strategy is initially
  activated.
- How to improve the reactive adaptation of activated strategies, ie how to
  improve the reactive behaviour of the metareasoner.
- How to best support the different problem solvers in order to improve their
  problem solving performance, ie how to improve support for object-level
  learning.

In the following sections each of the above meta-level learning tasks is discussed in turn. The proposed meta-level learning has been demonstrated in practice through a hybrid knowledge-based system for the domain of breast cancer histopathology [7]. The examples used below are taken from this system. The particular hybrid system has been developed to assist histopathologists in the histological classification of a new breast cancer case. Such a classification is based on a number of diagnostic factors extracted from a manual microscopic analysis of breast biopsies. The system uses three different problem solvers, each capable of solving the given problem on its own, a rule-based solver, a case-based solver and a deep-model solver. The knowledge of the rule-based solver consists of different rules associating the most important nuclear and cytoplasmic features of breast cancer with relevant conclusions. The case-based solver uses previously experienced problem cases for reaching its conclusions and the deep-model solver uses a detailed description of the domain (collection of functional constraints) for its operation. The metareasoner of this system knows the characteristics of the three problem solvers, and the dependencies between them. For example, the rule-based solver is characterized by its time-efficient and approximate problem solving, the case-based solver by its detailed and more time consuming problem solving and the deep-model solver is characterized by its detailed and even more time consuming problem solving. All three problem solvers can work in a competitive/collaborative way. For example the rule-based solver can be supported by the case-based solver and the case-based solver can be supported by the deep-model solver. During problem solving the metareasoner is responsible for controlling the use and the communication of the three problem solvers.

3 Improving the planning of problem solving strategies

The performance of a hybrid system could be improved, if for every problem case the most appropriate problem solving strategy is initially selected. As mentioned in the previous section the planning of a solving strategy is based on meta-parameters describing the problem case and on problem solver characteristics. A problem solving strategy is planned by matching the required problem case meta-parameters against the characteristics of appropriate problem solvers. For example, if the time aspect is specified for some problem case, then a suitable strategy should aim to utilize those problem solvers that could come up with some solution faster than the others. Normally a combination of solvers would be used for achieving the desired results. During problem solving a *solving path*, tracing the whole activity in a detailed way, is kept by the metareasoner, for controlling the overall process. The results achieved through the execution of the planned strategy are recorded on the solving path. In order for the metareasoner to improve the planning of strategies, ie to improve its ability to select for a specific problem case the best strategy to be used, past, successful, solving paths are stored as successful strategic cases for future use. Thus, past successes in problem solving could be regarded as situations giving opportunities for learning. A paradigm, appropriate for the learning of successful strategic cases, is the

case-based one [1][2]. Future problem cases could be effectively solved by retrieving and adapting existing strategic cases. This way the metareasoner learns
from its accumulated experiences, so that successful solving paths are repeated,
rather than devising new strategies all the time. A strategic case is represented
as follows:

```
strategic-case#
list-of-problem-case-parameters:  <A list of required meta-parameters>
problem-solving-strategy:         <An appropriate problem solving strategy>
main-characteristics:             <Main characteristics of problem case>
hypothesis:                       <A first solution approximation>
result:                           <A result>
other-characteristics:            <Other characteristics of problem case>
```

The following example taken from the breast cancer diagnostic system illustrates how a problem solving path results in a successful strategic case to
be saved for future use. Suppose that the requirements for a new problem case
(list-of-problem-case-parameters) are for an approximate and a time efficient
solution. The metareasoner plans an appropriate problem solving strategy by
matching the problem case requirements against characteristics of the different
problem solvers. In this case let us assume that it decides that the utilization
of the rule-based solver is the most appropriate strategy. In order to focus the
behaviour of the system and hence to increase its performance, after initially
planning/selecting some strategy, a first approximation of the solution (hypothesis), based on the main piece of information (main-characteristics) describing
the problem in hand, is formulated by an auxiliary problem solver which is automatically invoked by the metareasoner. For example, if the main characteristic of
the problem case is the existence of the substance MUCIN, then the hypothesis
of the existence of a "Mucinous Carcinoma" is made. If the rule-based solver
comes up with a classification of "Mucinous Carcinoma", then the hypothesis is
accepted and the resulting solving path for the specific problem case is saved as
the following successful strategic case in a strategic case base.

```
strategic-case1
list-of-problem-case-parameters:  approximate, time-efficient solution
problem-solving-strategy:         rule-based-solver
main-characteristics:             existence of MUCIN
hypothesis:                       Mucinous Carcinoma
result:                           Mucinous Carcinoma
other-characteristics:            none
```

The next time a new problem case has similar meta requirements (time-efficient,
no-detailed diagnosis) as the already learned strategic case, the existing strategic case would be retrieved and the same strategy, ie the deployment of the
rule-based solver, would be followed. If the main and the other characteristics
of the new problem case are the same with those of the past case, then the
same first solution approximation (hypothesis) would be made. If during problem solving the selected strategy proves to be inappropriate for the new problem
case, the metareasoner would need to decide whether to continue or interrupt

the specific problem solving. An interrupt is chosen if all the suggested activation patterns of the problem solvers in the selected strategy do not result in an appropriate conclusion. In the event of a continuation of the specific problem solving, the metareasoner analyses the reasons of failure and decides about new strategic steps to be followed. For example the metareasoner may decide that the failed solver should be supported by another solver (a collaborator), or that a competitor solver should take over alltogether. The way the different reasons of failure are analysed and new strategic steps are suggested reflects the reactive behaviour of the metareasoner which is discussed in the next section. In the current context it is important that new strategic steps are suggested and undertaken for continuing the problem solving. In the above example it is possible that the activated rule-based solver failed to come to a conclusion because a satisfied rule antecedent (MUCIN-POOLS is absent) is inconsistent with the pursued hypothesis. A new strategic step could be that the case-based solver should take over the problem solving (the case-based solver behaves as a competitor to the rule-based solver). The retrieved strategic case should then be adapted to include the new information. If the adapted strategic case leads to an appropriate result, it would then be saved as a new strategic case as shown below.

```
strategic-case2
list-of-problem-case-parameters: time-efficient, no-detailed diagnosis
problem-solving-strategy:        case-based-solver
main-characteristics:            existence of MUCIN
hypothesis:                      Mucinous Carcinoma
result:                          Mucinous Carcinoma
other-characteristics:           MUCIN-POOLS absent
```

The strategic case base constitutes part of the knowledge of the metareasoner. Strategic cases are learned incrementally; initially the strategic case base is empty and cases are incorporated one by one during problem solving. Strategic cases are indexed on the basis of solution requirements (list-of-problem-case-parameters), the main and the other characteristics of the problem case. The retrieval of relevant strategic cases is carried out in two steps. In the first step the solution requirements are used to select the most relevant cases and in the second step the main and other characteristics of the input problem case are used to extract from the already selected strategic cases the most appropriate one to be used.

4 Improving the reactive behaviour of the metareasoner

The reactive behaviour of the metareasoner reflects its ability (a) to react to unexpected situations arising during the execution of a problem solving strategy, (b) to support activated problem solvers to overcome such situations, and (c) to adapt the given strategy in accordance with new events occurring during the resolution of the particular unexpected situations. During its operation, an activated problem solver may be faced with various difficulties, such as missing data or contradictory data. As a result it may be unable to continue its operation unless the encountered difficulties are resolved. In the first instance the problem solver will try to resolve the problematic situation by itself, through its own knowledge and reasoning abilities. If this fails, then in the second instance the problem solver will turn to the metareasoner for support by referring the unresolved problematic situation to the metareasoner. Hence during the execution of a problem solving strategy the metareasoner may be dynamically requested by activated problem solvers to support their decision making. The metareasoner should be able to react to requests from problem solvers by providing new strategic steps to be undertaken in order to continue problem solving. Suggested strategic steps resulting in a successful continuation of problem solving should be used to adapt the solving path and also be memorized for future use.

Overall this type of meta-level learning is concerned with how to improve the performance of the metareasoner regarding the handling of requests for support from the problem solvers, and the relevant adaptation of the pursued strategies. Requests coming from the different solvers are regarded as *impasses*[1]. In general, an impasse occurs when an activated problem solver is unable to continue problem solving and thus is unable to come up with an appropriate conclusion. Impasses could be described as requests for support to overcome occurred difficulties. The reactive behaviour of the metareasoner can be improved by memorizing successfully resolved impasses for future use. This information would give the specific strategic steps that had to be undertaken in order to resolve the given problematic situation and the results achieved. Impasses are of different types since there are different reasons as to why an activated problem solver cannot continue its problem solving. Every type needs to be interpreted differently. For each type of impasse a different reasoning method is activated by the metareasoner. Such methods take as input the occurred impasse and give as output the steps to be followed in order to resolve the given impasse. As mentioned above, before a problem solver sends an impasse to the metareasoner, it tries to resolve the given problematic situation by itself. If it manages to do so, then it could locally memorize the specific situation together with the appropriate answer. Otherwise, an impasse occurs that should be handled by the metareasoner.

In general, I_i represents an impasse of type T_i coming from solver S_i while attempting to justify hypothesis H_i. The metareasoner should be able to activate an appropriate method $\mathcal{M}$ to suggest steps for resolving the impasse. A successfully resolved impasse is associated with a triple (S_j, T_i, A_i) giving an answer A_i to the impasse I_i. Thus:

$$I_i = (S_i, T_i, H_i) \Longrightarrow (S_j, T_i, A_i)$$

---

[1] The idea of using the concept of an impasse in the context of learning is taken from the SOAR system [9][10]. The use of impasses in this system is simpler than in our system, because only one problem solver is involved in SOAR and occurred impasses are resolved by splitting a goal into multiple subgoals.

For example A_i could give a different hypothesis that was successfully justified by solver S_j. The next time the same impasse type would occur from any solver trying to justify the same hypothesis, the metareasoner would respond with the same triple (S_j, T_i, A_i) for continuing problem solving. Thus, successfully resolved impasses are saved for future use, in order to improve the reactive behaviour of the metareasoner.

The following example, also taken from the breast cancer system, illustrates the use of impasses as opportunities to improve the reactive behaviour of the metareasoner (see Figure 1). Given that for a specific problem case the rule-based solver is activated for justifying the hypothesis of "Mucinous Carcinoma" and the solver is unable to justify the hypothesis because of one satisfied rule antecedent, $F_i = PALPABLE\_LUMP$, having a value $V_i = absent$ that is not consistent with the hypothesis of "Mucinous Carcinoma". An impasse then occurs $I_i = (S_i, T_i, H_i)$, where: $S_i = rule\_based\_solver$, $T_i = ((F_i, V_i), inconsistency\_with\_hypothesis\_Mucinous\_Carcinoma)$, $H_i = Mucinous\_Carcinoma$. The metareasoner responds to this impasse by activating a method $\mathcal{M}$ suggesting the activation of the deep-model solver as an appropriate solving step for checking whether (F_i, V_i) implies the existence of a different hypothesis H_j. The deep-model solver concludes that the value of F_i implies the coexistence of Mucinous with Lobular Carcinoma. The given impasse is therefore successfully resolved through the answer (S_j, T_i, A_i), where: $S_j = deep\_model\_solver$, $T_i = ((F_i, V_i), inconsistency\_with\_Mucinous\_Carcinoma)$, $A_i = coexistence\_Mucinous\_with\_Lobular\_Carcinoma$. The impasse together with its answer is saved for future use. Consequently, the solving path of the specific problem case is adapted to include the use of the deep-model solver, the additional characteristic (PALPABLE_LUMP, absent) and the new hypothesis of the coexistence of Mucinous with Lobular Carcinoma (see Figure 1). Finally, the adapted problem solving path is saved as a new successful strategic case. If a suggested answer to a specific impasse does not result in a successful continuation of the problem solving, then the metareasoner could try to obtain another answer or it could declare the specific impasse as unresolved. An unresolved impasse results in an interruption of the problem solving.

5 Improving the performance of the problem solvers

A problem solver should be able to improve its reasoning mechanisms and to enhance its knowledge in order to increase its time efficiency and the correctness of its conclusions. For example a case-based solver enhances its knowledge by including new successfully solved problem cases in its case base. The metareasoner is responsible for supporting the different problem solvers in their learning efforts. This can be achieved by communicating back to the solvers new information learned dynamically during problem solving. Such information can arise, for example, through the successful resolution of impasses. A problem solver is

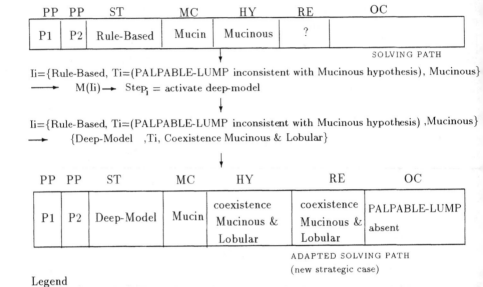

Ii={Rule-Based, Ti=(PALPABLE-LUMP inconsistent with Mucinous hypothesis), Mucinous}
⟶ M(Ii)⟶ Step₁ = activate deep-model

Ii={Rule-Based, Ti=(PALPABLE-LUMP inconsistent with Mucinous hypothesis) ,Mucinous}
⟶ {Deep-Model ,Ti, Coexistence Mucinous & Lobular}

PP	PP	ST	MC	HY	RE	OC
P1	P2	Deep-Model	Mucin	coexistence Mucinous & Lobular	coexistence Mucinous & Lobular	PALPABLE-LUMP absent

ADAPTED SOLVING PATH
(new strategic case)

Legend

PP = Problem case Parameter; ST = solving STrategy; MC = Main Characteristic
HY = HYpothesis; RE = REsult; OC = Other Characteristic

Fig. 1. Illustrating the resolution of an impasse

responsible for deciding how to utilize the communicated information, ie whether to use it for enhancing its factual knowledge or improving its reasoning mechanism. This is illustrated in the following example (see Figure 2). Let us suppose that for a given problem case the rule-based solver is activated for justifying the hypothesis of "Mucinous Carcinoma". The rule-based solver is unable to justify the hypothesis because the value for feature CUT-SURFACE-COLOUR does not belong to the expected set of values for that feature. Consequently an impasse occurs. The metareasoner tries to resolve the impasse by activating the deep-model solver. The answer of the deep-model solver is that the value brown assigned to the feature CUT-SURFACE-COLOUR does not violate the hypothesis of "Mucinous Carcinoma". This information is communicated by the metareasoner to the case-based solver. As a result the case-based solver creates a new case "Mucinous Carcinoma" in its case base with the relevant information. Additionally, the same information is transmitted to the rule-based solver. The rule-based solver adapts its rule sets to include the possibility that the feature CUT-SURFACE-COLOUR can obtain the value brown in the context of "Mucinous Carcinoma". Thus, the given information is used by both the rule-based and the case-based solvers for improving their knowledge.

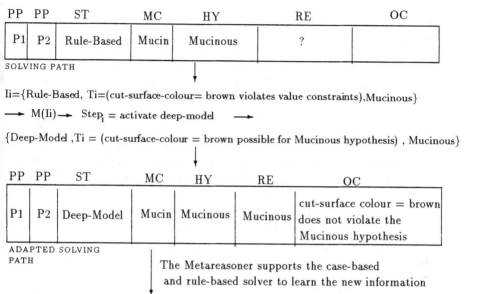

$Ii=\{\text{Rule-Based, Ti}=(\text{cut-surface-colour}= \text{brown violates value constraints}),\text{Mucinous}\}$

$\longrightarrow M(Ii) \longrightarrow \text{Step}_i = \text{activate deep-model} \longrightarrow$

$\{\text{Deep-Model ,Ti} = (\text{cut-surface-colour} = \text{brown possible for Mucinous hypothesis}) , \text{Mucinous}\}$

PP	PP	ST	MC	HY	RE	OC
P1	P2	Deep-Model	Mucin	Mucinous	Mucinous	cut-surface colour = brown does not violate the Mucinous hypothesis

ADAPTED SOLVING PATH

The Metareasoner supports the case-based and rule-based solver to learn the new information

A) Save in the case-base of the case-based solver a new problem case with the classification Mucinous Carcinoma with cut-surface-colour = brown

B) Add the possibility of cut-surface-colour = brown for the class Mucinous Carcinoma in the rules of the rule-based solver.

Legend

PP = Problem case Parameter; ST = solving STrategy; MC = Main Characteristic

HY = HYpothesis; RE = REsult; OC = Other Characteristic

Fig. 2. An example of improving the performance of the problem solvers

6 Related Work

Even though different research groups are presently working towards the development of knowledge-based architectures exploiting multiple problem solvers, only some of these efforts address the learning aspect [8]. Hybrid architectures addressing the learning aspect make only a weak reference to meta-level learning. For example within the ANALOG project [3][4][13] a knowledge modelling framework has been developed integrating different inference and learning methods. Learning is a kind of meta-level inferencing where successful and failed methods and impasses arising during problem solving are remembered for future use, but there is no planning of problem solving strategies. In the BOLERO hybrid system [11][12] the problem solving strategy to be followed is planned by a meta-level case-based solver, and is consequently executed by a rule-based solver. Important events occurring during the solving process are taken into consideration and new plans are constructed. Meta-level learning refers to the memorization of successful problem solving plans by the meta-level case-based solver. A limitation of BOLERO is that the planning of solving strategies is based on case factual knowledge and not on global meta-parameters of the problem cases. CHROMA [5][6] is a hybrid system integrating induction and case-based reasoning for problem solving. Meta-knowledge is used to select the most adequate reasoner for every case to be solved. This meta-knowledge depends only on some factual knowledge and not on meta-parameters of the current problem. This means that no problem solving strategies are planned or learned. A simple form of meta-level learning is exhibited by this hybrid system, where impasses arising during problem solving are stored for solving future cases. The idea of identifying different failure types occurring during problem solving and choosing appropriate strategies in order to avoid similar mistakes in the future shows also some similarities to the work done by [14][15]. In this work a meta-model is used to represent the system's reasoning, the decisions it took while performing the reasoning, and the results of the reasoning. If a difficulty or failure is encountered, the system introspectively examines its own reasoning processes to determine where the problem lies, and uses this introspective understanding to improve itself using the appropriate strategies.

7 Conclusions and further research

Learning constitutes an important aspect of a hybrid knowledge-based architecture. Learning can occur at the level of the different problem solvers or at the level of the metareasoner. The latter is referred to as meta-level learning. It reflects the ability of a hybrid system to improve its overall performance by improving the effectiveness of the tasks associated with the metareasoner. Such tasks are the planning of problem solving strategies, the reactive adaptation of chosen strategies and the support of object-level learning, ie learning at the level of the different problem solvers. In this paper we have concentrated on meta-level learning because of the significance of the metareasoner in a hybrid architecture. Through meta-level learning the knowledge of the metareasoner is continuously enhanced and furthermore the knowledge and reasoning mechanisms of the different problem solvers can be enhanced. Successfully applied strategies and also successfully resolved impasses are stored in different case bases for future use. The planning of problem solving strategies is improved by making use of past strategic choices and the reactive behaviour of the metareasoner is improved by using the impasse case base. Further research on meta-level learning for a hybrid system will address the issue of using not only successful but also unsuccessful problem solving strategies and impasses for improving the performance of the hybrid system.

478

Acknowledgement

The research reported here has been conducted in the context of project "Quantitative Immunohistochemical Assessment of Prognostic Factors in Carcinoma of the Breast" which is supported by the University of Cyprus.

References

1. Aamodt, A, 1993. *A case-based answer to some problems of knowledge-based systems*. In: E. Sandewall and C.G Jansson (eds.), proceedings of the Scandinavian Conference on Artificial Intelligence, IOS Press, pp 168-182.
2. Aamodt, A, 1994. *A knowledge representation system for integration of general and case-specific knowledge*. In: Proc. of IEEE TAI-94, International Conference on Tools with Artificial Intelligence.
3. Arcos, JL and Plaza, E, 1994. *Integration of learning into a knowledge modelling framework*. In: Lecture Notes in Artificial Intelligence, n. 867, Springer Verlag, pp 355-373.
4. Arcos, JL and Plaza, E, 1994. *A reflective architecture for integrated memory-based learning and reasoning*. In: Lecture Notes in Artificial Intelligence, n. 837, Springer Verlag, pp 289-300. pp 1-10.
5. Armengol, E and Plaza, E, 1994. *A knowledge level model of knowledge-based reasoning*. In: Lecture Notes in Artificial Intelligence, n. 837, Springer Verlag, pp 53-64.
6. Armengol, E and Plaza, E, 1995. *Integrating induction in a case-based reasoner*. In: Lecture Notes in Artificial Intelligence, n. 984, Springer Verlag, pp 3-17.
7. Christodoulou, E, 1994. *An integrated decision support system for the domain of breast cancer*. In: Proceedings of the International Conference Neural Networks and Expert Systems, Plymouth, UK, pp 433-441.
8. Christodoulou, E and Keravnou, E, 1996. *Integrating multiple problem solvers in knowledge-based systems*, to appear in the Knowledge Engineering Review.
9. Laird, J, Newell, A, Rosenbloom, P, 1987. *Soar: an architecture for general intelligence*. Artificial Intelligence, vol. 33, 1-64.
10. Laird, J, Rosenbloom, P, Newell, A, 1986. Chunking in SOAR: The anatomy of a general learning mechanism. Machine Learning, 1:11-46.
11. Lopez, B, 1993. *Reactive planning through integration of a case-based system and a rule-based system*. In: Proc. AISB, University of Birmingham, UK.
12. Lopez, B and Plaza, E, 1993. *Case-based planning for medical diagnosis*. In: Methodologies for intelligent systems: 7th International Symposium, ISMIS'93, Springer verlag, pp 90-105.
13. Plaza, E and Arcos, JL, 1994. *Flexible integration of multiple learning methods into a problem solving architecture*. In: Lecture Notes in Artificial Intelligence, n. 784, Springer Verlag, pp 403-406.
14. Ram, A, Cox, MT and Narayanan, S, 1992. *An architecture for integrated introspective learning*. In: Proc. of the 9th International Conference on Machine Learning, Workshop on Computational Architecture, Aberdeen, Scotland.
15. Ram, A and Cox, MT, 1994. *Introspective reasoning using meta-explanations for multistrategy learning*. In: R.S. Michalski and G. Tecuci (eds), Machine Learning: A Multistrategy Approach, Vol. IV, pp 349-377, Morgan Kaufmann.

A Framework for Building Cooperating Agents

Giordano Lanzola, Massimiliano Campagnoli, Sabina Falasconi and Mario Stefanelli
University of Pavia, Dept. of Informatics and Systems Science
Medical Informatics Laboratory
Via Abbiategrasso 209 - 27100 Pavia, Italy
{giordano,max,sabina,mario}@aim.unipv.it

Abstract. There is an increasing awareness in the AI community that the dissemination of Decision Support Systems in medical practice strictly depends on their seamless integration with those tools already available at clinical settings. In order to achieve that goal, this paper further elaborates on a previous research conducted by the same authors which identified the main components of a Distributed Hospital Information System based on Cooperating Software Agents. We propose a computational architecture supporting communication and the occurrence of multiple conversations among agents, thus effectively enforcing their cooperation. The architecture is being tested for implementing a prototype system able to coordinate the joint efforts of the several health care providers involved in managing patients affected by Acute Myeloid Leukemia.

1 Introduction

It's a common thought that AI applications in medicine have failed to achieve a widespread distribution in the daily practice despite the noteworthy performance which many of those are presently exhibiting [van Bemmel, 1993]. The chief reason of such a misfortune is concerned with the ill-conception that has caused to think of every Knowledge Based System (KBS) as a free-standing and completely self-contained application. According to that paradigm the user is asked to provide some input data and then wait for the resulting advice. Needless to say, the clerical duties concerned with entering the data, which often means duplicating those from the patient medical record, far outbalance the benefits achieved through the consultation and after few trials users soon loose their interests in using those tools. AI researchers should not loose sight of the settings where their systems are to be placed if a warmer acceptance is sought [Gardner and Lundsgaarde, 1994], thereby committing themselves to a substantial rethinking of the way KBSs are conceived. In fact, as Heathfield and Wyatt [1993] point out, it is now widely recognized that KBSs acceptance is closely related with organizational issues and human-computer interaction problems.

Furthermore, integrating KBSs within hospital settings has become even more complex given the emergence of countless hardware and software different products and it is no longer possibile to devise a set of modules to be used as the "standard" components of a single uniform distributed application. In order to increase the flexibility and the level of support provided by software systems we should start thinking of those as *autonomous agents*, possessing both the skills for solving a given set of tasks and the social ability to interoperate among each other [Jennings and Wooldridge, 1996]. Thus they are better referred to as *Software Agents* (SAs) which play the role of conceptual entities focused on the notions of *intelligence* and *autonomy* capable of reactively and/or pro-actively influencing a dynamic environment which necessarily includes other SAs. Intelligence refers to the SA capability of encapsulating an explicit model of the task to be solved, and exploiting it for shaping the strategies adopted during the problem solving process. Autonomy instead means that a SA must be able to accomplish the most part of its work without the direct intervention of humans, resorting to other agents populating the environment to get any information or knowledge required for solving the assigned tasks.

This paper builds on previous work by the same authors illustrating a methodology for designing Distributed Hospital Information Systems [Lanzola et al., 1996] and proposes a computational architecture facilitating their implementation. A protocol is defined based on a set of primitives for exchanging messages among agents which has been used for developing conventions and policies modeling the complex process by which agents ask their peers to provide services for them, as well as the willingness of the parties to fulfill or deny those requests. That architecture is being tested on a prototype system able to coordinate the joint efforts of the several health care providers involved in the management of patients affected by Acute Myeloid Leukemia.

2 The Multi-Agent Paradigm in Medicine

Designing a community of cooperating software agents in medicine requires the accomplishment of two different steps. On one side there is an *architectural* issue which is aimed at providing an abstract layout of the whole federation as seen from an outer perspective. Starting from a knowledge-level model of the task to be solved by the community a plan for its successful achievement is derived and any particular method to be adopted is subsequently made clear [Ramoni at al., 1992]. This is followed by an investigation concerning the nature of the knowledgeable and informational support to be provided by each agent and ends up with the operationalization of the methods within every single agent. There may be multiple criteria for shaping such an analysis according to which different methods may be involved. One may wish, for example, to take up the very same organizational model adopted in real life by humans, given that the available knowledge is already shaped to fit that model and no further structuring effort is required. A different choice may call for the homogeneity of the knowledge representation formalisms as well as the modularity of the resulting architecture in sight of maximizing shareability and reusability of the knowledge modules. No matter what criterion is adopted, the analysis results in the identification of the different characters taking part in the process of solving the high-level task so that all the different agents and their behaviors will be eventually tracked down.

A second step addresses instead the *functional* issue and is concerned with the suitable placement of each agent within the federation. Unlike the previous one this is more focused on an inner perspective, that is on how the whole community is perceived from every single agent and interoperability with other ones is achieved through a suitable coordination and planning of its own internal activities with those accomplished by other agents [Durfee et al., 1987; Shoham, 1993].

The problem may better be grasped by looking at Figure 1 which illustrates our computational model of a generic software agent and has been shaped on the KBS model since it subsumes a broad range of commonly used ones including database

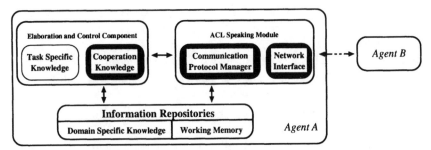

Figure 1. The computational architecture of a generic agent based on the KBS paradigm. Shaded boxes represent those whose design and implementation is being addressed in the paper.

management systems, decision support systems etc... From a computational point of view the architectural issue involves topics such as how to model and represent either Domain-Specific Knowledge and Task Specific Knowledge in order that the agent be able to accomplish the task for which it is meant. In fact, our previous research work has extensively addressed this issue both at the knowledge and computational levels [Lanzola and Stefanelli, 1993; Lanzola et al., 1996; Falasconi et al., 1996].

Thus, we are now in a position to address the functional issue which involves two separate but deeply intertwined topics. One is concerned with interconnecting SAs and enabling the exchange of information and knowledge among them through a suitable Agent Communication Language (ACL), while a second one addresses the problem of effectively modeling and representing cooperation knowledge within each agent. From a computational point of view we propose an implementation of the ACL Speaking Module and provide the primitives required for representing the Cooperation Knowledge, as indicated by the shaded boxes in Figure 1. The formalisms adopted for representing the cooperation knowledge have been designed for ensuring a smooth integration with those already available for shaping the agent internal problem-solving ability, thus augmenting it with the possibility of resorting to external supports. Nevertheless a special effort has been made for preserving the separation between the architectural and functional views as they emerge at the knowledge level also at the computational level. This resulted in a highly modular framework which is particularly suitable for enforcing the reusability of preexisting legacy systems which were developed as standalone modules.

3 The Agent Communication Language Speaking Module

In developing a suitable ACL for achieving interoperability among SAs we adopted the specifications provided by KQML [Finin et al., 1994] which have emerged as part of the Knowledge Sharing Effort (KSE), since that approach seemed to proficiently balance the expressive power of the language vs. its computational tractability. A KQML message is structured into a *performative* representing a primitive of the language, and a set of fields. The performative identifies the communicative act while the message fields carry its actual contents and help in defining an appropriate context for its interpretation (i.e. they specify the ontology, language, etc.). Decoupling the actual contents of the message being exchanged from the underlying conversational

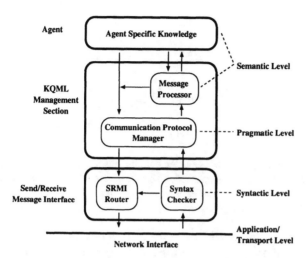

Figure 2. The architecture of the module implementing the Agent Communication Language (ACL) in the framework developed.

protocols adopted helps in developing a generic communication module which may be coupled with a wide set of already available applications turning those into SAs while preserving much of their internal coding and functionality.

Figure 2 illustrates the computational architecture of the module we are developing, and shows how it stands in between the network and the agent itself, extending the application/transport levels provided by the particular network technology adopted as defined by the OSI model, and addressing the syntactic, pragmatic and semantic levels.

More specifically the Send/Receive Message Interface (SRMI) preserves the independence of the higher levels from the application/transport levels which may be implemented using either the popular TCP/IP protocol suite as well as any other available one also including E-Mail. Incoming messages are received by the SRMI and must verify a syntax check before they are passed to the upper levels. This check only involves the KQML expression and is not aimed at analyzing the actual message which may only be interpreted by the Message Processor addressing the semantic level. Nevertheless it is useful to prevent the forwarding to the higher levels of a corrupted or misdelivered message or even if some of the KQML fields by themselves indicate that it may not be successfully interpreted by the recipient agent (i.e. the ontology and/or the language adopted for the message content are not supported by the recipient).

Whenever an incoming message fails to pass that check an error message is generated within the Syntax Checker and sent to the SRMI Router which subsequently dispatches it to the sender agent. The purpose of the SRMI Router is that of helping in properly dispatching any message to the right recipient. It acts as an interface between the agent and the network support by keeping track of the actual network addresses of any peer with which there is an ongoing conversation.

Messages verifying the syntactic test are passed to the KQML Management Section and first processed by the Communication Protocol Manager (CPM) where the

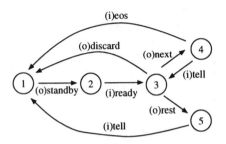

Figure 3. An ATN representing the states and the possible transitions in a conversation carried on between a physician agent and a database, as seen from the physician perspective. Each transition is labelled with the name of the performative causing its occurrence. The prefix (o) means that the message is an outgoing one, while (i) denotes an incoming message.

KQML performative is decoded in order to associate the message with the corresponding conversation. To accomplish that goal we used a formalism based on a set of Augmented Transition Networks (ATN) whose nodes represent the possible agent states with respect to the ongoing conversations and arcs joining them make explicit the only allowed transitions along with the relevant performatives.

Figure 3 shows a simple ATN where the initial state, that is the one signifying the absence of a conversation, is represented by node 1. That ATN may suitably represent a conversation initiated by a physician agent with a database which develops as follows. First the physician sends a message to the database asking it to retrieve all the available findings concerning a given patient. A new conversation is instantiated and its state, as it appears from the physician's perspective, moves to node 2. The message sent is based on the *standby* performative so the database doesn't reply with the requested data but caches those locally and when it is finished it notifies the physician and waits for its reaction. In fact, from the physician perspective when the conversation is in state 2 the only way for it to proceed will be toward state 3 upon the receipt of a message from the database based on the *ready* performative. The physician may then ask the database to transmit the first item in the list (*next*), send the remaining items at once (*rest*) or even discard those and drop the conversation (*discard*). If at some stage within a conversation an agent receives a message based on a performative which doesn't match the set causing the admissible transitions for that node, the conversation is dropped and the agent submitting the wrong message is notified by the CPM. The ability for each agent to carry on multiple conversations at the same time has been achieved by instantiating a separate ATN for each ongoing conversation.

Finally, the topmost module in the KQML Management Section is the Message Processor (MP) whose goal is to interpret the actual message contents and possibly make up the reply. To this aim MP must have access to the Agent Specific Knowledge and must be tightly coupled with it in order to activate the appropriate procedures required to accomplish the task implied by the incoming message contents. Its internal implementation is structured as shown in Figure 4. Basically, for each agent a set of specialized handler functions has been written, one for each performative referenced in the ATN representing possible transitions among conversation states. Those functions

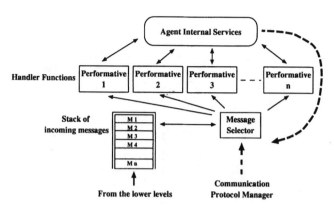

Figure 4. The computational architecture devised for implementing the Message Processor.

access the Agent Internal Services, represented by the topmost box in Figure 4, and must be written by fully exploiting the agent internal procedures.

Incoming messages are stored in a stack and picked up by the Message Selector (MS) in order to be dispatched to the appropriate handler function for their execution. The message selection policy enforced by MS may consist either in a very simple algorithm looking for the next available message, or may implement a more complex and adaptive logic. However, in the latter case also MS should be coupled with some of the agent internal functionality.

4 Representing Cooperation Knowledge Within Agents

A suitably designed ACL is essential for implementing a layered framework ensuring the independence from any particular agent type and from the platforms upon which the SAs themselves are built. However, the ability to interoperate with others and to exploit some kind of social behavior which must be exhibited by every SA cannot be enforced by the language alone. In fact, it is the SA Elaboration and Control Component as a whole which is responsible for deciding when a peer should be contacted and delegated the accomplishment of a given subtask or for devising the most appropriate strategy to be adopted while negotiating the terms for remotely executing that task.

According to the Jennings [1993] work in this area the agent delegating the accomplishment of a task is called the *manager* while the peer accepting to execute it is named the *contractor*. The whole process by which the contractor agent binds itself to the execution of the task is called *commitment*, in that the contractor becomes committed to executing the task on behalf of the manager. According to our view, SAs usually perform their problem solving activities following a task decomposition hierarchy, and they go on this way until they realize they are unable to cope with any given subtask. This may be caused either by the lack of knowledge and skills or by a shortage in the resources to be consumed for executing the task, in which case the agent tries to identify a possible contractor willing to solve that subtask on its behalf. It is important to point out that in a real scenario the contractor is dynamically selected by the manager at run time, possibly out of a set of several potential ones. Nevertheless, what makes an agent a potential contractor only depends on the organizational model

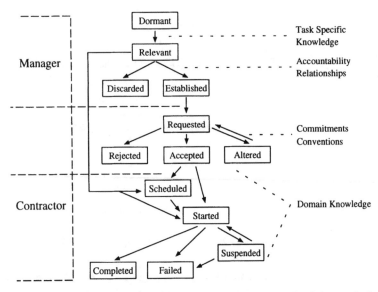

Figure 5. The network representing all the possible task states. In the right part the knowledge types responsible for the transitions are shown, while in the left side the agent role is marked.

adopted within the domain and is therefore known in advance. So, for every agent within a community there is a set of universally known relationships, called the *accountability* relationships, making explicit what tasks it is supposed to solve on behalf of which agents and what other tasks it may expect to delegate to others.

Whenever a manager selects a contractor for a given task it negotiates with it the terms for executing that task. However, in a dynamic environment the terms which have been negotiated are bound to change, which brings about the need of setting up some *conventions*, that is rules specifying when and how an agent plan should be reexamined.

Finally, to make explicit all the task states and knowledge chunks responsible for the transitions among those, we sketched the diagram shown in Figure 5 which has been adapted from Herbert's work [1994]. Within each agent the most part of the tasks are in the *dormant* state and are activated, that is made *relevant*, by the SA Task Specific Knowledge. Whenever an agent is able to accomplish a task and has the required resources, then that task is executed locally. Otherwise the agent becomes a manager and accountability relationships will be checked to find out contractors for the task which becomes *established*. *Request*ing the task marks the transition from the manager to the contractor, and commitments and conventions are responsible for negotiating the terms and conditions for its execution. Once the task becomes *accepted* it is the responsibility of the contractor Task Specific Knowledge to fulfill its execution.

In summary, enforcing cooperation among SAs and implementing the prototipical scenario described in the next section required modeling three different kinds of knowledge. First we had to make available to the whole agent community the accountability relationships which have been modeled as ternary relationships whose terms are the manager, the contractor and the task name. To this aim its instances have been represented as a set of triples collected in a globally accessible table.

Modeling Task Specific Knowledge, that is the one enabling every agent to solve the set of tasks for which it is planned, has been the easiest part of the game. As previously mentioned this is accomplished by means of a task decomposition hierarchy, and according to our past experience in building architectures for problem-solving, we had already developed a framework based on the metarule formalism for controlling task activation [Lanzola and Stefanelli, 1993]. A task decomposition approach is also useful in laying down the framework for enforcing cooperation among agents, since it makes explicit how the problem solving process of an agent develops and at which level an external support may be sought. Therefore, given the requirement of a smooth integration with the already existing framework implementing Task Specific Knowledge we decided to represent also Cooperation Knowledge by means of metarules. This required extending the set of the already available operators in order to support the new semantics. As a simple example of a cooperation rule let's consider the following one on the assumption that a peer agent (AGENT) is asking for the accomplishment of a given task (?TASK).

```
IF      ?TASK is requested by ?PEER
        AGENT is accountable to ?PEER for ?TASK
        ?TASK requires ?RESOURCE
        ?RESOURCE is available
THEN    AGENT commits to ?TASK for ?PEER
```

The rule is fired by the AGENT handler function implementing the *tell* performative whenever the contents of an incoming message include a request to accomplish a task. The first clause instantiates the two referenced variables with the true names as they appear in the message received, while the second one, based on the operator *is accountable*, checks if the receiving agent is actually accountable for executing ?TASK by accessing the global tables publishing those relationships. The third clause instantiates ?RESOURCE with any resource required for accomplishing the requested task as it emerges from the agent internal knowledge. Finally, if the required resources are available the THEN part is triggered causing the AGENT to become committed to ?TASK for ?PEER. The *commits* operator actually implements two different actions. It first schedules the execution of ?TASK by activating the metarule set, within the AGENT task decomposition tree, corresponding to the requested task. As a second effect however it causes CPM to send an acknowledgement message to the ?PEER, notifying it that the requested task has been accepted.

5 The Prototype Implemented

Given our experience in managing patients affected by Acute Myeloid Leukemia (AML) and the high number of professionals involved who contribute with different knowledgeable supports and personal skills to diagnosing and treating those patients we decided to focus on this specialty for implementing the prototype. The diagram shown in Figure 6 illustrates all the activities involved, and has been split into five horizontal slices corresponding to different interoperability scenarios ranging from the initial assessment of the symptoms reported to the General Practitioner, to the crucial phases

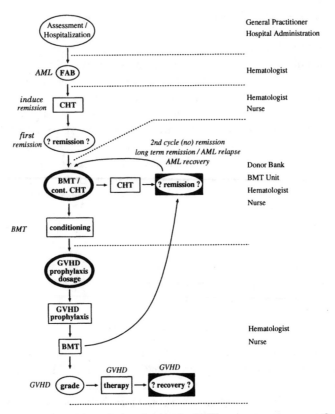

Figure 6. The diagram of the tasks involved in the AML management process. Ovals represent decision steps and fall into two different types. Thin ovals refer to diagnostic actions, while thick ones represent therapy planning actions useful for selecting the most appropriate treatment based on the patient data and the actual diagnosis. Rectangles refer to therapeutic actions, while the oval encapsulated in a black rectangle represents a monitoring action. The diagram has been partitioned into five horizontal slices corresponding to different interoperability scenarios according to the main actors involved, indicated in the right part.

of the AML therapy. For each slice the left side of the diagram shows the task sequence while on the right side the professionals taking part in that scenario are indicated.

Our effort is focusing on the implementation of several SAs, each one tailored to meet the specific needs of a different health care professional and enforcing his/her cooperation with other ones. We started modeling the last two slices of the diagram which concern the planning/administering of the main AML therapy and the monitoring/treatment for Graft Versus Host Disease (GVHD) which may ensue as a consequence of the Bone Marrow Transplantation (BMT) since they involve the highest number of professionals. In the rest of this section we shall provide a short description of the functionality of each agent as well as how it interoperates with others.

The *Ontology Server* (OS) encapsulates a representation of the domain structure concerning diseases and treatments related with AML management using the frame as the primary knowledge representation formalism. Entities are organized into a taxonomy of frames whose slots represent their features thereby giving rise to a huge semantic network [Lanzola et al., 1996]. Each disease has pointers to information concerning supportive and unsupportive findings, treatments, its typical evolution, and how it relates to AML whose management represents the high-level goal of our agent community. OS is therefore accessed by any other agent and provides the common semantics for exchanging and interpreting information and knowledge.

Different physician agents have been implemented, matching the different skills usually available with the humans involved in AML management. The *Hematologist* (HT) is responsible for assessing the patient state after administering an initial Chemoterapy (CHT) cycle, identified as LAM-87-M, which is meant to prepare him for the subsequent main therapy. That agent will be notified by the *Nurse Agent* (NA) reponsible for overseeing the fulfillment of the treatment plans when the LAM-87-M cycle comes to an end. From a computational point of view HT receives a message from NA, based on the *tell* performative, advertising it that the task LAM-87-M-CYCLE has been successfully completed for that patient, as indicated below:

```
(TELL:  :sender      NURSE
        :receiver    HEMATOLOGIST
        :content     (TASK-STATUS-CHANGE
                        :name        LAM-87-M-CYCLE
                        :patient     <patient id>
                        :new-state   COMPLETED))
```

According to its Task Specific Knowledge, HT will start planning the main therapy, and accessing the data available on the patient record it will be able to select between BMT or a different CHT. It is interesting to analyze the BMT selection, as in that case the therapy planning process cannot be carried out by HT alone, but relies on the cooperation with other agents and also includes a negotiation step. First HT will send a message to the *BMT Unit Agent* (BMTU), which is reponsible for performing BMT given the accountability rules, asking whether it accepts to execute that task.

BMTU must contact the *Donor Bank Agent* (BK) asking for all the available donors matching the required features. Upon receipt of the reply, and depending on the features of the donors found, BMTU will rank the suitability of performing BMT. Moreover, if BK has no suitable donors or fails to provide an answer within a given time limit BMTU adopts a proactive behavior and assumes that performing BMT cannot be fulfilled.

HT will receive the reply from BMTU indicating whether the task may be executed and upon which conditions, expressed in terms of treatment suitability. Of course this implies that both HT and BMTU make use of the same paradigm for expressing a treatment suitability. In our prototype we adopt a qualitative score signifying the probability of success which is ranked according to a small set of domain specific rules. Thus HT draws its conclusions and decides whether to delegate its actual accomplishment to BMTU or proceed instead with the CHT.

If BMT is performed the patient is likely to develop GVHD which must be prevented, monitored for its occurrence, and prompty treated at the outset. BMTU will therefore send a message to the *Database Agent* (DB), based on the *subscribe* performative, asking to be notified about any change concerning the GVHD state.

In our implementation DB is based on the classical relational model which makes use of tables and tuples. Its core has been implemented using a major commercial Relational DBMS to which an ACL speaking module has been linked. However DB has also been endowed with domain specific and task specific knowledge in order that whenever a request comes concerning some value not yet available, it will use the accountability relationships to identify which other agent is reponsible for collecting that observation. So, when BMTU subscribes to DB asking about GVHD state changes, DB will contact HT asking it to continuously look for a GVHD outset. Diagnosing GVHD relies on the values of several findings which include laboratory tests and clinical observations, and also depends on the results of simple diagnostic steps. Thus HT to fulfill that request will end up in asking DB to stay informed about those.

Finally this forces DB to contact other agents asking them to actually supply those data. In our implementation this step always ends up in rousing the NA which is the only one responsible for collecting data. However, the domain specific knowledge available within NA enables it to perform also some simple diagnostic steps, such as identifying if the patient is likely to be developing some infections. Besides storing the results of those inferences on DB, whenever NA detects an abnormal situation also sends out a message to the agent reponsible for treating it, as known by the accountability rules.

6 Conclusions

From the few available reports concerning the nature of human errors in health care settings it emerges that physicians make mistakes mainly because they are information overloaded and biased by their short term experience while making decisions. Nurses perform repetitive tasks and are prone to making mistakes whenever they accomplish a task similar to a standard one but with some slight deviations. Moreover most errors occurring in an ICU may be attributed to interoperation problems among health care professionals [Leape, 1994]. Hence there is an increasing demand for tools aimed at improving workflow management and planning, and increasing the cooperation among workers in the health care delivery process. However, although the rapid growth of Intra/InterNet based connectivity solutions has boosted work in the CSCW area causing the appearance of several commercial products, none of those may be considered as appropriate for medical applications, nor are they presently used in this area. On the whole we may observe that almost any tool has been implemented to solve a very specific task, so it implicitly encapsulates the task model to be adopted and doesn't provide any capability for customizing it.

To this aim a lot of research efforts are being spent in finding a more general and comprehensive approach to the problem, and a very interesting one has been proposed by Huang [Huang et al., 1995] which, stemming from Jennings work [Jennings, 1993], applies the multi agent paradigm to the delivery of health care services. In their approach an agent is seen as an entity including *domain specific*, *inferential* and *control knowledge*. However, that approach only sees an agent as an atomic entity able to accomplish some task and encapsulating all the required knowledge chunks. Therefore it's likely that enabling interoperability among two or more agents requires replicating part of that knowledge within all of them. Our approach on the contrary envisions the availability of some agents acting as servers [Lanzola et al., 1996] whose only goal is that of making available knowledge required for implementing other application agents. The issue may pushed up to the point that application agents might be regarded as personality modules which select the required knowledge chunks from the servers and only specify the strategy for applying it.

7 References

[Durfee et al., 1987] Durfee, E., Lesser, V. and Corkill, D. Coherent Cooperation Among Communicating Problem Solvers. *IEEE Transactions on Computers* 36(11):1275-1291, (1987).

[Falasconi et al., 1996] Falasconi, S., Lanzola, G. and Stefanelli, M. Using Ontologies in Multi-Agent Systems. *Proceedings of the KAW'96 Workshop* pp. 28-1/28-20, Banff (1996).

[Finin et al., 1994] Finin, T., Fritzson, R., McKay, D. and McEntire R. KQML as an Agent Communication Language. *Proceedings of the Third International Conference on Information and Knowledge Management*, ACM Press (1994).

[Gardner and Lundsgaarde, 1994] Gardner, R.M. and Lundsgaarde, H.P. Evaluation of User Acceptance of a Clinical Expert System. *Journal of the American Medical Informatics Association*, 1:42, 8-438, (1994).

[Heathfield and Wyatt, 1993] Heathfield, H. and Wyatt, J. Philosophies for the design and development of clinical decision support systems. *Methods of Information in Medicine*, 32:1-8, (1993).

[Herbert, 1994] Herbert, S. Informatics for Care Protocos and Guidelines: Towards a European Knowledge Model. In: *Health Telematics for Clinical Guidelines and Protocols* (Gordon, C. and Christensen, J.P. Eds.), IOS Press, (1994).

[Huang, 1995] Huang, J., Jennings, N.R. and Fox, J. An Agent-based Approach to Health Care Management. *Applied Artificial Intelligence: An International Journal*, Taylor & Francis London, 9 (4) (1995).

[Jennings, 1993] Jennings, N.R. Commitments and Conventions: The Foundation of Coordination in Multi-Agent Systems. *The Knowledge Engineering Review*, 8(3), 223-250, (1993).

[Jennings and Wooldridge, 1996] Jennings, N.R. and Wooldridge M.J. Software Agents. *IEEE Review*, January, 17-20, (1996).

[Lanzola and Stefanelli, 1993] Lanzola, G. and Stefanelli, M. Inferential Knowledge Acquisition. *Artificial Intelligence in Medicine*, 5, 253-268, (1993).

[Lanzola et al., 1996] Lanzola, G., Falasconi, S. and Stefanelli, M. Cooperating Agents Implementing Distributed Patient Management. *Proceedings of the MAAMAW-96 Conference*, LNAI 218-232, Springer-Verlag (1996).

[Leape, 1994] Leape, L.L. Error in Medicine. *Journal of the American Medical Association*, 272:23, 1851-1857 (1994).

[Ramoni et al., 1992] Ramoni, M., Stefanelli, M., Magnani, L. and Barosi, G. An Epistemological Framework for Medical Knowledge-Based Systems. *IEEE Transactions on Systems, Man, and Cybernetics*, 22(6):1361-1375 (1992).

[Shoham, 1993] Shoham, Y. Agent-Oriented Programming. *Artificial Intelligence* 60:139-159, (1993).

[van Bemmel, 1993] van Bemmel, J.H. Criteria for the acceptance of decision-support systems by clinicians; lessons from ECG interpretation system. *Proceedings of the AIME93 Conference*, pp. 7-10, (1993).

Adding Knowledge to Information Retrieval Systems in the World Wide Web

G. Mann, M. Schubert, V. Schaeffler

GSF - National Research Center for Environment and Health,
Institute for Medical Informatics and Systems Research,
D-85764 Neuherberg, Germany

Abstract: Common systems used to provide medical information on the World Wide Web have several shortcomings related to the quality of information retrieval and the maintenance of contents. In this paper a model of a knowledge-based information system is presented. The model provides a formalism for an explicit representation of domain knowledge. This domain knowledge is used to increase precision and recall of retrieval and for consistency checks. Additional knowledge concerning user types enables the system to generate user dependant views on information. Based on the model an architecture for a knowledge-based information system is described. A prototype is developed in the domain of ophthalmology.

1 Introduction

The importance of the World Wide Web (WWW) as a source of information in medicine is growing fast (cf. e.g. [Zelingher 1996]). For nearly all medical topics information is available. Compared to conventional media, such as books or journals, delivering information via the WWW is fast, and virtually no limitations exist regarding the amount of information that can be provided. Immediate update of information is possible, and the use of multimedia representation of information is supported. Basically, we can distinguish three approaches how information is provided. Type 1: In the majority of WWW-systems chunks of texts, images, video-sequences, and other multimedia information are clustered in pages and connected by 'hyperlinks'. In addition such 'hypermedia-systems' support search functions using key-words. In the WWW this type of information systems is mostly based on the 'Hypertext Mark-Up Language' (HTML) (cp. [Goldfarb 1990]) and search mechanisms. Type 2: Systems of this type store information in databases. Often the information is indexed by terms of a vocabulary (see [Cimino 1996] or [Okada, Yamashita, and Takahashi 1995]). Via HTML-based front-ends queries can be defined which usually contain key-words, i.e. terms of the vocabulary, and optional Boolean operators. These queries are processed by a server. Results are sent back to the user as HTML-pages.

Both types of systems have several shortcomings (cf. [Halasz 1988]). One set of problems is related to the quality of information retrieval, which is indicated by precision and recall. Precision is defined as the ratio of relevant information retrieved and the total amount of retrieved information. Recall is the ratio of relevant information retrieved and the total amount of information that is relevant. Using information retrieval by navigation in the information space only within smaller systems, good precision and recall can be achieved. Navigation also becomes very time consuming in larger domains. Navigation without appropriate guides is associated with the 'lost in hyperspace' phenomenon (for details cf. [Frisse, and Cousins 1990]). Information that is provided in systems of type 1 is either rather general, which reduces precision, or it is highly specialised. Specialised information systems either become confusing due to the size of the information space or, in case of smaller information spaces, the applicability is limited. Furthermore, he lack of formal structures for the representation of information is the cause of problems related to the maintenance of information. The use of information in different contexts leads to redundant representation in order to avoid fragmentation of information that would force users to collect small chunks of information via hyperlinks. Both, redundancy and fragmentation, create problems concerning the coherence and the consistency of information. Systems of type 2 can solve several problems linked to systems of type 1. Precision and recall can be improved by indexing information using controlled vocabularies. However, the expressive power of indexing and simple retrieval languages is limited. These limitations increase the granularity of information, which itself may lead to an increased redundancy.

The problems mentioned above can be solved by an explicit representation of knowledge of the corresponding domain and its use for retrieval (type 3). In the following a model is described that makes use of domain knowledge for information retrieval and information presentation. The architecture of a knowledge-based information system for the WWW, that is derived from the model, is presented.

2 Model

In the following the model, its properties, and implications related to authoring and maintenance are described. Especially five properties are essential for knowledge-based information systems:

1. Information systems should support not only the retrieval of rather general information about a medical subject, but also support the retrieval of highly specific information. For all queries retrieved information must be precise, and the recall must be high.
2. The information retrieval should be done automatically, but give the user the freedom to explore the information space.
3. The presentation of information must be flexible and support the needs of different types of users.
4. The representation of information about medical concepts must be uniform and restricted to one locus.
5. The maintenance of integrity and coherence must be supported.

2.1 Domain Model

Core of the knowledge-based information system is a model of the medical domain. For each domain specific models can be constructed. Some aspects of medical ontologies are rather general and can be used in different domains. To illustrate the functions of domain models and to explain, how domain models are constructed, we use a simplified example not related to a specific medical domain (see Fig. 1). The model contains concepts of the domain and relations among these concepts. In our example we want to store information about diagnosis, findings, therapies, follow-up, and diagnostic procedures. All concepts can be linked to terms of a controlled vocabulary.

An object oriented model is used for the description of domain models (for details cf. [Mann, Wormek, et al. 1996]). Object types provide generic structures for the description of properties of objects that represent medical concepts. Properties may be described by text, tables, images, sound, etc. Three different types of relations among objects are part of the model. We distinguish property relations, association relations, and complex relations (cf. Fig. 1). Property relations link two objects where an object A represents the description of properties of a second object B. The existence of object A depends on the existence of object B. An object of the type AETIOLOGY, for example, that is in a property relation with an object of the type DIAGNOSIS represents details about the aetiology of a specific diagnosis. Association relations are used for objects whose existence does not depend on each other. An example is the relation between an object B of the type diagnosis and an object C of the type ICD-10 whereby the latter contains the ICD-10 code for the diagnosis. The ICD-10 code can exist separately without a corresponding object of the type DIAGNOSIS. Complex relations are similar to association relations. The main difference is that the validity of complex relations can be restricted. Using properties of domain objects, conditions or 'medical contexts' are described. Only within a specific context a relation is valid. The representation of conditions for complex relations is based on propositional logic. It is

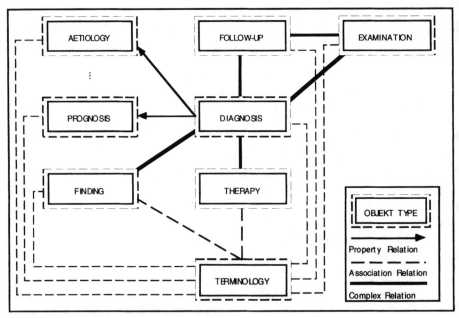

Fig. 1. A simplified domain model.

a three valued logic with the values *true, false,* and *unknown.* The truth tables are defined according to (cf. [Rosser, and Turquette 1952]). If a logic expression is evaluated to *true* or *unknown,* it is assumed, that the corresponding complex relation is valid for a given context. In case the result of an evaluation is *false,* the relation is invalid within the context (for details cf. chapter 2.2 and 2.4). For example the relation between an object *B* of the type DIAGNOSIS and an object *D* of the type THERAPY may only be valid for patients that have the diagnosis *B* and not the diagnosis *C* and not the finding *E.* In this example the complex relation defines contraindications for therapy *D.*

All information in the domain model that is relevant for accessing information is based on a standard terminology. That is the names of objects and the properties which are used to define conditions for complex relations refer to objects of the type TERMINOLOGY.

2.2 Retrieval Model

The retrieval model contains information that is necessary to process queries. Part of the retrieval model are query types. By selecting a query type a user defines a specific view on a domain model. Views are subsets of domain models which are described by 'retrieval trees' (cf. Fig. 2). Nodes of a retrieval tree are object types of a domain model

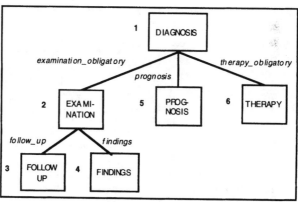

Fig. 2. Example of a retrieval tree for retrieval of diagnostic information.

with the corresponding sets of objects. Arcs of a retrieval tree are relations among objects. Root of a retrieval tree is always an object type that is in the focus of a query. Using relations of the domain model, other object types can be linked to the root of a retrieval tree. The example of a retrieval tree in Fig. 2 shows a query type that can be used to retrieve diagnostic information and additional information about examinations, prognosis, therapies, follow up, and findings that is related to retrieved diagnoses (cf. chapter 2.4).

With the selection of a query type a user also selects a template that is linked to the query type. Templates are the interfaces used to specify a query. A template consists of three parts:

1. A user type must be specified. Examples are 'diabetologist', 'ophthalmologist', 'optometrist', or 'patient'.
2. As explained, the selected query type corresponds with a retrieval tree and an object type that is the root of the retrieval tree. A user has to choose one or more objects out of the set of objects that belong to this object type. Referring

to our example (Fig. 2), a user has to define for which diagnoses information should be retrieved.

3. Part of a retrieval tree are complex relations that link object types. For each relation sets of properties are defined in the domain model, that are used to describe the conditions under which a complex relation is valid or not valid. These properties are presented to a user. If a user has information about a property, he can enter this information.

2.3 Layout Model

The layout model consists of a set of layout schemata, describing how information is presented to the user. Selection of a layout schema depends on the query type and the user type. Layout schemata consist of two sub-models. The first defines a projection on properties of retrieved objects. The resulting properties will be presented to the user. The second model defines

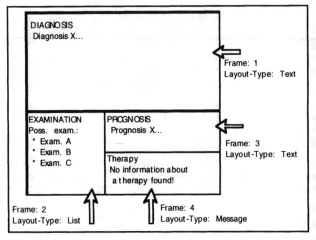

Fig. 3. Example of a layout.

structures that are used for presentation. Based on HTML-frames and sub-frames skeletons for HTML-pages are described. Each skeleton contains additional layout information as font size, colour, etc. All properties that will be presented to users are assigned to sub-frames (cf. Fig. 3). Now all information is available to fill the skeletons with retrieved information.

2.4 Task Model

Information retrieval can be described as a task that is divided into three subtasks: analysis task, execution task, and layout task.

- Retrieval starts with the analysis task. As explained in chapter 2.2 a user has to select a query type to perform a query. The query type is used to select a query type and a template. Using the template a user specifies the query. Information about the user type, objects he or she wants to retrieve and context information is entered (cf. Fig. 2, Fig. 4).

- The execution task identifies the object type which is the root of the retrieval tree. Out of the set of objects belonging to this type all objects are picked that are entered by the user (cf. point 2 in chapter 2.2). For these objects all complex relations that are part of the retrieval tree are identified. Using the context information provided by users it can be evaluated whether a complex relation is valid or not. As explained above a complex relation is only invalid when the condition evaluates to false. In case of missing context information it is assumed that the relation is valid. If the relation is valid, the path defined by the relation will be traversed, and following objects belong to the set of retrieved objects. This process is iterative and continued until the whole retrieval tree is traversed.

- The layout task uses knowledge from the layout model and the user type to perform a projection on properties of objects that have been retrieved. Based on knowledge represented in the layout model these properties are used to compose HTML-pages. Links (i.e. relations) that are present in the domain model, but are not part of a retrieval tree

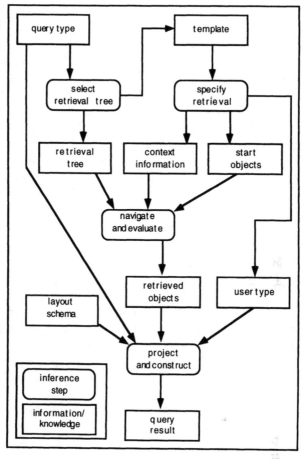

Fig. 4. Inference structure.

are presented in the HTML-pages. This enables users to start subsequent queries.

Provided the information in the domain model is valid and consistent, the retrieval process can guarantee, that only relevant and consistent information is retrieved.

2.5 Authoring and Maintenance

Authoring and maintenance of information depends on the formalisms that are used for the representation of information. The use of hypertext oriented representations is very similar to conventional linear texts. For medical authors hypertext oriented editors can be provided, which can be used like conventional text editors. Therefore, information that is already available in books or journals can easily be converted and used in WWW-based information systems. The disadvantage is, that no mechanism can be provided to check integrity and coherency of information.

Information systems based on formal models of the domain are more restrictive. The author has to use pre-defined schemata to represent medical information. On the one hand the freedom of authors is restricted, on the other hand formal structures provide information that can be used for checks (cf. [Musen, Fagan, et al. 1987]). For example, with a schema that defines properties of a diagnosis it can easily be checked, whether an author has omitted information about a diagnosis. By using formal domain models a separate representation of different properties of a medical concept does not lead to negative aspects of fragmentation of information, since all information is located within one object. As known from database systems, referential integrity can be controlled. Together with information that is not longer valid, e.g. a drug that is not longer available, all references to this information can be removed automatically. Knowing the relations of an object (i.e. a medical concept) to other objects, the system can provide the author a view on the information. The view includes the concept the author is dealing with and the complete set of related concepts. Association relations among objects of the domain model and objects that represent a standardised vocabulary can be used to retrieve objects.

3 Architecture

For the realisation of a knowledge-based information system for the WWW the authors have developed a client server architecture (cf. Fig. 5). The system's user-front-end is a frame-capable WWW browser (not presented in Fig. 5). This browser has access to a WWW server and is linked via a 'Common Gateway Interface' (CGI) to a client system. The client system receives all information related to a query and starts a session. Within a session, which may include several queries, the client uses the medical context defined in the first query of a session. A session is finished, when the user either quits the communication or defines a new context. The client provides all functions necessary to perform the inference steps that have been specified in the task model. Inference steps are either queries (e.g. selection of a retrieval tree), processing of retrieved data (e.g. identification of the start object in a retrieval tree) or a combination of both (e.g. navigation in the object space and evaluation of complex relations). Information and knowledge necessary for the execution of tasks is either part of a query or stored in a multimedia database.

The knowledge is organised in three different databases. The database for retrieval knowledge represents a mapping of query types on retrieval trees and templates. The database for domain knowledge contains the objects of the medical domain and their relations. Layout schemata are stored in the database for layout knowledge. An additional database stores information about users and their accounts. For realisation the database system 'MATISSE' was selected. Within the client system inference steps and additional control knowledge are encoded in C++. Communication with the database is via an application programming interface (API) supporting retrieval functions which are either based on a navigation language that is specific for MATISSE or on SQL. Another part of the API are functions that are used in the inference step 'project and construct' for the composition of HTML-pages.

An information server consists of a set of client systems that can perform requests for information of several users in parallel. MATISSE has an excellent performance when handling huge amounts of multimedia objects. Only the WWW browser has to be installed on the user's computer. All other components of the knowledge-based information system can be installed on a central server. MATISSE supports distributed data management.

Not presented in Fig. 5 are components of the authoring system. It enables authors to build and maintain the contents of the information system. Based on the client API editors are implemented to add, delete or change objects. To adopt the knowledge-based information system to other domains, the schema (e.g. the description of object types and relations) of the domain model has to be changed. Consecutively, the authors must change the description of query types, retrieval trees, etc. This process will be supported by the authoring system. A meta model (not presented in this paper) describes the dependencies of the schema of the domain model on the one hand and the contents of the retrieval model and the layout model on the other hand.

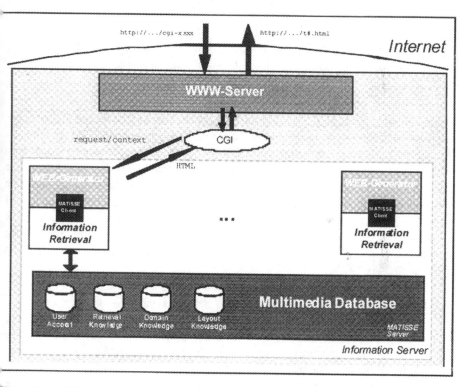

Fig. 5. Architecture of the knowledge-based information system.

4 Discussion

Everybody who uses the WWW as a source of medical information realises the need of improved retrieval mechanisms. Correlated with the increasing amount of information provided by the WWW the precision of retrieval is decreasing and the user has no information about the recall. Meanwhile, several initiatives exist to solve these problems. Some focus on the development of information broker services that collect and provide medical information. This can only be a temporary solution. Since they use the same techniques as presently used on the WWW, these services will face the same problems as the information increases. Developing improved search engines for the WWW is no solution, either. Using 'intelligent' information retrieval mechanisms requires an explicit representation of domain knowledge and the information that has to be retrieved. Otherwise retrieval is restricted to pattern matching on a syntactic level.

The model presented by this paper is based on a representation which makes aspects of the knowledge explicit. Access to information is improved by using a controlled vocabulary. Depending on the quality of the vocabulary, the recall of information can be controlled. The use of context information and corresponding knowledge represented in complex relations supports high precision of retrieved information. Still most information contained in knowledge-based information systems is represented as text, image or an other format. This information can not be used for an improved retrieval. However, the authors believe that a threshold exists where the additional effort for an explicit representation of knowledge exceeds the benefit that can be achieved. The convenience of automatic information retrieval and its restrictions does not tie the user. He/she can still navigate in the object space by following relations in the domain model.

In 1992 Cimino et al. (cf. [Cimino, Elkin, and Barnett 1992]) described a different approach to solve the problems connected to hypertext representation. The information space is split into a concept space and a text space. In the text space sections of text are hierarchically linked. These sections replicate traditional structures of medical text books. Elements of text sections are linked to nodes of the concept space. The concept space is a semantic network of concepts and links among concepts. The concept space has the function of a guide. Although the addition of a concept space to hypertext can solve the problem of disorientation in hyperspace it has some limitations. Only simple query mechanisms exist, and no context information can be used for information retrieval.

Another solution is proposed by Fikes and co-workers. They propose a computer-based information broker providing access to heterogeneous information sources (cf. [Fikes, Farquhar, and Pratt 1996]). Knowledge of the domain and the terminology used by information sources is part of the information broker system. The broker system provides a single interface to define queries. By using knowledge of information sources these queries can be transformed into queries of the source system. A limitation of usage in medicine is caused by the fact that representation of most medical information is not based on a standard terminology. Therefore, a computer-based information broker struggles with all the problems related to medical language processing like the existence of synonyms, homonyms, and the vagueness of medical terms. However, this approach can easily be applied to information systems that already support structured representation of information and the use of a standardised terminology. Therefore, it should be possible to link a knowledge-based information system as proposed in this paper to a computer-based information broker.

Knowledge-based information systems require a radical change of the authoring process compared to text books or representations based on hypertext. Information about medical concepts has to be precisely located. It must be contained within one object or a small set of objects. On the other hand there is no possibility to represent 'isolated' information. Chunks of information are accessed via relations of the corresponding medical concept to other medical concepts. Therefore, all information that can be accessed by traversing a path in the object space must be consistent and coherent. However, this problem can only partly be solved by authors and editors. The inconsistency and incoherence of medical knowledge itself will remain. Until now, the model has no features to deal with this issue.

Within the project 'Telematics in Ophthalmology' (OPHTEL) a knowledge-based information system is developed that is based on the approach presented in this paper. The information system will provide information to ophthalmologists, diabetologists, and patients. A prototype of the system is released in spring 1997. It contains reference information for the classification of fundus images. Other modules related to diabetic retinopathy and glaucoma will follow.

Acknowledgement: The work has been carried out in the framework of the OPHTEL-project. OPHTEL is part of the Telematics Application Programme and funded by the European Union under ref. HC 1036. The authors want to thank C. Birkmann for the comments on the English language.

Literature

Cimino, J.J. (1996): Linking Patient Information Systems to Bibliographic Resources. *Methods of Information in Medicine* **35**, 122-126.

Cimino, J.J., Elkin, P.L., Barnett, G.O. (1992): As We May Think: The Concept Space and Medical Hypertext. *Computer and Biomedical Research* **25**, 238-263.

Fikes, R., Farquhar, A., Pratt, W. (1996): Information Brokers: Gathering Information from Heterogeneous Information Sources. In: Stewman, J.H. (ed.) *Proceedings of the Ninth Florida Artificial Intelligence Symposium (FLAIRS '96)*, Key West, Florida.

Frisse, M.E., Cousins, S.B. (1990): Guides for hypertext: an overview. *Artificial Intelligence in Medicine* **2**, 303-314.

Goldfarb, C.F. (1990): *The SGML Handbook*. Clarendon Press: Oxford.

Halasz, F. (1988): Reflections on notecards: Seven issues for the next generation of hypermedia systems. *Communications of the ACM* **31** (7), 836-852.

Mann, G., Wormek, A., Satomura, Y., Suzuki, T., Takabayashi, K., Yamazaki, S., Kraut, U. (1996): An Object Oriented Method for the Development of Knowledge-Based Systems in Medicine. In: Lee, J.K., Liebowitz, J., Chae , M.Y. (ed.) *Proceedings of The Third World Congress on Expert Systems, Seoul 1996*, **234-243**. Cognizant Communication Corporation: New York.

Musen, M.A., Fagan, L.M., Combs, D.M., Shortliffe, E.H. (1987): Use of a domain model to drive an interactive knowledge-editing tool. *International Journal Man-Machine Studies* **26**, 105-121.

Okada, Y., Yamashita, Y., Takahashi, T. (1995): Multimedia search system for a textbook of urology in Japanese. *Medical Infomatics* **20** (4), 343-348.

Rosser, J.N., Turquette, A. (1952): *Many Valued Logic*. North Holland: Amsterdam.

Zelingher, J. (1996): Preventive Medicine Recommendations on the Internet. *M.D. Computing* **13** (3), 204-206.

Learning from Data Through the Integration of Qualitative Models and Fuzzy Systems

R. Bellazzi[1], L. Ironi[2], R. Guglielmann[2], M. Stefanelli[1]

[1] Dipartimento di Informatica e Sistemistica - Università di Pavia, Pavia, Italy
[2] Istituto di Analisi Numerica - C.N.R., Pavia, Italy

Abstract. This paper presents a method for the identification of the dynamics of non-linear patho-physiological systems by learning from data. The key idea which underlies our approach consists in the integration of qualitative modeling methods with fuzzy logic systems. The major advantage which derives from such an integrated framework lies in its capability both to represent the structural knowledge of the system at study and to exploit the available experimental data, so that a functional approximation of the system dynamics can be determined and used as a reasonable predictor of the patient's future state. As testing ground of our method, we have considered the problem of identifying the response to the insulin therapy from insulin-dependent diabetic patients: the results obtained are presented and discussed in the paper.

1 Introduction

The prediction of the evolution over time of the patient's state plays a crucial role both in a diagnostic and therapeutic medical context. A traditional approach to such a problem deals with both the formulation of mathematical models of the dynamics of patho-physiological systems and the simulation of their behaviour [2]. Such models, which are generally described by Ordinary Differential Equations (ODE), are computationally tractable with classical methods which allow us to derive, either analitically or numerically, meaningful predictions of the behaviour of the considered system. But, for the medical domain, quantitative model formulation may be not successfully applicable due to the incompleteness of the available knowledge about either the functional relationships between variables or the numerical values of model parameters, which could be not identifiable both for the lack of adequate experimental settings and for the impossibility of measuring "in vivo" the values of a few variables. Approaches recently proposed to cope with difficulties in model building are represented by qualitative modeling methods [6]. Such methods allow us to describe the dynamics of a system through Qualitative Differential Equations (QDE), where functional relationships and numeric values are respectively defined in terms of regions of monotonicity and of their ordinal relations with landmark values. Given a set of QDEs which model a dynamical system and an initial state, qualitative descriptions of the behaviours of the system are derived through qualitative simulation.

Whereas qualitative predictions of a patho-physiological system behaviour may be properly exploited in the testing phase of diagnostic reasoning [3], they are almost always inadequate to be used in a therapy planning context as the effects of different therapies are required to be quantitatively investigated.

As alternative to conventional mathematical modeling, the so-called non-parametric approaches, that are able to describe the dynamics of a real system from input-output data, have been proposed. Neural networks, multi-variate splines and fuzzy logic systems are the most known approximation schemes used for learning an input-output relation from data [4, 5, 9]. Although these approaches are successfully applied in a variety of domains, they are affected by two main drawbacks: first, the identification result does not exploit any structural knowledge; second, the model identification usually requires a large amount of data and is often extremely inefficient.

This paper describes a method which integrates both mathematical and non-parametric modeling frameworks. Our goal deals with the definition of a robust and efficient method for non-linear dynamic system identification, which exploits both the available a priori knowledge, namely the structural and human expert, and the experimental one. Among the non-parametric approaches, fuzzy logic systems seem to be the most suitable ones as they are capable of conjugating experimental data analysis and prior knowledge representation through a rule-base predefined by the human expert. When such a base is not available or poorly defined the fuzzy inference is extremely inefficient. Our method aims at solving the problem of the construction of a meaningful rule-base: Fuzzy Rules (FR) are automatically generated by encoding the knowledge of the system dynamics captured by its structural knowledge represented by qualitative models. As qualitative modeling formalism we have chosen QSIM because of both its expressive power to represent differential equations in case of incomplete knowledge and its reasonable predictive capacity. The basic steps of our method may be hence summarized as follows:

- formulation and simulation of a qualitative model of the system at study;
- automatic generation of the set of FRs from the outcomes of the simulation;
- generation of the Fuzzy System (FS) which correspond to the FRs;
- parameter estimation of the FS from a set of experimental data.

We have applied our method to the identification of the dynamics of the Blood Glucose metabolism in insulin dependent diabetic patients. In particular, we faced the problem of predicting the Blood Glucose Level (BGL) time course in response to different exogenous perturbations, such as meals and conventional insulin therapies. In such a clinical context the experimental data usually come from the home-monitoring of patients: their low-quality and the high complexity of the system motivate the use of the approach we have implemented.

2 Background

This section recalls the basic concepts and definitions of both QSIM [6] and fuzzy systems [9] which are relevant to a clear and formal description of our method.

2.1 Basic concepts of QSIM

The central inference within QSIM is qualitative simulation: given a set of QDEs which model a system and an initial state, a qualitative description of all of its possible behaviours (QBs) is provided. A *system* S is modeled by a set $\{x_i\}_{i=1}^{m}$ of state *variables*, real-valued continously differentiable functions of time, and a set of *constraints* that relate them.

The qualitative magnitude of each $x_i(t)$ is defined with respect to a finite ordered set $L_i := \{l_j\}_{j=1}^{k}$, called *quantity space*, whose elements l_j are landmark values that represent real qualitative distinctions for the behaviour of $x_i(t)$. Each set L_i is associated with the set of distinguished time-points T_i, which represents the set of instants where x_i takes on a landmark value.

Definition 1. The qualitative magnitude of $x_i(t)$, $qmag(x_i, t)$, is defined by either a landmark value or an open interval between two landmarks:

$$qmag(x_i, t) := \begin{cases} l_j & \text{if } x_i(t) = l_j \\ (l_j, l_{j+1}) & \text{if } x_i(t) \in (l_j, l_{j+1}) \end{cases}$$

Definition 2. The direction of change of $x_i(t)$, $qdir(x_i, t)$, is the sign of its time derivative and can be either decreasing, steady or increasing, i.e. $qdir \in \{-, 0, +\}$.

Definition 3. The qualitative value of $x_i(t)$, $QV(x_i, t)$, is defined by the pair $< qmag, qdir >$.

Definition 4. The qualitative state of S at time t, $QS(S, t)$, is the set of the qualitative values at time t of all the system's variables, which are consistent with the constraints.

Definition 5. A qualitative behaviour QB of S over the time set $T = \cup_i^m T_i = [t_0, t_n]$ is defined by the sequence:

$$QB = \{QS(S, t_0), QS(S, t_0, t_1), QS(S, t_1), ..., QS(S, t_{n-1}, t_n), QS(S, t_n)\},$$

where $QS(S, t_{n-1}, t_n)$ is the qualitative state of S at (t_{n-1}, t_n).

The QSIM constraint notation has a clear correspondence with ODEs by making explicit all the functions and operators in the equation. Therefore, constraints which express arithmetic and time derivative operators are defined. The functional relationships between variables are not explicitly specified but just described in terms of monotonicity regions. For example, the M^-/M^+ constraints express a relation of strict decreasing and increasing monotonicity, respectively; whereas the S^-/S^+ constraints describe functions which are monotonic decreasing/increasing over an interval and take constant values outside that interval.

2.2 Basic concepts of Fuzzy Systems

A Fuzzy System (FS) is a system which exploits fuzzy concepts for reasoning about a set of objects. Despite the theory on fuzzy sets is quite complex, for the purposes of this paper we will define FS through some simple ingredients.

The *Universe of discourse* (U) is the collection of objects that we would like to reason about.

A *Fuzzy set* F in U is a generalization of the concept of ordinary set. F is characterized by a membership function $\mu_F : U \to [0, 1]$; $\mu_F(u)$ represents the degree of membership of $u \in U$ to the set F.

A *linguistic variable* is a variable whose values are words in natural language, and that can be represented through a collection of fuzzy sets. For example, the continuous variable Blood Glucose Level (BGL) may be described with the linguistic terms Low, Normal, High, Very High. Each value of its universe of discourse may be hence assigned a degree of membership to the fuzzy set which corresponds to such linguistic terms.

A *Fuzzy Rule Base* (FRB) is the knowledge base that we use to reason about the objects in U. In particular, a FRB is a collection of rules of the kind:

IF x_1 is F_1 and ... and x_n is F_n THEN y is G

where $F_1, \ldots, F_n$ and G are fuzzy sets and $x_1, \ldots, x_n$ and y are linguistic variables. For example, if we want to express a rule that forecasts the linguistic value of the linguistic variable BGL, using the linguistic level of the (linguistic) variable *insulin*, we may write:

IF *insulin* is High THEN BGL is Low

As the goal of this paper is the approximation of continuous functions from $\Re^n \to \Re$, we make inferences on the values of an output variable y defined on $V \in \Re$ using a FRB with n input variables defined on $U_i \in \Re$, such that $U = U_1 \times \ldots \times U_n$. This means that each continuous variable must be properly *fuzzified*. The *fuzzification* operation performs a mapping from $x_i \in U_i$ into a fuzzy set. In this paper we will exploit the *singleton fuzzifier*, that transforms a real number $x_i \in U_i$ into a fuzzy set with membership function defined over U_i, such that it is equal to 1 in x_i and to 0 elsewhere. Given a quantitative measure of the inputs, this measure is fuzzified, and it is considered as an input of all the rules in the FRB.

In order to perform inferences, it is necessary to resort to a machinery that gives a precise interpretation of the terms is, and and THEN that appears in a fuzzy rule. For our purposes, it is sufficient to say that it is possible to select a *Fuzzy Inference Engine* (FIE), in which the fuzzy logic principles are used to map fuzzy sets in U into fuzzy sets in V. In particular, we chose FIE such that, given an input in U, we obtain a collection of M fuzzy sets as outputs, where M is the number of rules of the FRB. For the purpose of function approximation, we must transform into a real number the output of the application of FIE. This is done through the *defuzzification* operation. In this paper, we have chosen the *Center Average Defuzzifier* [9]. We will exploit a class of FS useful for function approximation. Such a class is derived by choosing properly the FIE as in [9], and taking all the membership functions as Gaussian. In that case the FS assumes a convenient mathematical form:

$$f(\mathbf{x}) = \frac{\sum_{j=1}^{M} \hat{y}_j [\prod_{i=1}^{n} exp(-(\frac{x_i - \hat{x}_i^j}{\sigma_i^j})^2)]}{\sum_{j=1}^{M} [\prod_{i=1}^{n} exp(-(\frac{x_i - \hat{x}_i^j}{\sigma_i^j})^2)]} \tag{1}$$

with $\mathbf{x} = \{x_1, \ldots, x_n\}$. Such an expression allows us to interpret the non-linear function approximation problem with FS as the process of identifying a set of free parameters $(\hat{y}_j, \hat{x}_i, \sigma_i)$ of a known non-linear function from a set of data. Moreover, the FS (1) is known to possess some desirable properties, like the capability of approximating any continuous function with an arbitrary degree of accuracy [9]. Other useful properties can be found in [7, 9].

3 Description of the method

The method we propose is grounded on the exploitation of a correspondence between elements of QSIM and fuzzy formalisms, as singled out by Fig. 1.

At a first level, namely the modeling one, the quantity space L_i associated with x_i finds its correspondence with the universe of discourse U_i of x_i. The set L_i contains all the significant distinct qualitative magnitude values ($qmag$) of x_i; whereas the linguistic values which x_i can assume, i.e. the linguistic names of the membership functions μ which define the fuzzy sets, are associated with elements of U_i. For the sake of clearness, let us consider again as example the variable BGL. Its universe of discourse may correspond to the quantity space (0 BGL_N BGL_{VH}), where BGL_N and BGL_{VH} are landmarks respectively associated with the terms (or, equivalently with their related μ) Normal and Very High, and the intervals (0, BGL_N), (BGL_N,BGL_{VH}) with the terms Low and High.

At a second level, more related to the system behaviour, a mapping between simulated qualitative predictions and fuzzy rule-bases can be defined. Each simulated QB is represented by a sequence of qualitative states of the system, where each state is a m-tupla of the qualitative values of each individual system variable. Given N input variables x_i ($N \leq m$), the output variable y, and a QB, the method generates a FRB in the following steps:

1. consider the totally ordered set $T' = \{t_0, (t_0, t_1), t_1, \ldots (t_{n-1}, t_n), t_n\}$, and $\forall t \in T'$ consider $QS(S, t)$;
2. from $QS(S, t)$, draw out the qualitative values of input and output variables, namely $QV(x_i, t)$ and $QV(y, t)$;
3. from $QV(x_i, t)$ and $QV(y, t)$, draw out its related $qmag$, i.e. $qmag(x_i, t)$ and $qmag(y, t)$;
4. build the subset $\overline{T} \subseteq T'$, $\overline{T} = t_0 \cup \{t_k \in T' | \exists i, qmag(x_i, t_k) \neq qmag(x_i, t_{k-1}), k = 1, \ldots, \overline{k}\}$, where $\overline{k}$ is the cardinality of T'
5. $\forall t_k \in \overline{T}$, consider the membership functions μ_i and $\overline{\mu}$ which are associated with $qmag(x_i, t_k)$ and $qmag(y, t_k)$, respectively, (necessarily, $qmag(y, t_{k+1})$ if $\cup_i^N \{x_i\} \cup \{y\} \neq \emptyset$);
6. generate a rule R where x_i are the antecedents, y the consequent, μ_i and $\overline{\mu}$ the fuzzy sets.

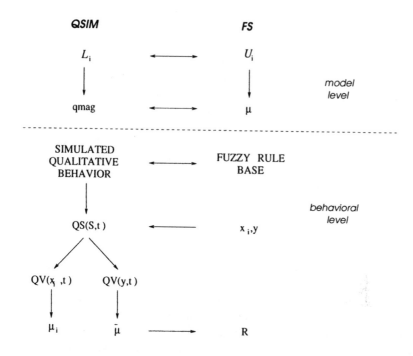

Fig. 1. Analogies between the QSIM and FS formalisms. Bi-directional arrows indicate a semantic correspondence, whereas the other ones have the usual meaning.

Obviously, the number of rules generated in correspondence with each QB cannot be greater than the cardinality of $\overline{T}$. Identical rules may happen to be generated as variables may have the same *qmag* at different time-instants: in such a case we group the equivalent rules and keep only one of them as representative of an input-output relation. At the current definition of our method, the resulting FRB is not guaranteed to be minimal: the problem of the generation of a FRB whose rules are univocally determined is still under study. Moreover, let us remark that QSIM may produce a quite large set of behaviours. Therefore, only behaviours which show significant distinctions in the subset of input-output variables are taken out of the produced behaviour tree to cope with the problem of the generation of a meaningful minimal set of fuzzy bases made up of rules univocally determined.

From an operational point of view, the construction of the FS to be used for the approximation of a set of data proceeds through five main phases. The phase 1 deals with the definition of the structural and behavioural knowledge of the system, that is the patho-physiological knowledge. More precisely, all relevant system variables together with its respective quantity spaces, and the contraints on the values those variables can take on must be defined. Then, an initial state of the system, which may describe a perturbation on the system, has to be provided to simulate all possible behaviours of the system. In parallel (phase 2), the input-output variables of the fuzzy system have to be specified, and for each of them the linguistic correspondence of the fuzzy elements (U, μ) with their quantity spaces defined in the QSIM model has to be stated. The choice of a fuzzy inference engine, as well as the fuzzification and defuzzification methods complete the definition of the fuzzy environment. The prior structural knowledge on the system captured by a selected QB (phase 3), properly integrated with the fuzzy knowledge given by the expert, is exploited to automatically build (phase 4) rules whose antecedents x_i and consequent y are the input and output variables to be used to identify the dynamics of the system. Finally, the generated rules, interpreted in accordance with the machinery specified at phase 2, initialize the FS (phase 5) which learns from the data an accurate input-output relation to be used as a predictive tool.

4 An application

In order to test the proposed methodology in a clinically significant context, we have studied the problem of identifying the response to conventional insulin therapy of insulin-dependent diabetic (IDDM) patients.

A Qualitative Model (QM) of glucose/insulin interaction in IDDM patients has been derived on the basis of the patho-physiological knowledge, and on a number of quantitative and qualitative models described in the literature [1, 3, 8].

The qualitative model exploited in our work is based on the compartmental structure shown in Fig. 2. Insulin (i) controls the plasma glucose (g) through two different mechanisms: the regulation of the g elimination (g_{out}) and the modulation of the net hepatic glucose balance $(nhgb)$, a variable that accounts for the liver capability of releasing or up-taking glucose.

From a qualitative point of view, it is possible to represent the insulin distribution in the body (i), which can vary from 0 to a maximum value (I_{max}), with a triangular or trapezoidal signal. Under this assumption the system may be described by a single qualitative differential equation:

$$\frac{dg(t)}{dt} = nhgb(t) + g_{in}(t) - g_{out}(t) - g_{ren}(t) \qquad (2)$$

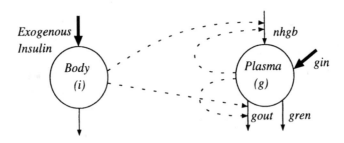

Fig. 2. The compartmental structure of the qualitative model of Insulin/Glucose dynamics. Continuous lines represent flows of matter, while dashed lines represent control signals.

where:

1. $g_{in}(t)$ is a triangular shaped input function, which represents the exogenous glucose intakes (meals). The quantity space is defined as $(0\ G^*)$, where G^* is the maximum quantity of absorbable carbohydrates.
2. $nhgb(t) = M^-(i) + S^-(g)$. $nhgb$ decreases when either g or i increases. Furthermore, the influence of the variable g saturates at a certain threshold value, indicated as GS. Finally, for each value of g, $nhgb > 0$ if $i = 0$. Following these limitations, the derived quantity space is $(L\ 0\ HBG\ UP)$, where L is the minimum negative value, $HBG = M^-(0) + S^-(GS)$, and $UP = M^-(0) + S^-(0)$.
3. $g_{ren} = M^+(g - GN)$. g_{ren} describes the renal elimination of glucose, and has quantity space $(0\ GN)$.
4. $g_{out} = M^+(i) + M^+(g)$. g_{out} is a monotonic increasing function of both g and i. The quantity space of this variable is $(0\ Max)$;

The quantity space of g may be hence defined, by ordering its previously introduced landmarks, as $(0\ GS\ GN)$.

As we are interested in the dynamics of g, we will consider a NARX (Nonlinear AutoRegressive eXogenous input) model of the glucose/insulin dynamics in IDDM patients. The FS has a rule-base in which the antecedents are the variables $g(t), di(t), dg_{in}(t)$, and the consequent is $g(t + 1)$. For what concerns the inputs, we decided to take the derivative of the input signals (di and dg_{in}), since the information on the slope is more reliably derived in clinical practice than the input signals themselves. As qualitative value of both di and dg_{in} we consider their sign, and therefore their quantity spaces are both defined as $(MINF\ 0\ INF)$, where $MINF, INF$ denote $-\infty$ and ∞, respectively. The linguistic levels of the variables were defined, as described in Table I.

Table I

g	
Qualitative Value	Linguistic Value
(0,GS)	Very-Low
GS	Low
(GS,GN)	Normal
GN	High
(GN,INF)	Very-High

dg_{in}, di	
Qualitative Value	Linguistic Value
(MINF,0)	Negative
0	Zero
(0,INF)	Positive

By exploiting the physiological knowledge available, and in particular referring to the studies presented by Lehmann and Berger [8, 1], we initialized the membership functions of the fuzzy systems. Such functions are Gaussian whose parameters are derived in accordance with the physiological knowledge. For example, the membership function associated with the linguistic value High of the variable g has its mean located in 180 mg/dl that corresponds to the renal threshold of glucose GN. Once that both the QM and the FS have been defined, it is necessary to assess the qualitative simulation and to set up the test-benchmark for evaluating the overall identification machinery.

509

5 The experiment

The scheme used for FS identification is shown in Fig. 3. At the current stage

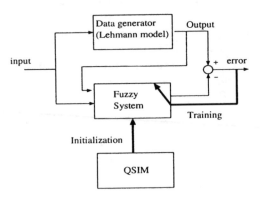

Fig. 3. The FS identification scheme.

of the work, the method has been tested on simulated data. The IDDM patient response was simulated by using the model proposed by Lehmann [8]. The evaluation of the method was performed on two different data sets: a training data set (TD-set) and a validation data set (VD-set). The TD-set has been obtained by simulating the patient response to an injection of regular insulin followed by a meal over a period of 24 hours, with a sampling time of 15 minutes, in different pathological conditions. The VD-set contains the data derived from a simulation of the patient response to a typical daily insulin protocol, composed by two injections of NPH insulin and three injections of regular insulin, followed by a meal, over a period of 24 hours, with a sampling time of 15 minutes. We generated a qualitative simulation of the IDDM patient response to a regular insulin injection, followed by a meal. Within the generated behaviour tree, five classes of equivalent behaviours have been identified, and the FRB which corresponds to a representative in each class has been automatically written. The five FSs have been ranked on the basis of their capability of forecasting the TD-set without any identification procedure, using the Akaike Information Criterion score (AIC). We have hence applied two different identification algorithms on the FS with the best AIC score:

Algorithm 1: Back-Propagation (BP)
The TD-set has been used to train and cross-validate the FS derived from QM (FS-QM) exploiting the back-propagation algorithm. The performances of the FS-QM have been compared (through Mean Absolute Error (ME) calculation) to the ones of a FS initialized by using only the data (FS-Black-Box, FS-BB), as proposed by Wang [9]. The more important results derived are described below:

1. In all the different situations considered, the FS-QM converges more quickly than the FS-BB to the ME minimum. Figure 4 shows the ME as a function of

510

the backpropagation loops, when experimental noise ($\pm 10\%$ of the generated value) is added to the data. As expected, if the number of backpropagation loops is sufficient, the two approaches have nearly equivalent performances.

2. Once the FS has been identified using the TD-set, we have exploited it to simulate and to forecast the VD-set. In this case, the FS-QM has a better performance than the FS-BB, independently of the back-propagation loops number and of the number of available data. Table IV shows the ME obtained in the forecasting phase as a function of the sampling rate.

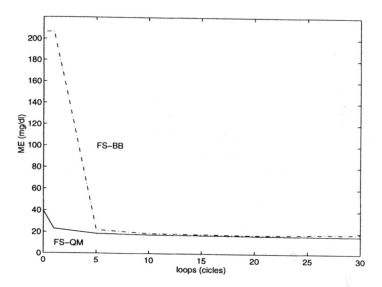

Fig. 4. The plot shows the ME as a function of backpropagation loops: FS-QM is denoted by the continous line (-), FS-BB by the dashed one (-.-). The results are obtained on the TD-set.

Table IV

Sampling rate:	ME (mg/dl)		
	1/1	1/2	1/4
FS-QM	9.5954	8.7310	9.7803
FS-BB	10.3319	14.5030	32.6714

Algorithm 2: Linear Least Squares (LS)
The advantages which derives from our method are not limited to a faster convergence of the back-propagation algorithm. Let us observe that a FS described by equation 1 can be conveniently rewritten as:

$$f(\mathbf{x}) = \sum_{j=1}^{M} \hat{y}_j \, \Phi_j(\mathbf{x}) \tag{3}$$

where

$$\Phi_j(\mathbf{x}) = \frac{\prod_{i=1}^{n} exp(-(\frac{x_i - \hat{x}_i^j}{\sigma_i^j})^2)}{\sum_{j=1}^{M}[\prod_{i=1}^{n} exp(-(\frac{x_i - \hat{x}_i^j}{\sigma_i^j})^2)]}$$

The functions $\Phi()$s are called Fuzzy Basis Functions (FBF); the FS is hence viewed as a linear combination of such FBFs. If the parameters $\hat{x}_i^j$ and σ_i^j are assumed to be known, it is sufficient to estimate the linear parameters $\hat{y}_j$ to predict the patients behaviour. The potential of such an approach is evident: a non-linear estimation problem is transformed into a linear one. In general, the drawback consists in the need of a careful construction of the FBFs: as in our method the FBFs are derived from the patho-physiological knowledge on the domain, their meaningfullness is guaranteed. Fig. 5 shows the results of the identification process of the patient response obtained by using the LS algorithm on the VD-set.

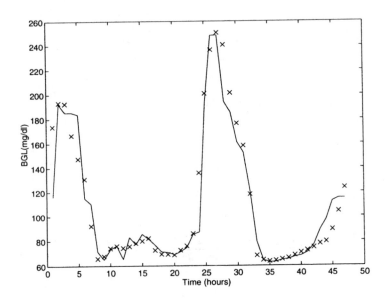

Fig. 5. Results obtained on the VD-set with 12 FBF by using the LS algorithm (ME=9.57 mg/dl). The data are indicated by x.

512

6 Conclusions and Future work

Medical applications are often characterized by problems of a two-fold nature: (i) the physician has usually a deep patho-physiological knowledge on the patients behaviour; (ii) it is not possible to measure all the quantities necessary to completely assess the patient's state. As a consequence, although a lot of mathematical models of physiological systems are available, their identification is usually problematic. Hence, it is necessary to resort to non-parametric strategies with a consequent loss of the available prior information on the domain.

This work represents a valuable answer to the above presented problems: it describes a novel approach to the identification of non- linear dynamic systems, which integrates fuzzy systems and qualitative models. The simulations obtained from a set of qualitative differential equations are used to automatically encode the available knowledge in a fuzzy rule-based system; such a system is then tuned to a set of experimental data. The results obtained show that the presented framework generates fuzzy systems that may be used for a quick and reliable identification of non-linear systems. At the current stage of this work, we have used simulated data instead of the real ones as our aim has been a preliminary evaluation of the method: obviously, the good results obtained so far need to be confirmed on real data sets. Moreover, further work has to be carried out both for a better formalization of the method and for a precise definition of its applicability.

References

1. M. Berger and D. Rodbard. Computer simulation of Plasma insulin and glucose dynamics after subcutaneous insulin injection, *Diabetes Care*, 12 (1989) 725-736.
2. E.R. Carson, C. Cobelli, and L. Finkenstein. *The Mathematical Modeling of Metabolic and Endocrine Systems*. Wiley, New York, 1983.
3. L. Ironi, M. Stefanelli, and G. Lanzola. Qualitative models in medical diagnosis. *Artificial Intelligence in Medicine*, 2:85–101, 1990.
4. J. Jang. Anfis: Adaptive network based fuzzy inference system. *IEEE Trans. on Systems, Man and Cybernetics*, 23:665–685, 1993.
5. T. Khannah. *Foundations of neural networks*. Addison-Wesley, Reading, MA, 1990.
6. B. J. Kuipers. *Qualitative Reasoning: modeling and simulation with incomplete knowledge*. MIT Press, Cambridge MA, 1994.
7. H.M. Kim, J.M. Mendel. Fuzzy Basis Functions: Comparison with Other Basis Functions, *IEEE Trans. Fuzzy Systems*, 3 (1995) 158-168.
8. E.D. Lehmann and T. Deutsch. A physological model of glucose–insulin interaction in type 1 diabetes mellitus. *Biomedical Engineering*, 14:235–242, 1992.
9. L.X. Wang. *Adaptive Fuzzy Systems and Control*, Prentice hall, Engelwood Cliffs, N.J., 1994.

Case-Based Reasoning and Statistics for Discovering and Forecasting of Epidemics *

M. Bull   G. Kundt   L. Gierl

University of Rostock, Department for Medical Informatics and Biometry
Rembrandtstr. 16/17, D-18055 Rostock, Germany
{mathias.bull|guenther.kundt|lothar.gierl}@medizin.uni-rostock.de

Abstract. We describe the methodology of an early warning system which fulfills the following tasks. (1) discovering of health risks, (2) forecasting of the temporal and spatial spread of epidemics and (3) estimating of consequences of an epidemic w.r.t. the personnel load and costs of the public health service. For mastering this three tasks methods from artifical intelligence and statistics are applied.

Keywords: case-based reasoning, statistics, forecasting, discovery, epidemics

1   Introduction

For ensuring a high level of human disease prevention, physicians and pharmacists need information on current health risks as well as on outbreaks and spreads of diseases. There is reason to believe that the number and incidence of emerging diseases and the risks of re-emerging diseases are increasing (migration, population growth, rapid transport, new food technologies, environmental changes etc.).

The public health surveillance is a complex problem of multiparametric time courses of diseases, pathogens, resistances, health services etc. in a geographical region [10]. Statistical methods are partially applicable to problems of disease clusterings either in time or in space but not appropriate to examine the time-spatial dynamics of communicable diseases (see [7]). Especially, there are observable time-spatial patterns of the spread of diseases which are complicate to describe by means of statistics (cf. [7, p.433]). For monitoring complex processes in time and space on other domains (cf. [4],[6],[9]) the successful applications used case-based techniques. Case-based reasoning (CBR) is a cyclical paradigm of the artifical intelligence for solving problems by analogical reasoning and for learning new problem-solution pairs through experiences. The CBR-cycle [1] consists of four stages: *retrieve* the most similar case or cases; *reuse* the retrieved case or cases to solve the problem by analogical reasoning; *revise* the proposed solution; *retain* the parts of this experience likely to be useful for future problem solving.

An interesting combination of statistics and CBR is implemented in the expert system Air Quality Predictor [6]. The problem of managing and retrieving large-scale case bases is discussed in [5]. In ICONS [9] we prognose probable course continuations of the kidney function of intensive care patients by CBR and abstractions of multiparametric time courses. Now, we combine methods of statistics, CBR, knowledge discovery and data mining (KDD) for an early warning system [2].

---
* supported by the DFN-Verein (German society for the national research net) and the AOK Mecklenburg-Vorpommern (General health insurance company)

2 Problem Description

We divide the considered geographical region in a finite number of disjoint geographical units, here called *locations*. For our project we have chosen the ZIP-code districts because this dissection includes implicitly facts on the demography and the infrastructure. Further, we choose a reasonable time period τ (for organisational reasons $\tau=$ one week) and divide the time scale in equidistant time steps. A finite number of consecutive time steps (of the time period τ) is called a *time interval*.

By a *scenario* we understand a concept which describes the public health situation and the load of the health service in the considered region during a period. More precisely, for each location a scenario s includes (i) each new case of illness given by an anonymous patient record, (ii) the load of the health service, and (iii) contextual information (weather and season, holiday seasons) which arise during a period τ.

A *scenario sequence* σ is a finite sequence of scenarios. We also denote a scenario sequence by the concatenation of its elements, e.g. $\sigma = s_0 s_1 \ldots s_n$ where s_i is a scenario. So we are able to describe the course of any epidemic by a scenario sequence since it keeps all information on the public health situation during a time interval. Furthermore, we define inductively a similarity metric sim on the set of all scenario sequences, i.e. at first we define similarity metrics on all elementary sets and then similarity metrics on sets of structured objects by using the metrics of its components.

By a *health risk* we understand an observable changing of the public health situation which may cause an epidemic. So we have the following main problems.

Discovering of Health Risks
Given: σ current scenario sequence
Question: Does there exists a health risk ?

Forecasting a Scenario
Given: σ current scenario sequence
Question: How does the successor scenario of σ looks like ?

Estimating the Consequences for Health Care Resources
Given: σ current scenario sequence
Question: What are the consequences for health care workers, for the pharmaceutical industry and for the over all costs ?

In the following we denote the case base by Σ which contains some scenario sequences describing the course of past epidemics. Let $\sigma = s_0 s_1 \ldots s_m$ be the current scenario sequence.

3 Discovering of Health Risks

We want to detect a health risk as soon as possible *to warn* whereas in epidemiological studies the aim is *to prove* a causal relationship of disease and exposition. Thus, the discovery of a health risk is based on the detection of suspicious changes in the health situation which could be an accumulation of illnesses of undetermined origin or an accumulation of resistances to antibiotics within a time period or a certain area. A frequent false-positive reaction of the system must be avoided. Therefore, it must be possible to improve the sensitivity and specificity of the system. The system works as follows.

Discover suspicious changes in the current scenario sequence. By using methods of KDD [3] the current scenario sequence σ is explored. Moreover, existing techniques of Scientific Visualisation can be applied to show temporal and spatial dependencies and correlations of the data contained in the current scenario sequence σ.

Retrieve the scenario sequences with similar onsets and epidemic courses. The system looks for a scenario sequence σ' which starts with a subsequence similar to the current scenario sequence σ and terminates in a dangerous scenario.

Reuse the retrieved scenario sequences to warn. If there is such a scenario sequence σ' then the system has to warn or alarm of an epidemic depending on severity degree of the detected health risk. The severity degree of a health risk is characterized by the incidence, by the population density of the location where the outbreak occurs, by the quality of a prevention, by the quality of a therapy, and by the course of the illness.

$$
\begin{array}{l}
\text{retrieved scenario sequence} \qquad\qquad\qquad\quad \nearrow\!\text{epidemic scenario}\\
\quad\text{from the case base } \Sigma \quad \longrightarrow \sigma' = s'_0 s'_1 \ldots s'_m s'_{m+1} \ldots s'_{m+k}\\
\qquad\qquad\qquad\qquad\qquad\qquad\qquad\qquad\quad \Downarrow warning\\
\text{current scenario sequence} \quad \longrightarrow \sigma \;=\; \underbrace{s_0 s_1 \ldots s_m}\boxed{\,!\,}\\
\qquad\qquad\qquad\qquad\qquad\qquad\quad \text{similar subsequences}
\end{array}
$$

Revise the warning. The quality of the discovery of health risks is evaluated by monitoring of the succeeding scenarios.

Retain the useful scenario sequences. If a scenario sequence led to an epidemic and has not been discovered by the system then this sequence will be stored in the case base.

4 Forecasting of a Scenario

The prediction of a regional health situation means to forecast a future scenario. We use the following steps.

Retrieve the most similar scenario sequences. The system retrieves all scenario sequences $\sigma' s'_{m+1} = s'_0 s'_1 \ldots s'_m s'_{m+1}$ from the case base Σ so that the differences between σ' and the current scenario sequence σ are minimal, i.e. for all $\sigma'' s'' \in \Sigma$ it holds $sim(\sigma, \sigma'') \leq sim(\sigma, \sigma')$.

Reuse the retrieved scenario sequences to forecast a scenario. By using the retrieved sequences $\sigma' s'_{m+1}$ the system adapts the scenario s'_{m+1} to a forecast scenario $\tilde{s}$. Here, we use background knowledge about demographic structures, several statistical models of epidemics [8] and the defined threshold values of epidemical levels. The resulting data will be stored in the case base and will be available for graphical presentation on the user interface.

$$
\begin{array}{l}
\text{similar scenario sequence}\\
\quad\text{from the case base } \Sigma \quad \longrightarrow \sigma' s'_{m+1} = s'_0 s'_1 \ldots s'_m s'_{m+1}\\
\qquad\qquad\qquad\qquad\qquad\qquad\qquad\qquad \Downarrow adaptation\\
\text{current scenario sequence} \quad \longrightarrow \sigma \qquad = s_0 s_1 \ldots s_m \boxed{\,?\,}\\
\qquad\qquad\qquad\qquad\qquad\qquad\qquad\qquad\quad \searrow \text{forecast scenario } \tilde{s}
\end{array}
$$

Revise the forecast scenario. After a time period τ we know the scenario s_{m+1}. In comparing the forecast scenario $\tilde{s}$ with the scenario s_{m+1} the system evaluates the forecast mechanism.

Retain the useful scenario sequences. If there are too many differences between these scenarios the system has to integrate the new scenario sequence σs_{m+1} in the case base or the inference mechanism must be changed. In the latter case, an expert (e.g. epidemiologist, biostastician) has to execute a working cycle with the system. This working cycle contains the modification of the threshold values and of the metrics, the visualisation of the multiparametric data of the current scenario sequence and those in the case base, and the forecast of a scenario (as a simulation step). This cycle is executed until the difference of the current scenario and the forecast senario is within a tolerance range.

5 Estimation of Consequences for the Health Care Resources

Based on discovered risks and the forecast scenario, monetrary and medical consequences can be estimated. Furthermore, the demands on intensive care beds, the required nursing care or the amount of vaccines can be concluded. Length of stay, probable surgery, lethal cases and further consequences can also be deduced. From consumables, departmental care rates etc. the expected costs for a case induced by the epidemic can be estimated.

References

1. Aamodt, A. ; Plaza, P. : *Case-Based Reasoning: Foundational Issues, Methodological Variations, and System Approaches.* AI Communications 7(1) 1994, 39-59
2. Bull, M.; Gierl, L.: *Architecture of an Early Warning System for Regional Health Risk.* Rostocker Informatik Berichte (1996)19, 5-18
3. Fayyad, U. M. ; Piatetsky-Shapiro, G.; Smyth,P. ; Uthurusamy, R.: *Advances in Knowledge Discovery and Data Mining.* MIT Press, 1996
4. Jones, E.K. ; Roydhouse, A. : *Iterative Design of Case Retrieval Systems.* Victoria University of Welligton, New Zealand, Technical Report CS-TR-94/6, see also: Proc.of the AAAI-94, Workshop on Case Based Reasoning, Seattle, Washington, 1994
5. Kitano, H.; Shimazu, H.; Shibata, A.: *A Methodology for Building Large-Scale Case-Based Systems.* in: Proceedings of the AAAI-93, Washington, 1993
6. Lekkas, G.P.; Arouris, N.M.; Viras, L.L.: *Case-Based Reasoning in Environmental Monitoring Applications.* Applied Artificial Intelligence, Vol. 8, 1994, 349-376
7. Marshall, R.J.: *A Review of the Statistical Analysis of Spatial Patterns of Disease.* J. R. Statist. Soc. A (1991) 154, Part 3, 421-441
8. Rothman, K.J.: *Modern Epidemiology.* Little Brown, Boston, Toronto 1986
9. Schmidt, R.; Heindl, B.; Pollwein, B.; Gierl, L.: *Abstraction of Data and Time for Prognoses of the Kidney Function in a Case-Based Reasoning System.* in J. Brender, J.P. Christensen et al.(eds.): Proc. of Medical Informatics Europe '96, IOS Press, Technology and Informatics, Vol. 34, Part A, 570-574
10. Thomas, R.J.: *Geomedical Systems.* London, New York 1992

Knowledge Refinement of an Expert System Using a Symbolic-Connectionist Approach

J. Santos[1], D. Lorenzo[1], S. Gomez[1], J. Heras[2] and R. P. Otero[1]

[1] Dept. Computación, Fac. Informática
Universidade da Coruña
E-15071 A Coruña, Spain
[2] Orthopaedic Surgery and Trauma Dpt.
Hospital General de Galicia
E-15701 Santiago de Compostela, A Coruña, Spain

Keywords: Machine Learning, Expert Systems in Medicine, Knowledge Refinement, Neural Networks

1 Introduction

TKR-tool [4] is an expert system (ES) for Total Knee Replacement that gives advice and assists patient management at every stage of the TKR process from pre-operatory and post-operatory evaluation to patient follow-up. The system has been evaluated at the Hospital General de Galicia in Santiago de Compostela (Spain) and it is being used on a daily practice basis.

The success of this ES has motivated us to study the inclusion of machine learning techniques for refining and/or generating new knowledge in accordance with the ES. When faced with real ESs usually one of the methods alone - symbolic learning, qualitative learning even connectionist learning- is not sufficient even when we have selected a particular portion of the system [6]. We have selected a representation widely used in medicine that is *scoring systems*. As we will show a symbolic-connectionist approach may perform well in the refinement of this representation.

The practical use of scores in medicine comes from the fact that they provide with an intuitive and easily interpretable way of evaluating the clinical situation of a patient, e.g., quantifying the expected risk and so on. Besides they are also useful as they allow for comparison with different studies and other authors.

Some of the scoring systems managed by TKR-tool ES are the patient's category of the American Knee Society [5] and the clinical scoring systems of the Hospital for Special Surgery, the American Knee Society, and the Rush Presbiteriam Medical Center-Chicago [2] and the evaluation of Polyethylene risk failure.

Scores quantify the importance of each feature -and even of each label from a set of ordered labels of each feature- with respect to the overall risk to predict. Thus, the intensity of the class is expressed as a weighted summation of the intensities of each influencing feature.

Symbolic learners associate a set of tests (*atribute, value*) to each class that allows to classify examples from a set of categories. However, they assign the same weight to each test and to each variable. Even in the most simple case -i.e., the class is the summation of the values of the features- a symbolic learner would tend to simply list the instances belonging to each category (range).

Neural networks seem more appropiated for this task. Connectionist learners modify the weights associated to each input until it perfectly distinguishes each level of the output variable. However they are usually considered as black boxes because it is difficult to interpret the results of learning.

This led us to consider a symbolic-connectionist approach which combines the efficiency of connectionist learning with the comprehensibility of symbolic methods. The key issue consists of limiting the topology of the neural net so as to make easier the interpretation of the net weights. This supposes that the initial structure of the net must somehow resemble the structure of the initial problem [3, 9], or in other words, we inject knowledge by establishing an adequate network architecture for this facility of interpretation.

2 Connectionist architecture

The neural architecture we present here is a multilayer perceptron with four hidden layers, where we limit the number of the hidden nodes in order to make possible the interpretation of the final weights. The two first hidden layers include a set of nodes whose combination function is a weighted addition of the previous layer outputs. These nodes do the same additions as physicians do to determine the punctuation levels, weighting each of the symbolic labels (previously translated into a numerical value). The net is not totally connected between the input nodes and the first hidden layer because the contribution to risk of the several features is assumed to be independent (as usual).

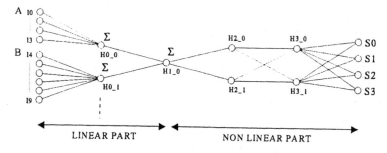

Fig. 1. Network used for the determination of the score levels

We applied the backpropagation learning procedure [7] to this not fully connected net. Input variables are encoded as binary vectors (with the bit corresponding to each value set to one). The first hidden layer accounts for the conribution to risk of each feature and for the internal ordering of each feature's labels. Node H1-0 of the second hidden layer calculates the overall contribution to the risk.

These nodes only calculate summations, therefore making a linear transformation. From these values a non-linear classification is determined in the scoring levels, and therefore we need a network structure that makes this non-linear transformation. To this aim, we have used two more hidden layers that apply the sigmoid function to the summation. Finally, the output units represent the scoring levels and they can be interpreted in a symbolic way.

The final aim is a net trained with the examples and their associated scores provided by an expert, that expresses through the weights of the linear subnet the weighting that must be applied to each of the symbolic labels of a variable.

As to the training, we only need to consider the different contributions to the final network error in each of the hidden nodes which will be fixed by its combination and transfer functions, whereas the variation of each weight in the negative direction of the error gradient will be different depending on the derivatives of these functions. Thus, we have an heterogeneous network with different training equations in each connection, although the algorithm we have used is backpropagation in the whole network. In this sense, the linear part of the network uses as data for training the error provided in the non-linear part.

3 Interpretation of the network

The system has been tested on a set of data of a representative example. In the training, we have used a momentum term and a random reading of the training vectors, given that in the training file they are ordered by their corresponding scoring levels. In our example the categories are not linearly distributed, so it is important to previously balance the number of examples of each category, e.g., by duplicating examples, thus, the presence of these examples is stressed.

In the linear part of the network there are many possibilities with different configurations of weights that provide the same result. Furthermore, a little change in the weights of the linear part modify the summation in the node H1-0, thus, it modifies greatly the non-linear transformation that must be carried out by the non-linear part of the network. This suggests that the changes in the linear part must be smaller than in the non-linear part, through different training coefficients so that the non-linear part is able to adapt to little changes in the linear part.

Finally, we can take the exact values of the weights returned by the network to form a symbolic expression or we can simply provide an indication of the relative weight of each variable's level to each scoring level. The thresholds to be included in the symbolic expression can be found by analyzing the levels of the node that accounts for the summation of the contributions (H1-0) in the changes of the output scoring level.

The definition and training of the network was carried out by Nettool [8], an environment for the connectionist-symbolic hybrid systems. The process of building the network, training it and the final interpretation is made with the same representation of the TKR expert system, and allows to overcome the problems associated with the two different methods we have worked on.

4 Conclusions

In this paper we have shown how to solve a real connectionist learning problem with a symbolic interpretation for the refinement of *scoring systems* and *risk evaluation systems*. This is a significant issue not easily manageable by classical symbolic methods [1] that are specially oriented to static domains. This has lead us to implement a symbolic-connectionist approach which combines the efficiency of connectionist learning with the comprehensibility of symbolic methods.

The network structure combines a linear part that does the same additions as physicians do to determine the weighted contributions of input variables and a non-linear transformation that determine the punctuation levels. The output units represent the scoring levels and they can be interpreted in a symbolic way. The system is currently validated with more real data, and it is being used to refine the scoring and risk evaluation systems of other hospitals by training the net with a set of local patients.

References

1. P. Clark and T. Niblett. The CN2 induction algorithm. *Machine Learning*, 1988.
2. Edwall F.C. The knee society total knee arthroplasty roentgenographic evaluation and scoring system. *Clinical Orthopaedics*, (248):9–12, 1989.
3. L.M. Fu. Knowledge-based connectionism for revising domain theories. *IEEE Transactions on Systems, Man and Cybernetics*, 23(1):173–182, 1993.
4. J. Heras and R.P. Otero. TKR-tool: An expert system for total knee replacement management. *Artificial Intelligence in Medicine Europe. Lecture Notes in Artificial Intelligence*, (934):444–446, 1995.
5. Insall J.N., Dorr D.D., Scott R.D., and Scott W.N. Rationale of the knee society clinical rating system. *Clinical Orthopaedics*, (248):13–14, 1989.
6. R. P. Otero, D. Lorenzo, and P. Cabalar. Applying induction in temporal expert systems. *IJCAI-Workshop on Data Engineering for Inductive Learning*, 1995.
7. D.E Rumelhart, G.E. Hinton, and R.J. Williams. Learning internal representations by error propagation. *Parallel Distributed Processing, Explorations in the Microestructure of Cognition, MIT Press, Cambridge*, 1:318–362, 1986.
8. J. Santos, R.P. Otero, and J. Mira. Nettool: A hydrid connectionist-symbolic development environment. *From Natural to Artificial Neural Computation, J. Mira and F. Sandoval (Eds.), Lecture Notes in Computer Science*, (930):658–665, 1995.
9. G. Towell and J.W. Shavlik. Refining symbolic knowledge using neural networks. In *Machine Learning, A Multistrategy Approach*, volume 4, chapter 15, pages 405–429. Morgan Kauffman Publishers, 1994.

Integrated Decision Support: The DIADOQ Computer-Based Patient Record

Wolfgang Moser[1], Thomas Diedrich[2] and DIADOQ[*]

[1] GSF - National Research Center for Environment and Health,
MEDIS - Institute for Medical Informatics and Health Services Research,
Ingolstädter Landstr. 1, 85764 Neuherberg, Germany
e-mail: moser@gsf.de
[2] DFI - Diabetes Research Institute, Auf'm Hennekamp 65, 40225 Düsseldorf,
Germany

Abstract. The DIADOQ project aims at assuring the quality of care for Diabetic patients by means of task specific decision support for clinically relevant problems in diagnosing, therapy planning, and monitoring of Diabetes. As a first step a knowledge-based CPR system for Diabetes outpatient clinics has been developed, utilising simple textbook presentations up to inferences by causal-probabilistic networks.

1 Introduction

The medical knowledge for an optimised Diabetes care is largely available (e.g. NIDDM and IDDM consensus guidelines [3,4]). Nevertheless, problems in the management of Diabetes patients occur. This is mainly due to difficulties in the application of the available knowledge at the appropriate time. A major step towards the goals of the St. Vincent Declaration [6] can be expected by computer-based patient record (CPR) systems for clinical routine integrating the available knowledge.

The DIADOQ project aims at assuring the quality of care for Diabetic patients by means of task specific decision support for clinically relevant problems in diagnosing, therapy planning, and monitoring of Diabetes. In order to achieve the constant availability of the knowledge bases and guidelines, a CPR system for Diabetes outpatient clinics has been developed, supporting both routine work and knowledge-based decision support.

---

[*] DIADOQ - Optimised Care Through Knowledge-based Quality Assurance: Diabetes Mellitus. The organisations involved are: Diabetes Research Institute, Düsseldorf; GSF - MEDIS Institute, Neuherberg; Institute for Diabetes, Karlsburg; University Hospital of Erlangen-Nürnberg, Nürnberg; IMIB - Institute for Medical Informatics and Biometry, Dresden; Department of Diabetes, München-Bogenhausen; Boehringer Mannheim GmbH, Mannheim; Institute for Mathematics, Ludwig Maximilians University, München. DIADOQ is part of the German MEDWIS (Medical Knowledge-bases) research programme.

2 CPR System

The conceptual model of the CPR is based on the "Clinical View of the Common Basic Specification" [1]. A controlled vocabulary is maintained in a frame-based concept system. The vocabulary enables the structured recording of nearly all patient data including history taking and physical examination. It is an extension of the EURODIABETA data-set [2] and currently comprises more than 2000 concepts.

The frame representation of the concepts forms the basis for the automatic generation of screen forms for user input and for data representation at system runtime. Each medical item of the CPR system keeps a reference to its corresponding concept. Laboratory concepts, for example, provide references to norm ranges. These can depend on the patient's age, gender, etc. They may be measured for different specimens (e.g. urine, blood) in different units (e.g. mmol/l, g/dl).

The CPR system adopts a problem-oriented medical record [8] as a natural model of the CPR for managing a chronic disease. Patient problems, organised in a problem list, provide a concise medical summary of the patient and serve as justifications of performed medical acts. Thus, the CPR system does not only record the medical data of a patient, but additionally keeps a record of justifications and acts leading to this data.

3 Integrated Decision Support

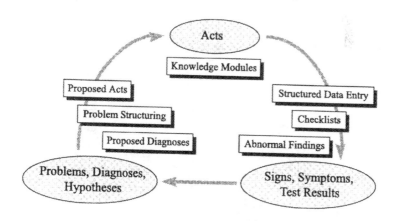

Fig. 1. Knowledge-based support in the DIADOQ CPR system

The possibility to represent the process of health care delivery in the medical record lays the foundation for the identification of steps where knowledge-based decision support beneficially could be applied [7].

In Figure 1 different functions supported by knowledge bases available in DIADOQ are indicated. This support employs methods ranging from simple textbook presentations up to inferences by causal-probabilistic networks (CPN) [5].

For example, the managing of the problem list is supported by an electronic medical textbook of relevant problems in the field of Diabetes. For each problem typical signs, symptoms, test results and sensible diagnostic medical acts are listed. These profiles have been elaborated by the DIADOQ Diabetes experts supported by a tool based on the controlled vocabulary and the underlying ontology of the knowledge base. Coupling the knowledge base to the data of a specific patient [8], possible explanations of patient problems and medical acts for further investigations are automatically proposed by the system.

Dedicated knowledge modules support the user during the performance of difficult medical acts. One such an example is a CPN built for the prognosis of nephropathy of IDDM patients. The foreground form in Figure 2 shows the result of the interaction with the CPN indicating the inclusion and exclusion criteria of the knowledge base, the used patient data from the medical record and the resulting probabilities displayed in a bar chart. In the background form of Figure 2 a patient's problem list and to-do list of medical acts are displayed in the main window of the CPR system. All interactions with knowledge modules are treated like any other medical act in the system.

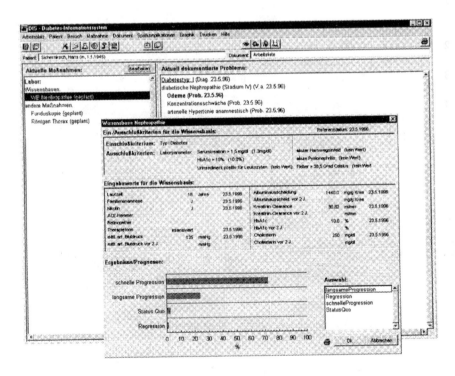

Fig. 2. Example forms of the DIADOQ CPR system

4 Conclusions

Analysis of the routine work has to be the starting point to define the scope of the required knowledge-based support. Only when persons involved in the delivery of care are supported in their daily routine, acceptance of information systems in general and knowledge bases in particular is achievable.

The DIADOQ CPR supports the explicit representation of the medical acts, facts and main inferences underlying the process of health care delivery. A controlled vocabulary is maintained by a frame-based concept system. This representation is the foundation for a consistent and comparable recording of patient data and for the flexible adaptation of screen forms to clinical contexts. The explicit and structured representation of the process of health care delivery enables the tight integration of knowledge-based decision support in the CPR system.

Currently the DIADOQ CPR system undergoes a first evaluation in two outpatient clinics. Thirty German Diabetes specialists will evaluate the system in the beginning of 1997. First evaluation results should be available in the first quarter of the next year.

References

1. Cairns T. et al. *The Clinical View of the Common Basic Specification: The COSMOS Project Clinical Process Model*, Version 2.0, NHS Information Management Centre, Birmingham, 1993.
2. EURODIABETA. Information Technology for Diabetes Care in Europe: The EU-RODIABETA Initiative. *Diabetic Medicine*, 7:536–560, 1990.
3. European NIDDM Policy Group (Ed.) *A Desktop Guide for the Management of Non-insulin-dependent Diabetes Mellitus (NIDDM)*. Kirchheim, Mainz, 1993.
4. European IDDM Policy Group (Ed.) *Consensus Guidelines for the Management of Insulin-dependent (Type 1) Diabetes*. Medicom Europe BV, Bussum, 1993.
5. Jensen F.V. *An introduction to Bayesian networks*. UCL Press Limited, London, 1996.
6. Krans H.M.J., Porta M., Keen H. (Eds.) *Diabetes Care and Research in Europe: The St. Vincent Declaration Action Programme*. World Health Organisation, Regional Office for Europe, Copenhagen; International Diabetes Federation, European Region, 1992.
7. Moser W., Böhm V., Böhmer K., Engelbrecht R., Brenner H.H. Integrated Development of a Knowledge-based CPR System for Quality Assurance in Diabetes Outpatient Clinics. In: Greens A.G., Peterson H.E., Protti D.J. (Eds.) *Proceedings of the 8th World Congress on Medical Informatics (MEDINFO)*, North Holland, 236–239, 1995.
8. Weed L.L. *Knowledge Coupling*. Springer Verlag, New York, 1991.

Author Index

Springer
and the
environment

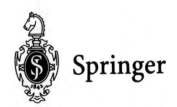

Springer

Lecture Notes in Artificial Intelligence (LNAI)

Lecture Notes in Computer Science